Hearing Assessment

a volume in the Perspectives in Audiology Series

Hearing Assessment

SECOND EDITION

Edited by WILLIAM F. RINTELMANN

ALLYN AND BACON

Boston London Sydney Toronto Tokyo Singapore

Copyright © 1991 by Allyn and Bacon
A Division of Simon & Schuster, Inc.
160 Gould Street
Needham Heights, Massachusetts 02194

Copyright © 1979 by PRO-ED, Inc.

Library of Congress Cataloging-in-Publication Data

Hearing assessment / [edited by] William F. Rintelmann. — 2nd ed.
    p.   cm.

    1. Audiometry. I. Rintelmann, William F.
RF294.H43   1990
617.8'9—dc20   90-8297
                                                                CIP

ISBN 0-205-13537-4

Chapter 5 is the work of the United States government and thus
not under copyright.

Printed in the United States of America

10 9 8 7 6 5 4 3   95 94 93 92

Perspectives in Audiology Series

contents

Preface   vii

Contributors   ix

preface

Less than five decades have elapsed since audiology emerged as a formal discipline, yet a vast body of knowledge and technical information has accumulated that focuses on the identification, assessment, and habilitation of auditory disorders.

The primary purpose of this book is to serve as a text for graduate-level audiology courses concerned with the assessment of the peripheral and central auditory systems. It should also be a useful reference for practicing audiologists, otolaryngologists, and other clinicians and scientists who are concerned with the assessment of hearing in its normal and disordered state.

The organization and content of this book provide the reader with both fundamental and specialized information concerning the clinical assessment of hearing and its disorders involving the peripheral and central auditory mechanisms. To this end some chapters present basic concepts, while several others deal with specialized topics.

Since the publication of the first edition of this text about ten years ago, methods used for the clinical assessment of hearing and auditory disorders have undergone substantial change. Applications to the field of audiology from technological advances in electronic instrumentation and especially microcomputers have contributed to an increased focus on electrophysiologic test procedures. By the same token certain behavioral so-called "classic site-of-lesion tests" have become largely obsolete. However, some basic tests (e.g., pure tone threshold measurement) and procedures (e.g., clinical masking) remain virtually unchanged except for improved instrumentation. Hence, in this second edition of *Hearing Assessment* certain chapters dealing with basic clinical audiology topics have been updated and retained. These include a chapter concerning pure tone audiometry, a chapter with extensive coverage of speech audiometry, and a chapter covering clinical masking. Three chapters from the first edition covering the topics of auditory adaptation, differential intensity discrimination, and recruitment are condensed to a single chapter in this second edition. These auditory phenomena are covered from a critical historical perspective because they provided the basis for several classic site-of-lesion tests for nearly two decades from the late 1950s through the latter part of the 1970s. By the same token the topics of acoustic immittance and auditory evoked responses have been expanded substantially from the first edition. Also, two new chapters are devoted to hearing assessment of newborns, infants, and young children, and one new chapter concerns the opposite end of the age continuum, namely, audiologic assessment of the elderly. This chapter includes the assessment of hearing handicap, the functional impact of hearing loss in the elderly, and management issues. Other topics that have been updated from the first edition include evaluation of central auditory disorders via behavioral testing techniques and assessment of pseudohypacusis via routine and special tests. This chapter includes a discussion of management strategies for children.

Also new to the second edition is a comprehensive chapter describing the clinical decision analysis process including measures of individual test performance, the formulation and use of test protocols, and methods for predicting protocol performance.

A chapter dealing with assessment of the vestibular system via the longstanding electronystagmography (ENG) test battery has been expanded and updated. This chapter also covers the most recent procedures of the rotational test and computerized dynamic posturography. Finally, as in the first edition of *Hearing Assessment*, the last chapter presents information concerning procedures and standards for the calibration of clinical test instruments.

All chapters contain extensive literature citations in the body of the text plus complete lists of references at the end of each chapter, thereby providing the reader with ready access to the classic and current literature. Also, many chapters contain numerous illustrations including examples of patient test results.

The editor is indebted to each of the authors for providing comprehensive and up-to-date coverage of their assigned topics and for their efforts to conform to the necessary space restrictions. Further, several other individuals contributed to the production of this text. Brian Blakley, MD, PhD, Gilmour Peters, PhD, and Sabina Schwan, MA provided valuable critiques of various chapters; Fred Bess, PhD, Frank Musiek, PhD, and Daniel Schwartz, PhD gave the editor helpful suggestions regarding the organization and content of the revised edition of this text; and Andrea Phillips provided secretarial assistance during various stages of the manuscript. Finally, my wife, Sandy, deserves a special note of thanks for her patience, understanding, and frequent encouragement during the period of over two years when this revision of *Hearing Assessment* was in progress.

William F. Rintelmann

contributors

Jane A. Baran, PhD
Associate Professor
Department of Communication
  Disorders
University of Massachusetts
Amherst, Massachusetts
and
Adjunct Associate Professor
Section of Audiology
Department of Surgery
Dartmouth-Hitchcock Medical
  Center
Hanover, New Hampshire

Fred H. Bess, PhD
Professor and Director
Division of Hearing and Speech
  Sciences
Vanderbilt University School of
  Medicine
and
Chief Executive Officer
Bill Wilkerson Center
Nashville, Tennessee

David G. Cyr, PhD
Director
Balance Disorders Clinic
The Boys Town National
  Research Hospital
and
Professor
Department of Otolaryngology
  and Human Communication
Creighton University School of
  Medicine
Omaha, Nebraska

John D. Durrant, PhD
Professor
Departments of Otolaryngology
  and Communication
University of Pittsburgh
and
Director
Center for Audiology
Eye and Ear Hospital of
  Pittsburgh
Pittsburgh, Pennsylvania

James W. Hall III, PhD
Associate Professor
Division of Hearing and Speech
  Sciences
Department of Otolaryngology
Vanderbilt University School of
  Medicine
and
Director of Audiology
Vanderbilt Hospital
Nashville, Tennessee

John T. Jacobson, PhD
Director of Audiology
Department of Otolaryngology
Head and Neck Surgery
University of Texas Health
  Science Center at Houston
Houston, Texas

Dan F. Konkle, PhD
Director
Department of Communication
  Disorders
The Children's Seashore House
and
Associate Professor of
  Audiology
Department of
  Otorhinolaryngology and
  Human Communication
University of Pennsylvania
  School of Medicine
Philadelphia, Pennsylvania

**Michael J. Lichtenstein, MD,
MSc**
Associate Professor of Medicine
  and Geriatrics
University of Texas Health
  Center—San Antonio
San Antonio, Texas

Susan A. Logan, MSc
Instructor
Division of Hearing and Speech
  Sciences
Vanderbilt University School of
  Medicine
and
Coordinator, Hearing Clinics
Bill Wilkerson Center
Nashville, Tennessee

Robert H. Margolis, PhD
Professor and Director of
  Audiology
Department of Otolaryngology
University of Minnesota
Minneapolis, Minnesota

Noel D. Matkin, PhD
Professor of Audiology
Department of Speech and
  Hearing Sciences
University of Arizona
Tucson, Arizona

William Melnick, PhD
Professor of Audiology
Department of Otolaryngology
The Ohio State University
University Hospitals Clinic
Columbus, Ohio

Frank E. Musiek, PhD
Professor of Otolaryngology
  and Neurology
Director of Audiology
Dartmouth-Hitchcock Medical
  Center
Hanover, New Hampshire

Wayne O. Olsen, PhD
Professor
Section of Audiology
Department of
  Otorhinolaryngology
Mayo Clinic and Mayo
  Foundation
Rochester, Minnesota

William F. Rintelmann, PhD
Professor and Chairman
Department of Audiology
Wayne State University School
  of Medicine
Detroit, Michigan

Jay W. Sanders, PhD
Professor Audiology Emeritus
Vanderbilt University School of
  Medicine
Bill Wilkerson Center
Nashville, Tennessee

Sabina A. Schwan, MA
Coordinator, Audiology Service
Harper Hospital
and
Adjunct Instructor, Department
  of Audiology, and
Associate in Otolaryngology
Wayne State University School
  of Medicine
Detroit, Michigan

Daniel M. Schwartz, PhD
Professor
Division of Bioelectrodiagnosis
  and Neural Monitoring
University of Pennsylvania
  Medical Center
Philadelphia, Pennsylvania

Jamie A. Schwartz, MA
Vice President
NeuroDynamics, Inc.
Newton Square, Pennsylvania

Janet E. Shanks, PhD
Audiology Section
Veterans Administration
  Medical Center
Long Beach, California
and
Assistant Professor in Residence
University of California
Irvine, California

Robert G. Turner, PhD
Director
Audiology and Speech Clinic
and
Associate Professor
Speech and Hearing Sciences
University of California–
  San Francisco
San Francisco, California

Laura Ann Wilber, PhD
Professor
Program in Audiology and
  Hearing Impairment
Department of Communication
  Sciences and Disorders
Northwestern University
Evanston, Illinois

Richard H. Wilson, PhD
Chief, Audiology Section
Veterans Administration
  Medical Center
Long Beach, California
and
Associate Professor
Division of Otolaryngology
University of California—Irvine
Irvine, California

Kenneth E. Wolf, PhD
Assistant Professor
Department of Otolaryngology
Drew University of Medicine
  and Science
and
Chief, Communication Sciences
  and Disorders
King/Drew Medical Center
Los Angeles, California

chapter one

Pure tone audiometry: Air and bone conduction

LAURA ANN WILBER

Contents

Initial concepts

Pure tone audiometry has become such an integral part of the audiologist's test battery that it is difficult to realize that the procedure did not exist until the latter part of the 19th century. In addition, normative threshold values for the pure tone audiometer did not officially exist in this country until 1951 when the American Standards Association published "Audiometers for General Diagnostic Purposes" (Document Z24.5, ASA, 1951).

Pure tone audiometry as we know it today probably began after the presentation in 1919 by C. C. Bunch and L. W. Dean (Bunch, 1943) of the "Pitch Range Audiometer" before the American Otologic Society. By 1922 Fowler and Wegel had developed the Western Electric 1A audiometer, which was the first commercially available vacuum tube audiometer existent in the United States (Bunch, 1943). In contrast, a standard procedure for threshold testing was not officially established until 1978 (ANSI, 1978).

1

Whisper tests

Physicians did test hearing, however, before the audiometer became commercially available. One of the first threshold tests of hearing probably was the "whisper" test. Whisper tests and tests using spoken voice are discussed in detail in Chapter 2 on speech audiometry. The procedure was used to try to determine whether the patient had normal hearing. Generally, the examiner used either spoken voice or whispered voice at a specified distance from the patient and determined whether the patient responded appropriately or not. The obvious problem with this type of procedure is that it is difficult to determine the level of one's voice or whisper. I have measured "whispers" from 20 dB to 65 dB sound pressure level (SPL) at 3 feet depending on the talker. It is also not possible to determine which ear is responding to the whisper or spoken voice. Despite its inadequacies we still receive forms from the government or insurance companies asking for results of "SV" (spoken voice) and "WV" (whispered voice).

As concern about the need for surgery or medical treatment of middle ear pathology became more prevalent, it was realized that it was necessary to determine the extent of the hearing loss and to differentiate hearing loss caused by problems in the external/middle ear versus those in the inner ear.

Tuning fork tests

One early technique is still in use today. Tuning fork tests were used to determine whether the patient had "normal" hearing at several frequencies. In addition, these tests were used because they enabled the physician to predict the probability of middle ear pathology. Tuning fork tests, which may have been used first simply to indicate more accurately whether the patient heard sounds equally well at different pitches, became critical in evaluating the possibility of a conductive component. Certain tuning fork tests are still commonly used today by otologists, some audiologists, and others as a quick method of assessing the probability of conductive pathology. Although most audiologists probably do not use tuning fork tests, they still need to be sufficiently familiar with them in order to discuss patient test findings, including tuning fork results, with otologists.

To administer the test, the examiner first strikes the tuning fork so that it emits a sound, usually on his or her own arm or leg or on some other object. The strength with which the tuning fork is struck influences the intensity of the sound from the fork. In addition, the material with which the tuning fork is made influences the intensity emitted and the length of time it takes for the tone to decay. We have found differences in intensity greater than 30 dB between fork presentations depending on the striking strength and the metal with which the tuning fork was made. Thus, hearing sensitivity with the tuning fork becomes difficult to quantify. It is possible for trained examiners to use tuning forks to estimate air conduction thresholds by determining the difference in seconds between the length of time the patient and the examiner heard the tone. This may be done at various test frequencies. It is also possible to use masking when testing. Most commonly, the Baranay Noise Box is used for tuning fork masking. The basic problem with the Baranay Noise Box is that its frequency response does not produce adequate masking, especially for high frequencies (see Chapter 3).

Table 1.1 describes five basic tuning fork tests in use today. The Schwabach has been used for both air and bone conduction, although it is commonly considered a measure of bone conduction. In this test the examiner's ability to consistently strike the fork must be relied on. The Schwabach and Rinne measure essentially the same thing by determining whether the sensorineural system is normal. The difference between the tuning fork and audiometric tests is that the tuning fork air-bone gap is normally classified as present or absent (except with highly experienced examiners who may be able to determine whether the gap is small, moderate, or large), whereas the audiometer allows the examiner to quantify the air–bone gap in decibels.

The Bing and Weber tests can be done using a bone vibrator and an audiometer in place of a tuning fork. The Gelle can be accomplished by changing air pressure in the ear canal with the probe from an acoustic immittance device and using the probe tone for the air-conduction Gelle. A bone vibrator (or tuning fork) may be used plus the air pressure change created by the acoustic immittance device for the bone-conducted Gelle.

In the hands of a careful and experienced examiner, tuning fork tests can provide a great deal of information about the probability, and even degree, of conductive pathology. However, these tests do not provide numerical threshold data. Only relative intensities for air and bone thresholds can be determined. The results can be reported and compared from one examiner to another, but only in a gross sense. With experience, an examiner may be able to delineate those persons who have normal hearing from those individuals with mild, moderate, or profound losses with or without conductive pathology.

Unfortunately, these tests are more susceptible to error than are audiometric tests. For example, the Weber will normally lateralize *either* to the ear with the better cochlear reserve *or* to the ear with the greater conductive component. However, for no apparent reason it may lateralize to an ear with poorer cochlear reserve or lesser conductive component.

TABLE 1.1
Tuning Fork Tests

Test	Definitions
Schwabach	A measure of bone conduction threshold. Place the tuning fork on the mastoid and determine the difference in seconds that the tone is heard by the examiner and the patient. If the patient hears it for a longer time, it is a prolonged Schwabach and conductive hearing loss can be assumed. If the patient hears it for a shorter time, it is a shortened Schwabach and sensorineural hearing loss can be assumed.
Rinne	Determine if the patient hears the tone longer by air conduction (AC) or bone conduction (BC). If the patient hears the tone for a longer time by BC than AC, the Rinne is negative and suggests a conductive (or mixed) lesion.
Bing	Occlude the ear with a finger. If the tone then appears louder, this indicates normal hearing or a sensorineural hearing loss. If the tone does not get louder, this indicates conductive hearing loss.
Weber	Place the tuning fork in the center of the forehead. If the patient hears the tone in the poorer ear, this indicates a conductive component, whereas if he or she hears it in the better ear, the loss is probably sensorineural. This test is usually done only with frequencies 256 Hz to 1024 Hz. (Note: The tone may lateralize to the ear with the greatest cochlear reserve regardless of conductive component.)
Gelle	Increase the air pressure in the auditory canal. In stapes fixation the increase of air pressure usually does not affect (or it decreases) loudness for bone conduction, but it does decrease loudness for air conduction.

Based in part on work reported by Tonndorf (1964).

The reason for this occurrence may be that the contour of the skull causes the tone to reach the cochlea quicker for one ear than the other (phase advance). We have seen instances in which the Weber, done audiometrically or with tuning forks, lateralizes to one ear at one frequency and to the other at another frequency. In addition, we have found instances in which the placement (i.e., forehead vs. dental) of the tuning fork or bone vibrator will affect the tonal lateralization.

Most tuning fork tests can be easily influenced by the manner in which the patient is questioned. For example, while doing the Bing, if the patient is asked if the tone appears to be louder after the ear is occluded than before, the examiner is more likely to get an affirmative response than if he or she simply asks the patient to tell what, if anything, happened to the tone when the ear was occluded. The latter is a preferable question because it is less likely to influence the response of the patient. Many patients in their desire to be cooperative are all too willing to respond in whatever way they believe the examiner expects or wishes.

Thus, with tuning fork tests it can be determined whether the patient hears better at one frequency than another, whether hearing is essentially normal or not, and whether conductive pathology is probable. Tuning fork tests can be done at any frequency for which a tuning fork is available, but generally they are done using either a 256- or 512-Hz tuning fork. It is extremely unlikely that the examiner will obtain positive Bing or Gelle results at frequencies above 512 Hz. Useful information may be obtained with the Schwabach or Rinne at higher frequencies, although it is usually somewhat more difficult to obtain reliable lateralization or air-bone differences with forks above 1024 Hz. Probably the 512-Hz fork is the most commonly used, although it is not quite as likely to produce a positive Bing as is the 256-Hz fork. Finally, it is generally best to draw conclusions with tuning fork tests only if two or more frequencies with at least two procedures have been tested.

Methods of threshold measurement

As suggested above, with the advent of pure tone audiometers it became possible to determine a patient's threshold of hearing. For a discussion of the audiometer and procedures for calibration, refer to Chapter 16. The audiometer can be used for speech testing and for special auditory tests; however, in this chapter we will discuss the use of the audiometer only as a device for obtaining pure tone thresholds for hearing.

Concept of threshold

The concept of threshold of hearing is both simple and complex. Clinicians (especially otolaryngologists and audiologists) tend to use one type of definition, whereas psychoacousticians use another type, which is slightly different. The American National Standards Institute defined the threshold of hearing as the "threshold of audibility" (ANSI, 53.20, 1973).

This document further states: "The threshold of audibility for a specified signal is the minimum effective sound pressure level of the signal that is capable of evoking an auditory sensation in a specified fraction of the trials" (p. 55, ANSI, 1973). The definition goes on to state that the characteristics of the test signal, of the procedure, and so forth should be defined.

The obvious problem is what is meant by "evoking an auditory sensation." If auditory sensation is viewed as a physiologic criterion, it is probably never met; whereas, if it is regarded as a psychologic criterion, it is conceivable that it could be attained. Strictly speaking in most audiologic testing, the threshold of audibility is probably not attained. In most audiologic test procedures a compromise is made between determining the faintest level at which an auditory sensation can be evoked and the level at which the examinee will *respond* to the presence of an auditory stimulus using available audiometric test equipment in a reasonable length of time. It is clear that the procedure that is used to measure "threshold" will determine to a large extent the value that will be obtained as threshold.

The level at which the examinee responds will be affected by whether (a) the test stimulus is presented in 1 dB steps (or any fraction thereof) or in 5 dB steps; (b) the signal appears in the presence of a defined noise or in "quiet"; (c) the patient indicates whether he believed a signal did or did not occur after a specific clue such as a light flash; (d) the criterion for definition of threshold (e.g., the level at which the examinee responds 50% of the time, more than 50% of the time, or some other specified percentage of the time); and/or (e) it is done by an examiner or computer system. These are, of course, only a few of the variables which may affect the outcome of threshold measurement.

The clinician and the psychoacoustician sometime engage in non-productive arguments in which the psychoacoustician informs the clinician, "You are *not* measuring threshold and you shouldn't say you are," whereas the clinician responds with equal fervor, "If I use the procedures which you outline it will take me a full day to get one threshold measurement for one frequency—and that one dB difference which I might get won't make a difference." It is beyond the scope of this chapter to decide which point of view, if either, is correct.

The working definition of *threshold of hearing* for the clinician should probably be the faintest level at which the patient will respond consistently (50% or more of the time) to the presence of an auditory signal using a specified technique. Some of these techniques are discussed later. It should be noted that the American Speech-Language-Hearing Association (ASHA) has developed a recommended procedure (ASHA, 1977) and the American National Standards Institute (ANSI) and the International Standards Organization (ISO) have produced standards for pure tone audiometric test procedures (ANSI, 1978; ISO, 1982, 1984). However, even when the standard procedure is used an examiner should realize that a "true auditory threshold" may not be obtained for the examinee.

As we leave the clinician and the psychoacoustician arguing as to whether the difference in an examinee's audiometric response and his or her true threshold of audibility differ by more than 5 dB, and whether any difference which may be obtained is "real" or "important," some discussion should be presented of the psychophysical procedures that have been used to obtain threshold of hearing for pure tones or tonal stimuli.

Psychophysical procedures

Despite the somewhat facetious remarks above, it is important to decide on the psychophysical procedure that will be used in determining threshold of hearing for pure tones by research subjects or patients. The contribution made by the psychoacousticians to our understanding of why patients respond as they do, and which procedures are most likely to elicit the most sensitive and reliable data, cannot be underestimated.

Before deciding which psychophysical method to use, the reasons for which the measurements are being made must first be considered. For example, some questions might involve whether the organism will respond to sound; in what way the organism will respond; to determining whether or not a patient has a hearing loss or not in a gross sense; determining the patient's specific hearing level for compensation purposes; or determining the probabilities of the patient having conductive pathology. Second, the nature of the specific stimulus which one plans to use must be considered: In this case, pure tones or tonal stimuli of varying intensities and durations. Third, the subject under investigation must be considered. For example, it would be inappropriate to expect a subject with severe muscular control problems to operate a switch with a rapidly changing continuous stimulus. The method that is used, therefore, must be appropriate to the subject, to the stimuli, and be able to answer the measurement question.

Stevens (1958, 1960) described seven procedures for determining *absolute threshold*. The absolute threshold is defined by ANSI as the "minimum stimulus that evokes a response in a specified number of trials (ANSI, 1973, p.1). Earlier, Stevens defined absolute threshold as "the value that divides the continuum of stimuli into two classes, those to which the organism reacts and those to which it does not" (Stevens, 1960, p. 33). Stevens's procedures are as follows: (a) single stimuli, (b) counting, (c) forced choice, (d) adjustment, (e) limits, (f) tracking, and (g) staircase. Although he pointed out that it was not possible to define absolute threshold absolutely since it shifts in time, he did describe procedures that might be used to try to determine the threshold of hearing for a given subject at a given point in time.

All of the above methods have been used alone, in combination, or in modified form to attempt to determine a subject/patient's threshold of hearing. Depending on the procedure, the stimulus (in this case a pure tone) is on either continuously or during discrete time intervals.

In the *single stimuli method* the tone is on or off at a particular intensity level, and the examinee is asked to indicate whether the tone is present. If the patient perceives that it is present, he or she may indicate yes by saying so, by pushing a button, by raising a hand, and so forth. If the patient does not perceive that it is present he or she will do nothing. *Threshold* is defined as the level at which the stimulus is correctly perceived as present 50% of the time. Another requirement such as 75% of the time may be used, but generally in clinical usage 50% is considered the threshold point.

If, instead of randomly presenting the stimulus at various intensities, it is varied in a systematic manner from levels above and below the threshold, it is called a *method of limits*. This may be done using either a continuous tone, as orginally described, or discrete tone bursts. The subject is instructed to indicate when he or she "just hears" the tone. A modification of this procedure is used in most clinical situations; it is described in more detail later in this chapter in the Conventional Procedures section. In the latter case, referred to as modified method of limits, the stimulus is increased in specified intensity intervals until the examinee indicates that he or she has heard it. The tone is then attenuated by a specified amount and again increased in discrete steps until the subject indicates that the tone is present.

The modified method of limits is not very different from the *staircase procedure* in which the intensity levels are also discrete and fixed. The response at a particular level during one trial will determine the level of the next trial. Specifically, if the stimulus did not elicit a response the intensity is increased by a fixed amount, whereas if a response was elicited it is decreased by a fixed-step interval. This technique is easily programmable so that the stimulus may be presented using a computer system.

In the procedures described above the examinee knows that a signal will occur, but he or she usually does not know *when*. In the *forced-choice method* the examinee knows when the stimulus may have been presented, but he or she does not necessarily know if it was. In this procedure during a fixed-time interval, which is usually defined by a light clue, the subject is required to indicate whether or not the stimulus was present. In a variation of this, the subject knows both that the tone was present and that it occurred during one of a series of time intervals (usually no more than four). In the latter case a signal such as a light flash is given, and the subject indicates in which discrete time interval the stimulus occurred. The forced-choice procedure was originally used with research subjects, but it is easily adaptable to most clinical situations with alert and cooperative patients.

Robinson and Watson (1972) indicated that the optimal time interval for a single-interval procedure is between 1 and 3 seconds. They further reported that in the multiple-interval procedure the time between successive observations is usually about half a second.

One more variant on the above procedures is the *counting method*. This was used at one time in classrooms when many children were tested simultaneously. A series of tones was presented through headsets to each of the children, and they were asked to indicate how many tones they heard during the time interval. In this case, the tones were attenuated in discrete steps; thus by comparing the number of tones perceived by the child against the number given, the examiner could decide the faintest level at which the child heard. The problem was that the child might lose count or copy from a neighbor. Another variant used today with difficult-to-test patients is to give one to three stimuli at a given intensity level. The patient is asked to indicate how many stimuli were heard. This often produces more reliable, if not more sensitive, threshold data.

Besides procedures that use discrete stimulus presentations, some methods use *constant stimuli*. In these procedures the stimulus is always present and the question is how faint it may be and still be perceived as audible by the examinee. In one procedure, the *method of adjustment*, the examinee controls an attenuator and adjusts the intensity of the tone until it is "just audible" (or in some cases, until it is "just inaudible"). The level to which the examinee adjusts the intensity is defined as threshold.

In another procedure, the method of limits described above using discrete stimuli, the stimuli may also be constantly on but systematically varied by the examiner. The examinee indicates when the tone is just audible, as it is increased and decreased in a specified range.

A variation on the continuous stimuli method of limits procedure is called *tracking* (more commonly called the "Bekesy" procedure today). It was described by von Bekesy (1947) and by Oldfield (1949). In this procedure the examinee presses a button or activates a switch for as long as he or she hears the tone and releases the button, or deactivates the switch when the tone disappears. The stimulus intensity is automatically increased or decreased dependent on the subject's action. It should be noted that in the original design described by von Bekesy, the stimulus frequency was changed automatically at the same time the intensity was increasing and decreasing.

With pathological subjects it is usually easier to determine threshold of hearing when the pure-tone frequency is fixed. This is because the time constants of the frequency change are such that the subject may not have reached threshold at one frequency before the next frequency is presented. If there is a dramatic difference in threshold (i.e., a sharp slope) from one frequency to another this often will not be reflected in the continuously varying frequency procedure.

Although all of the methods described above may be used with a clinical population, each procedure may not be equally effective for each individual. For example, the single-interval forced-choice procedure in which a stimulus may or may not occur during a fixed time interval normally produces very reliable and sensitive threshold data for research subjects. However, for *some* patients an uncertain time interval is thought to be of help clinically because it avoids predisposing the patient whose hearing level is unknown from responding when there is no stimulus. For example, it is not uncommon for both children and adults to establish their own rhythmic pattern of indicating the presence of a stimulus regardless of whether one was introduced. If the examinee is told that a signal may or may not occur in a given time interval, some patients will respond positively in each time interval. If this occurs, the clinician should either use a method of rewarding the patient only for a correct response, or use another forced-choice procedure, in which several time intervals transpire and the patient is asked in which interval the stimulus occurred. Again, some patients will either invariably pick a specific interval (e.g., the Number 2) or will become more concerned with guessing an interval than listening for a tone. The distinction may be that generally the research subject appears to interpret the important question as being whether he or she can respond correctly to the presence of a stimulus, whereas the patient with a hearing loss may respond in a completely different manner simply because this patient's goal is to define a level at which he or she can respond rather than to determine his or her ability to accomplish the task. If it is clear that the patient will not easily break a pattern response when a forced-choice technique is used, it may be necessary to vary time intervals, or to use another procedure.

As suggested above, when obtaining patient thresholds, the time interval between stimulus presentations for an alert, cooperating person is generally between 1 and 3 seconds. However, when the patient begins to respond at short time intervals such as once every 2 seconds regardless of the time of stimulus presentation, the time period between signal presentations may be expanded to 5 or 10 seconds. Finally, in clinical testing, an examiner will find some patients who appear to need several seconds before they are able to respond to the fact that a stimulus was presented. We have seen some patients who were consistently able to respond to the presence of a sound but who required a 5–10-second time interval between the end of the stimulus and the time when they were able to produce a response. Generally, this suggests the presence of some neurologic dysfunction.

In psychoacoustic signal detection experiments in which forced-choice procedures are used, it is common to establish a specific criterion level for the patient. The subject may be asked, for example, to respond when he is 90% sure that a stimulus has occurred during a given time interval. When a strict criterion is employed, it is expected that the response will *require* a greater intensity than it will if the subject is asked to respond if he or she thinks that there is a 10% probability of correctly indentifying the stimulus. In the latter instance the subject is likely to guess much more often and the level at which he or she responds will be fainter. Generally, the purpose of these experiments is not simply to define the level at which the subject can detect a signal but to determine probabilities of signal detection. Some experiments are designed to determine not only the listener's ability to discriminate the presence of a signal embedded in noise, but also his or her ability to adapt a particular strategy for responding to the presence of the stimulus. The display of data generated from these experiments is generally called a receiver operating characteristic (ROC) curve. This function relates the probability of a response being given when the signal is, in fact, absent. Egan, Greenberg, and Schulman (1961), for example, showed that there could be considerable difference in the probability curves that were generated, depending on whether the subject was instructed to be strict, medium, or lax in making a decision. Again, it is probably evident that there are many variations that can occur on this theme. For a further discussion of ROC curves, see Chapter 14.

The results of the experiments can be affected by (a) the time interval between stimulus presentation, (b) the level of the background noise in which the signal is embedded, (c) the percentage of time in which the signal is not present, (d) the intensity difference of the signal relative to the noise background from one time to another, and so forth. In addition, results will vary depending on the way in which the subject is instructed to respond. It has been demonstrated that after the subject is well practiced, experiments of this type yield extremely reliable data. If the instructions are precise, the subjects are well experienced, and other aspects of the procedure are consistent, the results will be highly predictable. It is somewhat more difficult to be certain whether procedures used in signal detection experiments will work as well with patients who have additional internal masking interference (such as tinnitus) as compared to research subjects who probably will not have additional internal stimulus interference possibilities.

The outcome of these experiments (or any threshold measurement procedure) can be affected in other ways such as by indicating to the examinee that he or she will be rewarded financially or in some other way if a particular percent correct criterion is achieved. If the subject is punished either by a mild electric shock or even by a signal light indicating that he or she was wrong, then the correct response percentage will also change. Some variations on these behavior modification techniques can be used effectively with patients. For example, in testing young children it is usually helpful to smile and nod enthusiastically when the child correctly responds to the presence of a tone. Likewise, it may be appropriate to frown or look dejected when the child responds to an absent sound. (*Note.* We do *not* recommend or condone the use of electric shock or any physically punitive procedure for children or other clinical patients as a reinforcer or as a punisher for incorrect response.)

In psychoacoustic experiments it also has been shown that the results can be dramatically affected by giving the subject false feedback information. If the examiner gives a light signal indicating the response was false when it was not, this can confuse the subject and will change the level at which he or she responds to the presence of the stimulus. The examiner should thus be careful not to give a subject false visual information. For example, if the clinician frowns in response to something occurring in the examining room at the same time that the patient is correctly responding to the presentation of a tone, this will confuse the patient and may result in false threshold estimations.

It should be remembered that signal detection theory, which has helped immeasurably to delineate psychophysical test procedure experiments and has provided a means to study the effect of variables, is actually a mathematical model designed to determine whether an electrical signal has occurred in the presence of noise. Originally these experiments were developed in electrical engineering (Tanner & Sorkin, 1972). Mathematical concepts may be used with human beings by asking that the human respond in the ways described above, but it should be remembered that it is infinitely easier to accurately detect the presence or absence of a signal in the presence of noise on an oscilloscope or with a computer than in a human's auditory system. The results from the machine are not as likely to be contaminated by human problems such as fatigue, desire to be rewarded, desire to confuse or confound the examiner, or by the constant change that appears to occur in a human's true auditory receptive ability.

Finally, criterion levels may be defined much more easily for electronic equipment than for humans. Every clinician is likely to have been confronted at one time or another with a patient who had been instructed very carefully to respond as soon as a tone was heard, but who did not respond consistently after repeated instructions and reinstructions. Just as the clinician becomes convinced that this patient has the largest threshold variation ever reported, the patient suddenly says, "Oh! You meant I should tell you every time I heard *that* itty bitty noise. Well, why didn't you tell me that's what you wanted me to listen to?" At this point the psychoacoustician generally has a distinct advantage over the clinician in that the former can walk out of the room and let the computer continue the test.

Conventional procedures

The majority of hearing tests for children and adults will be administered using so-called conventional procedures. For years the term *conventional* procedure has been used with no clear definition of what it meant. In recent years, most often it referred to manual audiometry using the modified Hughson-Westlake technique (Carhart & Jerger, 1959), which is essentially an ascending technique. In this procedure the examinee is asked to indicate when he or she hears the tone either by raising his or her hand or finger or by pushing a button. Briefly, with the manual procedure the examiner first familiarizes the examinee with the tone by producing the stimulus at a presumed supra-threshold level, or by gradually increasing the tone's intensity until the examinee responds. Then the tone is presented in short bursts of 1 to 2 seconds with silent intervals of varying length between tone presentations. The tone presentations are decreased in intensity until the examinee ceases to respond when it is presented. At that point, the intensity of the tone is increased. If the examinee responds when the tone is presented, the tone is lowered in intensity by 10 dB and then it is increased in 5-dB steps until the examinee again responds. This ascending procedure is repeated until the examinee responds 50% or more of the time at a given level. Given that most audiometer attenuators operate in 5-dB steps, in practice this level is quite often achieved when two out of three or three out of five correct responses are obtained at a given intensity level. A detailed description of the manual pure tone audiometry procedure is described in *Asha* (1977), and in the ANSI Standard 3.21 (ANSI, 1978). Working Group 3 (TC43/WG3) of ISO also developed a draft international standard for pure tone testing (ISO, 1984). This latter working group is developing a series of standard procedure documents. The first standard defined procedures to use in industrial testing, using automatic and manual threshold testing (ISO, 1982). The initial draft proposal of the manual procedure by the group differed from the Hughson-Westlake and was called a *bracketing procedure*. It more closely approximates an automatic procedure. As currently proposed, after familiarization, the tone is increased in specified steps and then decreased in specified steps. The faintest level at which the examinee responds to the tone on three ascending passes and on three descending passes is averaged to determine the threshold for hearing at a given frequency. The ascending technique described above was added as an alternate test procedure and is now considered equivalent to the bracketing procedure.

A systematic study was carried out by Arlinger (1979) to see if there was a substantial difference in the threshold values obtained with the two techniques outlined above. The results indicated that both procedures yielded similar thresholds. In any event, it is no longer sufficient for an examiner to say a "conventional" procedure was used. It is important to define specifically the procedure or to state that the ASHA, 1977, or ANSI, 1978, or ISO, 1984, procedure was used. All of the above standards and recommendations require that the examiner note on the audiogram (or report) if deviations from the described procedure were used. It is recognized that certain patients cannot be tested using any of the proposed or existent manual audiometric techniques and that special techniques must be used in these cases. In the latter instances, it is especially important to describe in detail the technique that was used.

Another "conventional" procedure for pure tone testing is self-recording (automatic) audiometry. It is outside the limits of this chapter to discuss the procedures for Bekesy audiometry as used for diagnostic purposes (see Chapters 12 and 13), but automatic machines are being used in increasing numbers to determine audiometric thresholds. In this procedure the examinee normally is asked to push a button when the tone is heard and to release the button when the tone fades away. The machine automatically decreases and increases the intensity of the tone as the button is pushed and released. Usually an X-Y plotter is attached to the attenuator output so that a graphic representation of the examinee's response may be obtained while increasing and decreasing the intensity of the sound. The midpoint of the ascending and descending patterns (Reger, 1952) or some other specific trace point is used to define the threshold level. It has been shown that the point on the tracing that one chooses to call 'threshold" can affect the correlation of these results with manual techniques (Harbert & Young, 1966). The problem of comparing manual to automatic thresholds has been discussed in detail by Rintelmann (1975), especially as applied to industrial hearing conservation procedures.

A second automatic technique is a preprogrammed computerized method. In one computerized procedure, the examinee presses a button if he or she thinks a sound has occurred. If the sound did occur the program calls for a fainter stimulus to be emitted at a discrete level. Attenuation may continue in discrete steps until the subject does not respond, at which time the intensity is increased. With the exception that this may be done with single tone bursts and discrete interval steps, the procedure is very much like the automatic procedure described above. In another preprogrammed computerized technique a tonal signal is presented at a predetermined intensity level. A light flashes and the subject responds by pushing a button to indicate whether he or she believes a tone presentation occurred or not. At certain randomly prescribed intervals the light will flash, but no tone will be presented. Again the subject must indicate whether he or she believes a tone occurred. The faintest level at which the subject correctly identifies a specified percentage of tonal stimuli is labeled "threshold." These procedures use the forced-choice technique discussed above. There are many variations on the above procedures. Currently an ANSI working group is trying to develop a standard for computerized audiometry. The ISO standard simply states that test results with a computerized system should yield thresholds that are the same as with the manual procedure (ISO, 1984).

No matter which of the techniques outlined above are used, it is clear that the examinee may respond at whatever suprathreshold level he or she desires or he or she may fail to respond at all, even when the tone is audible. The examinee's concept of "hearing the tone" will influence the obtained results. It is important that the examiner instruct the examinee in a manner likely to elicit the faintest response levels. For example, the examiner may say: "Be sure to push the button *as soon as* you hear the tone and let the button go *as soon as* it goes away. Remember, I want to find the *very faintest* level at which you can hear this tone." The examinee may be told to respond as soon as he or she hears the tone no matter how quiet it is, that it is all right to guess, and that he or she should indicate even if the hearing of the tone was only a possibility. If too many false positive responses occur, the examinee must be reinstructed.

Various techniques can be used for children or older persons who have difficulty in responding consistently to the stimulus. Patients who have tinnitus, regardless of age, often have difficulty, especially at high frequencies. Others have short attention spans. Others may forget the stimulus for which they are listening or the response which is expected. In these instances, the examiner may ask the patient to count the number of beeps (giving varying numbers of tonal stimuli usually 1 to 4, at a given intensity level) or to point to the ear in which he or she hears the sound. Assuming the patient can count or can point, these procedures may yield reliable threshold results. If the examinee wishes to deceive the examiner it is quite possible that he or she will respond only at suprathreshold levels. It is beyond the scope of this chapter to discuss ways in which this can be detected or the procedures to overcome it (see Chapter 12), but the clinician must always remember that it is possible that at a given time the examinee may not be responding at the faintest level at which he or she can hear.

Green (1972) described somewhat facetiously the "finger" test in which he discussed the height or way the finger is raised. In many instances an examiner truly can determine how close to threshold the examinee is by noting the alacrity and height to which the examinee raises his or her finger or hand. Although this particular observation is not always foolproof, the careful clinician will try to observe the examinee's behavior in order to gain more information about the examinee's probable reception of sound.

One 2-year-old whom we tested refused to raise his hand consistently, but he did say "no" firmly each time the tone was presented. It is the clinician's job to encourage, to cajole, and occasionally even to bully the examinee into responding as close as possible to his or her threshold of audibility.

The conventional procedures described above are highly repeatable, which is advantageous. It is not yet clear by how much the results of any of these "conventional" techniques will vary from the "true threshold of audibility" for a given examinee (the standard deviation is about 5 dB). For practical purposes, however, these techniques will enable the examiner to determine with a high degree of confidence whether the examinee has normal hearing, or a mild, moderate, severe, or profound hearing loss.

Procedures for conventional pure tone audiometry

After the examiner has chosen an appropriate method of measurement and basic stimuli, it is important to determine not only the amount of hearing loss but something of its nature. The most basic procedures for determining gross site of lesion (i.e., conductive or sensorineural) are the air- and bone-conduction tests. In this chapter each will be discussed separately, but it is important to remember that both must be administered to obtain the basic diagnostic information. It is also important to recognize that in addition to pure tone tests, the examiner will normally also administer acoustic immittance (see Chapters 4 and 5) and speech tests (see Chapter 2) to determine whether the loss is conductive or sensorineural.

Air-conduction tests

When obtaining behavioral air-conduction thresholds, a response to sound passed through the entire auditory pathway is being measured. Although when an examiner observes an infant, he or she may be misled into thinking that a child "hears" when in fact the sound may only be received at a subcortical level, in most instances the requirement of a specific voluntary action increases the probability that the patient has "heard" in the psychological sense (See Chapters 8 and 9). Thus, the examiner may believe with some degree of assurance that if the examinee responds to pure tone stimuli at normal threshold levels the basic auditory system is intact from the external ear to the auditory cortex. However, ability to respond to pure tones does *not* imply that the auditory system is undamaged. It will be shown in other chapters (Chapters 2 and 11) that in some retrocochlear lesions the subject may be able to respond to pure tones at normal threshold levels but may not be able to handle speech stimuli or complex tonal stimuli in a normal manner. Despite this problem, if the examinee makes consistent *voluntary* responses to sound stimuli, those sounds have probably reached the auditory cortex. With pure tone testing, the examiner is generally concerned with determining whether the patient has a peripheral hearing loss; that is, a loss at the level of the cochlea, middle, or external ear. Although in many instances damage to the VIIIth cranial nerve also will result in a pure tone hearing loss, its significance will not be discussed here.

Responses to pure tones at normal hearing levels only mean the examinee hears a sound at these normal intensity levels. A response at a normal intensity level does not indicate that the tone is necessarily received or perceived in a normal manner, that is, it may be distorted or it may have no tonal quality. It is, thus, important to try to determine *what* the examinee hears as well as how faintly he or she can respond. This usually can be learned by careful questioning at some time during the test session.

Air-conduction tests are administered either using earphones or in the sound field using loudspeakers or, as mentioned earlier, using tuning forks. In the next paragraphs we will be concerned with pure tone air-conduction testing using earphones or loudspeakers.

Earphone testing. At present there are no ANSI standards for earphones that are enclosed in circumaural cushions or enclosures (i.e., cushions that encircle the pinna as opposed to supra-aural cushions that rest on the pinna; ANSI, 1989; Zwislocki, Kruger, Miller, Niemoeller, Shaw, & Studebaker, 1988) so it will be assumed here that supra-aural cushions (MX41/AR) are used. A discussion of the importance of this distinction is given in Chapter 16 on calibration.

Insert earphones also have been suggested as a possible way to help control the problem of ambient noise and to assist in the solution of difficult masking problems by increasing interaural attenuation (Wilber,

Kruger, & Killion, 1988). The current ANSI standard (ANSI, 1989) does include interim Reference Equivalent Threshold Sound Pressure Level (RETSPL) values for calibration of insert receivers in its Appendix G. In addition, an ISO working group (TC/43 WG-3) is considering appropriate values for these earphones. Insert earphones currently are used by many clinicians, although they have not yet been accepted by some governmental bodies (e.g., for OSHA Occupational Hearing Conservation Programs), or some agencies (Zwislocki, Kruger, Miller, Niemoeller, Shaw, & Studebaker, 1988).

When an earphone is placed on or in an ear, it is important that the diaphragm be placed opposite the opening to the ear canal. Hair or anything else that can block the opening to the ear canal should be moved away. It behooves the clinician to visually inspect the examinee's ear canal to make sure there is no cotton or other object in the external ear. Sometimes persons who are in pain will put cotton in the ear canal, which, of course, will create or add to a hearing loss. If possible the ear should be cleared of cerumen. However, if the cerumen is not impacted and totally occluding the ear canal or touching the eardrum it appears to have little, if any, effect on hearing thresholds. Note: Removal of cerumen is especially important when using insert receivers. If threshold testing does reveal a conductive hearing loss and there appears to be cerumen, the patient should be referred to a physician for its removal and the test should be repeated after the cerumen has been removed. It is a mistake to fail to repeat the test after cerumen removal if a conductive loss was found. By repeating the test the examiner can determine whether the cerumen contributed to the initial test results.

Testing should be done in a room that is quiet enough to avoid masking by the ambient noise in the room. Table 1.2 shows the maximum sound pressure level (SPL) that may exist in a room in order to obtain thresholds as low as O-dB hearing level (HL). Note that ANSI (1977) values are lower for covered ears (earphones over both ears) than uncovered ones. If the examiner is doing bone-conduction or sound field testing (which will be discussed later), the uncovered values must be used as criterion values for room noise.

The covered values presume the use of supra-aural cushions. Although it is possible to obtain fainter and possibly more reliable thresholds in the presence of room noise using circumaural cushions (Villchur, 1970) the fact is that there are no current ASNI or ISO threshold standards for circumaural earphones. As mentioned above standards do now exist for insert receivers (ANSI, 1989).

When using supra-aural earphones, one should be sure that the earphone fits snugly over the ear and that the headband is adjusted appropriately. The earphones must be placed tightly over the ears or there will

TABLE 1.2
Acceptable Noise Levels in Audiometric Test Rooms
When Testing Is Expected to Reach "0" dB HL Re ANSI (1969)

	Frequency (Hz) Octave Band Level Measurements										
	125	250	500	750	1000	1500	2000	3000	4000	6000	8000
Under Earphones Only (in dB SPL)	34.5	23.0	21.5	22.5	29.5	29.0	34.5	39.0	42.0	41.0	45.0
Sound Field or Bone Conduction (in dB SPL)	28.0	18.5	14.5	12.5	14.0	10.5	8.5	8.5	9.0	14.0	20.5

From the ANSI Criteria for Permissible Ambient Noise During Audiometric Testing (ANSI, 1977).

be a low-frequency transmission loss (such as evidenced in open ear mold fittings), which will be reflected in the measured thresholds. Occasionally an examiner will encounter a patient whose head is too large for conventional headsets. In such an instance, two headsets may be used with the earphone from one headset on one ear and the other earphone from the same headset on the upper part of the head and vice versa. Although this is not a common problem, it does occur occasionally with unshunted hydrocephalic patients and others. Whether the head is large or small, it is infinitely better to use supra-aural earphones with a headband than to try to hold the earphone in place. The examiner's hand is unlikely to maintain consistent pressure against the pinna. A few manufacturers have provided earphone headbands for children, although these headbands are difficult to find. We know of no commercially available headbands for infants. It will behoove the clinician to have available at least one headset that is the appropriate size for children, otherwise the insufficient pressure exerted by the band holding the phone in place may allow escape of sound, creating the presence of an apparent low-frequency hearing loss and slippage so that the high frequencies are also in error.

In addition, when testing with supra-aural earphones, it is important to be sure that the pinna or ear canal does not collapse. In some instances when supra-aural earphones are placed on the ear, the ear canal or the pinna will collapse to occlude the external auditory meatus. This will not be visibly apparent since current cushions are not transparent. One can get some notion of this possibility by pushing on the pinna with one's fingers prior to putting on the earphones and observing whether the opening into the canal appears to collapse. If one finds an apparent conductive loss with a normal tympanogram or positive acoustic reflex, one should suspect the possibility of an occluded ear canal. If a collapsing canal is suspected one must use other procedures such as sound field testing, insert receivers, or some method of keeping the canal propped open. One procedure that seems to work quite well is to cut off the end of a plastic speculum and insert it into the ear canal to hold the canal open. Although sound will reflect off this plastic and might contribute to slightly different thresholds than those that would be obtained if the ear was not collapsing under the earphones, it appears to be a reasonable way of obtaining threshold measurements with persons who have collapsing canals.

Insert earphones may also be used to help control the problem of collapsing ear canals. When using insert earphones it is important to insert the tip deeply into the ear canal. If the tip extrudes from the canal opening, the advantages of the insert earphone (control of the problems of crossover, occlusion, and collapsing ear canals) will be lost.

When obtaining pure tone air-conduction thresholds one generally begins with a 1000-Hz tone. Although there is no compelling reason for starting at 1000 Hz (human sensitivity is slightly better at 2000 Hz, for example), some early studies by Harris (1945) and by Dadson and King (1952) indicated that test-retest reliability was slightly better at 1000 (or 1024) Hz than at the other frequencies tested. Perhaps for that reason 1000 Hz is the recommended starting point in both the ANSI and ISO standard procedures. After establishing a threshold one proceeds to the next highest octave frequency and so on through 8000 Hz, and then one establishes thresholds for the lower frequencies of 250 and 500 Hz. When testing children or others whose attention span is very short or who are difficult to test, one may wish to first obtain threshold values at 500 and 2000 Hz for each ear. Following those four thresholds, one may try to test the remaining frequencies. By finding thresholds for a high and low frequency, a basic impression of the examinee's response to sound can be gained. Albeit the information from two frequencies is not sufficient to make a full comment on the examinee's hearing, these frequencies will enable the examiner to make some statement regarding the probable hearing level of the patient and his or her probable communication problems.

Although it is not within the scope of this chapter to discuss speech audiometry (see Chapter 2), we have found it helpful to use the speech reception threshold results as guidelines for pure tone test expectations, especially in the case of young children. If the 1000-Hz threshold is considerably different than that obtained for speech, it is appropriate to test a frequency other than 1000 Hz to see if the second pure tone threshold is more compatible with the speech reception threshold. It should be expected that one of the frequencies of 500, 1000, or 2000 Hz will be within ± 5 to 10 dB of the speech reception threshold. Occasionally the speech reception threshold may be better than the thresholds for any of these three frequencies. However, if no pure tone threshold is within ± 5 dB of the speech reception threshold, one should suspect that the pure tone threshold results are inaccurate. The reason for the inaccuracy may be that the speech is more familiar and probably more interesting than pure tones or it may indicate a functional overlay (see Chapter 12).

It is important to be sure that one truly is testing through the earphones (not through speakers when the earphones are on) and that the appropriate earphones are used. It helps to ask the patient to raise the hand on the side that he or she hears the sound (or to point to the ear with the sound). However, often if all thresholds are obtained in this manner they will be approximately 5 dB poorer than thresholds obtained by simply asking the examinee to respond by raising a hand when he or she hears a tone. Apparently, it is difficult for many people to determine in which ear the sound is being heard very near—or at—their auditory threshold. In addition, the sound does not always have the same tonal quality near threshold that it does at suprathreshold levels. In any case, at some time during the test it is appropriate to ask the patient where he or she hears the sound to make sure that the earphones have not inadvertently been reversed.

When testing via earphone, one should expect the possibility of crossover if the air-conduction threshold is poorer than 40 dB HL. If the air-conduction threshold is 40 dB poorer than the bone-conduction threshold of the contralateral ear, crossover may occur; however, given that one normally tests air conduction in both ears before testing by bone conduction, it may initially be difficult to accurately determine bone-conduction threshold levels. Therefore, if responses occur at levels greater than 40 dB HL, the examiner should consider using masking. The necessity of, and procedures for, masking are discussed in detail in Chapter 3.

Sometimes it is difficult to teach young children to respond to the presence of the tone rather than to the presence of the masking noise. However, many children as young as 2 to 3 years of age can be taught this difference and will respond appropriately even when masking is used. A much more difficult problem is convincing a 2-year-old to use earphones. Many children in the 18- to 30-month-old age range do not like to have anything on their heads and object strenuously when earphones are placed on them. Some children can be persuaded to wear the ''hat'' or ''astronaut headphones''; others are not so easily persuaded. This usually is not a problem for children below 1 year of age, but it is difficult to find appropriate headbands for babies. When the child totally refuses earphones or they will not fit, sound field testing may be used.

It is wise to talk to the parents about the importance of testing via earphones, because only through earphone testing can the examiner be sure of the hearing in each ear. It is helpful to ask the parents to use headsets (such as stereo phones) with the child at home to get the child used to them. Wearing earphones can thereby become a pleasurable experience; hence on subsequent visits the child may permit earphone use even though initially he or she would not. See Chapter 9 for further discussion of testing infants and young children.

Sound field testing using warble tone and narrow band noises. If the patient cannot be tested by earphones, it may be necessary to use sound field testing in order to obtain an indication of the levels at which the patient hears the tones. It is not possible to use pure tones in the sound field in an audiometric test booth because of standing waves. These create an impossible calibration situation and in addition require the examinee's head to be held in a rigid position. Pure tones can probably be used in an anechoic chamber, provided that all reflecting surfaces, including the chair in which the patient sits, have been carefully padded in order to avoid any possibility of reflected sound. Normally, however, the examiner will be using an audiometric test booth and thus pure tones should not be used. Warble tones or narrow bands of noise may be used. As of this writing, there is no ANSI definition for warble tones or narrow band noise used for threshold testing. Basically, however, warble tones are pure tones with specific modulation rates; that is, the tone changes rapidly from the basic pure tone frequency to another above or below it in a specific manner (Delk, 1973; Staab & Rintelmann, 1972b). In contrast, a narrow band noise is either white noise that is filtered in a specific manner so that the center frequency is the nominal one for the band, or several discrete frequencies of equal intensity in a given band are produced. There are no normative values threshold for warble tones or for narrow band noise.

Some studies have been conducted using warble tones and/or noise in the sound field. Also, some investigations have made threshold level comparisons between pure tones and warble tones. An average of data presented by Staab (1971) and by Rintelmann, Orchik, and Stephens (1972), Staab and Rintelmann (1972a), Rudmose (1962), Morgan and Dirks (1974), Stream and Dirks (1974), and by Tillman, Johnson, and Olsen (1966) were combined to obtain values that may be appropriate for 0 dB HL warble tone threshold in the sound field (See Table 1.3). Other values have been proposed by Walker, Dillon, and Byrne (1984). Currently there are no ANSI or ISO sound field threshold recommendations, but both ASHA and ISO working groups are writing documents that will recommend threshold values for sound field testing.

In addition to the fact that there are no approved ANSI or ISO values, the numbers given in Table 1.3 should not be considered to represent normative data because, for example, there has been no definitive study to determine the appropriate modulation rate, the repetition rate, or any

TABLE 1.3
Sample SPL Values for "0" dB HL for Sound Field Warble Tones[a]

	Frequency (Hz)				
	250	500	1000	2000	4000
dB SPL	15	9	3	−3	−4

Data from studies by Morgan and Dirks (1974), Rintelmann et al. (1972), Rudmose (1962), Staab (1971), Staab and Rintelmann (1972a), Stream and Dirks (1974), and Tillman et al. (1966).
[a]Speakers at 45° azimuth.

of the parameters of the warble tone. Staab (1971) and Staab and Rintel-mann (1972a) did report an investigation in which 30 combinations of modulation ratios and frequency deviations were used with three trained listeners. The results obtained with those conditions led them to conclude that frequency deviations of up to ± 10% and modulation rates as rapid as 32 per second did not produce substantial differences between warble and pure tone thresholds. Whether these relationships are equally important for children is not yet known. Other studies by Dillon and Walker (1980, 1982) have also recommended characteristics of the sound field stimuli.

Some clinicians say that the warble tone should "sound interesting." This concept is almost impossible to define. In addition, a warble tone that is interesting to the clinician may not be equally interesting to the child. However, many audiometers are equipped with warble tone stimuli that at least prevent most of the problems of standing waves. Until nor-mative data are accepted, the clinician should establish his or her own threshold norms for each audiometer, given that they will vary in almost all parameters.

At the very least, it is necessary to make sure that there is no object between the loudspeaker and the ear of the patient and to try to eliminate reflecting surfaces in the sound room. The advantage of warble tone over narrow bands of noise was pointed out by Orchik and Rintelmann (1978) and Stephens and Rintelmann (1978). The latter study showed that for patients with flat hearing losses, warble tones and narrow bands of noise yield equivalent thresholds; however, if the patient has a high-frequency loss because of the spread of the noise band, the clinician will not get an accurate representation of the loss. That is, because a narrow band of noise as produced by current commercial audiometers has a spectrum that encompasses adjacent frequency bands at some point (6 to 20 dB fainter in most cases), the individual may respond to the noise from the adjacent frequency band rather than to the test band. Because the purpose of testing is to determine the nature and degree of loss, it appears clear that warble tones are preferable to narrow band noise. A further problem is that currently there is no standard bandwidth for a "narrow band" of noise used for threshold testing.

It is hoped that in the near future threshold values will be promulgated for warble tones and narrow bands of noise in the sound field. It is probably not important to use warble tones or narrow bands of noise under earphones, since most children who will wear earphones will respond equally well to warble tones or pure tones (Robinson & Vaughan, 1976). Warble tone stiumli may be used in the sound field with visual reinforcement audiometry (VRA), conditioned orienting response (COR), or play audiometry. Warble tone thresholds obtained in sound fields with play audiometry correlate well with pure tone thresholds obtained under earphones with the same child when he or she is older.

As mentioned earlier, one of the disadvantages of sound field testing is that the clinician cannot tell to which ear the patient is responding. Even when a child localizes to a particular side, it is not possible to be sure that the child hears in that ear. Generally, it is true however, that a child will respond a little more quickly and somewhat more consistently toward the side of the better ear.

When testing sound field audiometry it is important to place the examinee in the location at which the intensity of the sound was measured. One way to do this is to suspend a weight on a string in the test chamber at equal distance from each loudspeaker. The weight can be lowered to touch either the center of the patient's head (if necessary) or the microphone when it is used for calibration.

Finally, the examiner is again urged to use earphones whenever possible, because this will more accurately allow him or her to determine threshold values for each ear separately. It is recognized that in some instances children will refuse to wear earphones and will begin to cry so violently when earphones are forcibly put on or held against the ear that testing becomes impossible. In addition, it may not be possible to fit infants or very young children with headsets, so they may need to be tested in the sound field. As long as one realizes the limitations of sound field testing, it appears to be an acceptable procedure for tonal (although not pure tone) testing. See Chapter 9 for further discussion.

Bone-conduction tests

Bone-conduction theories.   Before von Bekesy's experiments, there was a question as to whether the auditory pathway for bone conduction was the same as for air conduction. Based on his work (Bekesy, 1932, 1960), it was recognized that the pathway is the same once sound reaches the cochlea. After that, investigators became concerned with determining how sound was conducted by bone conduction. Probably the most lucid explanation of bone-conduction hearing was presented by Tonndorf (1966).

Tonndorf described three modes of bone conduction as being (a) energy radiated into the external canal (sometimes known as osseotympanic) in which vibratory sound from the osseous portion of the canal is conducted into the external auditory meatus and thence through the tympanic membrane using the normal air-conduction pathway, (b) acceleration of the temporal bone (also known as inertial bone conduction) caused by both the inertial response of the ossicular chain (probably especially at the footplate of the stapes) and the inner ear fluids, and (c) distortional vibrations of the temporal bone (also known as compressional bone conduction), which sets up the traveling wave within the cochlea.

The normal ear probably makes use of all three modes in receiving the bone-conducted signal. However, the patient with a conductive lesion cannot (Tonndorf, 1964). If the problem is in the external ear, the first mode will be affected, because even if sound radiates into the external canal, it will not be carried through the tympanic membrane. The inertial and compressional aspects will probably not be affected by external ear pathology. But, if the patient has an ossicular fixation or ossicular discontinuity, he or she will lose Modes 1 and 2 to a greater or lesser extent, depending on where the ossicular abnormality occurs, and will be left only with the third, or compressional, bone conduction. Note also that the relationship between frontal bone and mastoid bone conduction threshold will vary depending on the presence and site of a conductive lesion. The fact that the "Carhart notch" (average bone conduction loss of 5 dB at 500 Hz, 10 dB at 1000 Hz, 15 dB at 2000 Hz, and 5 dB at 4000 Hz) found in cases of otosclerosis disappears after successful stapes surgery is one indication that the apparent hearing loss by bone conduction is an artifact. It probably reflects only a loss of the inertial and osseotympanic components of bone conduction which are restored when the ossicular chain is repaired.

Although it is true that one may never determine "true" cochlear reserve using conventional bone-conduction tests, one may obtain reliable estimates of it. Certainly, there will be an indication of whether there is a difference between the air-conduction and bone-conduction threshold (air-bone gap), which is indicative of conductive pathology and of the amount of gain in hearing that may be expected following successful middle ear surgery.

Bone-conduction test procedures. The most commonly used procedure for bone-conduction testing is mastoid placement. Two other techniques,

(a) frontal bone placement and (b) the sensorineural acuity level (SAL) procedure, also have been used. The latter test is not as widely used today as it was before the improvement of techniques of conventional bone-conduction testing, masking, and calibration.

It is interesting to realize that we have only had threshold values for bone conduction since 1966 when Lybarger published the HAIC (Hearing Aid Industry Conference) bone-conduction norms (Lybarger, 1966). These values were first incorporated into the Appendix of the ANSI Standard for Artificial Headbone Calibration in 1972 and revised in 1981, which is the current ANSI standard. This present standard (ANSI, 1982, S3.26-1981) gives threshold values for a Radioear B-71 (circular tip) bone vibrator used with a P-3333 headband. Also, specifications for a mechanical coupler (artificial mastoid or headbone) for calibrating bone vibrators used in audiometry have been published (ANSI, 1987, S3.13-1987). See Chapter 16 for further discussion of calibration. Before the HAIC and ANSI documents were published each clinic used a group of normal hearing listeners or persons with known sensorineural loss to determine the bone-conduction levels for each audiometer. This procedure was probably more often avoided than used because of the difficulty of obtaining enough threshold data on subjects, and because one was using "pure" sensorineural losses that probably were determined with the audiometer that the examiner calibrated—a bit of circular reasoning that always created some difficulty for some of us. With the development of the commercially available artificial mastoid (headbone), one major problem in bone-conduction testing (i.e., calibration) has been substantially lessened.

A second problem, masking, still exists but it is not as significant as it once was since our understanding of masking techniques has improved and since the use of narrow band and effective masking has become more routine (see Chapter 3). Finally, advances have been made in bone vibrators (i.e., those with more mass and more reliable electronic circuitry such as the Radioear B-71 and B-72) in the last few years, which enable us to obtain even more reliable and sensitive threshold data today. The procedures described below for testing via bone-conduction differ in detail but not in purpose. However, the basic problems mentioned above that preclude actual measurement of precise cochlear reserve exist in each method.

1. Mastoid bone conduction. Mastoid placement is most often used because it seems convenient, it is traditional, and it requires slightly less power to measure threshold with mastoid placement than with frontal bone placement; however, other differences are generally not significant. (Dirks, 1964a; Dirks & Malmquist, 1969). (Note: Although one may correctly calibrate to compensate for the intensity difference between mastoid and frontal bone placement, the characteristic of current vibrators do not allow the vibrators to be driven at equally high hearing levels because of distortion possibilities. The improvement in sensitivity with mastoid placement thus will enable the clinician to measure a wider range of hearing levels. This latter reason *may* be why most audiologists prefer to use mastoid placement. There is evidence that the newer vibrators, such as the Radioear B-72 [Dirks & Kamm, 1975] have greatly reduced the previous distortion problem.)

In the United States bone-conduction testing traditionally has been carried out by holding the vibrator in place on the mastoid process with a headband. Although we pay lip service to the fact that this should have a static force of approximately 500 grams, in fact the force is generally closer to 400 grams (Dirks, 1964b). Studies by Konig (1957) indicated that higher static pressures resulted in slightly more reliable thresholds. However, there is a point beyond which the patient will not allow the pressure to be increased. We have found, for example, that when using a pressure of 1,000 grams, even research subjects have difficulty in tolerating the physical pressure. There is a definite indentation on the head where the vibrator was located when testing is completed. A static force of 500 grams does not appear to be unduly uncomfortable for the majority of patients and is a practical, if not ideal, pressure.

Unfortunately, current commercially available headbands for vibrators do not allow the clinician to regulate and monitor static pressure. This becomes an even more difficult problem with the smaller heads of children. In the latter case pressures may not reach static force values of 250 grams. It should be mentioned that the solution in testing is *not* one of holding the vibrator by hand. Pressure will not be constant with this method either, and the stimulus output from the vibrator may be dampened.

In addition to the static pressure, the positioning of the vibrator on the mastoid process also will affect the bone-conduction threshold results. With the larger hearing aid type of vibrator (i.e., Radioear B-70A), placement does not always make a great deal of difference because this vibrator covers a large area of the mastoid. However, with the round tipped vibrators recommended by ANSI (1982, ANSI S3.26-1981; e.g., B-71) placement may make a considerable difference. To help control reliability, the clinician is advised to place the vibrator on the mastoid process, turn on the tone, and move the vibrator from place to place, asking the examinee at which place the tone appears to be the loudest. This place will sometimes vary from one frequency to another, so to avoid changing placement for each frequency, the examiner may use a specific frequency such as 500 Hz. It is, of course, difficult for young children and for some adults to indicate verbally at which place the tone appears loudest. In these cases, the clinician should simply find a convenient place on the mastoid for placement. Furthermore, the examiner must always be sure that the vibrator does not touch the pinna and that as much of the hair as possible is pushed away from under the vibrator. Obviously eyeglasses with temples that extend behind the pinna also must be removed.

The ear ipsilateral to the vibrator is left unoccluded and an earphone is placed on the contralateral ear for the purpose of masking. This is advisable because the currently used threshold values (ANSI, 1982) (ANSI S3.25-1981) were obtained using an open ear ipsilateral to the vibrator and contralateral masking. This was done because covering both ears could cause an occlusion effect in cases other than bilateral conductive loss, and because the fact of ≃ 0 dB intra-aural attenuation for bone conduction means that masking must be used whenever there is an air-bone gap. If the contralateral ear is covered with a masking phone, an occlusion effect will result unless the ear has a conductive hearing loss or masking is not used. The occlusion effect will result in a false impression of bone-conduction sensitivity given that it elevates low frequency thresholds (Dirks & Swindeman, 1967; Goldstein & Hayes, 1965; Huizing, 1960). Some clinicians prefer to obtain unmasked bone-conduction thresholds first and then repeat the test using appropriate masking if there is an air-bone gap of 5 to 10 dB at more than two frequencies. If there is no difference between the air-conducted and bone-conducted threshold there is no reason to mask. As mentioned earlier, normative threshold values for bone conduction were obtained using masked threshold data, because it was assumed that in most instances masking would be used and because it was realized that contralateral masking would slightly affect the obtained thresholds.

Whether the earphone is used contralaterally or ipsilaterally, enough masking to the contralateral ear must be provided to overcome the occlusion effect that will occur in the low frequencies. This effect can be as great as 25 dB at 500 Hz (Feldman, Grimes, & Shur, 1971). It should be emphasized, however, that the occlusion effect is highly variable and thus cannot be easily subtracted in the case of ears with conductive hearing loss (Dirks & Swindeman, 1967; Feldman et al., 1971). Normally an effective masking level of 30 dB will be enough to override the occlusion effect and to allow one to obtain accurate bone-conduction thresholds (Whittle, 1965). An explanation of this as well as other procedures for masking are given in detail in Chapter 3.

After the vibrator is in place and the pressure is judged, or measured, to be correct the procedure for testing bone conduction is essentially the same as for air conduction. Audiologists commonly use the ASHA- or ANSI-approved modified Hughson-Westlake technique. The patient is asked to respond when the tone is heard. The patient may need to be given additional instructions when masking is introduced. Bone-conduction testing may be done using automatic or manual audiometry, assuming apropriate calibration was performed.

As pointed out earlier the only advantage of mastoid placement is that it will enable the clinician to obtain slightly more sensitive threshold values than will frontal placement.

2. *Frontal bone.*   Frontal bone placement probably is more defensible as a technique than mastoid placement because it has been shown to be somewhat more reliable than mastoid placement (Dirks, 1964b; Studebaker, 1962) and because other possible contaminating factors mentioned below will not exist; however, it appears to be less popular with most clinicians. In this technique masking must always be used, because both cochlea are stimulated. Without masking it is not possible to know which ear was tested. In this technique the vibrator is placed in the center of the forehead and the examiner rarely has to worry about hair between the skin and the vibrator and never about touching the pinna. It is generally easier to obtain a static pressure that approximates 500 grams with currently available headbands using frontal placement (Dirks, 1964b).

The procedure for obtaining threshold is the same as for air conduction or bone conduction with mastoid placement except that masking must *always* be used in the contralateral ear. The results obtained are assumed to be from the unmasked ear.

After thresholds are obtained for one ear, masking is changed to the contralateral ear. In the United States the test ear generally is unoccluded. If both ears are occluded, the occlusion effect must be accounted for. However, as mentioned above, the ear with a conductive loss will have little or no occlusion effect, whereas the normal ear or ear with a sensorineural loss will have an occlusion effect. Because it may not be known in advance whether a conductive lesion exists, it is difficult to know whether to subtract the occlusion effect. Therefore, it seems more sensible to not cover the test ear. It should be mentioned that insert receivers can minimize the occlusion effect although they will not necessarily eliminate it.

3. *SAL.*   The third technique, Sensorineural Acuity Level (SAL) was developed by Jerger and Tillman (1960) at a time when it was critical for the surgeon to know as precisely as possible the acuity level of the sensorineural mechanism and when calibration and masking techniques were less precise. In the SAL technique white noise masking is introduced into the bone vibrator, which is placed on the forehead while hearing is tested by air conduction. Air-conduction thresholds are obtained with and without masking. The shift that occurs when masking is presented is called the SAL shift and is compared to the average shift obtained under the same conditions for a group of normal hearing subjects. The differ-

ence between the expected (local norms) and obtained shifts is the SAL threshold.

Problems with the SAL are as follows: (a) both ears are occluded, (b) some patients with sensorineural hearing loss have an abnormally large threshold shift with masking, and (c) difficulty in determining normative shifts. A useful application of the SAL, although not widely recognized, is in assessment of pseudohypacusis (see Chapter 12).

The three test procedures discussed above all have one common deficit. The cochlear reserve cannot be truly measured because the normal ear uses modes of bone conduction that the ear with a conductive component cannot. Thus these procedures will all underestimate the true level of the cochlear reserve to greater or lesser extents. Nonetheless, they all point to the probability of the presence or absence of conductive pathology. Finally, each of the three measures when properly used predict with high accuracy the expected postoperative air-conduction threshold. Because it is always important to know not only whether conductive pathology exists, but what may be expected for postoperative hearing levels, the latter is most helpful. Clearly, when the pathology has a serious morbidity probability (such as with cholesteotomas) the expected postoperative hearing levels are of little importance, but with pathologies not expected to cause serious illness or death (such as otosclerosis) it is very important to be able to predict with high probability the postoperative hearing levels.

Extended high-frequency audiometry

Another procedure, which can be used with either air conduction or bone conduction depending on instrumentation, is extended high-frequency audiometry. In this procedure one tests the hearing in the frequency range *above* 8000 Hz. High-frequency audiometry purportedly can reveal sensorineural hearing losses related to ototoxicity (Dreschler, van der Hulst, Tange, & Urbanus, 1985; Goldstein, Shulman, & Kisiel, 1987; Rappaport, Fausti, Schechter, & Frey, 1986; van der Hulst, Dreschler, & Urbanus, 1988), to noise exposure (Gauz, Smith, & Hinkle, 1986; Goldstein et al., 1987), or to other pathologies (Gauz et al., 1986; Goldstein et al., 1987; Rahko & Karma, 1986) before the hearing loss is evident in frequencies at or below 8000 Hz. Various investigators (Frank & Ragland, 1987; Gauz & Smith, 1985; Green, Kidd, & Stevens, 1987; Okstad, Laukli, & Mair, 1988; Stelmachowicz, Beauchaine, Kalberer, Langer, & Jesteadt, 1988) have studied the variability of the air and bone systems and found them to be comparable in variability to other systems, with only somewhat larger standard deviations in the higher frequencies. For example, Green et al. (1987) reported the standard deviations for their younger subjects as 2.5 dB in the 8-14 kHz range and 4.5 dB in the range above that. There also have been some attempts to establish normative threshold data for high-frequency test procedures but this has not yet been accomplished. Part of the problem relates to the fact that even more than at lower frequencies, age will influence the determination of a normal range of hearing. At the present time both ANSI and ISO have established groups to look at high-frequency audiometry both in terms of test equipment and in terms of possible normative data.

The specific test procedure to be used varies with instrumentation. In one case a probe tube is place down the ear canal. In another, high-fidelity circumaural earphones are used. In the third approach a large bone vibrator is used to transduce the signal. Because there are no standards for this procedure yet, the reader is advised to use the manufacturer's recommendations and proceed with caution. In theory the idea of high-frequency audiometry is excellent, but in practice there still appear to be some significant problems (calibration, normative data) that preclude its routine use at this time.

Concluding remarks

The unresponsive or difficult-to-test individual

The psychophysical procedures described earlier and the conventional procedures outlined above clearly require the cooperation of the patient because the examinee must respond by word or by manipulation of buttons or attenuators to indicate whether the stimulus is or is not heard. Although it is relatively easy to test the cooperating adult who wishes to know the faintest level at which he or she can hear, for the young child or patient who does not wish to respond the procedure is not so simple. It is difficult to test the uncooperative individual who wishes to make the clinician believe that his or her hearing is much worse than it is (see Chapter 12). It is also difficult to test an individual who is unable to communicate verbally with the clinician because of the lack of a verbal language system or because he or she uses a different language than the clinician. In the latter instance, gestures may be used effectively to describe what is wanted. Finally, it will be especially tedious to attempt to test the patient who appears not to notice or care whether the sounds that enter his or her environment are present or absent.

Despite the difficulty it is important to try to test the unresponsive or difficult-to-test individual using behavioral techniques. Although the electrophysiologic procedures (described in detail in Chapters 4-8) can give a great deal of information about the organism's ability to receive sound, the perception, or definition and usefulness of the reception can best be assessed with behavioral techniques. If electrophysiologic tests clearly demonstrate that the child or nonresponsive adult does not receive sound (at the level of the cochlea or higher), it probably is not necessary to do behavioral testing. However, if sound is received by the child's auditory system, it is important to know if it is usable. The difficult-to-test individual is considered to be one who because of maturation level, mental level, emotional well-being, or attitude is unable or unwilling to cooperate with the examiner using conventional test procedures. It must be remembered that this individual may be quite testable using special test procedures. However, in some instances it will be impossible to establish rapport and cooperation sufficient to allow the examiner to determine the threshold of hearing or even an approximation thereof. In these instances, one may need to use the electrophysiologic procedures described in Chapters 4-8. Also, see Chapters 8 and 9 for assessing hearing in the pediatric population via both electrophysiologic and behavioral techniques. Finally, refer to Chapter 10 for a discussion of hearing problems related to aging.

Variables and problems that influence measurement

Throughout this chapter some of the problems that may affect threshold measurements in a clinical population have been discussed. In addition to the currently insoluble problem of whether true auditory thresholds *can* be obtained with human subjects, there are specific factors that should be reemphasized.

First, with earphone placement it is imperative that the diaphragm of the earphone be opposite the opening of the ear canal, that the canal not collapse, and that there is no air leak between the cushion and the ear. If the earphone is off to one side of the canal, if the canal collapses, if headband pressure is insufficient, and so forth, the clinician will not obtain accurate measurement of the examinee's hearing threshold. It takes a little more time to make sure that the hair is not in front of the ear and that the earphone is properly placed, but without these precautions the measurement results may be meaningless.

Second, positioning the patient in the sound field must be done carefully. As pointed out, it is important that when two loudspeakers are used in a sound field, each ear should be an equal distance from the face of the loudspeaker. It is probably best to use 90° and 270° azimuth for sound field testing although 40° to 60° azimuth as well as 0° have been used. (In special procedures, such as hearing aid evaluations, the clinician may wish speakers to be at 0° and 180° azimuth relative to the listener's face.) Loudspeaker calibrations must be made at the place where the listener's head is expected to be. If the subject's head is not at the spot where the microphone was placed, the clinician will get an inaccurate representation of his or her threshold. In addition, if there is anything between the patient's ear and the loudspeaker (e.g., a parent's hand, the examiner's body, or any other object) erroneous thresholds will be obtained. As far as is possible, the head of the listener should be in the same plane as the loudspeaker. It may be difficult to move the speakers up and down to compensate for the difference in height of the listener, but if this is feasible it should be done.

Third, bone vibrator placement must be carefully controlled. As mentioned earlier, the spot on the mastoid on which the vibrator is placed will change the threshold test results to some extent. The change can be as great as 10 dB. It is most important that the vibrator not touch the pinna. In addition, the pressure with which the vibrator is affixed to the mastoid process will change the threshold test result as well as the reliability of threshold measurements.

Fourth, extended high-frequency audiometry can be used with special earphones or a special bone vibrator to assess hearing above 8000 Hz. However, there are currently no ANSI or ISO standards for hearing level in the extended high-frequency range.

Fifth, besides proper use of test equipment, another variable that will influence threshold measurement is the attention of the subject. If the examinee is not interested in the stimulus, does not care to play the games suggested by the examiner, or is trying to simulate a hearing loss, the results will not be accurate. In the case of young children, and some adults, it may be necessary to interrupt the test procedure from time to time to reinstruct them and to reestablish rapport. If there is something else that is interesting in the sound room, such as toys, flashing lights, or other visual stimuli, children may become distracted and not pay attention. If the patient is frightened, concerned, or distrusts the examiner, threshold measurements are likely to be inaccurate. Many persons begin to lose attention when their threshold is approached and they need to be revived again (sometimes just giving a louder stimulus will renew attention).

In some instances when testing children as well as others who are unresponsive or difficult-to-test, the examiner will obtain consistent play responses at suprathreshold levels and inconsistent responses as threshold is approached. This is probably because the child's attention begins to wander since tones are not inherently interesting and so he or she must constantly be brought back to the task. Fatigue will affect the results for all patients. If the patient is tired or sleepy, if it is nap time for the child, the results will not be as accurate or as close to true threshold as might otherwise be obtained. In short, any physical, mental, or emotional factor that affects the human can affect his or her ability to respond to pure tones. This is true even if the examinee is concerned about the level at which he or she hears and wishes to cooperate. Despite these comments, it should be pointed out that with patience it is possible to reliably test subjects who are so sick that they are on gurneys, who are in intensive care units, or who throw tantrums when they first enter the test room.

In addition, physical factors that are environmental may also influence test results. Temperature and ventilation must be appropriately controlled. In one test room that it was necessary to use, the temperature sometimes reached or even exceeded 90°. Under those conditions some children yielded threshold test results that were as much as 15 dB poorer than they were at other times when the room was more comfortable. The precise effect that temperature, humidity, or ventilation has on a subject will, of course, vary from one subject to another and even from one time to another. Thus the clinician is well advised to try to obtain the most comfortable, pleasant atmosphere possible in order to enhance the probability of obtaining reliable and accurate threshold measurements.

Finally, the clinician should realize when trying to obtain thresholds for pure tones or other tonal stimuli, factors such as equipment, the ability and willingness of the patient to respond, the condition of the test environment, and the interest and competence of the examiner are of paramount importance. Failure to control any of these variables may prevent the clinician from obtaining accurate and reliable measurements of the patient's threshold of hearing for pure tones. However, lest the clinician doubt the possibility of ever obtaining worthwhile threshold measurements, it *is* true that if the examiner remembers the reason for the test and attends to the procedures for controlling appropriate variables, reliable and accurate audiometric threshold data can be obtained.

References

American National Standards Institute. (1989). *American National Standard specifications for audiometers* (ANSI S3.6-1989). New York: Author.

American National Standards Institute. (1972). *American National Standard for an artificial headbone for the calibration of audiometer bone vibrators* (ANSI S3.13-1972). New York: Author.

American National Standards Institute. (1973). *American National Standard psychoacoustical terminology* (ANSI S3.20-1973). New York: Author.

American National Standards Institute. (1977). *American National Standard criteria for permissible ambient noise during audiometric testing* (ANSI S3.1-1977). New York: Author.

American National Standards Institute. (1978). *Manual pure-tone threshold audiometry* (ANSI S3.21-1978; R86) New York: Author.

American National Standards Institute. (1982). *American National Standard reference equivalent threshold force levels for audiometric bone vibrators* (ANSI S3.26-1981). New York: Author.

American National Standards Institute. (1987). *American National Standard specification for a mechanical coupler for measurement of bone vibrators* (ANSI S3.13-1987). New York: Author.

American Standards Association. (1951). *Audiometers for general diagnostic purposes* (Z 24.5). New York: Author.

American Speech-Language-Hearing Association. (1977). Guidelines for manual pure-tone threshold audiometry. *Asha, 19,* 236–240.

Arlinger, S. D. (1979). Comparison of ascending and bracketing methods in pure tone audiometry. *Scandinavian Audiology, 8,* 247–254.

Bekesy, G. v. (1932). Zur theorie des horens bei der schallaufnahme durch knochenleitung [Theories of hearing by sound transmission through bone conduction]. *Ann Physik, 13,* 111–136.

Bekesy, G. von (1947). A new audiometer. *Acta Oto-Laryngologica. Stockholm, 35,* 411–422.

Bekesy, G. von. (1960). *Experiments in hearing.* New York: McGraw-Hill.

Bunch, C. C. (1943). *Clinical audiometry.* St. Louis: C. V. Mosby.

Carhart, R., & Jerger, J. J. (1959). Preferred method for clinical determination of pure-tone thresholds. *Journal of Speech and Hearing Disorders, 24,* 330–345.

Dadson, R. S., & King, J. H. (1952). A determination of the normal threshold of hearing and its relation to the standardization of audiometers. *Journal of Laryngology and Otology, 66,* 366–378.

Delk, J. H. (1973). *Comprehensive dictionary of audiology.* Sioux City, IA: Hearing Aid Journal.

Dillon, H., & Walker, G. (1980). The perception by normal hearing persons of intensity fluctuations in narrow band stimuli and its implications for sound field calibration procedures. *Australian Journal of Audiology, 2,* 72–82.

Dillon, H., & Walker, G. (1982). The selection of modulation waveform for frequency modulated sound field stimuli. *Australian Journal of Audiology, 4,* 56–61.

Dirks, D. (1964a). Factors related to bone conduction reliability. *Archives of Otolaryngology, 79,* 551–558.

Dirks, D. (1964b). Bone-conduction measurements. *Archives of Otolaryngology, 79,* 594–599.

Dirks, D., & Malmquist, C. M. (1969). Comparison of frontal and mastoid bone-conduction thresholds in various conductive lesions. *Journal of Speech and Hearing Research, 12,* 725–746.

Dirks, D. D., & Kamm, C. (1975). Bone vibrator measurements: Physical characteristics and behavioral thresholds. *Journal of Speech and Hearing Research, 18,* 242–260.

Dirks, D. D., & Swindeman, J. G. (1967). The variability of occluded and unoccluded bone-conduction thresholds. *Journal of Speech and Hearing Research, 10*, 232–249.

Dreschler, W. A., van der Hulst, R. J., Tange, R. A., & Urbanus, N. A. (1985). The role of high-frequency audiometry in early detection of ototoxicity. *Audiology, 24*, 387–395.

Egan, J. P., Greenberg, C. Z., & Schulman, A. I. (1961). Interval of time uncertainty in auditory detection. *Journal of the Acoustical Society of America, 33*, 771–778.

Feldman, A. S., Grimes, C. T., & Shur, I. B. (1971). *Studies of the occlusion effect*. New York: SUNY Upstate Medical Center.

Frank, T., & Ragland, A. E. (1987). Repeatability of high-frequency bone conduction thresholds. *Ear and Hearing, 8*, 343–346.

Gauz, M. T., & Smith, M. M. (1987). High-frequency Bekesy audiometry: VI. Pulsed vs. continuous signals. *Journal of Auditory Research, 27(1)*, 37–52.

Gauz, M. T., Smith, M. M., & Hinkle, R.R. (1986). The simplified HF E-800 high-frequency audiometer: Clinical applications. *Journal of Audiology Research, 26*, 121–134.

Goldstein, B., Shulman, A., & Kisiel, D. (1987). Electrical high-frequency audiometry: Preliminary medical audiologic experience. *Audiology, 26*, 321–331.

Goldstein, D. P., & Hayes, C. S. (1965). The occlusion effect in bone-conduction hearing. *Journal of Speech and Hearing Research, 8*, 137–148.

Green, D. M., Kidd, G., Jr., & Stevens, K. N. (1987). High-frequency audiometric assessment of a young adult population. *Journal of the Acoustical Society of America, 81*, 485–494.

Green, D. S. (1972). Pure tone air conduction thresholds. In J. Katz (Ed.), *Handbook of clinical audiology*. Baltimore: Williams & Wilkins.

Harbert, F., & Young, I. M. (1966). Amplitude of Bekesy tracings with different attenuation rates. *Journal of the Acoustical Society of America, 39*, 914–919.

Harris, J. D. (1945). Group audiometry. *Journal of the Acoustical Society of America, 17*, 73–76.

Huizing, E. (1960). Bone Conduction, the influence of the middle ear. *Acta Otolaryngologica (Supplement 155)*, 1–99.

International Standards Organization. (1982). *Acoustics: Pure tone air conduction threshold audiometry for hearing conservation purposes* (ISO/DIS 6189.2). Geneva: Author.

International Standards Organization. (1984). *Acoustics: Pure-tone audiometric test methods* (ISO/DIS 8253). Geneva: Author.

Jerger, J., & Tillman, T. W. (1960). A new method for the clinical determination of sensorineural acuity level (SAL). *Archives of Otolaryngology, 71*, 948–955.

Konig, E. (1957). *Variations in bone conduction as related to the force of pressure exerted on the vibrator*. Chicago: Beltone Translations.

Lybarger, S. (1966). Interim bone conduction thresholds for audiometry. *Journal of Speech and Hearing Research, 9*, 483–487.

Morgan, D. E., & Dirks, D. D. (1974). Loudness discomfort level under earphones and in the free field: The effects of calibration methods. *Journal of the Acoustical Society of America, 56*, 172–178.

Okstad, S., Laukli, E., & Mair, I. W. (1988). High-frequency audiometry: Comparison of electric bone-conduction and air-conduction thresholds. *Audiology, 27*, 17–26.

Oldfield, R. C. (1949). Continuous recoding of sensory thresholds and other psychophysical variables. *Nature, 164,* 581.

Orchik, D. J., & Rintelmann, W. F. (1978). Comparison of pure-tone, warble-tone and narrow-band noise thresholds of young normal-hearing children. *Journal of the American Auditory Society, 3,* 214–220.

Rahko, T., & Karma, P. (1986). New clinical finding in vestibular neuritis: High-frequency audiometry hearing loss in the affected ear. *The Laryngoscope, 96,* 198–199.

Rappaport, B. Z., Fausti, S. A., Schechter, M. A., & Frey, R. H. (1986). A prospective study of high-frequency auditory function in patients receiving oral neomycin. *Scandinavian Audiology, 15,* 67–71.

Reger, S. N. (1952). A clinical and research version of the Bekesy audiometer. *The Laryngoscope, 62,* 1333–1351.

Rintelmann, W. F. (1975). Manual and automatic audiometry. In J. B. Olishifski & E. R. Harford (Eds.), *Industrial noise and hearing conservation* (pp.625–644). Chicago: National Safety Council.

Rintelmann, W. F., Orchik, D. J., & Stephens, M. (1972). *A comparison of pure-tone and warble-tone thresholds: I. Effects of stimulus parameters. II. Effects of occlusion of nontest ear and changes in azimuth.* East Lansing: Michigan State University.

Robinson, D. E., & Watson, C. S. (1972). Psychophysical methods in modern psychoacoustics. In J. Tobias (Ed.), *Foundations of modern auditory theory* (pp. 101–131). New York: Academic Press.

Robinson, D. O., & Vaughan, C. R. (1976). Relative efficiency of warble-tone and conventional pure-tone testing with children. *Journal of the American Auditory Society, 1,* 252–257.

Rudmose, W. (1962). *Pressure vs. free field thresholds at low frequencies.* Copenhagen: Fourth International Congress of Acoustics.

Staab, W. J. (1971). *Comparison of pure-tone and warble-tone thresholds.* Unpublished doctoral dissertation, Michigan State University, East Lansing.

Staab, W. J., & Rintelmann, W. F. (1972a). *A comparison of pure-tone and warble-tone thresholds.* Paper presented at the ASHA convention, San Francisco.

Stabb, W. J., & Rintelmann, W. F. (1972b). Status of warble-tone in audiometers. *Audiology: Journal of Auditory Communication, 11,* 244–255.

Stelmachowicz, P. G., Beauchaine, K. A., Kalberer, A., Langer, T., & Jesteadt, W. (1988). The reliability of auditory thresholds in the 8- to 20-kHz range using a prototype audiometer. *Journal of the Acoustical Society of America, 83,* 1528–1535.

Stephens, M. M., & Rintelmann, W. F. (1978). Influence of audiometric configuration on pure-tone, warble-tone and narrow band noise thresholds for adults with sensorineural hearing losses. *Journal of the American Auditory Society, 3,* 221–226.

Stevens, S. S. (1958). Problems and methods of psychophysics. *Psychological Bulletin, 55,* 177–196.

Stevens, S. S. (1960). Mathematics, measurement and psychophysics. In S. S. Stevens (Ed.), *Handbook of experimental psychology.* New York: John Wiley.

Stream, R. W., & Dirks, D. D. (1974). Effect of loudspeaker position on differences between earphone and free-field thresholds (MAP and MAF). *Journal of Speech and Hearing Research, 17,* 549–568.

Studebaker, G. A. (1962). Placement of vibrator in bone-conduction testing. *Journal of Speech and Hearing Research, 5,* 321–331.

Tanner, W. P., Jr., & Sorkin, R. D. (1972). The theory of signal detectability. In J. Tobias (Ed.), *Foundations of modern auditory theory*. New York: Academic Press.

Tillman, T. W., Johnson, R. M., & Olsen, W. (1966). Earphone vs. sound-field threshold sound pressure levels for spondee words. *Journal of the Acoustical Society of America, 39*, 125–133.

Tonndorf, J. (1964). Animal experiments in bone conduction: Clinical conclusions. *Annals of Otology, Rhinology and Laryngology, 73*, 659–679.

Tonndorf, J. (1966). Bone conduction—Studies in experimental animals. *Acta Oto-Laryngologica, (Supplement 213)*, 132.

van der Hulst, R. J., Dreschler, W. A., & Urbanus, N. A. (1988). High frequency audiometry in prospective clinical research of ototoxicity due to platinum derivatives. *Annals of Otology, Rhinology and Laryngology, 97 (2 pt. 1)*, 133–137.

Villchur, E. (1970). Audiometer earphone mounting to improve intersubject and cushion-fit reliability. *Journal of the Acoustical Society of America, 48*, 1387–1396.

Walker, G., Dillon, H., & Byrne, D. (1984). Sound field audiometry: Recommended stimuli and procedures. *Ear and Hearing, 5*, 13–21.

Whittle, L. S. (1965). A determination of the normal threshold of hearing by bone conduction. *Journal of Sound Vibrations, 2*, 227–248.

Wilber, L. A., Kruger, B. A., & Killion, M. C. (1988). Reference threshold levels for the ER-3A insert earphone. *Journal of the Acoustical Society of America, 83*, 669–676.

Zwislocki, J., Kruger, B., Miller, J. D., Niemoeller, A. F., Shaw, E. A., & Studebaker, G. (1988). Earphones in audiometry. *Journal of the Acoustical Society of America, 83*, 1688–1689.

chapter two

Speech audiometry

WAYNE O. OLSEN

NOEL D. MATKIN

Contents

Introduction

Audiologic tests using speech stimuli are essential in evaluations of patients with hearing and communication problems because speech represents the class of sounds most important to effective daily function. Results from routine pure tone tests often do not reflect either the potential or the limitations in receptive auditory communication of adults and children with hearing losses. Speech audiometry offers a means to assess an individual's auditory perception of speech in a quasi-systematic manner.

The intent of this chapter is to acquaint the reader with a variety of audiometric speech test materials and test methods for both adults and children. The major delineations are measurements of threshold sensitivity for speech stimuli and auditory discrimination of speech at suprathreshold levels (word or nonsense syllable recognition and/or identification).

History

Speech in some form typically is used during an informal test of hearing because it is a readily available acoustic stimulus. Speech utterances with and without voice still are used in some physician's offices for the purpose of hearing screening. Notations often are made relative to the distances at which either whispered and/or voiced speech are heard.

Pfingsten in 1804 was probably the first investigator to report degree of hearing impairment based on speech tests (Feldmann, 1960). He divided speech sounds into three classes: vowels, voiced consonants, and voiceless consonants. Within each class, sounds were ranked according to intensity. Pfingsten categorized hearing disorders according to the speech sounds understood by his patients. In 1846, a classification of hearing impairments based upon the distance at which speech could be understood at "moderate" and at "normal" levels was devised by Schmalz (Feldmann, 1960). Wolf, in 1871, reported further refinements in his determination of the distances at which various speech sounds could be heard. He also noted that large differences in audibility of various speech sounds were not apparent with whispered speech; hence, whispered speech provided more uniform test stimuli (Feldmann, 1960).

Edison's invention of the phonograph in 1877 allowed for the first recorded presentation of test materials. Lichtwitz, in 1889, controlled the intensity of recordings made with a phonograph by speaking at a constant intensity, but at different distances from the sound pickup (Feldmann, 1960). Using the findings of Wolf, he devised an "acumetric scale" of test words, and, as early as 1889 predicted that equivalent lists in all languages should and would be developed. In other words, standardized speech tests to measure hearing impairments were advocated a century ago. However, other investigators were less enthusiastic, citing the limitation imposed by poor high-frequency response of the phonographs then available. Nevertheless, in 1904 Bryant described the use of a phonograph for clinical speech tests. He adjusted and controlled the output intensity with clamps on the rubber tubes that delivered the signal from the phonograph to the listener's ear (Feldmann, 1960).

Whereas efforts to this time were directed toward developing tests of sensitivity for speech, work begun in 1910 at the Bell Telephone Laboratories centered on the discrimination of speech sounds. Campbell and Crandall developed 50-item lists of nonsense syllables. Each list contained 5 consonant–vowel (CV), 5 vowel–consonant (VC), and 40 consonant–vowel–consonant (CVC) items; they called these 50-item lists "articulation lists" and used them to test telephone circuits (O'Neill & Oyer, 1966). Also in 1910, Barany developed tests of phonemic discrimination changing one phoneme at a time in his phoneme substitution words. In 1923, Lempert extended Barany's work with sets of words in which only one phoneme was changed, but the difference could be the vowels, the initial, or the final consonants of the words (Feldmann, 1960).

Jones and Knudsen apparently were the first to incorporate circuitry for speech testing into their pure tone audiometer in 1924, but the first use of speech tests for mass screening took place with the advent of the Western Electric 4-A audiometer (Fletcher, 1929). This unit utilized phonograph recordings of pairs of digits recorded with intensity decrements of 3 dB between succeeding pairs covering a range of 33 dB. The task of the listener was to write the numbers heard. The number of digits correctly reported was used to calculate a threshold for speech. Although not used clinically, this device was employed for group screening in schools to assess adequacy of hearing for speech.

McFarlan, as early as 1940, used the first 500 monosyllables from the Thorndyke lists and the first 50 monosyllables from the Gates list in his speech test. Although McFarlan used these words for determining speech thresholds rather than for suprathreshold testing as used later, it was an early use of monosyllables whereby selection was based on frequency of occurrence. It also is of interest that, for different purposes, he developed recordings using 50 words per list. Virtually all subsequent test lists developed since 1910 have incorporated 50 words to sample speech perception.

Since the latter part of the 1940s investigators have tended to separate auditory tests using speech stimuli into tests for determining speech thresholds and tests for assessing recognition or identification of speech at suprathreshold levels. Measurements of thresholds for speech are discussed in the next section.

Measures of sensitivity for speech

Although Steinberg and Gardner (1940) demonstrated good agreement between an average of pure tone thresholds for 512, 1024, 2048, and

4096 Hz and the level at which hearing-impaired subjects achieved "articulation of 40%" (40% correct) on "lists of detached monosyllables of the consonant-vowel-consonant type," it was Hughson and Thompson (1942) who demonstrated a direct correlation between the hearing loss for pure tones and for speech. Hughson and Thompson used Bell Telephone Intelligibility Sentences (Fletcher & Steinberg, 1929) and presented three sentences at each level in a descending and bracketing procedure to establish thresholds of intelligibility for speech. They found this procedure to be accurate within 1 to 2 dB. Referring to this procedure as a test of speech reception, Hughson and Thompson coined the term *speech reception threshold* (SRT). Recently the Committee on Audiologic Evaluation of the American Speech-Language-Hearing Association (1988) recommended use of the same acronym for *speech recognition threshold*. Both terms are used in the following discussion.

Test materials

The development of materials other than sentences for determining SRTs was reported by Hudgins, Hawkins, Karlin, and Stevens in 1947 with the use of spondaic words (spondees), that is, two-syllable words with equal stress on each syllable, as test items. Selection was based on familiarity, phonetic dissimilarity, normal sampling of English speech sounds, and homogeneity with respect to audibility. Normal distribution of speech sounds among the test items was not considered important, but homogeneity in audibility was considered crucial for two reasons. First, homogeneity of test words enhances the precision with which the SRT can be established and, second, it is desirable to establish a threshold for speech using as few test items as possible in the interest of time and listener fatigue.

On the basis of these criteria, 84 spondees were selected, divided into two lists of 42 words each, and incorporated into PAL (Harvard Psychoacoustic Laboratory) Tests No. 9 and No. 14. PAL No. 9 was recorded on phonograph discs with succeeding sets of six spondees recorded at a level that was 4 dB weaker than the preceding set of six items. PAL No. 14 used the same words, but with all test items recorded at a single intensity level. Employing these test materials, Hudgins et al. (1947) found the standard error of speech reception threshold measurements to be on the order of 2 or 3 dB. Carhart (1946a), having access to these word lists and the Bell Telephone Intelligibility Sentences, compared threshold relationships for patients who were administered pure tone and sentence tests and for other patients who were administered pure tone and spondee tests. The pure tone and speech recognition threshold relationships were found to be essentially equivalent for the two groups. Because tests using spondees were easier and more rapid to administer than were sentence tests, spondaic words quickly gained acceptance for determining speech recognition thresholds.

Modifications of the PAL No. 9 and No. 14 tests followed. Hirsh et al. (1952) reduced the list of 84 spondees by first removing those items that were judged to be unfamiliar. The remainder were recorded and presented to six normal listeners at levels ranging from +4 dB to −6 dB relative to their thresholds obtained with PAL No. 9. Words that were missed either once or not at all, or five or more times by all six listeners were considered to be too easy or too difficult and were deleted. These manipulations reduced the pool of words to 36 spondees. Subsequent experiments with this reduced sample of words indicated that some were more difficult than others, apparently depending on their intensity levels as monitored on a volume unit (VU) meter. Consequently, the easier words were reduced in level by 2 dB and more difficult words were increased in level by 2 dB for subsequent recordings on Central Institute for the Deaf (CID) W-1 and W-2 spondee tests. Otherwise, the words were recorded at a constant level on CID W-1; spondees were recorded in groups of three, with each succeeding group of three spondees being 3 dB weaker than the preceding set on CID W-2.

In spite of all these efforts and adjustments to derive a more homogeneous list of words, Hirsh et al. observed that different randomizations "of lists of words are not equal in difficulty unless each entire list is heard. When only part of the list is heard the difficulty of the list depends on which part is heard. For a given listener it cannot be said that all parts of the lists are equal in difficulty" (Hirsh et al., 1952, p. 327). These comments led to further attempts to increase the homogeneity of the test items (Beattie, Edgerton, & Svihovec, 1975; Beattie, Svihovec, & Edgerton, 1975; Bowling & Elpern, 1961; Conn, Dancer, & Ventry, 1975; Curry & Cox, 1966; Dubno, Dirks, & Morgan, 1984; Olsen, 1965; Young, Dudley, & Gunter 1982). Details of these studies differed in many respects, but in all experimental designs, each of the 36 spondees had an equal opportunity to be included in the homogeneous set.

The results of these studies are shown in Table 2.1. The 36 CID spondees are listed in the order of frequency of selection and the words selected as homogeneous in audibility by the various investigators are indicated. All 36 spondees were selected as being among the most homogeneous in at least one study. Only two were unanimously selected, seven were acceptable in at least six of the studies, and six more were judged suitable in five of the investigations. Overall, only 13 spondees were considered homogeneous in five or more of the studies; 20 of the 36 items selected as homogeneous were common to the results of four or more of the investigations. Appropriate selection and use of the most

TABLE 2.1
List of 36 CID Spondees and an Indication of Studies in Which Individual Words Were Judged To Be Homogeneous in Eight Investigations

Spondee	Bowling and Elpern (1961)	Olsen (1965)	Curry and Cox (1966)	Conn et al. (1975)	Beattie et al. (1975a)	Beattie et al. (1975b)	Young et al. (1982)	Dubno et al. (1984)	Times Selected
Northwest	x	x	x	x	x	x	x	x	8
Railroad	x	x	x	x	x	x	x	x	8
Playground	x		x	x	x	x	x	x	7
Birthday	x	x	x	x	x	x			6
Eardrum	x		x	x		x	x	x	6
Iceberg	x	x	x	x	x	x			6
Sidewalk	x	x	x	x			x	x	6
Drawbridge		x	x			x	x	x	5
Mousetrap	x		x	x	x		x		5
Padlock			x		x	x	x	x	5
Stairway	x		x	x	x	x			5
Toothbrush	x		x		x		x	x	5
Woodwork	x		x			x	x	x	5
Airplane	x	x	x	x					4
Armchair	x		x	x		x			4
Farewell	x		x	x	x				4
Hardware		x	x		x	x			4
Sunset	x		x	x	x				4
Whitewash	x	x	x			x			4
Workshop	x	x					x	x	4

(continued)

TABLE 2.1
(Continued)

Spondee	Bowling and Elpern (1961)	Olsen (1965)	Curry and Cox (1966)	Conn et al. (1975)	Beattie et al. (1975a)	Beattie et al. (1975b)	Young et al. (1982)	Dubno et al. (1984)	Times Selected
Cowboy	x	x	x						3
Doormat			x	x				x	3
Greyhound	x		x			x			3
Horseshoe	x				x	x			3
Inkwell			x		x		x		3
Mushroom			x	x	x				3
Oatmeal	x		x		x				3
Baseball		x					x		2
Grandson							x	x	2
Headlight		x			x				2
Hotdog	x	x							2
Hothouse		x				x			2
Schoolboy			x		x				2
Daybreak			x						1
Duckpond							x		1
Pancake	x								1

homogeneous words should improve both the precision and the reliability of the measurement when establishing speech reception thresholds. In that the selections of test items in Table 2.1 are based on threshold tests in quiet, it is worth noting that Wilson, Hopkins, Mance, and Novak (1982) and Wilson, Shanks, and Koebsell (1982) have suggested 10 words for use in a special masking test using spondees. They recommended that the words "armchair, headlight, horseshoe, hot dog, inkwell, mushroom, northwest, oatmeal, sidewalk, and toothbrush" be used for tests of masking level differences (MLD) for speech. These 10 words yielded the largest MLDs.

Digits also have been used to determine thresholds for speech. Robinson and Koenigs (1979) compared thresholds for spondees and digits (1, 2, 3, 4, 5, 6, 8, 9) are found that thresholds for the two types of material were similar for normal hearing subjects. In contrast, Wilson and Gaeth (1976) found thresholds for digits to be 4 to 10 dB better (lower dB HL) than for spondees among hearing-impaired persons, dependent upon the audiometric configuration. Based on results from 130 patents, Rudmin (1987) reported that "When digit SRTs were used to predict the Fletcher average, random predicted error (standard error) was less than 5 dB" (p. 18). (The Fletcher pure tone average for predicting speech recognition thresholds is described later.)

Methods

A number of procedures have been described for determining speech reception thresholds using spondees. Most are variations of the technique described in 1947 by Hudgins et al. Recall that on PAL No. 9 recordings, consecutive groups of six spondees were recorded at an intensity level 4 dB below the preceding group of six. Given the successively lower level of each group of words, each word could be considered as having a value of two-thirds of a dB. To determine the threshold derived from administration of PAL No. 9, Hudgins et al. provided a table giving numbers of correct responses and the equivalent decrease in decibels. The examiner simply subtracted the latter value from the starting level to obtain the speech reception threshold expressed in dB.

The strategy suggested by Hirsh et al. (1952) for use with CID W-2 is essentially identical to that originally described by Hudgins et al. The only difference is that each word can be counted as the equivalent of 1 dB because successive groups of three words are 3 dB weaker on his recording. Hence, in establishing a speech recognition threshold, the number of correct responses is simply subtracted from the starting level. In order to reach a threshold level corresponding to a 50% criterion, half of the 3-dB first step, 1.5 dB, is added to the resultant value. Some investigators have suggested that thresholds be sought with a descending approach (ASHA, 1988; Chaiklin, 1959; Chaiklin & Ventry, 1964; Hirsh et al., 1952; Hudgins et al., 1947; Martin & Stauffer, 1975; Tillman & Olsen, 1973; Wilson, Morgan, & Dirks, 1973) or a descending and bracketing technique (Hopkinson, 1972; Jerger, Carhart, Tillman, & Peterson, 1959; Newby, 1958). Others have suggested an ascending approach (ASHA, 1977; Chaiklin, Font, & Dixon, 1967). (See appendix for details.) Investigations that have compared ascending and descending techniques for speech recognition thresholds generally have shown that slightly better thresholds are obtained with a descending approach (Huff & Nerbonne, 1982; Robinson & Koenigs, 1979; Wall, Davis, & Myers, 1984).

It is worth noting that Wilson et al. (1973) reported that the statistical basis for the Hudgins et al. (1947), Hirsh et al. (1952), Tillman and Olsen (1973), and American Speech-Language-Hearing Association (1988) procedures had been derived as early as 1908 by Spearman, and independently in 1931 by Karger (Finney, 1952). It is given in the formula

$$T_{50\%} = i + \tfrac{1}{2}(d) - \frac{d(r)}{n}$$

where $T_{50\%}$ = threshold, i = initial test intensity, d = decrement, r = correct responses, and n = number of words per dB decrement. Where d = n (e.g., 2 words per 2-dB decrement, or 5 words per 5-dB decrement), d and n cancel and the formula can be reduced to

$$T_{50\%} = i + \tfrac{1}{2}(d) - r$$

The $\tfrac{1}{2}(d)$ term takes into account the initial one-half step correction suggested by Hudgins et al. (1947), Hirsh et al. (1952), Tillman and Olsen (1973), and the American Speech-Language-Hearing Association (1988). Wilson et al. (1973) also demonstrated that the same procedure could be used with five words per 5-dB decrement with equivalent results being obtained.

Given the variety of procedures recommended for establishing speech reception thresholds with spondees, it is to be expected that wholly different methods would be suggested for determining speech thresholds with materials other than spondees or digits. Falconer and Davis (1947) obtained speech reception thresholds with PAL No. 9 and also asked listeners to adjust the level of recorded continuous discourse to the lowest intensity at which they could understand the talker, that is, the threshold of intelligibility for continuous discourse (TICD). Similarly, Dahle, Hume, and Haspiel (1968), Haspiel and Havens (1966), LeZak, Siegenthaler, and Davis (1964), Rubin and Ventry (1972), and Speaks, Parker, Harris, and

Kuhl (1972) asked their listeners to adjust the signal intensity to the level at which the speech stimuli were just intelligible. Speaks et al. (1972) also instructed subjects to adjust the speech levels for 25%, 50%, or 75% intelligibility. Falconer and Davis (1947) found the SRTs and TICDs to be essentially equal in terms of intensity levels and repeatability. However, they cautioned that the latter procedure is more subjective since it relies upon the judgment of the listener; the speech reception threshold procedure with spondees is more objective in that it requires a correct response from the listener. Chaiklin (1959) found thresholds for perception of running speech (TPRS) to be about 3 dB poorer (higher dB HL) than speech recognition thresholds. Because of the subjective nature of the task, thresholds for perception of running speech, or thresholds for intelligibility of continuous discourse have received little clinical application in determining thresholds for speech.

In most of the work described above, recorded materials have been used. However, it should be noted that Beattie, Forrester, and Ruby (1977), Carhart (1946a), and Creston, Gillespie, and Krahn (1966) have demonstrated that speech reception thresholds established by monitored live voice (MLV) procedures are reliable. Given the flexibility of monitored live voice testing as compared to the use of recorded materials it is not surprising that Martin and Pennington (1971), Martin and Forbis (1978), and Martin and Sides (1985) consistently found MLV to be used more commonly than recorded materials in clinical settings. However, standardization of test materials and procedures requires use of recorded test materials.

Relationship to pure tone thresholds

The relationship between thresholds for pure tones and for speech was noted as early as 1929 by Fletcher. He proposed that the average of pure tone thresholds for 512, 1024, and 2048 Hz (pure tone average, PTA) be used as a predictor of sensitivity for speech. After comparing speech reception thresholds to various methods and weightings of pure tone thresholds as predictors of the SRT, Carhart (1946a) noted that simple averaging of 512-, 1024-, and 2048-Hz thresholds was clinically expedient and adequate.

Later Fletcher (1950) suggested that the average of the two best thresholds for the octave frequencies of 500 to 2000 Hz (Fletcher average) was the better predictor of threshold sensitivity for spondees. Since then various predictive methods and weightings of pure tone thresholds have been proposed and evaluated (Carhart, 1971; Carhart & Porter, 1971; Graham, 1960; Harris, Haines, & Myers, 1956; Quiggle, Glorig, Delk, & Summerfield, 1957; Siegenthaler & Strand, 1964). Extensive analysis of a large array of clinical data has been completed by Carhart; Carhart and

Porter (1971) observed that the best single pure tone predictor for speech recognition thresholds was the threshold at 1000 Hz for all but those patients with marked high-frequency hearing losses. Later Carhart (1971) proposed averaging the 500- and 1000-Hz thresholds and subtracting 2 dB from this value as the closest predictor of the SRT.

The most important contribution of a speech recognition threshold is its indication of the accuracy of the pure tone findings. An unexplained discrepancy of more than 6 dB between the pure tone average and the speech reception threshold for a given patient indicates that these threshold measurements must be questioned (Carhart, 1960). For a variety of reasons some patients respond during pure tone testing at levels well above their actual thresholds, yet these same individuals yield speech recognition thresholds indicating much better hearing sensitivity for spondaic words. Some individuals fail to understand the examiner's instructions to respond to the very weak tones they hear, whereas others deliberately exaggerate hearing losses. (For further discussion of pseudo-hypacusis see Chapter 12.) Whatever the reason, large discrepancies (> 6 dB) between one of the pure tone averages mentioned above and the SRT immediately should alert the clinician to question the accuracy of the pure tone results. Further instructions for the patient, repeated pure tone testing, and further evaluation are necessary to resolve the discrepancy.

Conn, Ventry, and Woods (1972) suggested that use of an ascending approach during speech recognition threshold testing enhances discrepancies between thresholds for pure tones and speech, but large discrepancies also are readily observed using a descending approach for speech thresholds. The basis for such discrepancies apparently is the difference in loudness between pure tones and speech when presented at equal hearing levels (Ventry, 1976). Responses to speech will occur at lower intensity levels if the patient's response is based on a loudness judgment rather than on threshold sensitivity.

Because of the expected close relationship between speech recognition thresholds and pure tone thresholds in the 500- to 2000-Hz frequency region, it is important that speech reception thresholds be sought with a systematic method using predetermined criteria to establish the threshold level. Otherwise, there is a risk of the examiner inadvertently adjusting the presentation levels of the speech stimuli to obtain agreement between the SRT and a pure tone average.

Speech detection thresholds

The preceding discussion has been concerned with speech recognition thresholds, that is, the minimum intensity level at which 50% of the speech sample can be understood. But speech can be detected at intensity levels considerably lower than the levels at which 50% of a speech sample is understood. This difference is on the order of 8 to 9 dB (Beattie, Edgerton, & Svihouec, 1975; Beattie, Svihouec, & Edgerton, 1975; Chaiklin, 1959; Thurlow, Silverman, Davis, & Walsh, 1948). The lowest intensity level at which the listener reports detection or awareness of speech even though the words cannot be understood is referred to either as a *speech detection threshold* (SDT) or a *speech awareness threshold* (SAT). The American Speech-Language-Hearing Association Committee on Audiologic Evaluation (1988) recommends using the term *speech detection threshold* for this measurement. Speech detection thresholds are of value when testing individuals who, for some reason, are unable to repeat words as required for an SRT. Once again, levels at which speech stimuli are detected can be compared to the pure tone thresholds if one keeps in mind the 8- or 9-dB difference between speech recognition thresholds and speech detection thresholds. The audiometric configuration of the patient under study also must be considered because the SDT may be related more closely to the best pure tone threshold in the 250- to 4000-Hz range when the hearing configuration sharply slopes or rises.

Bone-conduction thresholds for speech

The discussion above has assumed that the speech stimuli were delivered via air conduction. But just as pure tone stimuli can be presented via either air conduction or bone conduction, speech stimuli also can be presented to the listener through either mode. Numerous investigations have demonstrated the value of speech tests presented by bone conduction (Edgerton, Danhauer, & Beattie, 1977; Goetzinger & Proud, 1955; Hahlbrock, 1962; Johnson & Bordenink, 1978; Karlsen & Goetzinger, 1980; Kasden & Robinson, 1973; Merrell, Wolfe, & McLemore, 1973; Srinivasson, 1974). Such tests are particularly useful when testing those children or adults for whom it is difficult to elicit reliable responses to pure tone stimuli. A comparison of thresholds for speech delivered by air and bone conduction provides clinically useful information relative to the type of hearing loss in such instances. Also, for some patients masking can be delivered to the nontest ear for speech tests even though masking for pure tone testing proves to be too difficult for them.

Masking

As in pure tone testing, it is necessary to mask the nontest ear when the speech signals being delivered to the test ear are sufficiently intense that the test stimuli are perceived in the nontest ear. Hence, when the speech recognition threshold for the test ear exceeds bone-conduction sensitivity in the opposite ear by a value greater than 40 dB, masking must be delivered to the nontest ear. Given that interaural attenuation is minimal, masking is necessary for SRT or SDT testing via bone conduction if the clinician is to establish the response as being isolated to a single ear. The occlusion effect of the masking earphone must be taken into account for bone-conduction speech tests just as for pure tone tests via bone conduction. Klodd and Edgerton (1977) found mean occlusion effects for bone-conducted speech stimuli delivered at the mastoid and forehead to be 6 dB and 9 dB, respectively. For a few subjects, occlusion effects of 20 dB were observed.

As in masking for pure tones, the effectiveness of the masking noise used during speech audiometry must be known. Empirical measurements in which speech and masking noise are mixed in the same earphone are easily accomplished. One simply delivers noise of a known level to the ears of normal listeners and then adjusts the level of the speech to the intensity just below the level at which spondees are intelligible or detectable, depending on whether the interest is in determining effective masking levels for SRT or SDT measures. It has been our experience that the sound pressure level of white noise must be approximately 20 dB more intense than the speech in order to mask it insofar as speech detection thresholds are concerned. The overall level of speech spectrum noise (white noise low pass filtered at 1000 Hz with a 9 dB/octave roll-off) can be about 4 to 6 dB less intense than white noise for equivalent masking levels. In any event, the clinician should determine empirically the noise levels necessary for masking speech with a particular audiometer and set of speech test materials.

Central masking effects for speech, in which the threshold in the test ear is elevated by the presence of even low levels of noise in the nontest ear, are minimal. Frank and Karlovich (1975) and Martin, Bailey, and Pappas (1965) observed central masking effects on the order of 1 to 3 dB for noise levels at sensation levels of 20 to 60 dB. (For further discussion of masking for speech signals, refer to Chapter 3.)

Modifications for pediatric speech thresholds

The use of conventional procedures, as described above, is appropriate when establishing speech thresholds for many children of school age. However, test procedures and materials that were developed for use with adults may not be appropriate in many instances. The effects of various hearing impairments during early childhood upon receptive language development, as well as the relatively short attention span of young children or those with developmental disabilities, explains the need for a battery of pediatric tests scaled in terms of difficulty. The restricted expressive language skills of many young hearing-impaired youngsters further complicates matters when selecting appropriate response modes for speech audiometry with them. The use of reinforcement to maintain optimal response behavior also merits consideration.

Materials. The need for modifying routine procedures when assessing younger children was recognized relatively early in the history of speech audiometry (McFarlan, 1940). For example, the use of 25 directions containing common nouns rather than spondees when establishing thresholds was recommended by Keaster in 1947. Alternate modifications, such as the use of spondee picture cards or familiar toys requiring pointing rather than a verbal response, were suggested in subsequent articles by Meyerson (1956), Siegenthaler, Pearson, and LeZak (1954), and Sortini and Flake (1953). Lists of spondaic words considered to be within most children's vocabularies have been published and are used by many clinicians (Newby, 1958; American Speech-Language-Hearing Association, 1988). Many of these spondees can be pictured or represented by miniature objects.

Although the use of familiar spondaic words with associated picture cards is one modification, Siegenthaler and Haspiel (1966) have published test materials, designated TIP (threshold by the identification of pictures), in which monosyllabic rather than bisyllabic words are employed. Monosyllabic words also are used when a young child is asked to point to familiar body parts. The TIP procedure was carefully evaluated before publication, and pointing to body parts is appealing in its simplicity. However, the use of monosyllabic words that lack both homogeneity and redundancy may limit the precision with which a threshold can be established.

Methods. Regardless of the test materials used, it is recommended that a preliminary step in determining an SRT for children is first, to familiarize the youngster with the test stimuli through bisensory input (audition and vision) and then, to eliminate those words that are not within the child's vocabulary. Obviously, using either picture or object pointing rather than a verbal response will require that the number of test items be limited to 12 or fewer. Otherwise, the visual scanning task and the demands upon memory become unwieldy. Furthermore, clinical experience has revealed that the use of a carrier phrase such as "point to" or "show me" often focuses the child's attention on the auditory task at hand. Finally, it is more expedient to work in 5-dB or 10-dB steps when establishing an SRT for a youngster whose attention span is limited. The length of time that "difficult-to-test" children will cooperate for such measurements often can be extended by incorporating not only social but visual or tangible reinforcements into the test approach (Martin & Coombs, 1976).

With the growing emphasis on early identification of handicapped children, an increasing number of youngsters who are essentially nonverbal are being seen for audiologic evaluations. Because of marked language deficits in such cases, it is not feasible to establish a speech reception threshold. As an alternative, determination of a speech detection threshold is more realistic. Any of the behavioral conditioning techniques used during pure tone audiometry (visual reinforcement audiometry, VRA; tangible reinforcement conditioning audiometry, TROCA; or conditioned play audiometry) can be used to establish a minimal response level to repetitive speech utterances such as "ah/oh" or "ba/ba/ba." As with conditioned pure tone audiometry, the reliability of the speech measures depends on such variables as ease of conditioning, rate of extinction, and the response ratio selected to represent threshold. Another limitation that must be recognized is that when the configuration of the hearing loss is either sharply sloping or rising, the relationship between the SDT and the average pure tone loss for the speech frequencies (500–2000 Hz) may be poor. As mentioned earlier, the SDT often relates most closely to the best single pure tone threshold within the frequency range of 250-4000 Hz.

If a child's age or presence of additional disabilities precludes successful conditioning, it often is necessary to reduce the complexity of the procedure and to establish a minimum response level to speech through behavioral observation audiometry. When assessing infants or difficult-to-test children, it is recommended that the term *minimal response level for speech* be used; this term implies that some improvement in speech recognition may be seen with maturation and auditory experience. Because rapid extinction of responses to repeated stimulus presentations is encountered with unconditioned behavior, as ascending rather than descending approach is strongly recommended. Careful determination of the intensity level at which the initial response is elicited is the critical observation during such unconditioned behavioral testing.

Because measurements of speech detection with very young children frequently are carried out in a sound field rather than under earphones, it must be kept in mind that the minimal response level to speech presented via loudspeakers may only reflect hearing sensitivity in the better ear. Furthermore, the presence of either a significant high-frequency or low-frequency hearing loss can never be ruled out on the basis of a response to a broad spectrum stimulus such as speech. In other words, clinicians must exercise caution when interpreting such information because the audiometric configuration cannot be inferred from speech audiometric findings.

Franklin (1977) reported on the use of tape-recorded speech stimuli, specifically "ah, clap, clap," spoken by a female, band-pass filtered at 250, 500, 1000, 2000, and 4000 Hz, to test infants or difficult-to-test patients. By such filtering she suggested that these materials were frequency specific and allowed measurement of audiometric configuration with stimuli that, because they retained speech qualities, gained attention from infants or other patients for whom testing with tone or narrow band noise stimuli was unsuccessful. Measurements of the stimuli by Surr, Siedman, Schwartz, and Mueller (1982) and by Koval and Stelmachowicz (1983), however, revealed that the filtered spectra were quite broad and that energy peaks were not necessarily at the indicated octave frequencies. In further evaluation of these test materials with cooperative adult patients, both groups of investigators also found marked underestimation of hearing loss for patients with sloping or rising audiometric configurations. Koval and Stelmachowicz (1983) concluded "that in their present form, the Speech-Band Audiometry tapes cannot be used to obtain valid frequency-specific threshold information, particularly in the presence of rising or sloping audiometric configurations" (p. 329). Similarly, Surr et al. (1982) cautioned that their "results cast substantial doubt on the advisability of using speech-band audiometry in its present form as an aid in pediatric evaluations or in assessment of characteristics of amplification" (p. 250).

Utilization of bone conduction to establish a threshold for speech with young children for whom detailed information regarding bone-conduction sensitivity for pure tones is not attainable provides valuable information. In a minimum of testing time, it can be determined whether there is a significant difference in the speech recognition thresholds obtained via air conduction and bone conduction. As described further on in this chapter, empirical calibration to determine an 0-dB reference level is essential if this technique is to be used. Furthermore, establishing a speech detection threshold rather than an SRT via bone conduction can be quite misleading. Children with severe and profound hearing losses may respond to vibrotactile rather than to auditory perception of the test stimuli at relatively low intensity levels.

The determination of either an SRT or an SDT is strongly recommended as a routine clinical procedure when evaluating children. Obviously, the specific approach taken for such testing should be modified after careful consideration of the child's level of function. Suggested guidelines for establishing thresholds for speech are presented in Table 2.2. An analysis of the methods and test materials successfully used for speech threshold testing may serve to highlight not only the child's auditory sensitivity but the level of auditory function. As with adults, the relationship between pure tone and speech audiometric findings is of primary

TABLE 2.2

General Guidelines for Speech Threshold Testing of Children

Approximate Level of Function[a]	Type of Measurement	Test Stimuli	Response Task	Type of Reinforcement
10 years or more	Conventional speech reception threshold	Spondee list	Verbal	Verbal (intermittent)
5 to 10 years	Conventional speech reception threshold	Children's spondee list	Verbal	Verbal (intermittent)
30 months to 6 years	Modified speech reception threshold	Selected children's spondees	Picture or object pointing often with verbal	Social, visual and/or tangible (40%–100% schedule)
Less than 3 years	Speech detection threshold	Repetitive speech utterance	Conditioned	Play, visual or tangible (100% schedule)
Limited	Speech detection threshold	Repetitive speech utterance	Unconditioned response	None

[a]Dependent on cognitive, motor, and language development and attending behavior.

interest. A marked discrepancy between the average pure tone thresholds and the speech reception threshold may be one of the first clues that a nonorganic hearing loss is present. Exaggerated hearing levels are a phenomenon encountered among school-aged children as well as adults (see Chapter 12).

Calibration

The American National Standards Institute Specifications for Audiometers (ANSI, 1969a) includes requirements for calibration of speech signals as well as pure tones. In the main, the ANSI standard calls for: (a) a VU meter with a response time from its resting position to 99% of its reference, 0 dB point, in 270 to 330 ms and an overshoot of 1.0 to 1.5% (American National Standards Institute, 1954) to monitor speech input levels; (b) a relatively flat frequency response, ±5 dB re the output at 1000 Hz across the frequency range 200 through 4000 Hz (and no more than 10 dB above 1000 Hz for frequencies below 200 Hz or above 4000 Hz for recorded or live voice presentation; (c) harmonic distortion no greater than 5.6%; (d) an intensity range of 0 to 100 dB (in steps of 2.5 dB or less); and (e) intensity level accuracy of ±3 dB.

Because speech fluctuates in intensity and is difficult to measure in actual sound pressure level (SPL), the calibration level for speech is specified relative to a 1000-Hz pure tone. Hence, "the sound pressure level of a speech signal at the earphone is defined as the rms sound pressure level . . . of a 1000-Hz signal adjusted so that the VU meter deflection produced by a 1000 Hz signal is equal to the average peak VU meter deflection produced by the speech signal" (ANSI, 1969a, p. 15). The standard reference level for speech as measured with a 1000-Hz tone is 20 dB SPL for the earphones that are conventionally provided with audiometers. Thus the reference level for speech at 0 dB HL is 20 dB SPL. This level is based on a variety of studies demonstrating that the average intensity level at which young normal hearing subjects correctly repeat 50% of the spondees presented to them via earphones is 20 dB SPL. Less intensity is required to establish speech recognition thresholds in sound field listening conditions. According to the data of Dirks, Stream, and Wilson (1972) and Tillman, Johnson, and Olsen (1966), 7.5 dB less intensity is needed to obtain speech reception thresholds in a sound field than under earphones when the loudspeakers are located at an azimuth of 45° relative to the listener's head. The difference is on the order of 4 to 4.8 dB less when the loudspeaker is at 0° azimuth (directly in front) of the listener (Breakey & Davis, 1949; Dirks et al., 1972; Stream & Dirks, 1974). Because a 1000-Hz pure tone cannot be used for measurement of the signal level in a sound field unless an anechoic sound field condition exists, Dirks et al. (1972) and Tillman et al. (1966) recommended use of speech spectrum noise for calibration of speech levels in the sound field.

Standard calibration values for bone-conducted speech stimuli are not available at this time. Empirical calibration comparing speech recognition thresholds obtained via air conduction and via bone conduction for normal hearers or sensorineural hearing loss subjects must be completed for each audiometer. Replacement of a bone vibrator for a given audiometer requires recalibration. The maximum level for bone-conducted speech tests with currently used bone vibrators and audiometers is no greater than 70 dB HL (Barry & Gaddis, 1978). (Refer to Chapter 16 for further discussion of calibration.)

Summary

From this review, it is apparent that equivalent results can be obtained from speech recognition threshold tests that require responses to sentences or spondees and threshold tests in which the listener adjusts the intensity of speech to the lowest level that continuous discourse can be just understood. Given that thresholds for spondees are more easily established and are more objective, use of spondaic words is the method of choice when determining thresholds for speech. To improve the homogeneity of the spondaic test items, the sample size was decreased from 84 to 36. Recent studies suggest that homogeneity would be improved with a further reduction of the sample of test items.

It is generally recommended that listeners be familiarized with the spondees before beginning speech recognition threshold testing (Tillman & Jerger, 1959). Most procedures for obtaining an SRT suggest a descending approach. Although test words are more commonly presented via monitored live voice, standardization requires use of recorded materials.

The close relationship between pure tone (500–2000 Hz) and speech recognition thresholds serves as an excellent index of the accuracy of the pure tone findings. This is one of the most important reasons for routinely determining speech recognition thresholds in clinical settings. SRTs that are considerably better (>6 dB) than the pure tone average indicate the need for further evaluation.

Assessment of a child's ability to detect (SDT) or to recognize (SRT) speech stimuli in addition to determining auditory sensitivity for various pure tones yields face validity to the pediatric test battery. Information regarding a child's response to speech often is more meaningful to parents and educators than is a discussion of pure tone sensitivity.

The reference level for speech presented via earphones is 20 dB SPL as measured for a 1000-Hz tone adjusted to the same VU meter reading as the average peaks of the speech signal. The reference sound pressure level in a sound field is on the order of 12.5 dB for loudspeakers at a 45° azimuth and 16 or 17 dB for a loudspeaker at 0° calibrated with speech spectrum noise.

Suprathreshold measures of speech recognition

Measurements of recognition of speech samples at intensity levels well above threshold are important to engineers concerned with apparatus for communication and to audiologists working with patients who have hearing problems. That speech understanding cannot be predicted from pure tone threshold findings has been demonstrated repeatedly. For example, Young and Gibbons (1962) noted that although there was some degree of association between scores obtained from tests of speech understanding presented at suprathreshold levels and pure tone thresholds for hearing-impaired subjects, the relationship was not strong enough to allow accurate prediction of speech understanding from the pure tone audiogram. Similarly, Elliot (1963), after analyses of 18 variables (13 based on pure tone thresholds), reported that none of the variables or their combinations satisfactorily predicted scores for tests of speech understanding. In agreement with the proposal of Kryter, Williams, and Green (1962), Harris (1965) found some relationship between threshold sensitivity averaged across 1000, 2000, and 3000 Hz and understanding of speech. Yoshioka and Thornton (1980) evaluated three methods of predicting scores for the CID W-22 word lists. The largest negative correlation between scores for suprathreshold speech tests and pure tone thresholds were for 1000 Hz, 2000 Hz, and the 500–2000 Hz pure tone average (the greater the hearing loss, the lower the percent correct score on the speech test). Marshall and Bacon (1981) observed some relationship between the combination of threshold sensitivity at 2000 Hz and age (actually age squared) and scores for CID W-22 word lists. However, the variability was sufficiently large that they agreed with Harris (1965) who stated that "probably no formula can ever be derived with slight enough error so that prediction of the DS [discrimination score for speech] of an individual ear may reach a satisfactory confidence level" (p. 829).

Similarly, attempts to relate speech processing abilities of impaired auditory systems to deficiencies in frequency or temporal resolution capabilities have not been wholly successful. Although some statistical relationships between scores on some tests of speech understanding at suprathreshold levels and selected measures of frequency and temporal resolution have been observed, the correlations generally have not been robust; variability has been substantial (Bonding, 1979; DiCarlo, 1962; Humes, 1983; Preminger & Wiley, 1985; Tyler, Summerfield, Wood, & Fernandes, 1982; Tyler, Wood, & Fernandes, 1982).

Hence, assessment of auditory recognition or identification of words, nonsense syllables, or phonemes is a necessary part of clinical evaluation of hearing impairments and associated communication difficulties. Inferences regarding a patient's ability to understand speech cannot be derived from indirect means at the present time. This lack of indirect measurement of speech perception abilities no doubt is due, in part, to the acoustic complexity of speech and to the complex processing of this acoustic information by the auditory system. Before beginning a discussion of various tests developed for assessing speech understanding at suprathreshold levels, a brief consideration of the acoustic content of speech is in order.

Speech spectra

Given the extreme complexity of the acoustic variations in connected speech from moment to moment, utterance to utterance, and talker to talker, it is indeed remarkable that the peripheral auditory mechanism and central auditory nervous system can code the incoming signals into neural impulses that ultimately are stored as a meaningful symbol system. Not only are there major variations in the intensity level, frequency content, and temporal pattern of repeated utterances of the same sounds in a single word by one individual, but variations from one individual to another are even greater. Furthermore, the characteristics of the same phonemes change as a function of the surrounding speech sounds, as a function of context and emotion, and as a function of the force exerted by the talker, that is, whether he or she is whispering, speaking normally, or shouting. In spite of this variability and complexity, speech signals heard by human beings are received, encoded, stored, retrieved from storage for comparison with other incoming stimuli, and related to the new events with astonishing speed and accuracy.

Figure 2.1 shows a plot of the intensity, frequency, and temporal characteristics of one sentence as spoken by one talker. This figure displays a conventional speech spectrogram revealing the frequency content on the ordinate and the time domain on the abscissa. The intensity of the various frequency components at a given time is indicated by the shading within the display; the darker the shading, the more intense is that particular portion of the speech signal at that moment. Energy in broad frequency regions occurs simultaneously, sometimes gradually shifts from one frequency region to another, sometimes changes suddenly.

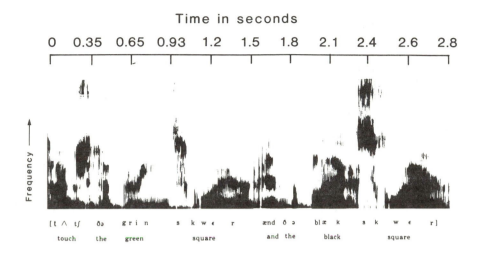

Figure 2.1. Speech spectrogram of sentence. (Courtesy of M. McNeil and University of Colorado, Denver)

Figure 2.2 shows a display of the same recording of the same sentence in a three-dimensional display developed by a Real Time Analyzer. The intensity is shown by the amplitude of the bars and the frequency content and time display are plotted on the other two dimensions. It is these relationships among frequency, intensity, and temporal variables that, despite their inconsistency over time, over conditions, and over talkers are, nevertheless, sufficiently consistent that they can be coded into the symbol system of speech.

A different manner of plotting speech spectra is shown in Figure 2.3. This representation is based on measurements of the sensation levels of one-third octave bands of speech presented in a sound field to normal hearing subjects (Pascoe, 1978) and is plotted on an audiogram format (Pascoe, 1980). For conversational speech having an overall level of 65 dB SPL, the three lines from top to bottom represent the levels that the speech sounds exceed the indicated levels 90%, 50%, and 10% of the time, respectively (Olsen, Hawkins, & Van Tasell, 1987; Pascoe, 1980). Skinner's (1988) representation of speech in Figure 2.4 for the same overall level of 65 dB SPL is similar but about 10 dB higher. The center solid line indicates the levels exceeded by speech 50% of the time; the bottom and top lines are at levels 12 dB stronger and 18 dB weaker to reflect speech peaks and speech minima, respectively, thereby representing a 30-dB dynamic range for speech spectra. Interestingly when the speech spectrum sug-

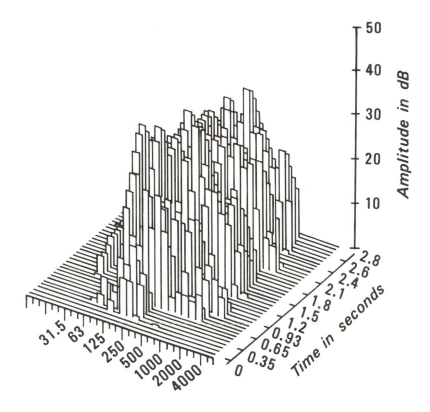

Figure 2.2. Three-dimensional plot of sentence shown in Figure 2.1. (Courtesy of M. McNeil and University of Colorado, and Veterans Administration, Denver)

gested by Cox and Moore (1988) for speech at an overall level of 70 dB SPL is converted to an audiogram format using CID values for sound field thresholds (Skinner, 1988) as a reference for 0 dB HL, the levels fall along the dashed line in Figure 2.4.

Figure 2.5 shows the same outline for speech spectra as does Figure 2.3, and the frequency regions for the voice fundamental, formants, and sibilants are indicated also. In addition, the approximate levels and frequency regions for some of the classes of speech sounds are shown. (See Olsen et al., 1987, for other estimates of speech spectra converted to an audiogram format.)

Representations of speech spectra relative to an audiogram as in Figures 2.3, 2.4, and 2.5 are very useful when counseling patients and their families about the receptive communication difficulties they are

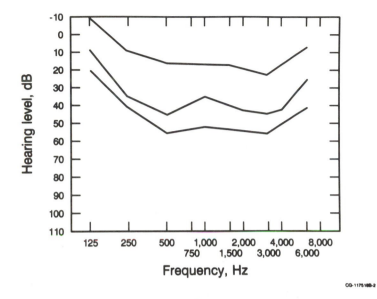

Figure 2.3. Representation of speech spectrum on audiogram format. Top, middle, and bottom lines indicate levels exceeded by speech energy 90%, 50%, and 10% of time for speech having overall level of 65 dB SPL. (Adapted from Pascoe, 1980)

encountering because of the filtering effect imposed by hearing impairments. After all, the complaints of hearing-impaired individuals are associated with their difficulties in hearing and understanding speech, not their inability to detect certain pure tones below a given intensity level. A graph of the long-term average of speech spectra converted to appropriate intensity relationships relative to an audiogram can be plotted on a transparency and used as an overlay on the audiogram. Superimposing this information often helps patients to understand, to some extent, the relevance of seemingly meaningless pure tone thresholds to their problems in perceiving and understanding speech. This approach also can be productive when discussing habilitation plans for hearing-impaired children with teachers and other clinicians. (Obviously, the graph does not illustrate problems in speech understanding created by distortion related to sensorineural damage.)

Definitions of selected terms

As mentioned earlier, the first materials designed for measurement of auditory recognition or identification of speech sounds were developed

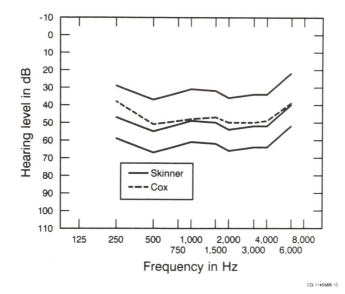

Figure 2.4. Speech spectra adapted from Skinner (1988) and Cox and Moore (1988). Middle solid line indicates levels exceeded by speech 10% of time for speech having overall level of 65 dB SPL. Bottom and top lines +12 dB and −18 dB re middle line. Dashed line indicates speech spectrum at overall level of 70 dB SPL from Cox and Moore (1988). CID reference sound field threshold levels (Skinner, 1988) subtracted from Cox and Moore data to convert to audiogram format for comparison purposes.

at the Bell Telephone Laboratories in 1910. These so-called "articulation lists" were used to evaluate the adequacy of telephone circuits for speech transmission. Curves plotting performance in terms of percent correct as a function of some variable, for example, intensity, came to be known as *articulation functions*. However, because the term *articulation* has an alternate meaning to those concerned with speech and hearing processes, the label *performance-intensity (PI) function*, suggested by Speaks and Jerger (1966), is more appropriate and now more commonly used.

Along the same line, Owens and Schubert (1968) recommended that the term *speech intelligibility* be applied to discussions concerning speech production, reproduction, and transmission systems, that is, the intelligibility of speech produced, reproduced, amplified, and transmitted.

Through common usage *speech discrimination* has come to mean an assessment of an individual's ability to understand speech, usually monosyllabic words, at suprathreshold levels. In the field of psychology, however, the term *discrimination* refers to differentiation among stimuli as "same" or "different." In that context audiology's use of the terminology

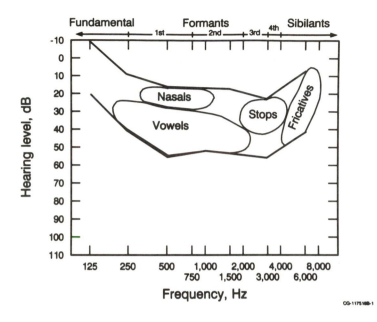

Figure 2.5. Speech spectrum from Figure 2.3. Location and classes of sounds within spectrum adapted from Tyler (1979). Estimates of frequency regions for fundamental, formants, and sibilants adapted from Liden (1954).

speech discrimination is inappropriate. More appropriate labels might be *recognition* or *identification* preceded by a descriptive term of the test items, thereby describing the test items and the task. This terminology is used in the remainder of this chapter. *Monosyllable recognition* or *word recognition* are the labels used to describe tests in which the listener repeats (or writes) the word heard following each presentation without being given a specific set of test items from which to select a response. If nonsense syllables are used, then the label becomes *nonsense syllable recognition*. Such tests are *open ended* in that restrictions in responses are not given to the listener. *Identification* is the term applied to *closed response* tests in which the task of the listener is to select a response from a given set of items visually displayed at the time of the presentation of the test item. The terms *phoneme, nonsense syllable, word,* or *sentence* precede the label *identification* to describe whether the possible selections differ only in one phoneme, whole nonsense syllables, whole words, or sentences, respectively.

Kruel, Bell, and Nixon (1969) contended that "only the actual recordings of the spoken lists of words can be considered to be the *test material*" (p. 281; emphasis added). In their view, the word lists in and of themselves should not be considered as the test material but rather as an identified group of words. These comments have merit; as pointed out later in this discussion, even though identical lists may be used, different test results are obtained when test materials are prepared at different facilities with different talkers.

Monosyllables: open-ended sets

Although lists of 50 nonsense syllables (CV, VC, and CVC items) were used to assess speech intelligibility in the early work at Bell Telephone Laboratories, most tests that were subsequently developed to evaluate suprathreshold speech intelligibility or speech understanding have employed monosyllabic words.

In 1939 Fry and Kerridge described five lists of 25 consonant-vowel-consonant words each, called Word Tests for Deaf People. Each list contained all but four sounds of English spoken language. The lists of words were to be spoken by a friend or relative in a quiet room at an agreed upon distance. The listener closed her or his eyes and responded to each word. Four points were given for each word, one per sound or phoneme, and one point was allowed if a response was made but was in error for all the sounds of the spoken item. Fry and Kerridge advised that any person whose score was less than 35% should be tested with a list from their sentence test (described later in this chapter) to allow the listener the advantage of context.

Criteria for development of test lists were described well by Egan in 1948. In Egan's words, "all or nearly all of the fundamental sounds into which speech can be analyzed should be represented in each list of test items [and] . . . the relative frequencies of occurrence of these fundamental speech sounds should reflect their distribution in normal speech" (p. 957). "If test lists are to be sensitive to small differences in intelligibility as well as convenient to use, the test items must be fairly closely distributed along a scale of difficulty, [and] . . . the distribution of difficulty should be sufficiently wide to embrace the requisite range as determined by the conditions under which the lists will be used" (pp. 960–961). With these goals in mind, Egan attempted to construct lists of monosyllables that were equal in average difficulty, equal in range of difficulty, and of equal phonetic composition, employing English words in common usage. The phonetic composition of the lists was based on Dewey's (1923) count of sounds in a sample of 100,000 words in newsprint. Egan noted that attempts to satisfy these criteria using lists of 25 words were not successful. Furthermore, strict adherence to the desired phonetic content with lists of 50 words was not possible either. For example, 25% of the words in Dewey's sample of 100,000 words begin with short vowel sounds, but there are only 40 common monosyllables beginning with a short vowel. Also, the frequency of occurrence of final sounds in the lists do not exactly follow the pattern suggested by Dewey's sample. Nevertheless, Egan developed 20 lists of "phonetically balanced" monosyllables, which came to be known as the Harvard PB-50 lists.

Hirsh et al. (1952) modified the PB-50 lists by reducing the vocabulary from 1,000 words to 200 familiar words and incorporating them into four lists of 50 words each. Five judges rated the words in terms of familiarity; only the more familiar words were selected for inclusion as test items. Of the 200 words used, 190 are among the 4,000 most common words of the Thorndike and Lorge (1944) lists. Each list of 50 items was rigidly balanced phonetically based on both Dewey's count and on a study of telephone conversations in New York City by the Bell Telephone Company (French, Carter, & Koenig, 1930). The lists were labeled CID W-22 word lists and are widely used in clinical settings.

A somewhat different set of criteria in the form of phonemic rather than phonetic balancing of word lists was used by Lehiste and Peterson (1959) in their development of monosyllabic word lists. It was their contention that because speech sounds are strongly influenced by the other speech sounds occurring around them, articulation of a speech sound is rarely physically identical to a previous utterance. Therefore, according to Lehiste and Peterson, it is not possible to have word lists that are phonetically balanced. In their definition, phonetic is the study of the physiologic and physical properties of speech sounds; accordingly only phonemic balancing is possible. A first order of balancing would be to have each initial consonant, each vowel, and each final consonant appear with the same frequency of occurrence in each list. After analyzing the balance within the Harvard PB-50 lists, Lehiste and Peterson set out to develop word lists that were phonemically balanced more precisely. The frequency of occurrence was determined for each initial consonant (C), vowel (labeled syllable nucleus [N] by Lehiste and Peterson), and final consonant (C) in the Thorndike and Lorge list of 1,263 such monosyllables. Using this frequency of occurrence as their guide, they developed 10 lists with 50 different CNC words in each list. In 1962, Peterson and Lehiste revised their word lists so all but 21 of the words had a frequency of occurrence greater than five per million. The reason for this revision was that "in clinical testing an untrained listener is confronted with an unknown message set. Although the word lists commonly used in this type of testing constitute a restricted and well-defined corpus for the experimenter, the listener is in fact comparing the words he hears with a large vocabulary of the English language contained in his memory . . . thus in clinical testing, word frequency is probably a very significant factor" (p. 62).

As Hirsh et al. (1952) had reduced the original Harvard PB-50 lists from 20 lists to four lists, the 10 lists of the Lehiste and Peterson were reduced to two lists (Tillman, Carhart, & Wilber, 1963) and subsequently expanded to four lists (Tillman & Carhart, 1966) in an effort to achieve lists of 50 CNC items that conformed more closely to the phonemic balance sought by the original investigators. These lists of words, labeled Northwestern University Auditory Test No. 6 (NU No. 6), have gained some popularity recently in research and clinical use.

"High-frequency" word lists for use in evaluation of high-frequency hearing losses and hearing aid selection procedures have been described by Gardner (1971) and Pascoe (1975). Gardner's lists consist of two lists of 25 monosyllables each using only voiceless plosives [p, t, k], the fricatives [s, f, ǝ], and the aspirate [h] with a single vowel [I], for example, "kits." In Pascoe's list of 50 monosyllables, 63% of the consonants are voiceless fricatives, affricates, aspirates, and plosives, the rest being voiced plosives [b, d, g], and nasals [m, n]. The vowels in Pascoe's list are [I, aI] and [ou] as in "hits," "wine," and "road." Other than the reports of Gardner (1971), Pascoe (1975), Dennison and Kelly (1978), Skinner, Karstaedt, and Miller (1982) and Skinner and Miller (1983), we are unaware of other current reports dealing with the use of these test lists for evaluating communicative difficulties or for hearing aid selections.

Fry (1961) revised and expanded the lists he and Kerridge described in 1939. The new lists consist of 10 lists of 35 monosyllables, 30 consonant-vowel-consonant, and 5 consonant-vowel or vowel-consonant items, for a total of 100 phonemes in each list. The frequency of occurrence of the various consonants and vowels is the same in each list. Either 100 phonemes or 35 words can be scored, but Fry recommended phoneme scoring.

Boothroyd (1968) described so-called isophonemic word lists with 10 words rather than 35 words per list. All of the test items are of the consonant-vowel-consonant type and the 15 lists are phonemically balanced with respect to one another. The same 20 consonants and 10 vowels occur once in each list. The phonemes chosen were those occurring most frequently in the CVC words, but obviously no attempt was made to relate the frequency of individual phonemes in the lists to their frequency of occurrence in spoken English. Boothroyd also recommended scoring each phoneme; hence, 30 phonemes are scored in each list of this test rather than just the 10 words. According to Boothroyd, one of the advantages of scoring phonemes rather than words is that the phoneme scores give a more valid estimate of the subject's ability to recognize the acoustic features of speech sounds.

Papers presented by Olsen, Van Tasell, and Speaks (1982a, 1982b, 1983, 1986a, 1986b) have demonstrated the feasibility of developing equivalent lists and pairs of lists for clinical use. Presentation of two lists of 10 words each can be accomplished quickly and allows scoring of the same 30 phonemes twice to provide a quick check on the consistency of the patient's scores for two equivalent lists. If scores are similar, within predetermined criteria, they can be averaged and considered a reasonable estimate of the patient's performance. If dissimilar, additional 10-word lists can be administered to obtain a better estimate of the patient's phoneme recognition. Such procedures are in keeping with the Hughes, Arthur, and Johnson (1979) recommendation that two or more 50-word lists be presented to obtain a more stable estimate of a patient's word-recognition performance. However, using two or more 50-word, or even 25-word lists, to attain stable performance, or to plot word recognition performance as a function of intensity, becomes very time-consuming and fatiguing for the patient in a clinical setting. An obvious advantage of the shorter 10-word lists is the considerable reduction in testing time. A list can be administered in less than 1 minute. Thus it becomes possible to present two or more such lists at a single level to achieve an indication of stability of performance, or at several intensities to plot performance-intensity functions relatively quickly (Walker & Boothroyd, 1987).

Five subsets of items differing in degree of difficulty for a Speech Discrimination Scale (SDS) were suggested by Beykirch and Gaeth (1978). Less difficult items were digits (1, 2, 3, 4, 5, 6, 8, 9) followed by "easy letters" (A, B, H, J, K, L, X), "hard letters" (C, E, F, G, N, P, T, V), "easy words" (eat, good, job, kid, love, our, smile, there), and "hard words" (dab, flop, heap, most, need, ode, thigh, vamp). Presentation of these materials to patients who yielded word recognition scores of 76% to 80%, 50% to 66%, or 24% to 30% for 100 items of NU No. 6 revealed, as expected, different performance-intensity functions for the different materials. Interestingly, the functions were similar for the three groups of patients but were shifted to higher sensation levels for those with poorer word recognition scores.

Nonsense syllables: open-ended sets

Edgerton and Danhauer (1979) described bisyllabic test materials using consonant–vowel–consonant–vowel (CVCV) nonsense syllables. Twenty consonants and 10 vowels are used. The test lists consist of 25 CVCV items each, randomized six times. At 55-dB sensation level above SRT a group of normal hearing subjects attained mean scores on the order of 95%, 90%, 86%, and 66% for vowels, phonemes, consonants, and whole bisyllable recognition, respectively. Mean performance values for a group of patients with sensorineural hearing losses were approximately 80%, 72%, 62% and 24% for vowels, phonemes, consonants, and bisyllables, respectively. In agreement with Fry (1961) and Boothroyd (1968), they concluded that their data did not support use of bisyllable scoring and "that while the data supported the use of both phoneme and consonant scoring for nonsense stimuli, phoneme scoring was clearly superior" (Edgerton & Danhauer, 1979, p. 75). Edgerton and Danhauer also indicated that "Nonsense syllables are optimal stimuli for discrimination testing because they can be easily combined into equivalent lists, are low in information redundancy, and are relatively insensitive to familiarity effects" (p. 36). However, they cautioned that these bisyllable lists "must be tested more extensively on much larger normal and hearing-impaired subject samples before the clinical usefulness of this type of stimulus can be established with certainty" (p. 74).

Monosyllables: closed-response sets

Within the past few years the use of multiple-choice, or closed-response, test lists for clinical assessment of word or phoneme identification has attracted some attention. As mentioned earlier, Barany and Lempert reported such efforts in the early 1900s (Feldmann, 1960). Interest in the United States is an outgrowth of the work of Black (1957), and more directly that of Fairbanks (1958). Five lists of rhyming monosyllables with 50 items per list are used in the Fairbanks rhyme test. Only the initial consonant differs in a set of five rhyming words, but the initial consonants are not given on the response sheet. Hence the response task of the listener is to write the initial consonant for the stem provided on the answer sheets. As such, the Fairbanks rhyme test actually is not a classic "closed-message" or "closed-response" test. However, it is not an open set either, because the listener is only required to recognize the initial consonant of each test item based on perception of the initial consonant and vowel transition. Thus the Fairbanks rhyme test probably is more correctly labeled as a phoneme recognition, actually a consonant recognition test.

House, Williams, Hecker, and Kryter (1965) developed the Modified Rhyme Test (MRT) by expanding the Fairbanks test into six lists and incorporating the differentiation of final and initial consonants. Each list includes 50 items requiring identification of 25 initial and 25 final consonants. Rather than completing the word by adding the appropriate symbol, as in the Fairbanks rhyme test, entire words are printed on the response sheets. The task of the listener is to select the monosyllabic word presented from a set of six items such as: "sing, sit, sin, sill, sip, sick" for final consonant identification, or "vest, rest, nest, test, best, west" for initial consonant identification. As such, the MRT might be called a phoneme or consonant identification test.

Kruel et al. (1968) prepared tape recordings of the modified rhyme test for clinical use. In order to increase the range of difficulty for these test materials, a background of bandpass filtered pink noise (3 dB/octave fall 400 to 4000 Hz and approximately 20 dB/octave drop below 150 Hz and above 5000 Hz) was mixed with the words. In a normative study with these materials, normal hearing adult subjects yielded scores of 96%, 83%, and 75% in quiet, and at signal-to-noise ratios of +12 dB and +8 dB, respectively.

Griffiths refined the MRT further in 1967. In Griffiths's test lists each word within a given set differs from another word in the same set in only one of the distinctive features characterizing speech sounds, that is, manner of articulation, place of articulation, or voicing. For example, in a given set of "cup, cub, cut, cud, cuff," the items "cup" and "cub," and "cut" and "cud" differ only in voicing, "cut" and "cup," and "cub" and "cud" differ only in place of articulation, and "cuff" differs from the others in manner of articulation. Griffiths's basis for developing word lists of this type was that earlier work had demonstrated that listener confusions in manner of articulation, place of articulation, and voicing were essentially independent; therefore, word sets of minimal contrasts ("rhyming minimal contrasts" as labeled by Griffiths) should enhance the diagnostic utility of the test. The rhyming minimal contrasts test is made up of 250 monosyllables (150 of the words from the modified rhyme test and 100 new items), arranged in five 50-word lists. The initial consonant is the variable in 25 sets and the final consonant is the variable in the other 25.

McPherson and Pang-Ching (1979) carried Griffiths idea a step further in the description of their Distinctive Feature Discrimination Test (DFDT). The DFDT consists of four lists of 50 CNC words in each list, 25 with the initial consonant as the variable, and 25 with the final consonant as the variable phoneme. The rhyming error responses for each stimulus differ by one, two, or three distinctive features in terms of voicing, nasality, affrication, duration, and place of articulation. For example, for the stimulus word "cuff," the three error selections given are "cup," which differs in affrication, "cut," which differs in affrication and place, and "cud," which differs in voicing, affrication, and place. Scoring can be simply correct or incorrect, or weighted with one point for a one-feature error, two points for a two-feature error, and three points for a three-feature error.

Development of a closed-response format for the CID W-22 word lists was reported by Schultz and Schubert in 1969. For each of the 50 words in each of the four CID W-22 lists, the test word and four alternative choices are available on the answer sheets provided to the listeners. The response task is to mark the item presented each time. Whereas only the initial and final consonants differ in a given set in the MRT and minimal rhyming contrasts lists, various sets in the Multiple-Choice Discrimination Test (MCDT) of Schultz and Schubert include foils allowing for confusion of either the initial consonant or final consonant in the same set. In their report Schultz and Schubert considered this version of the MCDT to be a prototype and indicated that a vowel substitution version of the MCDT was under construction. We are not aware of subsequent reports dealing with further development and modification of the MCDT.

A closed-response test that includes vowel confusions as well as initial and final consonants was described by Pederson and Studebaker in 1972. Called the University of Oklahoma Closed Response Speech Test, it is a minimal contrast test consisting of three independent subtests. The variable phonemes differ in place of articulation. Twenty initial consonant items are used four times in a subtest, yielding an 80-item subtest. Similarly, 20 final consonant items are used four times in an 80-item final consonant subtest. The vowel subtest uses eight vowels repeated eight times for a 64-item subtest. The repetition of the test items is designed to increase reliability when analyzing confusions made by listeners. The University of Oklahoma Closed Response Speech Test appears to be the only such test in which vowel and consonant confusions are considered.

Another closed-response test, called the California Consonant Test (CCT) was developed by Owens and Schubert (1977). Composed of 100 items with three foils for each, there are 36 initial consonant and 64 final consonant test words per list. The format and words incorporated into this test are the product of a long-term study by Owens and co-workers (Owens, Benedict, & Schubert, 1971, 1972; Owens & Schubert, 1968, 1977; Owens, Talbott, & Schubert, 1968). Decisions regarding the final test format and selection of test words were based on extensive studies employing hearing-impaired listeners as subjects and biserial correlations of the test items. Items selected for inclusion in the CCT were those that hearing-impaired patients did not hear clearly and those that were confused with two or three other phonemes. Work by Schwartz and Surr (1979) has indicated that the CCT is more sensitive to high-frequency hearing losses than is NU No. 6. Givens and Jacobs-Condit (1981) and Townsend and Schwartz (1981) observed some consistency in errors made by hearing-impaired persons on the CCT in terms of more errors for place and manner of articulation than for voicing and nasality. Errors are more frequent for final consonants (Givens & Jacobs-Condit, 1981; Owens, 1978; Owens & Schubert, 1977). Owens (1978) and Givens and Jacobs-Condit (1981) also suggested that patterns of errors observed on the CCT can be used in planning and implementing aural rehabilitation strategies.

A picture identification test for adult patients unable to respond orally or in writing was developed by Wilson and Antablin (1980). Two hundred CNC word with three rhyming alternates that could be illustrated easily were selected from the Thorndike and Lorge (1944) lists. Four lists of 50 words each were assembled to conform to the Lehiste and Peterson (1959) criteria for phonemic balance. The four pictures on a plate differ in the final phoneme for 183 sets, the initial phoneme for 17 sets. Based on their comparisons of these test materials and NU No. 6 materials with normal and hearing-impaired subjects, Wilson and Antablin concluded that the Picture Identification Task can provide "a good estimate of word recognition performance . . . [for] many nonverbal adults who are unable to respond to conventional speech audiometry techniques" (Wilson & Antablin, 1980, p. 236).

Nonsense syllables: closed-response sets

Lists of seven to nine CV and VC syllables presented in a closed-response format were described by Resnick, Dubno, Hoffnung, and Levitt (1976) and Levitt and Resnick (1978). Voiced consonants with the vowel [a] are incorporated into three lists, unvoiced consonants followed vowels [a], [u], or [i] in three other lists, and unvoiced consonants followed by [a] make up another list of the nonsense syllable test (NST). Because the vowels are constant within a given subtest or list, the task of the listener becomes one of phoneme or consonant identification. Items included in each list are those most frequently confused with one another by normal hearing and hearing-impaired individuals. In their investigations using NST materials Dubno and Dirks (1982) and Dubno, Dirks, and Langhofer (1982) found that responses from hearing-impaired subjects were highly reliable. They noted that voiced versus voiceless consonant confusions, and nasal versus nonnasal confusions were rare, that place errors were more common than errors in manner of articulation, and that fricatives were more likely to be confused with plosives. Overall, place errors constituted about 49% of the errors, manner errors accounted for about 22% of the confusions, and about 29% of the misidentifications were errors of both place and manner of articulation. More errors occurred for final consonants.

Another closed-response nonsense syllable test, the Distinctive Feature Difference (DFD) test, was described by Feeney and Franks (1982). The consonants having an error probability of 0.3 or greater from the data of Owens and Schubert (1968) were selected. The 13 consonants [p, b, t, d, k, f, v, θ, s, ʃ, tʃ, dʒ] are inserted in nonsense syllables having the same intervocalic context, for example, [ˆbIl], [ˆpIl], and so forth. Seven features for each phoneme (high, back, anterior, coronal, continuant, voice, and strident) are scored. A correct response is given 7 points, but a response of [d] for [t] (voicing error) would receive 6 points, [b] for [t] (place and voicing errors) would score 5 points, [v] for [t] (place, voicing, and manner errors) would earn 3 points, and so on. Feeney and Franks concluded that these test materials and procedures appeared to be promising but must be evaluated in clinical situations and through further research.

Sentences: open-ended sets

One of the frequent and valid criticisms of monosyllabic word tests for assessing speech understanding is that the test items are presented in a way that does not represent everyday speech. The concern is that oral communication is conducted via phrases and sentences, not single words. Hence, the contention is that sentences should be used for determining an individual's ability to understand speech. It long has been understood that a large sample of sentences would be needed for such tests, because significant learning effects occur with repeated use of sentences.

As mentioned earlier, Fry and Kerridge (1939) prepared sentence tests for patients who obtained scores of 35% or less on their word lists. These "Sentence Tests for Deaf People" consisted of five lists of "short commonplace" sentences. There were 25 sentences per list with four to seven words per sentence. A correct sentence received a score of four points; one point was deducted for each error, but inaccuracies for "the" and "a" were ignored.

Watson and Knudsen (1940) prepared phonograph records of 25 phrases such as "Listen to . . . ," "Try to hear . . . ," and so forth, followed by three monosyllables such as "bite, rim, let," or "bet, men, ring," and so on. The task of the listener was to write down the last three words; only selected phonemes in each word were scored. However, normative data were not published, and the phonograph records and the word lists were not released (Harris, 1980).

Use of lists of "nonsense sentences" such as "The river rolled over on its back" and "Soft coal is hard to eat" was proposed by McFarlan in 1945. Details of scoring procedures were not given. In his publication McFarlan also briefly reviewed a number of other tests, nonsense syllables, open- and closed-response sets of monosyllables, and other sentence tests described prior to 1945. Most of the references cited are available in few, if any libraries. Therefore, McFarlan's article serves as an important review of early audiometric speech tests in addition to those summarized here.

Ten years later Silverman and Hirsh (1955) described their CID Everyday Sentences. They constructed 100 sentences of 2 to 12 words in length to represent "everyday American speech." Ten sentences are incorporated in each list of the 10 lists with 50 key words being considered as the test items in each list. Scoring is based on the correct recognition of key words, but the task of the listener is to repeat the entire sentence. Although these CID sentences have been used in various research activities, they have not received widespread clinical use.

Fry (1961) developed 10 lists of 25 sentences each, with 100 words being scored in each list. Scoring can be either for each complete sentence or "main words" in each sentence. Interestingly, Fry commented that very little additional information is gained when counting each word as correct or incorrect as opposed to considering each sentence as a whole correct or incorrect.

A different approach, in which only the last word of the meaningful sentence is considered as the test item, was initiated by Kalikow, Stevens, and Elliot (1977). Each of eight lists contains 50 sentences of five to eight words (six to eight syllables) in length. The task of the listener is to repeat (or write) the last word of each sentence. A unique feature of these test lists is that the key words for 25 of the sentences are considered to be high-predictability items and the other 25 are low-predictability items. High predictability suggests that the key word is predictable from the sentence context, whereas the low-predictability key word is not. Each of the test words is used twice; high-predictability items in one list are used as low-predictability words in a companion list. For example, "He caught the fish in his net" and "Paul should know about the net" represent, respectively, high-predictability and low-predictability use of the word "net" in two different lists. Tape recordings of these sentences have been prepared with the sentences on one channel and the babble of 12 voices reading continuous text on the second channel. Thus the user can mix the test sentences and babble at various signal-to-babble ratios. Because the intent is that the babble is to serve as noise against which the sentences are heard, and thereby more closely simulating everyday listening conditions, this test has been labeled the SPIN (Speech Perception In Noise) test by Kalikow et al. (1977). Morgan, Kamm, and Velde (1981) and Bilger, Neutzel, Rabinowitz, and Rzeczowski (1984) found that all forms of the SPIN test were not equal in difficulty. Morgan et al. suggested discarding some of the lists. Bilger et al. suggested that the best items from all forms should be selected to produce new forms that are equivalent in difficulty. Using this strategy, Bilger (1984) reported eight forms for the Revised SPIN test. He noted that with this revised version, the reliability of Form 2 was slightly lower than the reliability of the other seven forms. He suggested that, when possible, use of Form 2 and its cognate, Form 1, might be avoided.

Test materials that use the same words in isolation and in sentences in the German language were described by Niemeyer (1965). (Even though a test of this type is not available in English, a brief description is included here because the idea seems to have merit.) The test consists of eight groups of 10 sentences with four to six words per sentence. Each word is scored. Scoring each word results in efficient use of test time in that a full list of 10 sentences, that is, 50 words, can be administered in about 80 seconds. The same words can be presented singly in random order. In this way, an individual's ability to recognize words in isolation and to understand the same words with the aid of contextual clues can be determined.

Hagerman (1984) developed a similar sentence test in Swedish in which each word is scored. Each of 10 sentences is made up of five words consisting of a proper name, a verb, a number, an adjective, and a noun in that order. All of the words are not monosyllables. For example, "Karin gave two old buttons" and "Peter bought six new pencils" (Hagerman's translation) are two of the sentences. The test words were spoken without transitions between words and stored digitally. With computer recall any of the stored proper names, followed by any of the verbs, then any number, any adjective and any noun can be selected to construct meaningful sentences. Although substantial learning effects were observed when these materials were presented to hearing-impaired subjects in quiet, it was noted that the second presentation of the sentence materials yielded scores very similar to those obtained from presentation of a monosyllabic word list.

A different sentence test for patients having severe to profound hearing losses, and for cochlear implant patients was described recently by Danhauer, Beck, Lucks, and Ghadialy (1988). Three lists of 10 sentences and 10 questions, with a total of 140 syllables in each list, have been recorded on videotape. Obviously, the test can be administered as a test of auditory, visual, or auditory and visual recognition. Scoring is based on the number of correct sentences, number of syllables recognized, number of syllables correctly recognized, and number of statements correctly recognized as declarative sentences and as questions. Preliminary work has been completed, but the test must be evaluated further with hearing-impaired patients to establish its reliability and validity before it can be used clinically.

Sentences: closed-response sets

In an effort to circumvent the problems of learning contextual meaning, difficulties in developing equivalent sentences, and equivalent lists of sentences, and so on, Speaks and Jerger (1965) devised a method of assessing speech understanding using synthetic sentences. The sentences are synthetic in that words were selected at random from the 1,000 most common words in the Thorndike and Lorge (1944) list to form first-order approximations of sentences of designated lengths. Second-order approximations of sentences were formed by selecting one word at random, reporting it to an individual, then asking that individual to select a second word, reporting that second word to another person and asking him or her to select a third word, and so on. The word selected had to follow reasonably from the preceding word in the sentence and be from the 1,000 most common words of the Thorndike and Lorge list. Third-order synthetic sentences were generated by giving selected word pairs to an individual for her or his selection of a third word, then asking another individual for a fourth word after hearing only the second and third words of the sentence, and so on. "Forward march, said the boy a" is an example of such a synthetic sentence (Speaks & Jerger, 1965, p. 188). Again, the constraints were that the words selected were to be from the Thorndike and Lorge list and reasonably follow the preceding two words. In this way, 24 lists of 10 sentences each were developed, 9 first-order sets, 9 second-order sets, and 6 third-order sets. The third-order sets seem to have been used more than the other sets (Jerger, Speaks, & Trammel, 1968). In administering these test materials, the 10 sentences in a set are presented on a panel or answer sheet and the task of the listener is to identify the sentence presented. Speaks and Jerger (1965) named this test the Synthetic Sentence Identification (SSI) test.

In order to make the task more difficult, the same talker reading a story is recorded as competition on the second channel of the tape recording. This competition can be mixed at various levels with the sentences to vary the message-to-competition ratio (MCR). Martin and Mussel (1979) noted that pauses in the competition allowed perception of one or a few words in the sentences and, thereby, identification of the target sentence. Therefore, they added speech spectrum noise to the competition at a level 6 dB below the overall level of the continuous prose. The continuous noise filled in the pauses and made it more difficult for the subjects to identify the sentence on the basis of one or a few words, yet allowed perception of the story. According to the authors, adding the speech spectrum noise in this way did not compromise the principle of the original procedure.

The effect of a four-talker rather than a single-talker competing message on performance for SSI materials was evaluated by Beattie and Clark (1982). At like message-to-competition ratios, they found functions with a four-talker competing message similar to those obtained by Martin and Mussel when they added speech spectrum noise to the single-talker competition.

It should be noted that relatively large practice or learning effects have been observed for the SSI (Beattie & Clark, 1982; Dubno & Dirks, 1983; Speaks & Jerger 1965; Speaks, Karmen, & Benitez, 1967). All have suggested practice or training trials of various lengths to attain stability of performance. Also, Dubno and Dirks (1983) suggested that an SSI score for a given difficult condition should be based on responses to at least 30 sentences.

A different closed-set sentence format is incorporated in the Kent State University Word Identification Test devised by Berger (1969). Meaningful sentences are printed on answer sheets with five phonetically similar key words given in the middle or at the end of the sentence. Most of the word sets are monosyllables, but a few are bisyllables. An example of a test item is:

$$\text{He painted the } \begin{bmatrix} \text{door} & & \text{porch} \\ \text{store} & \text{gourd} & \text{board} \end{bmatrix} \text{ red.}$$

The listener's task is to determine which of the five words was used in a given sentence. Eight lists of equal difficulty with 13 sentences in each were constructed. The sentences are ordered by difficulty within each list. Such ordering allows for a unique scoring system: the number of the sentence in which the error occurred is subtracted from 100. For example, if, in a given list, a listener made errors in sentences 8 and 13, their sum, 21, is subtracted from 100 for a score of 79%. (The minimum score a listener can achieve is 9%, given that the cumulative error total, if all items are missed, is 91.)

Berger, Keating, and Rose (1971) compared the performance on CID W-22 tests and Kent State University sentence tests for 228 patients having sensorineural hearing losses. As would be expected, the mean score for the open-set CID W-22 lists was lower, 69%, compared to 83% for the closed-set response Kent State University sentence lists. The correlation coefficient for the two sets of scores was low, 0.39.

Sergeant, Atkinson, and LaCroix (1979) have used Griffiths's word lists in the Naval Submarine Medical Research Laboratory Tri-Word Test of Intelligibility (NSMRL TTI), but present the test items in groups of three. The words were spoken in three word sets, not as "discrete productions." Three lists of 50 sets were recorded. The task of the listener is to mark the three items heard, one mark in each column in the 8-second silent interval between sets. The test items of one set are italicized in the example given below.

badge	bathe	*mat*
batch	base	fat
bass	*bayed*	that
bat	bays	rat
bash	beige	mat

Using this approach, Sergeant et al. indicated that 150 test items can be presented in 7 minutes, compared to about 5 minutes for 50 items when the words are presented as single items. Table 2.3 briefly summarizes the tests described above.

Speech test batteries for severe to profound hearing losses

A battery of tests described by Owens, Kessler, Telleen, and Schubert (1981), and Owens, Kessler, Raggio, and Schubert (1985) for assessment of speech processing capabilities of patients who suffer postlingual profound hearing losses, incorporates some of the tests described above. The minimal auditory capabilities (MAC) battery was designed for pre- and postsurgical evaluation of cochlear implant patients. The test battery consists of 14 tests of varying difficulty. Eight are multiple-choice identification or discrimination tests. One requires discrimination as to whether the inflection of the item is rising or falling to denote a question or statement. For another test, the listener identifies the accented word in a statement. A third test determines the ability to discriminate voice from speech modulated noise. In a fourth test, the listener states whether the spondees he or she hears are the same spondee repeated twice or two different spondees. Identifying vowels, initial consonants, and final consonants from closed-response sets are the tasks for three separate tests. Identifying a spondee from a set of four spondees is another closed-response test in the battery. Open-response tasks include recognition of environmental sounds, spondees, the last word in high-probability sentences from the SPIN test, and monosyllables from NU No. 6. CID sentences are presented under three conditions: without visual cues with the amplifier on, with visual cues with the amplifier on, and with visual cues with the amplifier off. Owens et al. (1981) recommend that less difficult tests be interspersed among the more difficult tasks. Although designed as a pre- and postsurgical test battery for cochlear implant patients, they suggest that the tests also can be used for evaluations of patients with severe to profound hearing losses, and for determination of their aural rehabilitation needs. Fifer, Stach, and Jerger (1984) agreed that this test battery was useful for evaluating and monitoring adults with profound hearing losses with hearing aids or cochlear implants. Based on their observations of 19 patients with severe to profound hearing losses, 9 whose onset was postlingual and 10 whose onset was prelingual, they concluded that the severity of the hearing loss was the major factor influencing performance on this battery, not the language skills associated with the age of onset of hearing loss, that is, prelingually or postlingually.

Modification of some of the tests from the MAC battery as well as some new tests were described by Tyler, Gantz, McCabe, Lowder, Otto, and Preece (1985) in the Iowa Cochlear Implant Test Battery. The medial

TABLE 2.3
A Guide to Selected Speech Recognition Tests

Type of Stimuli	Investigator (Year)	Task	Name	Items Per List	Alternate Forms	Commercial Recordings Available for Purchase
Monosyllables						
Open-set	Fry and Kerridge (1939)	Word or phoneme recognition	Word Tests for Deaf People	25	5	No
	Egan (1948)	Word recognition	PAL PB-50	50	20	Yes
	Hirsh et al. (1952)	Word recognition	CID-W-22	50	4	Yes
	Lehiste & Peterson (1959)	Word recognition	CNC Lists	50	10	No
	Fry (1961)	Word recognition or phoneme recognition	Fry Lists	35	10	Yes
	Tillman & Carhart (1966)	Word recognition	NU No. 6	50	4	Yes
	Boothroyd (1968)	Word recognition or phoneme recognition	Short Isophonemic Word Lists	10	15	No
	Beykirch & Gaeth (1978)	Number, letter, word recognition	Speech Discrimination Scale	8 numbers/ 16 letters & words	—	No
Closed-set	Fairbanks (1958)	Initial consonant identification	Rhyme Test	50	5	No
	House et al. (1965)	Initial & final consonants identification	Modified Rhyme Test	50	6	No
	Griffiths (1967)	Initial & final consonants identification	Rhyming Minimal Contrast	50	5	No
	Kruel et al. (1968)	Initial & final consonants identification in filtered noise	Modified Rhyme Test	50	6	Yes
	Schultz & Schubert (1969)	Initial & final consonants identification	Multiple Choice Discrimination Test (MCDT)	50	4	Yes (CID W-22)

(continued)

TABLE 2.3
(Continued)

Type of Stimuli	Investigator (Year)	Task	Name	Items Per List	Alternate Forms	Commercial Recordings Available for Purchase
Closed-set	Pederson & Studebaker (1972)	Initial & final consonants/vowel identification	Oklahoma University Closed Response Speech Test	80/64	5	No
	Owens & Schubert (1977)	Initial & final consonants identification	California Consonant Test	100	2	Yes
	McPherson & Pang-Ching (1979)	Initial & final consonants identification	Distinctive Feature Discrimination Test	50	4	No
	Wilson & Antablin (1980)	Word/picture identification	Picture Identification Task	50	4	Yes
Sentences Open-Set	Fry and Kerridge (1939)	Repeat sentences	Sentence Tests for Deaf People	25 sentences/ 100 words	5	No
	McFarlan (1945)	Repeat sentences	Nonsense Sentences			No
	Silverman & Hirsh (1955)	Repeat sentences	CID Everyday Sentences	10 sentences/ 50 key words	10	Yes
	Kalikow et al. (1977)	Repeat last word in sentence	Speech Perception in Noise Test (SPIN)	50	8	No*
	Fry (1961)	Repeat sentences	Fry Revised Sentences	25 sentences/ 100 words	10	Yes
	Bilger (1984)	Repeat last word in sentence	Revised SPIN Test	50	8	No*
Closed-set	Speaks & Jerger (1965)	Identify sentence from printed list	Synthetic Sentence Identification (SSI)	10	24	Yes

(continued)

TABLE 2.3
(Continued)

Type of Stimuli	Investigator (Year)	Task	Name	Items Per List	Alternate Forms	Commercial Recordings Available for Purchase
Closed-set	Berger (1969)	Select key word among five choices	KSU Speech Discrimination	13	8	Yes
	Sergeant et al. (1981)	Identify 3 individual words	Naval Submarine Medical Research Laboratory Tri-Test of Intelligibility	150	3	No*
Nonsense Syllable						
Open-set	Edgerton & Danhauer (1979)	Bisyllable or phoneme recognition	NST	25	2	Yes
Closed-set	Resnick (1976)	Initial and final consonants identification	CUNY NST	7 or 9	7	Yes
	Feeney & Franks (1982)	Middle consonant identification	Distinctive Feature Difference	13	1	No

*Contact authors for information regarding availability of tape recordings.

vowel, initial consonant, and final consonant tests are offered as color-videotaped audiovisual tests that can be administered in sound alone, vision alone, and sound and vision modes. Similarly, 30 sentences from the Bamford-Kowal-Bench sentences (Bench, Kowal, & Bamford, 1979) are videotaped and presented with and without context, that is, with and without pictures portraying the sentence topics. Twenty stimuli represent everyday environmental sounds in open-set and closed-set formats. Detection and/or identification of warning sounds in cafeteria noise (+6 dB S/N ratio) is another environmental sound test. In another task listeners are asked to indicate whether the stimulus word was one, two, three, or four syllables in length. Determination as to whether a given sentence was spoken by a female or by a male is one of the discrimination tests. In two other discrimination tests the listener must decide whether two presentations of the same sentence were spoken by the same talker or two different talkers, and whether a pair of different sentences were uttered by the same talker or two different talkers. Live voice presentation of 30 sentences read by the patient's spouse or someone familiar to the patient with and without visual cues constitutes another comparison. Identification of spondees from a closed set format and recognition of NU No. 6 monosyllables also are part of the Iowa Cochlear Implant Test Battery.

Factors affecting speech test results

Given the variety of test lists and materials developed for assessing speech intelligibility via some communication system, or the ability of a normal hearing or a hearing-impaired person to understand speech in various test situations, it is obvious that there is little agreement regarding use of test materials or procedures. Some factors that influenced the development of various tests and the results from some of these test are considered in this section.

Word familiarity.   One factor on which there is agreement in selecting test items is familiarity. Word familiarity was one of the major criteria considered by Hirsh et al. (1952) in their modification of the 20 Harvard PAL lists to four CID W-22 lists. The importance of word familiarity was demonstrated by Owens (1961) when he prepared word lists matched phonetically, but varied systematically with respect to word familiarity based on the Thorndike and Lorge count. He found that "lists characterized by greater familiarity, even to a slight degree, were significantly more intelligible" (p. 129). Epstein, Giolas, and Owens (1968) later confirmed Owens's findings. Schultz (1964b) noted that although 95% of the words in the CID W-22 lists are among the 5,000 most familiar words, the few words included that are among the 10,000 most familiar words contribute 14% of the error responses to the CID W-22 lists. It is worth noting that Elkins (1970) found the CNC lists of Lehiste and Peterson (1959) to be relatively uniform in word familiarity.

Word familiarity no doubt contributes to responses on multiple-choice closed-message sets too. Nixon (1973) administered the modified rhyme test as an open-response set and compared the responses obtained to the foil words given for the MRT. He noted that in many instances only one or two of the foils seemed to serve as possible alternatives, and in a few instances none of the alternatives was realistic, at least in terms of the responses yielded by listeners for open set administration of the MRT. Nixon commented that "in . . . measuring speech-sound discrimination ability, an important step is to develop foil words that have demonstrable perceptual relationships to the test word speech sounds" (pp. 665–666). He also cautioned that "Black (1968) has shown that the proportion of listeners writing a given word in a free-response test cannot be used to accurately predict the response probability of that word when it is used as an alternate stimulus in a multiple-choice test. Therefore, one cannot simply take written responses of listeners and use them as foils in a multiple-choice format without verifying that the words do, in fact, preserve some above chance probability for selection when used as foils" (p. 666).

Along the same lines, word predictability is a factor in word recognition in sentences. Duffy and Giolas (1974) and Giolas, Cooker, and Duffy (1970) noted that key words that were easy to predict in sentences increased the scores achieved, whereas difficult-to-predict key words decreased the scores. Based on their investigation in which subjects filled in missing key words in the CID sentences and revised CID sentences (Harris, Haines, Kelsey, & Clack, 1961), Giolas, Cooker, Duffy (1970) found that the key words in the revised CID sentences were less predictable than in the original version. They suggested that the less predictable version was probably preferable if test performance was to evaluate word recognition rather than speech understanding based on contextual clues. In an effort to evaluate both of these facets in speech understanding, Kalikow et al. (1977) incorporated both "high-predictability" and "low-predictability" items into the SPIN test.

List length—phonetic (phonemic) balance.   Although there is general agreement regarding the importance of the familiarity of words used in test lists, there is little agreement about the importance of phonetic or phonemic balance. As mentioned, Egan (1948) incorporated "phonetic" balance into the PAL PB-50 word lists, Hirsh et al. (1952) followed the phonetic balance criteria more closely, and Lehiste and Peterson (1959) and Peterson and Lehiste (1962) adopted phonemic balance criteria for their CNC lists, as did Tillman and Carhart (1966). Elkins (1970) subsequently confirmed that the CNC lists are well balanced to the English language based on the data of French et al. (1930) and Tobias (1959). It should be noted, however, that phonemic balance criteria have not been followed or even considered in the development of most of the multiple-choice or sentence tests.

A major criticism of the use of lists shorter than 50 words has been the absence of phonetic or phonemic balance in such lists (Grubb, 1963a, 1963b). (Recall that Egan, 1948, reported that phonetic balance was not achieved with 25-word lists.) Tobias (1964), on the other hand, questioned the importance of phonetic of phonemic balancing for clinically useful tests. Part of his argument is based on Grubb's own statements that, clinically, the Harvard PB lists (not extremely well-balanced phonetically) separate some types of hearing impairments better than do CID W-22 lists (which are well-balanced phonetically).

Whatever the arguments for or against the necessity of maintaining phonemic balance with 50-word lists, a number of investigators have studied the clinical utility of 25-word lists. The interest in using less lengthy lists is, of course, based on saving time and decreasing the fatigue of the listener and tester. Campanelli (1962), Elpern (1961), and Resnick (1962), in their comparisons of results from 25-word versus 50-word lists, arbitrarily divided 50-word lists between the 25th and 26th items or selected the 25 odd-numbered items and 25 even-numbered items to form two 25-word lists. In general, they observed good agreement between scores for the two 25-word lists and between half-list and full-list scores. Similar studies by Rintelmann and Associates (1974) also demonstrated equal scores for half-lists of NU No. 6 lists, except for one randomization of one list (List 3, Form A). In contrast, Jirsa, Hodgson, and Goetzinger (1975) and Schwartz, Bess, and Larson (1977) recommended against the use of half-lists of NU No. 6.

Both the Harvard PB-50 and CID W-22 lists have been divided into 25-word lists on the basis of frequency of occurrence of error responses by Burke, Shutts, and King (1965), Campbell (1965), Keating (1974), Margolis and Millin (1971), and Shutts, Burke, and Creston (1964). Deutsch and Kruger (1971) used point biserial correlation coefficients (correlating scores for each stimulus item with whole-list scores) to derive two equally difficult 25-word lists from two 50-word lists. In general, these investigations have shown relatively high correlations for results from two 25-word lists and for 25-word and 50-word list comparisons. If one is to derive two shorter lists from a longer list of test items, it is more reasonable to do so on the basis of item analyses of the words within the list than to divide a list arbitrarily at the halfway point, or on an even-odd-numbered item basis.

In their study of four of the Harvard PB-50 lists for the purposes of developing 25-word lists, Burke et al. (1965) reviewed the results from a number of presentations to hearing-impaired patients and on that basis arranged the words within the list in the order of difficulty. They then selected odd- and even-numbered words to form two equally difficult 25-word lists from one 50-word list. Keating (1974) followed a somewhat similar procedure using CID W-22 lists. There is, of course, no pretense of phonemic balance in such list development.

Rose, Schreurs, and Miller (1979) proposed a further reduction in the test lists based on data accumulated with the CID W-22 lists. They suggested that the most frequently missed 10 words of all the lists be used as a screening list to determine whether or not it is necessary to administer a longer list of words. If the listener correctly responds to these 10 words, or to possibly 8 of 10, then there is little need to administer longer lists of words because the listener already has responded correctly to the most difficult items. If 3 or more of these 10 most difficult words are missed, it is necessary to present longer lists to the listener.

Clinical experience has demonstrated the merit of this, or a similar, approach. When a patient correctly responds to the first 10 words of the lists derived by Keating (1974), it is rare that any of the subsequent words are missed. Even if one or two words are missed after the 10 have been responded to correctly, there is little significance clinically whether the word recognition score reported is 96% or 100%. In fact, it appears that when words are missed after the first 10 yielded correct responses, this often is attributable to lapses in attention rather than to misperception of the test word. Hence, following correct recognition of the first 10 words in lists such as those derived by Keating, one can legitimately terminate presentation of the list to a given patient.

Support for this approach has been provided by Hosford-Dunn, Runge, and Montgomery (1983) and Runge and Hosford-Dunn (1985) also working with CID W-22 lists in which the words were rank ordered in terms of difficulty. Runge and Hosford-Dunn recommended ''using lists that are rank ordered by difficulty and terminating testing after 10 words if no errors occur or after 25 words if there are no more than four errors'' (p. 361).

List length—binomial distribution and speech recognition. In this pursuit of shortening test lists and to make more efficient use of the clinician's and patient's time, there has been discussion of the binomial theorem, that is, the binomial distribution, as a statistical model to help determine the reliability of a given score. Such a statistical model can assist in determining the test length necessary for obtaining a satisfactorily reliable test result.

Hagerman (1976), Raffin and Schafer (1980), Raffin and Thornton (1980), and Thornton and Raffin (1978) have demonstrated that the binomial distribution can be used to assess the reliability of the speech test results of an indiviudal listener. The reliability of a score depends not only on the performance of the listener, but also, according to the binomial theorem, on the length of the test list.

The mean and standard deviation of the binomial distribution are determined by the probability of occurrence of a binary event and the number of such events sampled in a given test. In speech recognition testing the binary event is that the response can only be scored as correct or incorrect. For application of the binomial theorem to a pair of test results, it is assumed that scores obtained from administration of test lists can be considered members of a binomial distribution. Assumptions are that lists of test items can be represented as a random sample drawn from a larger pool of words and that the performance of the listener remains constant, not only in terms of basic speech understanding ability but also in terms of attentiveness and motivation. Given these assumptions, the standard deviation (SD) of the scores from repeated measurements of the same subject is, according to the binomial theorem, proportionally inverse to the square root of the number of test items. This statement accrues from the fact that the standard deviation of a binomial distribution is based on the formula:

$$SD = \sqrt{\frac{\begin{array}{c}\text{probability of a}\\\text{single binary}\\\text{event}\end{array} \times \begin{array}{c}\text{probability of}\\\text{a complimentary}\\\text{event}\end{array}}{\text{N of sample}}}$$

On this basis then, each doubling or halving of the sample size (length of lists for our purposes here) decreases or increases, respectively, the standard deviation by the square root of 2, that is, 1.414.

From this formula it is possible to plot the standard deviation of the binomial distribution for given sample sizes and for given probabilities of the binary event, as is done in Figure 2.6. Here it can be seen that standard deviations vary as a function of the sample size and as a function of the probability of the binary event being less than 100% or greater than 0%. The largest standard deviations occur for scores around 50%.

Such information can be carried a step further to determine confidence intervals for a given score, because confidence intervals are based on standard deviations around the "true" score. In Figure 2.7, curves for the

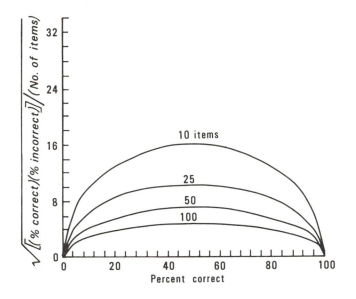

Figure 2.6. Standard deviation for binomial distribution of speech recognition scores as a function of the probabilities of a binary event.

95%, 90%, and 80% confidence limits have been drawn for 10-, 25-, 50-, and 100-item samples. Note that, given a 50-item list and a score of 80% in one test condition, the score on a second measurement would have to differ by more than 12 percentage points to achieve a 95% "critical difference" (Thornton & Raffin, 1978), that is, a difference sufficiently large that the probability of such a change occurring by chance is only 1 in 20 (5%). For 90% critical difference, the second score would have to differ from the original 80% score by more than 10% to exceed a 1 in 10 probability of the difference occurring by chance. A difference greater than 8% is necessary for a second score to reach an 80% critical difference in this instance, that is, 2 chances in 10 that a second score could differ from the original 80% score by as much as 8% by chance alone. Like derivations can be made from different scores and sample sizes of 10- to 100-item test lists from the curves drawn in Figure 2.7. For clinical use, tables can be developed for critical differences at various degrees of statistical significance for a variety of sample sizes of test items. The data used by Hagerman (1976) in his derivation of confidence intervals for the test materials employed in his investigation reveal ranges in confidence intervals that are similar to those shown here in Figure 2.7. It should be noted, however, that Dillon (1982) suggested that the variability in speech

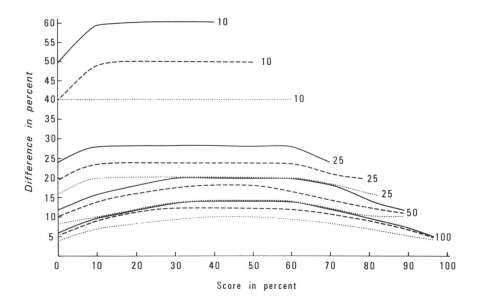

Figure 2.7. Critical differences for speech recognition scores. Two scores have to differ by values indicated by curves to reach 95% critical difference _____, 90% critical difference ---------, 80% critical difference .... Number of test items per list is parameter. Curves terminated at points for which score higher than 100% would be necessary to differ significantly from lower score. (Graph derived from table provided by K. Offord, Medical Statistics Department, Mayo Clinic.)

recognition scores may be greater than estimated by the binomial distribution.

Information such as that derived by Hagerman (1976) and by Thornton and Raffin (1978), Raffin and Schafer (1980), and Raffin and Thornton (1980), and summarized here in Figure 2.7, should be considered in clinical applications of speech recognition tests. Application of this concept indicates that the oft-repeated rule that a 6% or 10% difference in scores represents a clinically significant difference in speech understanding cannot be applied for the entire range of scores for all test situations. In addition, the practice of shortening test lists from 50 to 25 words when scores occur at other than the upper limits (e.g., 90% to 100%) or lower limits (e.g., 0% to 10%) is not appropriate unless one is willing to accept larger standard deviations for repeated tests. However, it would appear reasonable to use shorter lists when scores fall near the upper or lower limits of the range. What constitutes the upper and lower limits in scores for use of 25-, 50-, or 100-item (or longer) lists must be left to the discretion of the individual clinician in deciding what represents a "critical" or "noncritical" difference.

Given this information, it seems reasonable that the standard deviation and error of measurement would be reduced if each phoneme were scored in the monosyllabic lists as recommended by Fry (1961) and Boothroyd (1968). Such a procedure certainly increases the sample size. Along this line it is of interest that Hood and Poole (1977) reported that the 95% confidence interval derived from the standard deviations of their speech test results for 16 subjects decreased from ±12% to ±9.5% when scored for each phonemic element as opposed to whole words. Their analysis was based on plots of performance-intensity functions for fifteen 25-word lists.

Importantly, Studebaker (1985) derived rationalized arcsine units (raus) in order to linearize speech recognition scores in percent relative to the variance. As mentioned above, the largest standard deviations in the binomial distribution (and speech recognition scores) occur for scores around 50% and become smaller as scores approach 0% or 100%. Studebaker applied the arcsine transform to linearize the variability across a range of scores and added one step to the calculations to determine raus whose values are similar to percentage scores over an extended range, except at the extreme ends of the 0% to 100% scale. Tables can be derived for converting percentage scores to raus for various sample sizes of test items. Such use can simplify critical difference applications. Furthermore, because variability is linearized across the range of scores, raus are suitable for parametric statistical analyses.

Tape-recorded versus monitored live voice.   Use of tape-recorded test materials versus monitored live voice presentation of test lists in clinical situations is an ongoing controversy. Those (e.g., Northern & Hattler, 1974; Penrod, 1979) who urge use of only tape-recorded test materials argue that only then can consistency in presentation be maintained from one listener to the next and for repeated testing of the same patient. Those favoring use of monitored live voice presentation of test lists point out the greater flexibility afforded by this method and also cite reports in the literature demonstrating satisfactory test–retest reliability (e.g., Beattie, Svihovec, & Edgerton, 1978; Creston et al., 1966; Resnick, 1962). It is interesting to note, however, that Resnick (1962) found somewhat lower correlation coefficients ($r = .78$ to $.80$) for test–retest data obtained when using the same test lists but different talkers (monitored live voice presentation) than when the same talker presented different lists via monitored live voice to the subjects on a test–retest basis ($r = .88$ to $.94$). Creston et al. (1966), on the other hand, observed slightly lower test–retest correlation for the group of subjects to whom they presented tape-recorded test materials twice ($r = .70$) than for the group tested on two occasions with monitored live voice procedures ($r = .81$). The correlation coefficient for the group who heard tape-recorded test materials on one occasion and monitored live voice presentation on another was intermediate ($r = .75$).

Hood and Poole (1980) found marked differences in word recognition scores obtained with three different talkers. Some differences among recordings of the same materials by different talkers may be due to differences in the levels of the test items relative to the carrier phrase and calibration tones. Gengel and Kupperman (1980) observed that the test words were 5 to 8 dB stronger on disc recordings of CID W-22 words than on tape recordings of CID W-22 test materials (two different talkers). Similarly, Frank and Craig (1984) noted that the test words were 2.5 dB lower than the carrier phrase and calibration tone on one version of NU No. 6, but 3 dB above the carrier phrase and calibration tone of a different version of NU No. 6. Word recognition scores in a noise background differed by 24% to 28% for these two versions of NU No. 6. Manipulation of the data to adjust for the differences in level resulted in the two sets of scores being quite similar.

In another investigation using six different talkers (3 female, 3 male) Gengel and Kupperman (1980) obtained very similar word recognition scores in noise for two of the talkers, one male and one female, but results for the other four talkers differed from one to another. The differences in mean scores for three of the talkers differed substantially, as much as 26%. Although Beattie et al. (1978) noted similar scores for a tape-recorded version of NU No. 6 and the average of four talkers presenting the same test items via monitored live voice, differences in results for each of the talkers and the tape recording were not given. Brandy (1966) found that even tape recordings by one talker for three scramblings of one word list recorded on three separate days yielded different word-recognition scores, whereas a single recording of the lists copied and reordered into three different scramblings did not. Penrod (1979) noted differences in results among four talkers and also reported that a talker–listener interaction was observed. He concluded that, ''Large differences in scores . . . clearly reflect the need for standardized presentation'' (p. 348).

In busy clinical settings, it is clear that monitored live voice procedures are used more commonly than are recorded materials in clinical assessment of a patient's speech reception and word recognition abilities. The survey of clinical practices completed by Martin and Pennington (1971) indicated that almost 81% of 290 respondents used monitored live voice for speech reception threshold testing and almost 65% of 281 respondents employed monitored live voice for word-recognition tests. (The latter issue was not addressed in the Martin and Forbis, 1977, or Martin and Sides, 1985, surveys.) In the proposed guidelines for determining threshold levels for speech, the American Speech-Language-Hearing Association (1988) states that, "Either a recorded or monitored live voice technique can be used . . . (but) recorded presentation of the test material is . . . preferred . . . When monitored live voice is used, it should be noted with the test results" (pp. 86–87).

Carrier phrase versus no carrier phrase.   Another variable in speech recognition testing is the use or non-use of a carrier phrase preceding the test item. Phrases, such as "Say the word _____," "You will say _____," "The word is _____," "Say the _____ again," and "Write the word _____," are used not only to alert the listener to the upcoming test word but also to assist the talker in monitoring the speech intensity to the appropriate level on the VU meter. Generally the carrier phrase is spoken with sufficient effort to cause the desired deflection on the VU meter; the test words are then spoken with the same effort as the carrier phrase but without concern as to whether the test items cause the same deflection on the VU meter.

Martin, Hawkins, and Bailey (1962) raised the question of whether a carrier phrase is essential for word recognition testing. They found that the test scores were the same with and without the carrier phrase. Since then Gelfand (1975) and Gladstone and Siegenthaler (1971) have reported slightly poorer scores for word-recognition tests administered without a carrier phrase than with a carrier phrase. The difference was an average of four words per list when normal hearing subjects were tested at 5-dB sensation level (Gladstone & Siegenthaler, 1971) and 5% for sensorineural hearing loss patients (Gelfand, 1975). Martin et al. (1962) and Gelfand (1975) reported that about half of the sensorineural hearing loss subjects preferred that the carrier phrase precede the test word; most of the normal subjects and those with conductive hearing losses did not.

McLennan and Knox (1975) found no difference in word recognition scores obtained with and without the carrier phrase when the listeners controlled the word presentation for the latter condition. For the condition in which the subject controlled the word presentation, the tape transport mechanism automatically stopped after each word, and was activated again by the listener pushing a button when ready for the next stimulus. McLennan and Knox noted that this procedure reduced the length of time required for each list administration to about one-half that required for conventional presentation with the carrier phrase and a fixed-time interval between items. They also reported that most of their listeners preferred the test conditions in which the time of presentation of each item was controlled by the listener. Given the equality of scores observed by McLennan and Knox, this procedure appears to have merit. With the advent of digitized speech stimuli (Kamm, Carterette, Morgan, & Dirks, 1980) and the introduction of computers into audiometer technology, subject control of presentation of speech stimuli in a manner akin to that used by McLennan and Knox should not be difficult.

Presentation level. Given performance-intensity functions such as those shown in Figure 2.8, it is obvious that the presentation level of the words is a critical variable. Clinically, the most commonly used sensation levels (SL) are 25 to 40 dB SL (Martin & Sides, 1985). Twenty-five dB SL corresponds to the beginning of the plateau at which normal hearing subjects attain scores of 90% or better on most tests, and 40 dB sensation level represents a reasonably comfortable listening level for normal hearing persons. Most comfortable level for speech loudness and most comfortable listening level for comfortable speech understanding are at similar levels for normal hearing individuals and for persons with sensorineural hearing loss (Hochberg, 1975); however, most comfortable loudness (MCL) for speech and best speech understanding do not necessarily occur at the same levels for hearing-impaired persons. Ullrich and Grimm (1976) reported that of 10 sensorineural hearing loss patients, three attained their best word recognition scores at the same level as their most comfortable listening level, but seven others achieved scores 16% to 28% poorer at their most comfortable level compared to the scores they obtained at higher presentation levels. Similarly, for a group of patients having sensorineural hearing loss due to Ménière's disease, Clemis and Carver (1967) noted that "in not one patient in this test group did the MCL and PB max [maximum word recognition score] coincide" (p.617). Mean data for 45 subjects with sensorineural hearing loss tested by Posner and Ventry (1977) show MCL to be about 20 dB lower than the level at which the best speech recognition scores were observed. It appears that hearing-impaired individuals generally indicate most comfortable loudness level for speech at levels considerably lower than those at which they achieve their best speech scores. Taking a different approach, Kamm, Morgan, and Dirks (1983) compared levels suggested for maximum word recognition based on an adaptive procedure, and levels at which best performance was obtained when plotting performance-intensity functions using lists of monosyllables. The adaptive procedure satisfactorily identified the level of best performance for 19 of 25 subjects with sensorineural hearing losses. However, the authors also pointed out that "arbitrary selection of a 95 dB SPL speech presentation level also would have resulted in measurement of maximum performance for . . . 20 of the 25 hearing-impaired subjects" (p. 208).

The present writers do not advocate a specific level for administration of speech test materials, but presentation at more than one level is encouraged. Recalling the importance of 2000 Hz to speech understanding, as reviewed earlier in this section, a stronger recommendation is that the threshold at 2000 Hz be considered in selecting one of the presentation levels. For persons with high-frequency hearing losses, one list of words should be presented at hearing levels at least a few dB above the pure tone threshold at 2000 Hz, if possible. The dramatic improvement in scores frequently observed when speech presentation levels are increased just a few dB to reach and exceed the threshold obtained at 2000 Hz attests to the contribution of the acoustic energy in the 2000-Hz frequency region for correct recognition or identification of monosyllabic words.

One other point worthy of mention here is that the level at which the test materials are presented and the bone-conduction thresholds of the nontest ear also must be considered during speech recognition testing at suprathreshold levels. Whenever the test items will be delivered at a level that exceeds the bone-conduction thresholds of the opposite ear by more than 40 dB, masking must be delivered to the nontest ear in order to assure that the responses are attributable to the test ear.

Differences among test materials. Figure 2.8 compares performance-intensity functions for three different recordings of NU No. 6, two versions of CID W-22, one version of the Harvard PB-50 test lists, and one of the synthetic sentence lists. Note that all curves are similar in that percent correct increases as a function of sensation level; however, none of the curves directly superimposes upon another. The linear portions of the curves reveal an increase in percent correct word recognition at the rate of 5.6%/dB for the original version of NU No. 6 (Tillman & Olsen, 1973), and 4.5% for another version of NU No. 6 (Wilson, Coley, Haenel, & Browning, 1976). Causey, Hermanson, Hood, and Bowling (1983) also observed a 4.5%/dB slope for the Maryland NU No. 6 test recorded with a female talker. (The talker for the NU No. 6 utilized by Wilson et al. was a male.) Using their own recording of NU No. 6, Rintelmann and Associates (1974) obtained a performance-intensity function with a slope of 5.0%/dB. A comparison of NU No. 6 and CID W-22 test materials spoken by the same individual revealed performance-intensity functions of 4.2% and 4.6%/dB, respectively (Beattie, Edgerton & Svihovec, 1977). The Harvard PB-50 function has a more gradual slope, 3.8%/dB. From these data for normal hearing subjects, it is clear that different test materials yield different performance-intensity functions. Note also that the linear portion of each curve ends with a plateau or flattening of the function at scores of 90% or greater. The plateau occurs at sensation levels ranging from 16 to 32 dB. Clearly, the steepest performance-intensity function is for the synthetic sentences.

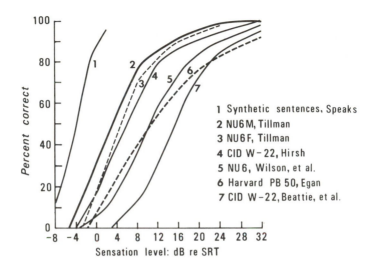

Figure 2.8. Performance-intensity functions for various speech recognition materials.

Steeper functions are obtained for words presented in meaningful sentences than for monosyllables in isolation in both open or closed sets, because of the additional length of the test items and, hence, the number of cues available to the listener (Miller, Heise, & Lichten, 1951; Niemeyer, 1965; O'Neill, 1957). That the difference in results depends on the manner of presentation is further highlighted by the Smaldino and Myers (1971) results for synthetic sentences administered as a closed set and as an open set in a white noise background. Conditions for which 87% correct identification of synthetic sentences was obtained in a closed set format yielded scores of only 12% when the same listeners were required to write as many words as they could understand when the sentences were administered as open-set tests.

In their comparison of responses to Harvard PB-50 test lists and modified rhyme test lists, Kryter and Whitman (1962) found scores for the open set Harvard lists to be about 25% lower than for the closed response modified rhyme test. They attributed this difference to the larger word set (1,000 words) of the Harvard tests relative to the 300 words in the modified rhyme test.

Although the data summarized above were obtained from normal hearing samples, it should be noted that performance-intensity functions and other comparisons have been made when various test materials have been presented to sensorineural hearing loss subjects also. For example, Causey et al. (1983), Tillman and Carhart (1966), and Wilson et al. (1976) have reported that the slope for NU No. 6 test materials is less steep and the plateau occurs at higher sensation levels for persons with sensorineural hearing impairments. The data of Kopra, Blosser, and Waldron (1968) indicated essentially equal slopes for normal hearing and for sensorineural hearing loss subjects responding to CID W-22 and Fairbanks rhyme test materials in quiet; however, the average scores for the sensorineural subjects did not reach 90% at 32 and 40 dB SL as did the scores for the normal subjects. Also of interest in the findings of Kopra et al. is the virtually identical performance-intensity functions for the two types of test materials. Northern and Hattler (1974), on the other hand, noted that sensorineural hearing loss subjects demonstrated a very steep performance-intensity function for synthetic sentences, but reached their maximum performance at 10 dB SL, whereas normal hearing subjects attained 100% correct identification at 20 dB SL.

In comparing performance of sensorineural hearing loss subjects for synthetic sentences and for monosyllables, Speaks, Jerger, and Trammel (1970a) noted relatively similar performance-intensity functions for synthetic sentences mixed with a competing speech message at 0-dB signal-to-competition ratio and for monosyllables in quiet. However, as pointed out by Speaks et al., this similarity was most apparent for the group of subjects with relatively flat sensorineural hearing losses. The groups with sloping high-frequency hearing losses attained poorer scores for the monosyllables than for the synthetic sentences. Similarly, Miner and Danhauer (1976) obtained scores of 41%, 50%, and 38% for synthetic sentences at a message-to-competition ratio of −10 dB (5 male, 4 female multitalker babble) for normal hearing subjects, for flat sensorineural hearing loss, and for sloping sensorineural hearing loss subjects, respectively. The same groups attained scores of 74%, 36%, and 51%, respectively, for the modified rhyme test in the same babble competition at a 0-dB message-to-competition ratio. Based on these findings Miner and Danhauer (1976) concluded that "the SSIT [synthetic sentence identification test] and the MRT [modified rhyme test] are two significantly different tests and should not be used interchangeably" (p. 66).

Orchik, Krygier, and Cutts (1979) found scores for CID W-22 and NU No. 6 test materials for their sample of sensorineural hearing loss subjects to differ slightly; the CID W-22 scores were about 6% higher. Causey et al. (1983) reported scores for CID W-22 materials to be about 13% higher than scores for Maryland CNC materials (Peterson and Lehiste lists) presented to 62 hearing-impaired patients. Interestingly, scores on the Maryland NU No. 6 (female talker) and the Maryland CNC (male talker) materials were very similar, 76% and 77%, respectively.

Using the modified rhyme test, Northern and Hattler (1974) found that sensorineural hearing loss subjects attained scores on the order of 54% to 59% for the two versions of the modified rhyme test designed by Kruel et al. (1969) to yield scores of 75% and 83% for normal hearing subjects. The decreased performance of the sensorineural loss subjects on this test was anticipated, but not the similarity in performance for the two signal-to-noise ratios. Results akin to these were reported earlier by Elkins (1971). Curiously, the normal subjects tested by Elkins and by Northern and Hattler did not achieve average scores of 83% and 75% for these two signal-to-noise ratios either. Their results were 8% to 12% below the expected scores.

From the above review, it is clear that different results are obtained when different test materials are administered to the same subjects. Hence, it is important to describe carefully the speech test materials and test conditions employed in gathering speech recognition data. This statement applies not only to experimental investigations, but also to clinical settings in which these materials are used for evaluation and rehabilitation purposes.

Background competition. The preceding description of test materials, their application, and comparison among various investigations frequently have alluded to presentation against a background of noise, the speech babble of a number of talkers, or the background competition of a single talker. The rationale for mixing some background competition (noise or other speech) is twofold. First, it makes the test more difficult. Second, and more important, speech communication in everyday life situations most commonly takes place against background competition of some sort. Hence, it seems only appropriate that tests administered for assessing an individual's ability to hear and understand speech should include background noise or speech competition as well. Interestingly, Surr and Schwartz (1980) and Danhauer, Doyle, and Lucks (1986) reported that adding background noise competition to the California consonant test, or to the bisyllabic nonsense syllable test did not separate the performance of normal and sensorineural hearing loss groups any more than presenting these tests in quiet. However, there is abundant evidence that the presentation of other test materials against a background of noise or other speech enhances the sensitivity of the test in detecting and demonstrating communication difficulties experienced by hearing-impaired individuals. Cohen and Keith (1976) and Liden (1967), for example, demonstrated that low-pass filtered noise mixed with monosyllabic words sharply diminished the word recognition scores for their sensorineural hearing loss subjects as compared to the diminution in performance experienced by their normal hearing control groups. Background competition in the form of speech from one or more talkers has been used by Aniansson (1974), Findlay (1976), and Lovrinic, Burgi, and Curry (1968), among others, to assess communication difficulties of hearing-impaired persons. The findings of these studies are consistent in revealing markedly greater decreases in scores for hearing-impaired listeners than for normal hearing subjects. Of interest is the observation by Findlay (1976) that when CID W-22 word lists were presented against a background of speech spectrum noise or against the background babble of three male and three female talkers, the separation in the performance of the normal and hearing-impaired subjects was more distinct for the speech babble competition.

Dirks, Morgan, and Dubno (1982) used an adaptive procedure (Bode & Carhart, 1974; Levitt, 1971; Levitt & Rabiner, 1967; Levitt & Resnick, 1978) to determine the signal-to-noise ratios necessary to reach preselected performance criteria. Test items were maintained at constant sound pressure levels but the intensity of competing speech babble was adjusted after each correct or incorrect response to find the signal-to-babble ratios necessary for 50% correct response. A 29.3% correct response level was determined by increasing the level of the competition after a correct response and decreasing the intensity of the competition after two consecutive incorrect responses. To locate the 70.7% correct response point on the psychometric function, the speech babble was decreased after an incorrect response and increased after two consecutive correct responses. Using this approach Dirks et al. (1982) observed that virtually all of their sensorineural hearing-impaired subjects required a more favorable signal-to-noise ratio than did the normal hearing subjects to attain preselected performance criterion levels of 29.3%, 50%, and 70.7% correct.

Dubno et al. (1984) also demonstrated that more favorable signal-to-babble ratios were needed for persons with hearing losses to achieve a 50% correct performance criterion on SPIN materials. Furthermore, they were able to demonstrate that older subjects matched with younger subjects in terms of hearing sensitivity required more favorable signal-to-noise ratios than did their younger counterparts.

However, adding noise background to a set of test materials is not without its drawbacks. Equivalence of lists may be lost when noise is added to a test condition (Loven & Hawkins, 1983). The type of noise, test materials, and hearing loss can have different effects and interactions on performance as well (Van Tasell & Yanz, 1987). These data warrant consideration when speech tests in noise are used in clinical settings.

Error analysis. There is some evidence that important information can be gained from error analysis of the subject's responses. When such analyses have been completed for responses obtained from hearing-impaired persons, several patterns emerge: The errors for consonants are more frequently substitutions than omissions; omissions are more common for the final consonant than for the initial consonant (Oyer & Doudna, 1959); voicing errors are rare, but errors do occur for both place and manner of articulation (Owens & Schubert, 1968, 1977); vowel errors do occur, at least for open-set materials (Oyer & Doudna, 1959; Schultz, 1964a); fewer vowel errors have been noted in closed message sets (Owens et al., 1968; Owens et al., 1971); and general but not strong relationships between errors and configuration of hearing loss have been reported (Bilger & Wang, 1976; Owens et al., 1972; Sher & Owens, 1974). Walden, Schwartz, Montgomery, and Prosek (1981) observed differences in the number of errors when CV syllables were presented to normal and hearing-impaired subjects having unilateral hearing losses even though the signal presented to the normal ear was shaped to match the hearing loss and loudness experience of the impaired ear. The performance of the impaired ear was about 20% poorer, but the patterns of errors were reasonably similar for the impaired ear and the normal ear receiving a signal stimulating what was heard in the ear with the sensorineural hearing loss.

Fabry and Van Tasell (1986) used both selective filtering and filtered masking noise to simulate a hearing loss in the normal ear matching the hearing sensitivity of the impaired ear for their unilateral hearing loss subjects. They found that for three of their six subjects the error patterns were very similar for the impaired ear and the ear in which a like hearing loss was simulated regardless of which method was used to simulate the hearing loss; for one subject, filtering the signal to the normal ear yielded error patterns similar to those of the impaired ear but masking the normal ear did not. Neither filtering the signal nor masking the normal ear produced error patterns similar to those of the impaired ear for two of their subjects. These results emphasize again the heterogeneity of results for patients with sensorineural hearing losses, but an encouraging note also is found in their observation that filtering did successfully simulate the unilateral hearing loss for four of their six subjects. Fabry and Van Tasell (1986) suggested that "if selective attenuation [filtering] of speech signals in normal ears can produce error patterns similar to those of impaired ears, then selective amplification without additional signal processing may improve speech recognition in some hearing impaired individuals" (p. 177).

Unfortunately, errors made by some hearing-impaired patients are not the same from time to time according to Oyer and Doudna (1959) and Owens and Schubert (1977). Possibly such inconsistency in errors led Egolf, Rhodes, and Curry (1970) to report that no clear-cut error pattern was observed for hearing-impaired subjects. Observations of inconsistencies in errors also led Gengel (1973) to comment that a closed response set per se does not reduce the variability in the performance of some sensorineural hearing-loss subjects. He reported that large and similar variability was observed regardless of whether the words were heard once or up to four times before the hearing-impaired subjects were required to respond. Findings that errors made by a given subject were not the same from time to time on the closed-set California consonant test led Owens and Schubert (1977) to state that the hearing-impaired subjects were "guessing . . . [and] narrowing their choice by elimination processes not necessarily related to hearing. This behavior tends to weaken suppositions that ear pathology might consistently cause one phoneme to sound like another, although the question must be explored in depth with various kinds of hearing loss" (p. 466).

Although many investigators have presented their error analyses in tables in the form of confusion matrices, that is, frequency of occurrence of specific substitutions for the various sounds under study, Stevenson (1975) and Stevenson and Martin (1977) devised a graph system for plotting confusion matrices. An example of their method of plotting confusion matrices is shown in Figure 2.9. The place of articulation is shown on the abscissa and the manner of production is on the ordinate. The aspirate [h] (not shown in Figure 2.9) and affricates [tʃ] and [dʒ] have been grouped with stops because their confusions occur more frequently across place of articulation (Stevenson, 1975). The lines and arrows indicate the frequency of occurrence of specific confusions. Numbers can be added to indicate specific confusions in proportion to the number of presentations. Dots or other notations at the symbol can be used to show omissions. To these writers at least, such a plot is easier to follow and displays confusion matrices in a more interesting form than confusion matrices in table form.

Scoring responses. Most of the error analyses of the type described above are based on closed-set tests in which the listener writes or marks the response on an answer sheet. Of course, the examiner can tape record or write the listener's oral responses to open-set materials and complete error analyses from such recordings. Obviously with the latter procedure, the error analyses are based on the examiner's aural monitoring and interpretation of the subject's responses, and another variable is added to the test situation. It is this addition of another difficult-to-control variable that led Lovrinic et al. (1968) and Northern and Hattler (1974) to advocate that responses be obtained in written or marked form on answer sheets. Their recommendations are based in part on the work of Merrell and Atkinson (1965) and Nelson and Chaiklin (1970); both investigations reported errors in scoring of up to 16% and 20%, respectively, when scores based on aural monitoring of responses were compared with written responses for the

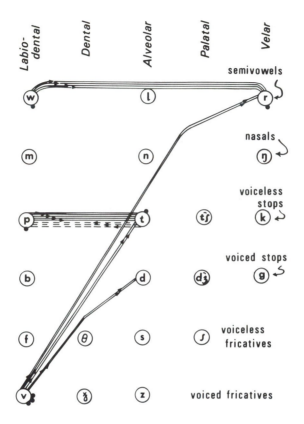

Figure 2.9. Format for plotting consonant confusion matrix. (Adapted from Stevenson, 1975.)

same test administrations. The most common errors were incorrect responses accepted as correct. Not addressed in these investigations were the specific errors made by the auditors scoring the oral responses. As suggested by Owens and Schubert (1977), it is virtually impossible to differentiate [f] from [θ] and [v] from [ð] with auditory cues alone. It is necessary for the auditor to watch the talker's lips to differentiate "thin" from "fin" or "than" from "van" when these words are spoken in isolation. Even though it is recognized that auditory monitoring of the listener's responses adds another variable in word recognition test results, the oral response mode is used most commonly in clinical situations because of its convenience.

Application of suprathreshold tests

The primary purposes of suprathreshold speech tests are to evaluate hearing difficulties encountered by hearing-impaired individuals and to provide some data for differential diagnostic purposes. Because virtually all speech test materials described in this chapter were developed primarily to assess communicative difficulties of hearing-impaired persons, that application is considered first.

Social adequacy index and hearing handicap scales. The intent in the development and use of the various tests using speech stimuli has been to determine the extent of an individual's handicap for hearing and understanding speech on the basis of a score (or scores) achieved on a given test. Early efforts along this line were reported by Silverman, Thurlow, Walsh, and Davis (1948) in their description of the Social Adequacy Index (SAI). Their value for the SAI was based on the average of word-recognition scores obtained at soft, average, and loud conversational levels with Rush Hughes recordings of the PB-50 word lists developed by Egan (1948). After analysis of a large set of data, they concluded that an average score of 94% for the test lists administered at the three levels was within normal limits, 67% indicated some difficulty in hearing and understanding speech, and 33% was minimally adequate. Davis (1948) modified this procedure by developing a social adequacy index table based on a speech reception threshold determined with spondees and a single word recognition score obtained at a level sufficiently intense to be on the plateau of maximum word recognition performance. It should be kept in mind that the social adequacy indexes of Silverman et al. and Davis were based on the relatively difficult Rush Hughes recordings and the gradually sloping performance-intensity function associated with these materials (Figure 2.8). Attempts to apply these social adequacy index values to less difficult test materials and their steeper performance-intensity functions, such as CID W-22 or NU No. 6 materials, yield overly optimistic indications of ability to hear and understand speech (Carhart, 1965).

The Social Hearing Index (SHI) described by Niemeyer (1965) is very similar to Silverman et al.'s SAI, except that it is based on sentence materials (described earlier) and gives different weights to scores obtained at three presentation levels. The formula for Niemeyer's SHI is:

$$\text{SHI} = \frac{2\text{SD}_{50} + 3\text{SD}_{65} + \text{SD}_{80}}{6}$$

where SD_{50}, SD_{65}, and SD_{80} represent scores for sentence test materials at 50, 65, and 80 dB SPL, respectively. The greatest weight is given to the score at 65 dB SPL because it represents normal conversational level for speech, whereas 50 dB SPL corresponds to speech in a quiet room, and speech at 80 dB SPL occurs only in exceptional conditions. Niemeyer did not report any data representing normal, mild impairment, or severe impairment in social hearing, but it would seem that this approach could be used with various test materials and developed to have clinical utility.

An early effort to relate word recognition scores to hearing difficulties as judged by hearing-impaired individuals was reported by High, Fairbanks, and Glorig in 1964. They developed a Hearing Handicap Scale (HHS) based on a questionnaire in which the patient rates his or her ability to hear and understand speech in various listening situations as being (a) almost always, (b) usually, (c) sometimes, (d) rarely, or (e) almost never. Although relatively high correlations were observed between results from the HHS and speech reception thresholds as well as 500 to 2000 Hz thresholds, correlations between the HHSs and word recognition scores obtained with CID W-22 test materials and the Fairbanks rhyme test were low. Low correlations between scores obtained from various test materials and the HHS were found by Blumenfeld, Bergman, and Millner (1969) and Speaks et al. (1970a, 1970b) too. It should be noted, however, that Tannahill (1979) found that changes in HHS results correlated with improvement in word recognition scores when test materials were presented at conversational levels without and with hearing aids.

A similar 21-item questionnaire, the Social Hearing Handicap Index (SHHI), has been described by Ewertsen and Birk-Nielsen (1973). Respondents are required to answer only "yes" or "no" to each question rather than make a judgment on a 5-point scale.

A Hearing Measurement Scale (HMS) composed of 42 items was devised by Noble and Atherly (1970). This scale also uses a 5-point rating scale for various listening situations. Initially designed for a direct interview format, the HMS also can be administered as a paper-and-pencil questionnaire (Noble, 1979). It correlates most closely with speech reception thresholds, followed by hearing sensitivity for high-frequency pure tones and word recognition scores (Noble & Atherly, 1970). McCartney, Maurer, and Sorenson (1976), however, noted significant relationships between results of the HHS and the HMS to audiometric measurements of auditory deficits for elderly subjects. These observations and their own investigations of the hearing measurement scale with elderly patients led to the development of the Hearing Handicap Inventory for the Elderly (HHIE; Ventry & Weinstein, 1982; Weinstein & Ventry, 1982). The 25 items (or 10 items for the screening version of the HHIE-S) are answered "yes," "sometimes," or "no" in either an interview or paper-and-pencil format; reliability is slightly higher with the interview format, and its use is recommended when possible (Weinstein, Spitzer, & Ventry, 1986).

Perceived reduction in hearing handicap by hearing aid wearers and their spouses after 1 year of hearing aid use was noted by Newman and Weinstein (1988) in their administration of this questionnaire to hearing-impaired subjects and a like version to their spouses. Lichtenstein, Bess, and Logan (1988) found the HHIE-S to be a valid test for identifying elderly patients having hearing impairments.

Sanders (1975) devised separate profile questionnaires for rating communicative performance in a home environment, occupational environment, social environment, and school environment. Respondents indicate the degree of difficulty encountered in various situations on a 4-point scale and frequency of occurrence on a 3-point scale.

A longer questionnaire, the Hearing Performance Inventory (HPI) was described by Giolas, Owens, Lamb, and Schubert in 1979. Its 168 items are scaled 1 to 5, from "almost always" to "almost never" and covers six categories: understanding speech (with and without visual cues), intensity factors of speech, response to auditory failure, social (group conversational situations), personal (hearing loss influence on social situations), and occupational (hearing impairment effects on occupational settings). Demorest and Walden (1984) demonstrated the validity and reliability of this hearing performance inventory. The 168 items were reduced to 90 by Lamb, Owens, and Schubert in 1983. Modifications of this questionnaire to a 74-item scale as a Performance Inventory for Profound and Severe Hearing Loss (PIPSL) was described by Owens and Raggio (1988).

A considerably shorter Self-Assessment of Communication (SAC) and Significant Other Assessment of Communication (SOAC) was described by Schow and Nerbonne (1982). The 10 items deal with various communication situations, feelings about communication, and reaction of others to the hearing impairment. Oja and Schow (1984) reported good correlation between self-assessment of communication and significant other assessment of communication questionnaires.

Demorest and Erdman (1986, 1987) reported their development of the Communication Profile for the Hearing Impaired (CPHI). The 145 items are categorized in terms of communication performance, communication importance, communication environment, communication strategies, and personal adjustment. Part 1 is scaled in terms of importance, Part 2 is scaled in terms of frequency of occurrence, and Part 3 responses are "agree," "disagree" in nature.

As mentioned above, results from these scales generally correlate more closely with measures of hearing sensitivity than with scores from tests of speech understanding presented at suprathreshold levels (Blumenfeld et al., 1969; Hawes & Niswander, 1985; High et al., 1964; Lutman, Brown, & Coles, 1987; Rowland, Dirks, Dubno, & Bell, 1985; Speaks et al., 1970a, 1970b; Weinstein & Ventry, 1983). Tyler and Smith (1983) suggested that correlations between data from questionnaires or inventories, threshold, and suprathreshold speech tests may be mediated by their common dependency on thresholds for pure tones and that such questionnaires do provide complimentary information. Furthermore, Lamb et al. (1983) indicated that the inventory approach can be of therapeutic value. The patient is encouraged to confront problems associated with hearing loss and consider strategies, some of which are suggested by statements in the inventory, to help overcome some of their communication problems. As stated by Hawes and Niswander (1985), "the amount of difficulty a client reports is often inconsistent with the amount of difficulty that would be predicted based on the audiogram alone. Many factors, in addition to the psychophysically measured hearing loss, will determine the impact of hearing loss on the client's life. Hearing handicap scales offer a method of systematically assessing that impact" (p. 96).

Hearing aid selection and counseling. Just as some of the earliest test lists were developed and used to evaluate the intelligibility of speech transmitted by telephone, so too have speech recognition tests been used to evaluate hearing aid performance, beginning with the work of Hartig and Newhart in 1936 and Holmgren in 1939. Carhart (1946b) described a systematic approach using speech tests (spondees, monosyllables in quiet and in noise) and other listening situations to assist in selecting suitable hearing aids for hearing-impaired veterans. Portions of the procedure described by Carhart continue to be used in some clinical settings, but not without controversy. Many professional workers agree with Schwartz (1982), Schwartz and Walden (1983), Shore, Bilger, and Hirsh (1960), and Walden, Schwartz, Williams, Holum-Hardegen, and Crowley (1983) that currently used word recognition test results are neither sufficiently sensitive nor satisfactorily consistent to demonstrate differences in the performance of various hearing aids. Some researchers (e.g., Hayes, Jerger, Taff, & Barber, 1983; Jerger & Hayes, 1976; Jerger, Malmquist, & Speaks, 1966) have suggested that sentence-type test materials presented against background competition should be used to demonstrate benefit from hearing aid use in test situations. The recommendation that background noise or competing speech be added to speech recognition test conditions for hearing aid evaluations has been made often (Beattie & Edgerton, 1976; Berry, 1939; Bleeker & Huizing, 1953; Carhart, 1946b, 1967; Carhart & Thompson, 1947; Davis et al., 1946; Ewertsen, 1966; Fest, 1944; Gerber & Fisher, 1979; Hallpike, 1934; Holmgren, 1939; Mueller, 1953; Olsen, 1970; Olsen & Carhart, 1967; Olsen & Tillman, 1968; Orchik & Oyer, 1972; Orchik & Roddy, 1980; Tillman, Carhart, & Olsen, 1970). Gerber and Fisher (1979), Orchik and Oyer (1972), and Orchik and Roddy

(1980) have suggested that the use of background competition is more critical than a particular test stimulus. Orchik and Roddy concluded that, "The indication is that, given the appropriate level for the primary signal and the appropriate MCRs [message-to-competition ratios], any speech discrimination test can be used . . . in clinical hearing aid evaluations" (p. 406).

Seavertson and McLennan (1983) have suggested that measurement of response time during speech recognition tests could be more sensitive to differences in performance than percent correct scores. Such findings are in accord with those of Hecker, Stevens, and Williams (1966), Jerger and Thelin (1968), and Pratt (1981). Such assessments are possible given instrumentation allowing patient control of the rate at which test items are presented as described by McLennan and Knox (1975), or presentation of digitized speech test materials via a computer (Kamm et al., 1980).

Cox and co-workers (Cox, Alexander, & Gilmore, 1987; Cox, Alexander, Gilmore, & Pusakulich, 1988; Cox & McDaniel, 1984) have described use of connected discourse for intelligibility rating of different hearing aids or listening conditions. The connected speech test (CST) consists of passages on various topics. The listener is informed of the topic, and sentences are presented one at a time with the listener repeating the entire sentence as she or he heard it. Key words are scored in each sentence with a total of 25 words being scored for each passage. Pairs of passages are presented (scoring 50 key words) to attain reasonable stability of scores. Cox et al. (1988) concluded that their connected speech test "is uniquely suited to measurement of hearing aid benefit in that it has content validity (conversationally produced connected speech), good sensitivity and a large number of equivalent forms" (p. 206).

Use of procedures such as mentioned above, administration of a speechreading test with visual cues alone, auditory cues alone, or both (Dodds & Harford, 1968), and utilization of some measure of social adequacy, hearing handicap or hearing performance scales, or questionnaires developing profiles of communicative problems encountered by the hearing-impaired individual in home, work, and social environments should be of assistance in understanding the difficulties in communication experienced by hearing-impaired persons. The combination of such information is vital to appropriate counseling, to the planning and conduct of audiologic habilitative programs, and to the assessment of progress and improvement in communication.

Importantly, measures of speech understanding can be compared to prediction of speech understanding based on the articulation index (ANSI, 1969b):

> The articulation index (AI) is based on . . . the effective proportion of the
> normal speech signal that is available to a listener conveying speech intelli-

gibility. AI is computed from acoustical measurements or estimates of the speech spectrum and the effective masking spectrum of any noise which may be present along with the speech at the ear of the listener . . . The AI presumes to predict the relative performance of communication systems operating under given conditions when testing with a given group of typical talkers and listeners and when training and other listener-talker proficiency factors are kept constant or controlled for different tests by proper experimental procedures. (pp. 6, 23)

Aniansson (1974), Dirks (1982), Dugal, Braida, and Durlach (1978), Humes, Dirks, Bell, Ahlstrom, and Kincaid (1986), Kamm, Dirks, and Bell (1985), Ludvigsen (1987), Pavlovic (1984, 1988), and Pavlovic, Studebaker, and Sherbecoe (1985) have applied the AI concept to results obtained from groups of patients with sensorineural hearing losses responding to a variety of test materials. Agreement between observed and predicted scores has been reasonably good on a group basis. As would be expected, predictions for individual subjects were not always accurate because of individual variability. As emphasized earlier in this chapter, scores on tests of speech understanding can vary considerably from one patient to the next despite similar audiometric configurations.

Observations regarding speech recognition performance and predictions based on the articulation index are relevant to the various prescriptive techniques for hearing aid selection. The goal of these procedures is to provide as much of the speech spectra as possible in the usable auditory area between the patient's pure tone hearing thresholds and loudness discomfort levels. Some prescriptions use mathematical formulas based on threshold sensitivity alone (Byrne & Dillon, 1986; Byrne & Tonisson, 1976; Libby, 1986; Lybarger, 1944); others are based on measurements of thresholds and loudness discomfort levels (Berger, Hagberg, & Rane, 1977; McCandless & Lyregaard, 1983; Schwartz, Lyregaard, & Lundh, 1988), thresholds and upper limits of comfortable loudness (Cox, 1985, 1988), or thresholds, most comfortable listening levels, and loudness discomfort levels (Pascoe, 1978; Skinner, 1984, 1988; Skinner, Pascoe, Miller, & Popelka, 1982). Such procedures can be used to select gain, frequency response, and maximum output characteristics for the amplifier, which can of course be modified somewhat based on the hearing aid user's report on speech intelligibility and sound quality, and/or results from one or more tests of speech recognition.

Diagnostic implications from speech recognition test results. As mentioned earlier, data obtained from word recognition tests administered at suprathreshold levels are considered to yield some differential diagnostic information also. However, differential results obtained from conventional speech test materials presented at one or two sufficiently intense levels with good quality reproduction are, at best, only generally suggestive of site of peripheral pathologies. (Speech tests for detecting deficits in the central auditory system are discussed in Chapter 11.) In general, persons having hearing losses due to conductive pathologies generally attain word recognition scores on the order of 90% or better when undistorted test materials are presented at sensation levels of 25 dB or greater. Scores of 80% or lower at like sensation levels usually suggest some sensorineural involvement. However, scores higher than 80% should not be considered to preclude sensorineural hearing loss; many individuals having sensorineural hearing loss impairments achieve perfect or nearly perfect scores for monosyllabic word lists presented in quiet. Individuals having VIIIth nerve lesions may achieve word recognition scores near 0% even in quiet, but again some patients with VIIIth nerve tumors attain perfect or near perfect scores (Bess, 1983; Johnson, 1968, 1979; Liden, 1954; Olsen, Noffsinger, & Kurdziel, 1975; Schuknecht & Woellner, 1955; Walsh & Goodman, 1955). Furthermore, some hearing impairments due to cochlear pathologies also result in very poor understanding of speech at suprathreshold levels. Hence, it is obvious that results from speech recognition tests administered in quiet do not clearly differentiate sensory from neural involvements in the peripheral auditory system.

As mentioned earlier, mixing monosyllabic test items with noise increases the difficulty of some test materials and thereby sensitizes the test somewhat. Some patients having VIIIth nerve tumors demonstrate excess decrease in scores for monosyllables mixed with white noise (Katinsky, Lovrinic, & Buchheit, 1972; Olsen et al., 1975). However, some individuals with cochlear hearing losses also experience marked difficulty in correctly recognizing monosyllables mixed with white noise (Cooper & Cutts, 1971; Keith & Talis, 1970; Olsen et al., 1975; Ross, Huntington, Newby, & Nixon, 1965; Shapiro, Melnick, & Ver Muelen, 1972). Thus, a marked decrease in scores for monosyllabic words administered in white noise does not specifically differentiate cochlear from neural lesions either.

A word recognition test procedure that differentiates between cochlear and VIIIth nerve lesions somewhat more successfully was reported by J. Jerger and S. Jerger (1971). Their procedure consists of presentation of monosyllabic word lists at a number of intensity levels up to a maximum level of 110 dB SPL. The intent is to demonstrate the rollover phenomenon, that is, successively higher scores as the test materials are presented at successively greater intensity levels until a maximum score is reached, followed by poorer scores at still greater intensity levels. A rollover ratio is then determined by subtracting the poorest score (PB-min) obtained above the rollover point from the best score (PB-max) and dividing the result by the PB-max score:

$$\text{Rollover ratio} = (\text{PB-max} - \text{PB-min})/\text{PB-max}$$

According to Jerger and Jerger, the highest rollover ratio they observed for a patient with a cochlear hearing loss was 0.40, whereas the lowest ratio observed for VIIIth nerve lesion patients was 0.45. Dirks, Kamm, Bower, and Bettsworth (1977) confirmed the findings of Jerger and Jerger in that all but one of the cochlear lesion patients in their sample yielded rollover ratios less than 0.45, whereas all five of the VIIIth nerve lesion patients demonstrated rollover ratios greater than 0.45. PB-min was consistently observed at 100 dB HL by Dirks et al. Based on their findings, Dirks et al. cautioned that the rollover ratio is restricted if all scores are low and that the accuracy of the PB-max score is critical. They recommended that smaller intensity increments in stimulus presentation be used near PB-max levels and that each clinic establish a rollover ratio based on the specific test material used. Bess, Josey, and Humes (1979) and Meyer and Mishler (1985) have confirmed the importance of the latter recommendation. Bess et al. found that a rollover ratio of 0.25 for their NU No.6 test materials separated most of the cochlear and the VIIIth nerve tumor patients in their sample. Meyer and Mishler, using a different set of NU No. 6 recordings, reported that a rollover ratio of 0.35 best separated the VIIIth nerve tumor and the cochlear hearing loss patients in their sample.

Gang (1976) and Shirinian and Arnst (1980) reported that high rollover ratios are obtained for elderly persons also. Jerger and Jerger (1971) and Dirks et al. (1977) noted similar findings. However, J. Jerger and S. Jerger (1976) and Shirinian and Arnst (1980) disagreed with Gang's conclusion that such results limited the clinical utility of the rollover ratio; the points they stressed are that rollover should be expected given the suspected neural involvement for some elderly individuals and that such auditory test results are specific to site of involvement, not to etiology.

Modifications of suprathreshold speech recognition tests for children

The assessment of a young child's ability to understand speech is an essential feature of a comprehensive audiologic evaluation. Such measurements require consideration of numerous variables. Otherwise, the results from such tests may have little meaning when considering audiologic classification, educational placement, and/or habilitation. In addition to those variables routinely considered when testing adults, the selection of test materials within a child's receptive vocabulary competency, the designation of an appropriate response task, and the use of reinforcement are primary facts that affect the reliability and validity of pediatric measurements. Furthermore, it must be kept in mind that, unlike adults, the results obtained during measures of speech recognition and comprehension may reflect the child's level of auditory development at the time of the test rather than maximum potential for auditory processing. In fact, improvement in speech perception over time may serve as one indicator of the appropriateness of a child's habilitation and education programs.

Every attempt must be made to select stimuli that fall within the child's receptive vocabulary. Otherwise scores will not only reflect limitations in auditory recognition abilities but also the language delay imposed by the hearing loss. Unfortunately, establishment of definitive guidelines for selection of pediatric test materials is difficult because research with children, as well as the development of alternate test materials, is still limited.

With respect to the use of conventional adult lists of phonemically balanced monosyllabic words, clinical investigations by McNamee (1960) and by Sanderson-Leepa and Rintelmann (1976) revealed that scores for normal hearing youngsters continue to improve during the elementary school years. Hence, it appears that scores approximating those achieved by adults may not be attained by normal hearing children until they are approximately 10 to 12 years of age. For younger children the number of unfamiliar monosyllabic words incorporated into the test lists may be related to the child's age. Thus if one takes a conservative approach, it appears that the use of adult lists of speech recognition materials may rarely be indicated when working with children having significant bilateral hearing impairments and concomitant language deficits.

Monosyllables: open-ended sets.   Three lists of phonemically balanced words selected from the spoken vocabulary of kindergartners (PBK-50) were devised by Haskins in 1949. The monosyllabic words incorporated into the lists were selected on the basis of the International Kindergarten Union vocabulary lists and are representative of speech observed for children entering the first grade. A similar approach was taken by Watson in England, resulting in the generation of the Manchester Jr. (MJ) lists, which consist of four lists of phonemically balanced monosyllables considered to be in the vocabulary of children who are 6 years of age or older (Ewing, 1957).

The PBK-50 lists have been used widely. Yet the receptive vocabulary level of the particular child under audiologic study often is not ascertained before administering these materials. Consequently, the PBK-50 scores may be depressed in that they reflect language deficits as well as problems in auditory recognition. Evidence that use the PBK-50 words does not yield maximum word recognition scores is found in the data published by Sanderson-Leepa and Rintelmann (1976). They found that normal hearing preschoolers, at 3½ years of age, yielded scores substantially lower than did older children. Thus it is recommended that the clinician exercise caution in administering this test unless there is relatively good assurance that the receptive vocabulary age of the youngster is at least equivalent to that of a normal hearing kindergartner.

Another major limitation in the use of the Haskins PBK-50 lists is that only three equivalent lists are available. Unfortunately, in those situations where the child's performance is to be assessed without and with hearing aids, and/or auditory training systems, as well as different acoustic environments, there is a good possibility that a significant learning effect will accrue with repeated administration of the same test materials.

Monosyllables: closed-response sets.   Because many hearing-impaired youngsters' receptive language skills do not approximate those of a normal 6-year-old, alternate speech materials must be available for clinical use. One such test is the Word Intelligibility by Picture Identification (WIPI) materials (Lerman, Ross, & McLaughlin, 1965; Ross & Lerman, 1970). Although the four lists of 25 monosyllabic words are not phonemically balanced, an attempt was made by the authors to assure that different distinctive features were included in the selection of the test items. The WIPI test kit includes picture plates with six illustrations per plate. An obvious advantage of this test is that the problem of poor speech production by the child can be circumvented by using a pointing response task. Although extensive analysis of the vocabulary included in the WIPI test lists has not been published, clinical experience and the findings contained in the unpublished study by Schwartz (1971) suggest that normal hearing children below 4 years of age encounter a number of words in the WIPI test that are not within their recognition vocabulary. The Sanderson-Leepa and Rintelmann (1976) study corroborates Schwartz's findings in that normal hearing youngsters at age 3½ years manifested a significant number of errors, especially on Lists 3 and 4. On the basis of the data available, it appears that use of the WIPI materials is most appropriate for those youngsters with receptive vocabulary ages of 4 years and older.

A more recent test designed for use with young children and commercially recorded is the Northwestern University Children's Perception of Speech Test (NU-CHIPS; Elliot & Katz, 1980). The word lists represent 50 monosyllabic test items randomized four times. During the development of this test, these words were found to be familiar to 3-year-old research subjects with normal hearing. As with the WIPI test, the child identifies the test item via picture identification. Important to the use of word/picture identification tasks is that the pictures be readily identified by the youngster. Dengerink and Bean (1988) found five test items in NU-CHIPS and seven test items in the WIPI test were not identified correctly in two test conditions by 5% or more of their sample of 40 5-year-old children. These observations support clinical experience that an incorrect response may reflect either the child's difficulty in visually recognizing the test item or confusion regarding the authors' intended concept conveyed by the picture. Thus it is important during clinical assessment to determine whether an error response represents a visual or an auditory misperception. Interestingly, Mackie and Dermody (1986) successfully used NU-CHIPS materials and the adaptive procedure of Levitt and Rabiner (1967) (mentioned earlier in this chapter) to obtain 50% performance levels for children as young as 3 years of age.

Because both the WIPI and NU-CHIPS tests use a closed- rather than open-set response task, it is not surprising that the scores for these tests often are 10 to 20 percentage points higher that those obtained from administration of PBK-50 word lists to children with sensorineural hearing impairments. Therefore, it is advisable that audiologic reports include not only the scores obtained, but also the specific test materials used.

Another commercially available word identification test that incorporates picture identification is the Discrimination by Pictures (DIP) Test (Siegenthaler & Haspiel, 1966). This measure was designed to be administered to young children with pictures selected for easy identification by preschoolers. The stimuli consist of 48 pairs of familiar monosyllabic words that differ in distinctive features. No attempt was made to achieve phonemic balance. Unfortunately, only two items are pictured on each response plate; hence, there is a 50% probability of correct response by chance alone.

The Manchester Picture Vocabulary Test, which contains six lists of 20 monosyllabic words, has been devised for use with children having significant linguistic retardation. Each test word is illustrated on a response card containing six pictures (Watson, 1967). Apparently this test has not been widely studied in this country.

An informal approach to the assessment of word recognition ability is a viable alternative for those children whose language is quite limited. One procedure that has proven useful clinically is to choose a number of miniature toys whose monosyllabic names are within the child's vocabulary, for example, car, shoe, chair, ball. Suggestions by parents and preschool teachers are particularly valuable when selecting such test stimuli for a child. Because the procedure is not standardized, scores should be recorded in terms of number of correct responses relative to the number of stimulus items rather than as a percentage correct score. Despite the obvious limitations of such informal testing, differences between ears, as well as differences without and with hearing aids can be highlighted by this approach.

Another useful technique when evaluating children with extremely restricted language competence is the administration of a test requiring the recognition of familiar environmental sounds through picture pointing. Clinical experience with the Sound Effects Recognition Test (SERT), described by Hieber, Matkin, and Skalka (1975), has revealed that many youngsters with very limited ability to understand words may reveal surprisingly good ability to identify familiar environmental sounds. Such information often is useful when describing to parents and teachers the importance of hearing aid use, even in those instances where speech processing abilities are quite limited.

By careful selection of test materials, it is possible in most cases to obtain important information with respect to auditory recognition of test stimuli even though adult test materials cannot be used. Unfortunately, habilitation and educational programs frequently are designed after consideration of only information regarding hearing sensitivity. By using a battery of test materials suitable for children at different developmental stages, it is often possible to provide audiologic information regarding the child's ability to utilize residual hearing in addition to describing the degree, type, and configuration of the hearing loss.

Sentences: open-ended sets.   Although lists of words are used most commonly when assessing speech perception of both children and adults, the use of monosyllabic words embedded into sentences also has been explored. Blair (1976) developed six lists of 25 sentences equated in syntactical difficulty. Two monosyllabic test items are incorporated into each sentence. His selection of test words was based on an earlier analysis of the Peterson and Lehiste (1962) lists by Hieber (1974), who substituted alternative words for those items not typically found within the vocabulary of children in the early elementary school years. Phonemic balance, however, was maintained.

Bench, Kowal, and Bamford (1979) have developed an open-set response sentence test based on language samples elicited from hearing-impaired children aged 8 to 15 years. Twenty-one lists of 16 sentences with 50 words in each list have been devised. Not all key words are monosyllables, but sentence length is limited to seven syllables, for example, "The dog sleeps in a basket."

Sentences: closed-response sets.   Weber and Reddell (1976) incorporated the WIPI test items into meaningful sentences appropriate for use with younger children. The task of the listener is to identify the picture corresponding to the sentence.

A more recent development is the Pediatric Speech Intelligibility Test (PSI) for use with children having a linguistic age of 3 to 6 years (S. Jerger & J. Jerger, 1982; S. Jerger, J. Jerger, Alford, & Abrams, 1983; S. Jerger, J. Jerger, & Lewis, 1981; S. Jerger, Lewis, Hawkins, & J. Jerger, 1980). All test items in the word and sentence portions of the test were observed in the spontaneous and elicited speech of young children. The test materials consist of 20 monosyllabic words divided into four lists of five words each, and 10 sentences for each of two syntactic constructions. The response task is to identify the picture corresponding to the word or sentence heard. The test items are administered in the presence of competing sentences (different talker) at a variety of message-to-competition ratios. This test procedure is intended to evaluate children with suspected central nervous system lesions as well as those with peripheral hearing impairments.

Although the use of sentence materials has obvious limitations in the typical clinical setting, the fact that short-term auditory memory as well as speech perception are tapped may resemble more closely the listening demands encountered in many educational and social situations than does single word recognition or identification.

Predicting an individual's ability to understand speech on the basis of pure tone findings is even more difficult for children than for adults; developmental factors as well as the degree of auditory impairment affect children's performance at suprathreshold levels. Erber and Alenecewicz (1976), in a study of speech recognition abilities of 160 severely hearing-impaired children, found that the relationship between the average pure tone hearing loss and speech understanding was poor for those children with hearing losses in the range of 95- to 100-dB HL.

A better understanding of a child's strengths and limitations with respect to auditory function may be obtained by using a test battery that incorporates stimuli representing different levels of difficulty. For example, one such test is the Children's Auditory Test (CAT) developed by Erber (1977), in which spondees, trokees, and monosyllables are used. One use of this battery with children having profound hearing losses is to differentiate those who can perceive spectral components of speech from those who are limited to recognition of time and intensity patterns (Plant, 1984). Similarly, a battery requiring recognition of familiar environmental sounds, selected spondees, and monosyllables can be used to highlight differences in auditory performance among children with similar audiograms (Matkin, 1977).

Presentation level. Another variable that merits consideration in the administration of pediatric speech materials is the selection of an appropriate sensation level for the presentation of test items. Analysis of the

Sanderson-Leepa and Rintelmann (1976) data suggests that a sensation level of 32 dB is appropriate for normal hearing children. Examination of a relatively large number of clinical records indicates that relatively high speech recognition scores are attained at sensation levels of 36 to 40 dB by children having mild to moderate hearing losses. One notable exception occurs when a child has a precipitous high-frequency hearing loss. Often the maximum speech recognition score is not obtained unless the degree of impairment at 2000 Hz is considered when selecting the presentation level (Matkin, 1968). Ideally, information in the high-frequency region should be audible if the clinician's goal is to determine maximum performance. At the same time one must take cognizance of the report by Erber and Witt (1977), which revealed that in the cases of severe and profound hearing losses, best scores are achieved at sensation levels considerably lower than those typically used in a routine audiologic evaluation. Specifically, they found that severely hearing-impaired youngsters achieved their best scores at an average sensation level of 30.6 dB relative to speech detection threshold. An average sensation level of 21.6 dB above speech detection threshold was sufficient for those children with profound hearing losses to achieve their best scores.

Other considerations. In those cases where recognition of speech is limited through auditory processing alone, it is often worthwhile to repeat such measurements, giving the child the opportunity to both "look and listen." Such bisensory scores are especially useful if obtained while the youngster is wearing amplification. Obviously, the child whose scores are quite high when given the opportunity to process speech information in both visual and auditory modes is a better candidate for placement in an oral/aural classroom or for mainstreaming in a regular school setting. In contrast, when relatively low bisensory scores are obtained, the potential benefits of supplementing sensory input with alternate forms of visual communication should be considered when developing an individual educational plan (IEP).

Although various modes of reinforcement (i.e., play, tangible, or visual) can be used in conditioning young children for pure tone audiometry, research is limited with respect to the effect of systematic reinforcement on speech recognition scores obtained by young children. Smith and Hodgson (1970) found that both normal hearing and hearing-impaired youngsters obtained significantly higher mean scores under conditions of systematic reinforcement. Furthermore, younger subjects in the control (nonreinforced) groups demonstrated some deterioration in performance as the number of test lists increased. Because audiologists frequently administer several speech tests during a pediatric audiologic evaluation, the use of reinforcement seems appropriate. Data in Smith's (1970) dissertation suggest that the effectiveness of the reinforcement is particularly noteworthy for preschool-age children. Furthermore, reinforcement probably is most effective when the task is difficult.

The many variables mentioned earlier that affect speech recognition test results for adults also affect test results for children. In addition, test materials within the youngster's receptive vocabulary must be selected, an appropriate response must be found, and use of reinforcement must be considered. When all these factors are kept in mind, important information about a child's current auditory reception and perception of speech can be obtained. Such insights are vital to planning educational placement and habilitation programs and in counseling parents and others concerned with the youngster's education and habilitation needs. (See Chapter 9 for further discussion of assessment of hearing loss in young children.)

Summary

This chapter has dealt with test materials, test conditions, and test procedures used for clinical measurement of speech recognition. Obviously, use of test stimuli having the complexity of speech results in a number of variables that are difficult to specify and control. Nevertheless, much useful information concerning an individual's hearing loss and communicative problems can be obtained from speech recognition tests. It is hoped that audiologists engaged in clinical and research activities, and others in related specialties interested in audition, speech science, or speech perception will seriously consider and study these variables and problems further. Through such efforts, improved test materials and procedures will be developed and more meaningful information will be obtained.

References

American National Standards Institute. (1954). *Volume measurements of speech and program waves* (ANSI C16.5-1954). New York: Author.

American National Standards Institute. (1969a). *American National Standard specifications for audiometers* (ANSI S3.6-1969). New York: Author.

American National Standards Institute. (1969b). *Methods for Calculation of the Articulation Index* (ANSI S3.5-1969). New York: Author.

American Speech-Language-Hearing Association Committee on Audiometric Evaluation. (1977). Guidelines for determining threshold level for speech. *Asha, 19,* 241–243.

American Speech-Language-Hearing Association Committee on Audiologic Evaluation. (1988). Guidelines for determining threshold level for speech. *Asha, 30,* 85–89.

Aniansson, G. (1974). Methods for assessing high frequency hearing loss in everyday listening situations. *Acta Oto-Laryngolica,* (Supplement, 320), 1–50.

Barry, S. J., & Gaddis, S. (1978). Physical and physiological constraints on the use of bone-conduction speech audiometry. *Journal of Speech and Hearing Disorders, 43,* 220–226.

Beattie, R. C., & Clark, N. (1982). Practice effects of a four-talker babble on the synthetic sentence identification test. *Ear and Hearing, 3,* 202–206.

Beattie, R. C., & Edgerton, C. (1976). Reliability of monosyllabic discrimination tests in white noise for differentiating among hearing aids. *Journal of Speech and Hearing Disorders, 41,* 464–476.

Beattie, R. C., Edgerton, B. J., & Svihovec, D. V. (1975). An investigation of Auditec of St. Louis recordings of Central Institute for the Deaf spondees. *Journal of the American Audiology Society, 1,* 97–101.

Beattie, R. C., Edgerton, B. J., & Svihovec, D. V. (1977). A comparison of the Auditec of St. Louis cassette recordings of NU-6 and CID W-22 on a normal hearing population. *Journal of Speech and Hearing Disorders, 42,* 60–64.

Beattie, R. C., Forrester, P. W., & Ruby, B. K. (1977). Reliability of the Tillman–Olsen procedure for determination of spondee threshold using recorded and live voice presentations. *Journal of the American Audiology Society, 2,* 159–162.

Beattie, R. C., Svihovec, D. V., & Edgerton, B. J. (1975). Relative intelligibility of the CID spondees as presented via monitored live voice. *Journal of Speech and Hearing Disorders, 40,* 84–91.

Beattie, R. C., Svihovec, D. A., & Edgerton, B. J. (1978). Comparison of speech detection and spondee thresholds for half- versus full-list intelligibility scores with MLV and taped presentations of NU-6. *Journal of the American Audiology Society, 3,* 267–272.

Bench, J., Kowal, A., & Bamford, J. (1979). The BKB (Bamford–Kowal–Bench) sentence lists for partially-hearing children. *British Journal of Audiology, 13,* 108–113.

Berger, K. W. (1969). Speech discrimination task using multiple choice key words in sentences. *Journal of Auditory Research, 9,* 247–262.

Berger, K. W., Hagberg, E. N., & Rane, R. L. (1977). *Prescription of hearing aids: Rationale, procedures, and results.* Kent, OH: Herald.

Berger, K. W., Keating, L. W., & Rose, D. E. (1971). An evaluation of the Kent State University Speech Discrimination Test on subjects with sensorineural loss. *Journal of Auditory Research, 11,* 140–143.

Berry, S. (1939). The use and effectiveness of hearing aids. *The Laryngoscope, 49,* 912–942.

Bess, F. H. (1983). Clinical assessment of speech recognition. In D. F. Konkle & W. F. Rintelmann (Eds.), *Principles of speech audiometry* (pp. 127–201). Baltimore: University Park Press.

Bess, F. H., Josey, A. F., & Humes, L. E. (1979). Performance intensity functions in cochlear and eighth nerve disorders. *American Journal of Otolaryngology, 1,* 27–31.

Beykirch, H., & Gaeth, J. (1978). A comparison of speech discrimination scores by using PB-50 lists and speech discrimination scale with hearing impaired adults. *Journal of Auditory Research, 18,* 153–164.

Bilger, R. C. (1984). Speech recognition test development. In E. Elkins (Ed.), *Speech recognition testing by the hearing impaired ASHA reports, 14,* 2–15.

Bilger, R. C., Neutzel, J. M., Rabinowitz, W. M., & Rzeczowski, C. (1984). Standardization of a test of speech perception in noise. *Journal of Speech and Hearing Research, 27,* 32–48.

Bilger, R. C., & Wang, M. D. (1976). Consonant confusions in patients with sensorineural hearing loss. *Journal of Speech and Hearing Research, 19,* 718–748.

Black, J. W. (1957). Multiple-choice intelligibility tests. *Journal of Speech and Hearing Disorders, 22,* 213–235.

Black, J. W. (1968). Response to multiple choice intelligibility tests. *Journal of Speech and Hearing Research, 11,* 453–466.

Blair, J. C. (1976). *The contributing influences of amplification, speechreading, and classroom environments on the ability of hearing impaired children to discriminate sentences.* Unpublished doctoral dissertation, Northwestern University, Evanston, IL.

Bleeker, G. F., & Huizing, H. C. (1953). Speech audiometry and selection of hearing aids. *Proceedings of the First International Congress of Audiology* (Leiden), 116–120.

Blumenfeld, V. G., Bergman, M., & Millner, E. (1969). Speech discrimination in an aging population. *Journal of Speech and Hearing Research, 12,* 210–217.

Bode, D. L., & Carhart, R. (1974). Stability and accuracy of adaptive tests of speech discrimination. *Journal of the Acoustical Society of America, 56,* 963–970.

Bonding, P. (1979). Frequency selectivity and speech discrimination in sensorineural hearing loss. *Scandinavian Audiology, 8,* 205–215.

Boothroyd, A. (1968). Developments in speech audiometry. *Sound, 2,* 3–10.

Bowling, L. S., & Elpern, B. S. (1961). Relative intelligibility of items on CID Auditory Test W-1. *Journal of Auditory Research, 1,* 152–157.

Brandy, W. T. (1966). Reliability of voice tests in speech discrimination. *Journal of Speech and Hearing Research, 9,* 461–465.

Breakey, M. R., & Davis, H. (1949). Comparisons of thresholds for speech: Words and sentence tests; receiver vs. field and monaural vs. binaural listening. *The Laryngoscope, 59,* 236–250.

Bryant, W. W. (1904). A phonographic acoumeter. *Archives of Otolaryngology, 33,* 438–443.

Burke, K. S., Shutts, R. E., & King, W. P. (1965). Range of difficulty of four Harvard phonetically balanced word lists. *The Laryngoscope, 75,* 289–296.

Byrne, D., & Dillon, H. (1986). The National Acoustics Laboratory (NAL) new procedure for selecting the gain and frequency response of a hearing aid. *Ear and Hearing, 7,* 257–265.

Byrne, D., & Tonisson, W. (1976). Selecting the gain of hearing aids for persons with sensorineural hearing impairments. *Scandinavian Audiology, 5,* 51–59.

Campanelli, P. A. (1962). A measure of intra-list stability of four PAL word lists. *Journal of Auditory Research, 2,* 50–55.

Campbell, R. (1965). Discrimination test word difficulty. *Journal of Speech and Hearing Research, 8,* 13–22.

Carhart, R. (1946a). Monitored live voice as a test of auditory acuity. *Journal of the Acoustical Society of America, 17,* 339–349.

Carhart, R. (1946b). Tests for selection of hearing aids. *The Laryngoscope, 56*, 780–794.

Carhart, R. (1960). The determination of hearing loss. *Department of Medicine and Surgery Information Bulletin—Audiology, IB10-115*, 1–18.

Carhart, R. (1965). Problems in the measurement of speech discrimination. *Archives of Otolaryngology, 82*, 253–260.

Carhart, R. (1967). The advantages and limitations of a hearing aid. *Minnesota Medicine, 50*, 823–826.

Carhart, R. (1971). Observations on the relations between thresholds for pure tones and for speech. *Journal of Speech and Hearing Disorders, 36*, 476–483.

Carhart, R., & Porter, L. S. (1971). Audiometric configurations and prediction of threshold for spondees. *Journal of Speech and Hearing Research, 14*, 486–495.

Carhart, R., & Thompson, E. A. (1947). The fitting of hearing aids. *Transactions of the American Academy of Ophthalmology and Otolaryngology, 5*, 354–361.

Causey, G. D., Hermanson, C. L., Hood, L. J., & Bowling, L. S. (1983). A comparative evaluation of the Maryland NU-6 auditory test. *Journal of Speech and Hearing Disorders, 48*, 62–69.

Chaiklin, J. B. (1959). The relation among three selected auditory speech thresholds. *Journal of Speech and Hearing Research, 2*, 237–243.

Chaiklin, J. B., Font, J., & Dixon, R. F. (1967). Spondaic thresholds measured in ascending 5 dB steps. *Journal of Speech and Hearing Research, 10*, 141–145.

Chaiklin, J. B., & Ventry, I. M. (1964). Spondee threshold measurement: A comparison of 2- and 5-dB steps. *Journal of Speech and Hearing Disorders, 29*, 47–59.

Clemis, J. D., & Carver, W. F. (1967). Discrimination scores for speech in Ménière's diseases. *Archives of Otolaryngology, 86*, 614–618.

Cohen, R. L., & Keith, R. W. (1976). Use of low-pass noise in word recognition. *Journal of Speech and Hearing Research, 19*, 48–54.

Conn, M. J., Dancer, J., & Ventry, I. M. (1975). A spondee list for determining speech reception threshold without prior familiarization. *Journal of Speech and Hearing Disorders, 40*, 388–396.

Conn, M., Ventry, I. M., & Woods, R. W. (1972). Pure tone average and spondee relationships in simulated hearing loss. *Journal of Auditory Research, 12*, 234–239.

Cooper, J. C., Jr., & Cutts, B. P. (1971). Speech discrimination in noise. *Journal of Speech and Hearing Research, 14*, 332–337.

Cox, R. M. (1985). Aural rehabilitation: A structured approach to hearing aid selection. *Ear and Hearing, 6*, 226–239.

Cox, R. M. (1988). The MSU hearing instrument prescription procedure. *Hearing Instruments, 39*(1), 6, 8, 10.

Cox, R. M., Alexander, G. C., & Gilmore, C. (1987). Development of the connected speech test (CST). *Ear and Hearing, 8* (Supplement), 119S–126S.

Cox, R. M., Alexander, G. C., Gilmore, C., & Pusakulich, K. M. (1988). Use of the connected speech test (CST) with hearing-impaired listeners. *Ear and Hearing, 9*, 198–207.

Cox, R. M., & McDaniel, D. M. (1984). Intelligibility rating of continuous discourse: Application to hearing aid selection. *Journal of the Acoustical Society of America, 76*, 758–766.

Cox, R. M., & Moore, J. N. (1988). Composite speech spectrum for hearing aid gain prescriptions. *Journal of Speech and Hearing Research, 31*, 102–107.

Creston, J. E., Gillespie, M., & Krahn, C. (1966). Speech audiometry: Tape vs. live voice. *Archives of Otolaryngology, 83*, 14–17.

Curry, E. T., & Cox, B. P. (1966). The relative intelligibility of spondees. *Journal of Auditory Research, 6,* 419–424.

Dahle, A., Hume, W. G., & Haspiel, G. S. (1968). Comparisons of speech Bekesy tracings with selected clinical auditory measures. *Journal of Auditory Research, 8,* 125–129.

Danhauer, J. L., Beck, D. L., Lucks, L. E., & Ghadialy, F. B. (1988). A sentence test for audiologic assessment of severe and profound losses. *Hearing Journal, 41,* 7, 26, 28–29, 32–33.

Danhauer, J. L., Doyle, P. C., & Lucks, L. E. (1986). Effects of signal-to-noise ratio on the nonsense syllable test. *Ear and Hearing, 7,* 323–324.

Davis, H. (1948). The articulation area and social adequacy index for hearing. *The Laryngoscope, 58,* 761–778.

Davis, H., Hudgins, C. C., Marquis, R. J., Nichols, R. H., Jr., Peterson, E., Ross, D. A., & Stevens, S. S. (1946). The selection of hearing aids. *The Laryngoscope, 56,* 85–163.

Demorest, M. E., & Erdman, S. A. (1986). Scale composition and item analysis of the communication profile for the hearing impaired. *Journal of Speech and Hearing Research, 28,* 515–535.

Demorest, M. E., & Erdman, S. A. (1987). Development of the communication profile for the hearing impaired. *Journal of Speech and Hearing Disorders, 52,* 129–143.

Demorest, M. E., & Walden, B. E. (1984). Psychometric principles in the selection, interpretation, and evaluation of communication self-assessment inventories. *Journal of Speech and Hearing Disorders, 49,* 226–240.

Dengerink, J. E., & Bean, R. E. (1988). Spontaneous labeling of pictures on the WIPI and NU-CHIPS by 5-year-olds. *Language, Speech, and Hearing Services in Schools, 44,* 144–152.

Dennison, L. B., & Kelly, B. R. (1978). High-frequency consonant word discrimination lists in hearing aid evaluation. *Journal of the American Auditory Society, 4,* 91–97.

Deutsch, L. J., & Kruger, B. (1971). The systematic selection of 25 monosyllables which predict the CID W-22 speech discrimination score. *Journal of Auditory Research, 11,* 286–290.

Dewey, G. (1923). *Relative frequency of English speech sounds.* Cambridge, MA: Harvard University Press.

DiCarlo, L. M. (1962). Some relationships between frequency discrimination and speech reception performance. *Journal of Auditory Research, 2,* 37–49.

Dillon, H. (1982). A quantitative examination of the source of speech discrimination score test variability. *Ear and Hearing, 3,* 51–58.

Dirks, D. D. (1982). Comments regarding "speech discrimination ability in the hearing impaired." In G. A. Studebaker & F. H. Bess (Eds.), *The Vanderbilt hearing aid report* (pp. 44–50). Upper Darby, PA: Monographs in Contemporary Audiology.

Dirks, D. D., Kamm, C., Bower, D., & Bettsworth, A. (1977). Use of performance-intensity functions for diagnosis. *Journal of Speech and Hearing Disorders, 42,* 408–415.

Dirks, D. D., Morgan, D. E., & Dubno, J. R. (1982). A procedure for quantifying the effects of noise in speech recognition. *Journal of Speech and Hearing Disorders, 47,* 114–123.

Dirks, D. D., Stream, R. W., & Wilson, R. H. (1972). Speech audiometry: Earphone and sound field. *Journal of Speech and Hearing Disorders, 37,* 167–173.

Dodds, E., & Harford, E. (1968). Application of a lipreading test in hearing aid evaluation. *Journal of Speech and Hearing Disorders, 33,* 167–173.

Dubno, J. R., & Dirks, D. D. (1982). Evaluation of hearing-impaired listeners using a nonsense-syllable test. I. Test reliability. *Journal of Speech and Hearing Research, 25,* 135–141.

Dubno, J. R., & Dirks, D. D. (1983). Suggestions for optimizing reliability with the synthetic sentence identification test. *Journal of Speech and Hearing Disorders, 48,* 98–103.

Dubno, J. R., Dirks, D. D., & Langhofer, L. R. (1982). Evaluation of hearing-impaired listeners using a nonsense-syllable test. II. Syllable recognition and consonant confusion pattern. *Journal of Speech and Hearing Research, 25,* 141–148.

Dubno, J. R., Dirks, D. D., & Morgan, D. E. (1984). Effects of age and mild hearing loss on speech recognition in noise. *Journal of the Acoustical Society of America, 76,* 87–96.

Duffy, J. R., & Giolas, T. G. (1974). Sentence intelligibility as a function of key word selection. *Journal of Speech and Hearing Research, 17,* 631–637.

Dugal, R. L., Braida, L. D., & Durlach, N. I. (1978). Implications of previous research for the selection of frequency-gain characteristics. In G. Studebaker & I. Hochberg (Eds.), *Acoustical factors affecting hearing aid performance* (pp. 379–403). Baltimore: University Park Press.

Edgerton, B. J., & Danhauer, J. L. (1979). *Clinical implications of speech discrimination testing using nonsense stimuli.* Baltimore: University Park Press.

Edgerton, B. J., Danhauer, J. L., & Beattie, R. C. (1977). Bone conduction speech audiometry in normal subjects. *Journal of the American Audiology Society, 3,* 84–87.

Egan, J. (1948). Articulation testing methods. *The Laryngoscope, 58,* 955–991.

Egolf, D. B., Rhodes, R. C., & Curry, E. T. (1970). Phoneme discrimination differences between hypacusics and normals. *Journal of Auditory Research, 10,* 176–179.

Elkins, E. (1970). Analyses of the phonetic composition and word familiarity attributes of CNC word intelligibility lists. *Journal of Speech and Hearing Disorders, 35,* 156–159.

Elkins, E. (1971). Evaluation of modified rhyme test results from impaired- and normal-hearing listeners. *Journal of Speech and Hearing Research, 14,* 589–595.

Elliot, L. L. (1963). Prediction of speech discrimination scores from other test information. *Journal of Auditory Research, 3,* 35–45.

Elliot, L. L., & Katz, D. R. (1980). *Northwestern University—Children's perception of speech (NU-CHIPS).* St. Louis: Auditec of St. Louis.

Elpern, B. (1961). The relative stability of half list and full list discrimination tests. *The Laryngoscope, 71,* 30–36.

Epstein, A., Giolas, T. G., & Owens, E. (1968). Familiarity and intelligibility of monosyllabic word lists. *Journal of Speech and Hearing Research, 11,* 435–438.

Erber, N. P. (1977). Evaluating speech-perception ability in hearing-impaired children. In F. H. Bess (Ed.), *Childhood deafness causation, assessment and management* (pp. 173–181). New York: Grune & Stratton.

Erber, N. P., & Alenecewicz, C. M. (1976). Audiologic evaluation of deaf children. *Journal of Speech and Hearing Disorders, 41,* 256–267.

Erber, N. P., & Witt, L. H. (1977). Effects of stimulus intensity on speech perception by deaf children. *Journal of Speech and Hearing Disorders, 42,* 271–277.

Ewertsen, H. (1966). The fitting of hearing aids in Danish rehabilitation centers. *International Audiology, 5,* 385–391.

Ewertsen, H. W., & Birk-Nielsen, H. (1973). Social hearing handicap index. *Audiology, 12,* 180–187.

Ewing, A. W. G. (1957). Speech audiometry for children. In A. W. G. Ewing (Ed.), *Education guidance and the deaf child* (pp. 278–296). Washington, DC: Volta Bureau.

Fabry, D. A., & Van Tasell, D. J. (1986). Masked and filtered simulation of hearing loss: Effects on consonant recognition. *Journal of Speech and Hearing Research, 29,* 170–178.

Fairbanks, G. (1958). Test of phonemic differentiation: The rhyme test. *Journal of the Acoustical Society of America, 30,* 595–600.

Falconer, G., & Davis, H. (1947). The intelligibility of connected discourse as a test for the threshold of speech. *The Laryngoscope, 57,* 581–595.

Feeney, M. P., & Franks, J. R. (1982). Test–retest reliability of a distinctive feature difference test for hearing aid evaluation. *Ear and Hearing, 3,* 59–65.

Feldmann, H. (1960). A history of audiology: A comprehensive report and bibliography from the earliest beginnings to the present. *Translations for the Beltone Institute for Hearing Research, 22,* 1–111. [Translated by J. Tonndorf from *Die Geschichtliche Entwicklung der Horprufungsmethoden, kuze Darstellung and Bibliographie von der Anfongen bis zur Gegenwart.* In H. Leicher, R. Mittermaiser, & G. Theissing (Eds.), *Zwanglose Abhandungen aus dem Gebiet der Hals-Nasen-Ohren-Heilkunde.* Stuttgart: Georg Thieme Verlag, 1960.]

Fest, T. B. (1944). Hearing aids: Recent developments. *Journal of Speech and Hearing Disorders, 9,* 135–146.

Fifer, R. C., Stach, B. A., & Jerger, J. F. (1984). Evaluation of the minimal auditory capabilities (MAC) test in prelingual and postlingual hearing-impaired adults. *Ear and Hearing, 5,* 87–90.

Findlay, R. C. (1976). Auditory dysfunction accompanying noise-induced hearing loss. *Journal of Speech and Hearing Disorders, 41,* 374–380.

Finney, D. J. (1952). *Statistical method in biological assay.* London: C. Griffen.

Fletcher, H. (1929). *Speech and hearing.* Princeton, NJ: Von Nostrand Reinhold.

Fletcher, H. (1950). A method of calculating hearing loss for speech from an audiogram. *Acta Oto-Laryngologica,* (Supplement 90), 26–37.

Fletcher, H., & Steinberg, J. C. (1929). Articulation testing methods. *Bell Systems Technical Journal, 7,* 806–854.

Frank, T. & Craig, C. H. (1984). Comparison of the Auditec and Rintelmann recordings of NU-6. *Journal of Speech and Hearing Disorders, 49,* 267–271.

Frank, T., & Karlovich, R. S. (1975). Effect of contralateral noise on speech detection and speech reception thresholds. *Audiology, 14,* 34–43.

Franklin, B. (1977). Split-band amplification and speech band audiometry. *Hearing Instruments, 28*(11), 18–20.

French, N. R., Carter, C. W., Jr., & Koenig, W., Jr. (1930). The words and sounds of telephone conversations. *Bell System Technical Journal, 9,* 290–324.

Fry, D. B. (1961). Word and sentence tests for use in speech audiometry. *Lancet, 2,* 197–199.

Fry, D. B., & Kerridge, P. M. T. (1939). Tests for the hearing of speech by deaf people. *Lancet, 1,* 106–109.

Gang, R. P. (1976). The effects of age on the diagnostic utility of the rollover phenomenon. *Journal of Speech and Hearing Disorders, 41,* 63–69.

Gardner, H. J. (1971). Application of high frequency consonant discrimination word list in hearing aid evaluation. *Journal of Speech and Hearing Disorders, 36,* 354–355.

Gelfand, S. A. (1975). Use of the carrier phrase in live voice speech discrimination testing. *Journal of Auditory Research, 15,* 107–110.

Gengel, R. W. (1973). On the reliability of discrimination performance in persons with sensorineural hearing impairment using a closed set test. *Journal of Auditory Research, 13,* 97–100.

Gengel, R. W., & Kupperman, G. L. (1980a). On the calibration of two commercially recorded versions of CID auditory test W-22. *Ear and Hearing, 1,* 229–231.

Gengel, R., & Kupperman, G. L. (1980b). Word discrimination in noise: Effect of different speakers. *Ear and Hearing, 1,* 156–160.

Gerber, S. E., & Fisher, L. B. (1979). Prediction of hearing aid user's satisfaction. *Journal of the American Auditory Society, 5,* 35–40.

Giolas, T. G., Cooker, H. S., & Duffy, J. R. (1970). The predictability of words in sentences. *Journal of Auditory Research, 10,* 328–334.

Giolas, T. G., Owens, E., Lamb, S. H., & Schubert, E. D. (1979). Hearing performance inventory. *Journal of Speech and Hearing Disorders, 44,* 169–195.

Givens, G. D., & Jacobs-Condit, L. (1981). Consonant identification in quiet and in noise with the normal and the sensorineural hearing-impaired. *Journal of Auditory Research, 21,* 279–285.

Gladstone, V. S., & Siegenthaler, B. M. (1971). Carrier phrase and speech intelligibility score. *Journal of Auditory Research, 11,* 101–103.

Goetzinger, C. P., & Proud, G. O. (1955). Speech audiometry by bone conduction. *Archives of Otolaryngology, 62,* 632–635.

Graham, J. T. (1960). Evaluation of methods for predicting speech reception threshold. *Archives of Otolaryngology, 72,* 347–350.

Griffiths, J. D. (1967). Rhyming minimal contrasts: A simplified diagnostic articulation test. *Journal of the Acoustical Society of America, 42,* 236–241.

Grubb, P. A. (1963a). Phoneme analysis of half-list discrimination tests. *Journal of Speech and Hearing Research, 6,* 271–276.

Grubb, P. A. (1963b). Considerations in the use of half-list speech discrimination tests. *Journal of Speech and Hearing Research, 6,* 294–297.

Hagerman, B. (1976). Reliability in the determination of speech discrimination. *Scandinavian Audiology, 5,* 219–228.

Hagerman, B. (1984). Some aspects of methodology in speech audiometry. *Scandinavian Audiology, 21,* 1–25.

Hahlbrock, K. H. (1962). Bone conduction speech audiometry. *International Audiology, 1,* 186–188.

Hallpike, C. S. (1934). Hearing aids and hearing tests. *Journal of Laryngology and Otology, 49,* 240–246.

Harris, J. D. (1965). Pure tone acuity and intelligibility of everyday speech. *Journal of the Acoustical Society of America, 37,* 824–830.

Harris, J. D. (1980). On the use of a three-words-per-item format in tests for the hearing of speech. *Journal of the Acoustical Society of America, 67,* 345–347.

Harris, J. D., Haines, H. L., Kelsey, P. A., & Clack, T. D. (1961). The relation between speech intelligibility and electroacoustic characteristics of low fidelity. *Journal of Auditory Research, 1,* 357–386.

Harris, J. D., Haines, H. L., & Myers, C. K. (1956). A new formula for using the audiogram to predict speech hearing loss. *Archives of Otolaryngology, 63,* 158–176.

Hartig, H. E., & Newhart, H. (1936). Performance characteristics of electrical hearing aids for the deaf. *Archives of Otolaryngology, 23,* 617–632.

Haskins, H. (1949). *A phonetically balanced test of speech discrimination for children.* Unpublished master's thesis, Northwestern University, Evanston, IL.

Haspiel, G. S., & Havens, R. M. (1966). Comparison of speech-Bekesy tracings with pure tone Bekesy thresholds. *Journal of Auditory Research, 6,* 235–237.

Hawes, N. A., & Niswander, P. S. (1985). Comparison of the revised performance inventory with audiometric meaures. *Ear and Hearing, 6,* 93–97.

Hayes, D., Jerger, J., Taff, J., & Barber, B. (1983). Relations between aided synthetic sentence identification scores and hearing aid use satisfaction. *Ear and Hearing, 4,* 158–161.

Hecker, M. H. L., Stevens, K. N., & Williams, C. E. (1966). Measurements of reaction time in intelligibility tests. *Journal of the Acoustical Society of America, 39,* 1188–1889.

Hieber, T. F. (1974). Analysis of Peterson and Lehiste lists for children. Unpublished data. Evanston, IL: Northwestern University.

Hieber, T. F., Matkin, N. D., & Skalka, E. (1975). *A preliminary investigation of a sound effects recognition task.* Paper presented at the annual convention of the American Speech and Hearing Association, Washington, DC.

High, W. S., Fairbanks, G., & Glorig, A. (1964). Scale for self-assessment of hearing handicap. *Journal of Speech and Hearing Disorders, 29,* 215–230.

Hirsh, I. J., Davis, H., Silverman, S. R., Reynolds, E. G., Eldert, E., & Benson, R. W. (1952). Development of materials for speech audiometry. *Journal of Speech and Hearing Disorders, 17,* 321–337.

Hochberg, I. (1975). Most comfortable listening for loudness and intelligibility of speech. *Audiology, 14,* 23–27.

Holmgren, L. (1939). Hearing tests and hearing aids. *Acta Oto-Laryngologica,* (Supplement 34), 1–164.

Hood, J. D., & Poole, J. P. (1977). Improving the reliability of speech audiometry. *British Journal of Audiology, 11,* 93–102.

Hood, J. D., & Poole, J. P. (1980). Influence of the speaker and other factors affecting speech intelligibility. *Audiology, 19,* 434–455.

Hopkinson, N. T. (1972). Speech reception threshold. In J. Katz (Ed.), *Handbook of clinical audiology* (pp. 143–156). Baltimore: Williams & Wilkins.

Hosford-Dunn, H. L., Runge, C. A., & Montgomery, P. A. (1983). A shortened rank-ordered word discrimination list. *Hearing Journal, 36,* 15–19.

House, A. S., Williams, C. E., Hecker, M. H. L., & Kryter, K. D. (1965). Articulation testing methods. Consonantal differentiation in a closed-response set. *Journal of the Acoustical Society of America, 37,* 158–166.

Hudgins, C. V., Hawkins, J. E., Jr., Karlin, J. E., & Stevens, S. S. (1947). The development of recorded auditory tests for measuring hearing loss for speech. *The Laryngoscope, 57,* 57–89.

Huff, S. J., & Nerbonne, M. A. (1982). Comparison of the American Speech-Language-Hearing Association and the revised Tillman–Olsen methods for speech threshold measurement. *Ear and Hearing, 3,* 335–339.

Hughes, E. C., Arthur, R. H., & Johnson, R. L. (1979). Test-retest variability in testing hearing of speech. *Journal of the American Auditory Society, 5,* 17–20.

Hughson, W., & Thompson, E. A. (1942). Correlation of hearing acuity for speech with discrete frequency audiograms. *Archives of Otolaryngology, 36,* 526–540.

Humes, L. E. (1983). Midfrequency dysfunction in listeners having high-frequency sensorineural hearing loss. *Journal of Speech and Hearing Research, 26,* 425–435.

Humes, L. E., Dirks, D. D., Bell, T. S., Ahlstrom, C., & Kincaid, G. E. (1986). Applications of the articulation index to the recognition of speech by normal hearing and hearing-impaired listeners. *Journal of Speech and Hearing Research, 29*, 447–462.

Jerger, J. F., Carhart, R., Tillman, T. W., & Peterson, J. L. (1959). Some relations between normal hearing for pure tones and for speech. *Journal of Speech and Hearing Research, 2*, 126–140.

Jerger, J., & Hayes, D. (1976). Hearing aid evaluation: Clinical experience with a new philosophy. *Archives of Otolaryngology, 102*, 214–225.

Jerger, J., & Jerger, S. (1971). Diagnostic significance of PB word functions. *Archives of Otolaryngology, 93*, 573–580.

Jerger, J., & Jerger, S. (1976). Comments on "The effects of age on the diagnostic utility of the rollover phenomenon." *Journal of Speech and Hearing Disorders, 41*, 556–557.

Jerger, J., Malmquist, C., & Speaks, C. (1966). Comparison of some speech intelligibility tests in the evaluation of hearing aid performance. *Journal of Speech and Hearing Research, 9*, 253–258.

Jerger, J., Speaks, C., & Trammell, J. (1968). A new approach to speech audiometry. *Journal of Speech and Hearing Disorders, 33*, 318–328.

Jerger, J., & Thelin, J. (1968). Effects of electroacoustic characteristics on speech understanding. *Bulletin of Prosthetics Research, 10*, 159–196.

Jerger, S., & Jerger, J. (1982). Pediatric speech intelligibility test: Performance intensity characteristics. *Ear and Hearing, 3*, 25–34.

Jerger, S., Jerger, J., Alford, B. R., & Abrams, S. (1983). Development of speech intelligibility in children with recurrent otitis media. *Ear and Hearing, 4*, 138–145.

Jerger, S., Jerger, J., & Lewis, S. (1981). Pediatric speech intelligibility test II. Effect of receptive language and chronological age. *International Journal of Pediatric Otorhinolaryngology, 3*, 101–118.

Jerger, S., Lewis, S., Hawkins, J., & Jerger, J. (1980). Pediatric speech intelligibility test I. Generation of test materials. *International Journal of Pediatric Otohinolaryngology, 2*, 217–230.

Jirsa, R. E., Hodgson, W. R., & Goetzinger, C. P. (1975). Unreliability of half-list discrimination tests. *Journal of the American Audiology Society, 1*, 47–49.

Johnson, C., & Bordenink, R. (1978). Bone conduction speech reception thresholds with the mentally retarded. *Journal of Auditory Research, 18*, 229–235.

Johnson, E. W. (1968). Auditory findings in 200 cases of acoustic neurinomas. *Archives of Otolaryngology, 88*, 598–603.

Johnson, E. W. (1979). Results of auditory tests in acoustic tumor patients. In W. F. House & C. M. Leutje (Eds.), *Acoustic tumors: Vol 1. Diagnosis* (pp. 209–224). Baltimore: University Park Press.

Jones, J. H., & Knudsen, V. O. (1924). Functional tests of hearing. *Journal of Laryngology, 39*, 1–16.

Kalikow, D. N., Stevens, K. N., & Elliot, L. L. (1977). Development of a test of speech intelligibility in noise using sentence materials with controlled word predictability. *Journal of the Acoustical Society of America, 61*, 1337–1351.

Kamm, C., Carterette, E. C., Morgan, D. E., & Dirks, D. D. (1980). Use of digitized speech materials in audiological research. *Journal of Speech and Hearing Research, 23*, 709–721.

Kamm, C., Dirks, D. D., & Bell, T. S. (1985). Speech recognition and the articulation index for normal and hearing impaired listeners. *Journal of the Acoustical Society of America, 77*, 281–288.

Kamm, C. A., Morgan, D. E., & Dirks, D. D. (1983). Accuracy of adaptive procedure estimates of PB-max level. *Journal of Speech and Hearing Disorders, 48*, 202–209.

Karlsen, E. A., & Goetzinger, C. P. (1980). An evaluation of speech audiometry by bone conduction in hearing impaired adults. *Journal of Auditory Research, 20*, 89–95.

Kadsen, S. D., & Robinson, M. (1973). Bone conduction speech discrimination in different pathologies. *Journal of Auditory Research, 13*, 268–270.

Katinsky, S. J., Lovrinic, J., & Buchheit, W. (1972). Cochlear findings in VIIIth nerve tumors. *Audiology, 11*, 213–217.

Keaster, J. (1947). A quantitative method of testing the hearing of young children. *Journal of Speech and Hearing Disorders, 12*, 159–160.

Keating, L. W. (1974). Error frequency in CID W-22 lists. Unpublished data. Rochester, MN: Mayo Clinic.

Keith, R. W., & Talis, H. P. (1970). The use of speech in noise in diagnostic audiometry. *Journal of Auditory Research, 10*, 201–204.

Klodd, D. A., & Edgerton, B. J. (1977). Occlusion effect: Bone conduction speech audiometry using forehead and mastoid placement. *Audiology, 16*, 522–529.

Kopra, L. L., Blosser, B., & Waldron, D. L. (1968). Comparison of Fairbanks Rhyme Test and CID Auditory Test W-22 in normal and hearing-impaired listeners. *Journal of Speech and Hearing Research, 11*, 735–739.

Koval, C. B., & Stelmachowicz, P. G. (1983). Clinical validity of speech band audiometry. *Journal of Speech and Hearing Disorders, 48*, 328–329.

Kruel, E. J., Bell, D. W., & Nixon, J. C. (1969). Factors affecting speech discrimination test difficulty. *Journal of Speech and Hearing Research, 12*, 281–287.

Kruel, E. J., Nixon, J. C., Kryter, K. D., Bell, D. W., Lang, J. S., & Schubert, E. D. (1968). A proposed clinical test of speech discrimination. *Journal of Speech and Hearing Research, 11*, 536–552.

Kryter, K. D., & Whitman, E. C. (1965). Some comparisons between rhyme and PB word intelligibility tests. *Journal of the Acoustical Society of America, 37*, 1146.

Kryter, K. D., Williams, C., & Green, D. M. (1962). Auditory acuity and the perception of speech. *Journal of the Acoustical Society of America, 34*, 1217–1223.

Lamb, S. H., Owens, E., & Schubert, E. D. (1983). The revised form of the hearing performance inventory. *Ear and Hearing, 4*, 152–157.

Lehiste, I., & Peterson, G. E. (1959). Linguistic considerations in the study of speech intelligibility. *Journal of the Acoustical Society of America, 31*, 280–286.

Lerman, J. W., Ross, M., & McLauchlin, R. M. (1965). A picture-identification test for hearing-impaired children. *Journal of Auditory Research, 5*, 273–278.

Levitt, H. (1971). Transformed up-down methods in psychoacoustics. *Journal of the Acoustical Society of America, 49*, 467–477.

Levitt, H., & Rabiner, L. R. (1967). Use of sequential strategy in intelligibility. *Journal of the Acoustical Society of America, 42*, 609–612.

Levitt, H., & Resnick, S. B. (1978). Speech reception by the hearing-impaired: Methods of testing and the development of new tests. *Scandinavian Audiology*, (Supplement 6), 107–130.

LeZak, R. J., Siegenthaler, B. M., & Davis, A. I. (1964). Bekesy-type audiometry for speech reception threshold. *Journal of Auditory Research, 4*, 181–189.

Libby, E. R. (1986). The ⅓-⅔ insertion gain hearing aid selection guide. *Hearing Instruments, 37*(3), 27–28.

Lichtenstein, M. J., Bess, F. H., & Logan, S. A. (1988). Diagnostic performance of the hearing handicap inventory for the elderly (screening version) against differing definitions of hearing loss. *Ear and Hearing, 9,* 208–211.

Liden, G. (1954). Speech audiometry, an experimental and clinical study with Swedish language material. *Acta Oto-Laryngologica* (Supplement 114).

Liden, G. (1967). Undistorted speech audiometry. In A. B. Graham (Ed.), *Sensorineural hearing processes and disorders* (pp. 339–357). Boston: Little, Brown.

Loven, F. C., & Hawkins, D. B. (1983). Interlist equivalency of CID W-22 word lists presented in quiet and in noise. *Ear and Hearing, 4,* 91–97.

Lovrinic, J. H., Burgi, E. J., & Curry, E. T. (1968). A comparative evaluation of five speech discrimination measures. *Journal of Speech and Hearing Research, 11,* 372–381.

Ludvigsen, C. (1987). Prediction of speech intelligibility for normal-hearing and cochlear hearing-impaired listeners. *Journal of the Acoustical Society of America, 82,* 1162–1171.

Lutman, M. E., Brown, E. J., & Coles, R. R. A. (1987). Self-reported disability and handicap in the population in relation to pure-tone threshold, age, sex, and type of hearing loss. *British Journal of Audiology, 21,* 45–58.

Lybarger, S. F. (1944). [Patent application SN 543, 278].

Mackie, K., & Dermody, P. (1986). Use of a monosyllabic adaptive speech test (MAST) with young children. *Journal of Speech and Hearing Research, 29,* 275–281.

Margolis, R. H., & Millin, J. P. (1971). An item-difficulty based speech discrimination test. *Journal of Speech and Hearing Research, 14,* 865–873.

Marshall, L., & Bacon, S. P. (1981). Prediction of speech discrimination scores from audiometric data. *Ear and Hearing, 2,* 148–155.

Martin, F. N., Bailey, H. A., Jr., & Pappas, J. J. (1965). The effect of central masking on threshold for speech. *Journal of Auditory Research, 5,* 293–296.

Martin, F. N., & Coombs, S. (1976). A tangibly reinforced speech reception threshold procedure for use with small children. *Journal of Speech and Hearing Disorders, 41,* 333–338.

Martin, F. N., & Forbis, N. K. (1978). The present status of audiometric practice: A follow-up study. *Asha, 20,* 531–541.

Martin, F. N., Hawkins, R. R., & Bailey, H. A. T. (1962). The non-essentiality of the carrier phrase in phonetically balanced (PB) word testing. *Journal of Auditory Research, 2,* 319–322.

Martin, F. N., & Mussell, S. A. (1979). The influence of pauses in the competing signal on synthetic sentence identification scores. *Journal of Speech and Hearing Disorders, 44,* 282–292.

Martin, F. N., & Pennington, C. D. (1971). Current trends in audiometric practices. *Asha, 13,* 671–677.

Martin, F. N., & Sides, D. (1985). Survey of current audiometric practices. *Asha, 27*(2), 29–36.

Martin, F. N., & Stauffer, M. L. (1975). A modification of the Tillman–Olsen method for obtaining speech reception threshold. *Journal of Speech and Hearing Disorders, 40,* 25–28.

Matkin, N. D. (1968). The child with a marked high frequency hearing impairment. *Pediatric Clinics of North America, 15,* 677–690.

Matkin, N. D. (1977). Hearing aids for children. In W. R. Hodgson & P. H. Skinner (Eds.), *Hearing aid assessment and use in audiologic habilitation* (pp. 145–169). Baltimore: Williams & Wilkins.

McCandless, G. A., & Lyregaard, P. E. (1983). Prescription of gain/output (POGO) for hearing aids. *Hearing Instruments, 34*(1), 16–17, 19–21.

McCartney, J. H., Maurer, J. E., & Sorenson, F. D. (1976). A comparison of the hearing handicap scale with standard audiometric measures on a geriatric population. *Journal of Auditory Research, 16,* 51–58.

McFarlan, D. (1940). Speech hearing and speech interpretation testing. *Archives of Otolaryngology, 31,* 517–528.

McFarlan, D. (1945). Speech hearing tests. *The Laryngoscope, 55,* 71–115.

McLennan, R. O., Jr., & Knox, A. W. (1975). Patient-controlled delivery of monosyllabic words in a test of auditory discrimination. *Journal of Speech and Hearing Disorders, 40,* 538–543.

McNamee, J. (1960). *An investigation of the use of CID Auditory Test W-22 with children.* Unpublished master's thesis, Ohio State University, Columbus.

McPherson, D. F., & Pang-Ching, G. K. (1979). Development of a distinctive feature discrimination test. *Journal of Auditory Research, 19,* 235–246.

Merrell, H. B., & Atkinson, C. J. (1965). The effect of selected variables upon discrimination scores. *Journal of Auditory Research, 5,* 285–292.

Merrell, H. B., Wolfe, D. L., & McLemore, D. C. (1973). Air and bone conducted speech reception thresholds. *The Laryngoscope, 83,* 1929–1939.

Meyer, D., & Mishler, E. T. (1985). Rollover measurements with Auditec NU-6 word lists. *Journal of Speech and Hearing Disorders, 50,* 356–360.

Meyerson, L. (1956). Hearing for speech in children: A verbal audiometric test. *Acta Oto-Laryngologica,* (Supplement 128), 1–165.

Miller, G. A., Heise, G. A., & Lichten, W. (1951). The intelligibility of speech as a function of the context of the test materials. *Journal of Experimental Psychology, 41,* 329–335.

Miner, R., & Danhauer, J. L. (1976). Modified rhyme test and synthetic sentence identification test scores of normal and hearing-impaired subjects listening in a multitalker noise. *Journal of the American Audiology Society, 2,* 61–74.

Morgan, D. E., Kamm, C. A., & Velde, T. M. (1981). Form equivalence of the speech perception in noise (SPIN) test. *Journal of the Acoustical Society of America, 69,* 1791–1798.

Mueller, W. (1953). The fitting of hearing aids as an office procedure. *The Laryngoscope, 63,* 581–592.

Nelson, D. A., & Chaiklin, J. B. (1970). Writedown versus talkback scoring and scoring bias in speech discrimination testing. *Journal of Speech and Hearing Research, 13,* 645–654.

Newby, H. A. (1958). *Audiology: Principles and Practice.* New York: Appleton-Century-Crofts.

Newman, C. W., & Weinstein, B. E. (1988). The hearing handicap inventory for the elderly as a measure of hearing aid benefit. *Ear and Hearing, 9,* 81–85.

Niemeyer, W. (1965). Speech audiometry with phonetically balanced sentences. *International Audiology, 4,* 97–101.

Nixon, J. C. (1973). Investigation of the response foils of the modified rhyme hearing test. *Journal of Speech and Hearing Research, 16,* 658–666.

Noble, W. G. (1979). The hearing measurement scale as a paper-pencil form: Preliminary results. *Journal of the American Auditory Society, 5,* 95–106.

Noble, W. G., & Atherly, G. R. C. (1970). The hearing measurement scale: A questionnaire for the assessment of auditory disability. *Journal of Auditory Research*, 10, 229–250.

Northern, J. L., & Hattler, K. W. (1974). Evaluation of four speech discrimination tests/procedures on hearing impaired patients. *Journal of Auditory Research Supplement*, 1–37.

Oja, G. L., & Schow, R. L. (1984). Hearing aid evaluation based on measures of benefit, use and satisfaction. *Ear and Hearing*, 5, 77–86.

Olsen, W. O. (1965). [Intelligibility of spondees]. Unpublished data. Evanston, IL: Northwestern University.

Olsen, W. O. (1970). Presbycusis and hearing aid use. *Journal of the Academy of Rehabilitative Audiology*, 3, 34–42.

Olsen, W. O., & Carhart, R. (1967). Development of test procedures for evaluation of binaural hearing aids. *Bulletin of Prosthetics Research*, 10(7), 22–49.

Olsen, W. O., Hawkins, D. B., & Van Tasell, D. J. (1987). Representations of the long-term spectra of speech. *Ear and Hearing*, 8 (Supplement), 100S–108S.

Olsen, W. O., Noffsinger, D., & Kurdziel, S. (1975). Speech discrimination in quiet and in white noise by patients with peripheral and central lesions. *Acta Oto-Laryngologica*, 80, 375–382.

Olsen, W. O., & Tillman, T. W. (1968). Hearing aids and sensorineural hearing loss. *Annals of Otology, Rhinology and Laryngology*, 77, 717–726.

Olsen, W. O., Van Tasell, D. J., & Speaks, C. E. (1982a). *Preparation of isophonemic word list and sentence materials.* Paper presented at the annual convention of the American Speech-Language-Hearing Association, Toronto, Canada.

Olsen, W. O., Van Tasell, D. J., & Speaks, C. E. (1982b). *Evaluation of isophonemic word list and sentence materials.* Paper presented at the annual convention of the American Speech-Language-Hearing Association, Toronto, Canada.

Olsen, W. O., Van Tasell, D. J., & Speaks, C. E. (1983). *Further evaluation of isophonemic word list and sentence materials.* Paper presented at the annual convention of the American Speech-Language-Hearing Association, Cincinnati, OH.

Olsen, W. O., Van Tasell, D. J., & Speaks, C. E. (1986a). *List equivalence of isophonemic word lists.* Paper presented at the annual convention of the American Speech-Language-Hearing Association, Detroit, MI.

Olsen, W. O., Van Tasell, D. J., & Speaks, C. E. (1986b). *Comparison of scores for words in isolation and in sentences.* Paper presented at the annual convention of the American-Speech-Language-Hearing Association, Detroit, MI.

O'Neill, J. J. (1957). Recognition and intelligibility test materials in context and isolation. *Journal of Speech and Hearing Disorders*, 22, 87–90.

O'Neill, J. J., & Oyer, H. H. (1966). *Applied audiometry.* New York: Dodd, Mead.

Orchik, D. J., Krygier, K. M., & Cutts, B. P. (1979). A comparison of the NU-6 and W-22 speech discrimination tests for assessing sensorineural hearing loss. *Journal of Speech and Hearing Disorders*, 44, 522–527.

Orchik, D., & Oyer, H. (1972). A modified traditional hearing aid evaluation. *Journal of Auditory Research*, 12, 8–13.

Orchik, D. J., & Roddy, N. (1980). The SSI and NU6 in clinical hearing aid evaluation. *Journal of Speech and Hearing Disorders*, 45, 401–407.

Owens, E. (1978). Consonant errors and remediation of sensorineural hearing loss. *Journal of Speech and Hearing Disorders*, 43, 331–344.

Owens, E. (1961). Intelligibility of words varying in familiarity. *Journal of Speech and Hearing Research*, 4, 113–129.

Owens, E., Benedict, M., & Schubert, E. D. (1971). Further investigation of vowel items in multiple-choice speech discrimination testing. *Journal of Speech and Hearing Research, 14*, 841–847.

Owens, E., Benedict, M., & Schubert, E. D. (1972). Consonant phonemic errors associated with pure tone configurations and certain kinds of hearing impairment. *Journal of Speech and Hearing Research, 15*, 308–322.

Owens, E., Kessler, D. K., Raggio, M. W., & Schubert, E. D. (1985). Analysis and revision of minimal auditory capabilities (MAC) battery. *Ear and Hearing, 6*, 280–290.

Owens, E., Kessler, D. K., Telleen, C. C., & Schubert, E. D. (1981, September). The minimal auditory capabilities battery (MAC). *Hearing Aid Journal, 34*, 9, 32, 34.

Owens, E., & Raggio, M. (1988). Hearing performance inventory for profound and severe loss (PIPSL). *Journal of Speech and Hearing Disorders, 53*, 42–56.

Owens, E., & Schubert, E. D. (1968). The development of consonant items for speech discrimination testing. *Journal of Speech and Hearing Research, 11*, 656–667.

Owens, E., & Schubert, E. D. (1977). Development of the California consonant test. *Journal of Speech and Hearing Research, 20*, 463–474.

Owens, E., Talbott, C. B., & Schubert, E. D. (1968). Vowel discrimination of hearing impaired listeners. *Journal of Speech and Hearing Research, 11*, 648–655.

Oyer, J. J., & Doudna, M. (1959). Structural analysis of word responses made by hard of hearing subjects on a discrimination test. *Archives of Otolaryngology, 70*, 357–363.

Pascoe, D. P. (1975). Frequency responses of hearing aids and their effects on the speech perception of hearing impaired subjects. *Annals of Otology, Rhinology and Laryngology Supplement, 23*, 1–40.

Pascoe, D. P. (1978). An approach to hearing aid selection. *Hearing Instruments, 29*(6), 12–16, 36.

Pascoe, D. P. (1980). Clinical implications of nonverbal methods of hearing aid selection and fitting. *Seminars in Speech Language and Hearing, 1*, 217–229.

Pavlovic, C. V. (1984). Use of the articulation index for assessing residual auditory function in listeners with sensorineural hearing impairment. *Journal of the Acoustical Society of America, 75*, 1253–1258.

Pavlovic, C. V. (1988). Articulation index predictions of speech intelligibility. *Asha, 30*(7), 63–65.

Pavlovic, C. V., Studebaker, G. A., & Sherbecoe, R. L. (1985). Articulation index based procedure for predicting speech recognition performance of hearing impaired individuals. *Journal of the Acoustical Society of America, 80*, 50–57.

Pederson, O. T., & Studebaker, G. A. (1972). A new minimal contrasts closed-response-set speech test. *Journal of Auditory Research, 12*, 187–195.

Penrod, J. (1979). Talker effects on word discrimination scores of adults with sensorineural hearing impairment. *Journal of Speech and Hearing Disorders, 44*, 340–349.

Peterson, G., & Lehiste, I. (1962). Revised CNC lists for auditory tests. *Journal of Speech and Hearing Disorders, 27*, 62–70.

Plant, G. (1984). A diagnostic speech test for severely and profoundly hearing-impaired children. *Australian Journal of Audiology, 6*, 1–10.

Posner, J., & Ventry, I. M. (1977). Relationships between comfortable loudness levels for speech and speech discrimination in sensorineural hearing loss. *Journal of Speech and Hearing Disorders, 42*, 370–375.

Pratt, R. L. (1981). On the use of reaction time as a measure of intelligibility. *British Journal of Audiology, 15,* 253–255.

Preminger, J., & Wiley, T. L. (1985). Frequency selectivity and consonant intelligibility in sensorineural hearing loss. *Journal of Speech and Hearing Research, 28,* 197–206.

Quiggle, R. R., Glorig, A., Delk, J. H., & Summerfield, A. B. (1957). Predicting hearing loss for speech from pure tone audiograms. *The Laryngoscope, 67,* 1–15.

Raffin, M. J. M., & Schafer, D. (1980). Application of a probability model based on the binomial distribution to speech discrimination scores. *Journal of Speech and Hearing Research, 23,* 570–575.

Raffin, M. J. M., & Thornton, A. R. (1980). Confidence levels for differences between speech discrimination scores. *Journal of Speech and Hearing Research, 23,* 5–18.

Resnick, D. M. (1962). Reliability of the twenty-five word phonetically balanced lists. *Journal of Auditory Research, 2,* 5–12.

Resnick, S. B., Dubno, J. R., Hoffnung, S., & Levitt, H. (1976). Phoneme errors on a nonsense syllable test. *Journal of the Acoustical Society of America, 58,* Supplement 1, 114.

Rintelmann, W. F., & Associates. (1974). Six experiments on speech discrimination utilizing CNC monosyllables. *Journal of Auditory Research, 2,* Supplement, 1–30.

Robinson, D. O., & Koenigs, M. J. (1979). A comparison of procedures and materials for speech reception thresholds. *Journal of the American Auditory Society, 4,* 227–230.

Rose, D. E., Schreurs, K. K., & Miller, K. E. (1979, Winter). A ten-word speech discrimination screening test. *Audiology and Hearing Education,* pp. 15–16.

Ross, M., Huntington, D. A., Newby, H. A., & Nixon, R. F. (1965). Speech discrimination of hearing impaired individuals in noise: Its relationship to other audiometric parameters. *Journal of Auditory Research, 5,* 47–72.

Ross, M., & Lerman, J. (1970). Picture identification test for hearing-impaired children. *Journal of Speech and Hearing Research, 13,* 44–53.

Rowland, J. P., Dirks, D. D., Dubno, J. R., & Bell, T. S.(1985). Comparison of speech-recognition-in-noise and subjective communication assessment. *Ear and Hearing, 6,* 291–296.

Rubin, M., & Ventry, I. M. (1972). The use of Bekesy audiometry in the measurement of intelligibility for connected discourse. *Journal of Auditory Research, 12,* 255–260.

Rudmin, F. (1987). Speech reception thresholds for digits. *Journal of Auditory Research, 27,* 15–21.

Runge, C. A., & Hosford-Dunn, H. L. (1985). Word recognition performance with modified CID W-22 word lists. *Journal of Speech and Hearing Research, 28,* 355–362.

Sanders, D. A. (1975). Hearing aid orientation and counseling. In M. Pollack (Ed.), *Amplification for the hearing impaired* (pp. 323-372). New York: Grune & Stratton.

Sanderson-Leepa, M. E., & Rintelmann, W. F. (1976). Articulation function and test-retest performance of normal-hearing children on three speech discrimination tests: WIPI, PBK 50, and NU Auditory Test No. 6. *Journal of Speech and Hearing Disorders, 41,* 503–519.

Schow, R. L., & Nerbonne, M. A. (1982). Communication screening profile: Use with elderly patients. *Ear and Hearing, 3,* 135–147.

Schuknecht, H. F., & Woellner, R. (1955). An experimental and clinical study of deafness from lesions of the cochlear nerve. *Journal of Laryngology and Otology, 69,* 75–97.

Schultz, M. C. (1964a). Suggested improvement in speech discrimination testing. *Journal of Auditory Research, 4,* 1–14.

Schultz, M. C. (1964b). Word familiarity influences in speech discrimination. *Journal of Speech and Hearing Research, 7,* 395–400.

Schultz, M. C., & Schubert, E. D. (1969). A multiple choice discrimination test (MCDT). *The Laryngoscope, 79,* 382–399.

Schwartz, D. (1971). *The usefulness of the WIPI-A speech discrimination test for preschool children.* Unpublished master's thesis, Central Michigan University, Mount Pleasant, MI.

Schwartz, D. M. (1982). Hearing aid selection methods: An enigma. In G. A. Studebaker & F. H. Bess (Eds.), *The Vanderbilt hearing aid report* (pp. 180–187). Upper Darby, PA: Monographs in Contemporary Audiology.

Schwartz, D. M., Bess, F. H., & Larson, V. D. (1977). Split half reliability of two word discrimination tests as function of primary-to-secondary ratio. *Journal of Speech and Hearing Disorders, 42,* 440–445.

Schwartz, D. M., Lyregaard, P. E., & Lundh, P. (1988). Hearing aid selection for severe-to-profound hearing loss. *Hearing Journal, 41,* 13–17.

Schwartz, D. M., & Surr, R. (1979). Three experiments on the California consonant test. *Journal of Speech and Hearing Disorders, 64,* 61–72.

Schwartz, D. M., & Walden, B. E. (1983). Speech audiometry and hearing aid assessment: A reappraisal of an old philosophy. In D. Konkle & W. F. Rintelmann (Eds.), *Principles of speech audiometry* (pp. 321–352). Baltimore: University Park Press.

Seavertson, J. M., & McLennan, R. O., Jr. (1983). Response time and percentage correct as measures of hearing aid performance. *Journal of Speech and Hearing Disorders, 48,* 409–414.

Sergeant, L., Atkinson, J. E., & Lacroix, P. G. (1979). The NSMRL tri-word test of intelligibility. *Journal of the Acoustical Society of America, 65,* 218–222.

Shapiro, M. T., Melnick, W., & Ver Muelen, V. (1972). Effects of modulated noise on speech intelligibility of people with sensorineural hearing loss. *Annals of Otology, Rhinology and Laryngology, 81,* 241–248.

Sher, A. E., & Owens, E. (1974). Consonant confusions associated with hearing loss above 2000 Hz. *Journal of Speech and Hearing Research, 17,* 669–681.

Shirinian, M. J., & Arnst, D. J. (1980). PI-PB rollover in a group of aged listeners. *Ear and Hearing, 1,* 50–53.

Shore, I., Bilger, R. C., & Hirsh, I. (1960). Hearing aid evaluation: Reliability of repeat measurements. *Journal of Speech and Hearing Disorders, 25,* 152–170.

Shutts, R., Burke, K., & Creston, J. (1964). Derivation of twenty-five word PB lists. *Journal of Speech and Hearing Disorders, 29,* 442–447.

Siegenthaler, B., & Haspiel, G. (1966). *Development of two standardized measures of hearing for speech by children* (Project No. OE-5-10-003). Washington, DC: U.S. Department of Health, Education and Welfare.

Siegenthaler, B., Pearson, J., & LeZak, R. (1954). A speech reception threshold test for children. *Journal of Speech and Hearing Disorders, 19,* 360–366.

Siegenthaler, B. M., & Strand, R. (1964). Audiogram-average methods and SRT scores. *Journal of the Acoustical Society of America, 36,* 589–593.

Silverman, S. R., & Hirsh, I. J. (1955). Problems related to the use of speech in clinical audiometry. *Annals of Otology, Rhinology and Laryngology, 64,* 1234–1244.

Silverman, S. R., Thurlow, W. R., Walsh, T. E., & Davis, H. (1948). Improvement in the social adequacy index of hearing following the fenestration operation. *The Laryngoscope, 58,* 607–631.

Skinner, M. W. (1984). Recent advances in hearing aid selection and adjustment. *Annals of Otology, Rhinology and Laryngology, 93,* 569–575.

Skinner, M. W. (1988). *Hearing aid evaluation.* Engelwood Cliffs, NJ: Prentice Hall.

Skinner, M. W., Karstaedt, M. M., & Miller, J. D. (1982). Amplification bandwidth and speech intelligibility for two listeners with sensorineural hearing loss. *Audiology, 21,* 251–268.

Skinner, M. W., & Miller, J. D. (1983). Amplification bandwidth and intelligibility of speech in quiet and noise for listeners with sensorineural hearing loss. *Audiology, 22,* 253–279.

Skinner, M. W., Pascoe, D. P., Miller, J. D., & Popelka, G. (1982). Measurements to determine the optimal placement of speech energy within the listener's auditory area: A basis for selecting amplification characteristics. In G. A. Studebaker & F. H. Bess (Eds.), *The Vanderbilt hearing aid report* (pp. 161–169). Upper Darby, PA: Monographs in Contemporary Audiology.

Smaldino, J. J., & Myers, C. K. (1971). *Differences between word intelligibility and sentence identification responses to "synthetic" sentences.* Groton, CT: Navy Submarine Medical Research Laboratory Report No. 683.

Smith, K. E. (1970). *An experimental study of the effects of systematic reinforcement on the discrimination responses of normal and hearing impaired children.* Unpublished doctoral dissertation, University of Kansas, Lawrence.

Smith, K. E., & Hodgson, W. (1970). The effects of systematic reinforcement on speech discrimination responses of normal and hearing impaired children. *Journal of Auditory Research, 10,* 110–117.

Sortini, A. J., & Flake, C. G. (1953). Speech audiometry testing for pre-school children. *The Laryngoscope, 63,* 991–997.

Speaks, C. (1967). Performance-intensity characteristics of selected verbal materials. *Journal of Speech and Hearing Research, 10,* 344–353.

Speaks, C., & Jerger, J. (1965). Performance-intensity characteristics of synthetic sentences. *Journal of Speech and Hearing Research, 9,* 305–312.

Speaks, C., & Jerger, J. (1966). Method for measurement of speech identification. *Journal of Speech and Hearing Research, 10,* 344–353.

Speaks, C., Jerger, J., & Trammell, J. (1970a). Comparison of sentence identification and conventional speech discrimination scores. *Journal of Speech and Hearing Research, 13,* 755–767.

Speaks, C., Jerger, J., & Trammell, J. (1970b). Measurement of hearing handicap. *Journal of Speech and Hearing Research, 13,* 768–776.

Speaks, C., Karmen, J. L, & Benitez, L. (1967). Effect of competing message on synthetic sentence identification. *Journal of Speech and Hearing Research, 11,* 390–396.

Speaks, C., Parker, B., Harris, C., & Kuhl, P. (1972). Intelligibility of connected discourse. *Journal of Speech and Hearing Research, 15,* 590–602.

Spearman, C. (1908). The method of "right and wrong cases" ("constant stimuli") without Guass's formulae. *British Journal of Psychology, 2,* 227–242.

Srinivasson, K. P. (1974). Bone conducted speech reception threshold. An investigation with the Oticon A 20 bone vibrator calibrated on the Bruel and Kjaer artificial mastoid. *Scandinavian Audiology, 3,* 145–148.

Steinberg, J. C., & Gardner, M. B. (1940). On the auditory significance of the term hearing loss. *Journal of the Acoustical Society of America, 11,* 270–277.

Stevenson, P. W. (1975). Responses to speech audiometry and phonemic discrimination patterns in the elderly. *Audiology, 14,* 185–231.

Stevenson, P. W., & Martin, M. C. (1977). Adaptive speech audiometry and speech discrimination space in hearing-impaired subjects. *Audiology, 16,* 110–123.

Stream, R. W., & Dirks, D. D. (1974). Effect of loudspeaker position on differences between earphone and free-field thresholds (MAP and MAF). *Journal of Speech and Hearing Research, 17,* 549–568.

Studebaker, G. A. (1985). A "rationalized" arcsine transform. *Journal of Speech and Hearing Research, 28,* 455–462.

Surr, R. K., & Schwartz, D. M. (1980). Effects of multi-talker competing speech on the variability of the California consonant test. *Ear and Hearing, 1,* 319–323.

Surr, R. K., Siedman, J. H., Schwartz, D. M., & Mueller, H. G. (1982). Effects of audiometric configuration on speech-band thresholds in sensorineural hearing loss subjects. *Ear and Hearing, 3,* 246–250.

Tannahill, J. C. (1979). The hearing handicap scale as a measure of hearing aid benefit. *Journal of Speech and Hearing Disorders, 44,* 91–99.

Thorndike, D. L., & Lorge, I. (1944). *The teacher's word book of 30,000 words.* New York: Columbia University Press.

Thornton, A., & Raffin, M. J. M. (1978). Speech discrimination scores modeled as a binomial variable. *Journal of Speech and Hearing Research, 21,* 507–518.

Thurlow, W. R., Silverman, S. R., Davis, H., & Walsh, T. E. (1948). A statistical study of auditory tests in relation to the fenestration operation. *The Laryngoscope, 58,* 43–66.

Tillman, T. W., & Carhart, R. (1966). *An expanded test for speech discrimination utilizing CNC monosyllabic words. Northwestern University Auditory Test No. 6.* Brooks Air Force Base, TX: USAF School of Aerospace Medicine Technical Report.

Tillman, T. W., Carhart, R., & Olsen, W. O. (1970). Hearing aid efficiency in a competing speech situation. *Journal of Speech and Hearing Research, 13,* 789–811.

Tillman, T. W., Carhart, R., & Wilber, L. (1963). *A test for speech discrimination composed of CNC monosyllabic words. Northwestern University Auditory Test No. 4.* (Technical Documentary Report No. SAM-TDR-62-135). Brooks Air Force Base, TX: USAF School of Aerospace Medicine.

Tillman, T. W., & Jerger, J. F. (1959). Some factors affecting the spondee threshold in normal-hearing subjects. *Journal of Speech and Hearing Research, 2,* 141–146.

Tillman, T. W., Johnson, R. M., & Olsen, W. O. (1966). Earphone versus sound-field threshold sound pressure level for spondee words. *Journal of the Acoustical Society of America, 39,* 125–133.

Tillman, T. W., & Olsen, W. O. (1973). Speech audiometry. In J. Jerger (Ed.), *Modern developments in audiology* (pp. 37–74. 2nd Ed.). New York: Academic Press.

Tobias, J. V. (1959). Relative occurrence of phonemes in American English. *Journal of the Acoustical Society of America, 31,* 631.

Tobias, J. V. (1964). On phonemic analysis of speech discrimination tests. *Journal of Speech and Hearing Research, 7,* 98–100.

Townsend, T., & Schwartz, D. M. (1981). Error analysis on the California consonant test by manner of articulation. *Ear and Hearing, 2,* 108–111.

Tyler, R. (1979). Measuring hearing loss in the future. *British Journal of Audiology Supplement, 2,* 29–40.

Tyler, R. S., Gantz, B. J., McCabe, B. F., Lowder, M. V., Otto, S. R., & Preece, J. P. (1985). Audiological results with two single channel cochlear implants. *Annals of Otology, Rhinology and Laryngology, 94,* 133–139.

Tyler, R. S., & Smith, P. A. (1983). Sentence identification in noise and hearing handicap questionnaires. *Scandinavian Audiology, 12,* 285–292.

Tyler, R. S., Summerfield, Q., Wood, E. J., & Fernandes, M. A. (1982). Psychoacoustics and phonetic temporal processing in normal and hearing impaired listeners. *Journal of the Acoustical Society of America, 72,* 740–752.

Tyler, R. S., Wood, E. J., & Fernandes, M. (1982). Frequency resolution of hearing loss. *British Journal of Audiology, 16,* 45–63.

Ullrich, K., & Grimm, D. (1976). Most comfortable listening level presentation versus maximum discrimination for word discrimination material. *Audiology, 15,* 338–347.

Van Tasell, D. J., & Yanz, J. L. (1987). Speech recognition threshold in noise: Effects of hearing loss, frequency response and speech materials. *Journal of Speech and Hearing Research, 30,* 377–386.

Ventry, I. M. (1976). Pure tone-spondee threshold relationships in functional hearing loss. *Journal of Speech and Hearing Disorders, 41,* 16–22.

Ventry, I. M., & Weinstein, B. E. (1982). The hearing handicap inventory for the elderly: A new tool. *Ear and Hearing, 3,* 128–134.

Walden, B. E., Schwartz, D. M., Montgomery, A. A., & Prosek, R. A. (1981). A comparison of the effects of hearing impairment and acoustic filtering on consonant recognition. *Journal of Speech and Hearing Research, 24,* 32–43.

Walden, B. E., Schwartz, D. M., Williams, D. L., Holum-Hardegen, L. L., & Crowley, J. M. (1983). Test of assumptions underlying comparative hearing aid evaluations. *Journal of Speech and Hearing Disorders, 48,* 264–273.

Walker, J., & Boothroyd, A. (1987). *Speech audiometry: Plotting P/I function in a clinically acceptable time.* Paper presented at the annual convention of the American Speech-Language-Hearing Association, New Orleans, LA.

Wall, L. G., Davis, L. A., & Myers, D. K. (1984). Four spondee threshold procedures: A comparison. *Ear and Hearing, 5,* 171–174.

Walsh, T. E., & Goodman, A. (1955). Speech discrimination in central auditory lesions. *The Laryngoscope, 65,* 1–8.

Watson, T. J. (1967). *The education of hearing-handicapped children.* Springfield, IL: Charles C. Thomas.

Watson, N. A., & Knudsen, V. O. (1940). Selective amplification in hearing aids. *Journal of the Acoustical Society of America, 11,* 406–419.

Weber, S., & Reddell, R. C. (1976). A sentence test for measuring speech discrimination in children. *Audiology and Hearing Education, 2,* 25, 30, 40.

Weinstein, B. E., Spitzer, J., & Ventry, I. M. (1986). Test-retest reliability of the hearing handicap inventory for the elderly. *Ear and Hearing, 3,* 128–134.

Weinstein, B. E., & Ventry, I. M. (1983). Audiologic correlation of hearing handicap in the elderly. *Journal of Speech and Hearing Research, 26,* 148–151.

Weinstein, B. E., & Ventry, I. M. (1982). Hearing impairment and social isolation in the elderly. *Journal of Speech and Hearing Research, 25,* 593–599.

Wilson, R. H., & Antablin, J. K. (1980). A picture identification task as an estimate of word-recognition performance of noverbal adults. *Journal of Speech and Hearing Disorders, 45,* 223–238.

Wilson, R. H., Coley, K. E., Haenel, J. L., & Browning, K. M. (1976). Northwestern University Auditory Test No. 6: Normative and comparative intelligibility functions. *Journal of the American Audiology Society, 1,* 221–228.

Wilson, R. H., Hopkins, J., Mance, C., & Novak, R. (1982). Detection and recognition masking-level difference for individual CID W-1 spondaic words. *Journal of Speech and Hearing Research, 25,* 235–242.

Wilson, R. H., Morgan, D. E., & Dirks, D. D. (1973). A proposed SRT procedure and its statistical precedent. *Journal of Speech and Hearing Disorders, 38,* 184–191.

Wilson, R. H., Shanks, J. E., & Koebsell, K. A. (1982). Recognition masking-level differences for 10 CID W-1 spondaic words. *Journal of Speech and Hearing Research, 25,* 624–628.

Wilson, W. C., & Gaeth, J. H. (1976). *Digits versus spondees for measurement of speech reception threshold.* Paper presented at the annual convention of the American Speech-Language-Hearing Association, Houston, TX.

Yoshioka, P., & Thornton, A. R. (1980). Predicting speech discrimination from the audiometric threshold. *Journal of Speech and Hearing Research, 23,* 814–827.

Young, L. L., Jr., Dudley, B., & Gunter, M. B. (1982). Thresholds and psychometric functions of individual spondaic words. *Journal of Speech and Hearing Research, 25,* 586–593.

Young, M. A., & Gibbons, E. W. (1962). Speech discrimination scores and threshold measurements in a non-normal hearing population. *Journal of Auditory Research, 2,* 21–23.

APPENDIX

Guidelines for Various SRT Procedures

Investigator	Initial Trial					Threshold Search				
	Method	Starting Level	Words Per Level	Step Size (dB)	Termination	Starting Level	Words Per Level	Step Size (dB)	Termination	Threshold Criterion
Hudgins et al. (1947) PAL No. 9	Descending					<24 dB above expected threshold	6	4	Administer at least 2 lists; if thresholds within 4 dB terminate tests; if not, continue	Count words correct and consult table for dB equivalent. Subtract from starting point, and average for 2 lists
Hirsh et al. (1952) CID W-2	Descending					<33 dB above expected threshold	3	3	Not stated	Subtract number of words correct from starting level and add 1.5 dB for 50% criterion
Newby (1958)	Descending and bracketing	15 to 20 dB above estimated threshold	3-4	5		Bracketing around level at which words were missed	1-2		Not stated	Level at which about ½ of spondees missed

(Appendix continues)

APPENDIX (Continued)

Investigator	Initial Trial					Threshold Search				Threshold Criterion
	Method	Starting Level	Words Per Level	Step Size (dB)	Termination	Starting Level	Words Per Level	Step Size (dB)	Termination	
Jerger et al. (1959)	Descending and bracketing	20 to 30 dB above estimated threshold	2–3	10	Level at which 2 consecutive words were missed	Bracketing around level at which words were missed	4	2	Not stated	Lowest level at which 2 out of 4 words are repeated correctly, or level at which 3 out of 4 are correct if next lower level yielded only 1 out of 4 correct
Chaiklin (1959)	Descending		5	5	Level at which 1 word was missed	5 to 6 dB above level at which word is missed in initial descent	3–6	2	When 4 words are missed at each of 3 consecutive levels	Lowest level at which 3 out of possible 6 words are repeated correctly (threshold search repeated 3 times)
Chaiklin and Ventry (1964)	Descending	25 dB above 2-frequency pure tone average	1	5	Level at which 1 word was missed	10 dB above level at which word is missed in initial descent	3–6	5	When 4 words are missed at 2 consecutive levels	Lowest level at which 3 out of 6 possible words are repeated correctly
Chaiklin and Ventry (1964)	Descending	25 dB above 2-frequency pure tone average	1	5	Level at which 1 word was missed	5 to 6 dB above level at which word is missed in initial descent	2–4	2	When 3 words are missed at 3 consecutive levels, or no words are repeated correctly at 2 consecutive levels	Lowest level at which 2 out of 4 possible words are repeated correctly

(Appendix continues)

APPENDIX (*Continued*)

| Investigator | Method | Initial Trial | | | | Threshold Search | | | | |
		Starting Level	Words Per Level	Step Size (dB)	Termination	Starting Level	Words Per Level	Step Size (dB)	Termination	Threshold Criterion
Chaiklin, Font, and Dixon (1967)	Ascending	−10 dB HL	1	10	Level at which 1 word was repeated correctly	Decrease 20 dB below level at which 1 word is repeated correctly	3-6	5	Level at which 3 out of possible 6 words are repeated correctly	Lowest level at which 3 out of 6 possible words are repeated correctly
Hopkinson (1972)	Descending and bracketing	20 dB above 1000-Hz threshold	1	2	Level at which words missed		Varies	2	Not stated	2 dB above lowest level at which any word is repeated
Tillman and Olsen (1973)	Descending	30 to 40 dB above expected threshold	1-2	10	Level at which 2 consecutive words are missed	10 dB above level at which 2 words are missed in initial descent	2	2	If less than 5 of 6 words are repeated correctly in first 3 steps, increase level 4 to 6 dB and begin new descent; terminate when 5 of 6 consecutive words are missed	Subtract number of words repeated correctly from starting level, and add 1 dB for 50% criterion

(Appendix continues)

APPENDIX (*Continued*)

Investigator	Method	Initial Trial Starting Level	Words Per Level	Step Size (dB)	Termination	Threshold Search Starting Level	Words Per Level	Step Size (dB)	Termination	Threshold Criterion
Wilson, Morgan, and Dirks (1973)	Descending	30 to 40 dB above expected threshold	1–2	10	Level at which 2 words are missed	10 dB above level at which 2 words are missed	2 or 5	2 or 5	If less than 5 of 6 words in first 3 steps (2 dB/step) or less than all 5 words (5 dB/step) are repeated correctly, increase level 4 to 10 dB and begin new descent; terminate when 5 of 6 words (2 dB/step) or all 5 words (5 dB/step) are missed	Subtract number of words repeated correctly from starting level, and add 1 dB (2 dB/step) or 2 dB (5 dB/step) for 50% criterion
Martin and Stauffer (1975)	Descending	50 dB HL unless incorrect response, then increase in 20-dB steps	1–2	10	Same procedure as used in Tillman and Olsen	16 dB above level at which 2 words are missed in initial descent	2	2	Same procedure and criteria as used in Tillman and Olsen	Same procedure and criteria as used in Tillman and Olsen

(*Appendix continues*)

APPENDIX (*Continued*)

| Investigator | Method | Initial Trial | | | | Threshold Search | | | | |
		Starting Level	Words Per Level	Step Size (dB)	Termination	Starting Level	Words Per Level	Step Size (dB)	Termination	Threshold Criterion
ASHA (1977)	Ascending	−10 dB HL	1	10	Level at which 1 word is repeated correctly	15 dB below level at which 1 word is repeated correctly in initial ascent	4	5	Level at which at least 3 words are repeated correctly; repeat again, beginning 10 dB below level at which at least 3 words are repeated correctly; repeat above process a third time	Lowest level at which ½ of words are repeated correctly in minimum of 2 ascending series
ASHA (1988)	Descending	30–40 dB	1–2	10	Level at which 2 consecutive words are missed	10 dB above level at which 2 words were missed	2 or 5	2 or 5	Same procedure and criteria as used in Wilson, Morgan, and Dirks	Same procedure and criteria as used in Wilson, Morgan, and Dirks

chapter three

Clinical masking

JAY W. SANDERS

Contents

Although auditory masking has been defined in various ways (Studebaker, 1973), it can be regarded, for clinical purposes, as the elevation in threshold of sensitivity for one signal (the test stimulus) by a second signal (the masking noise). The importance of appropriate and accurate masking in audiometry cannot be overemphasized. Without proper masking, test results can indicate a moderate conductive impairment in an ear with a profound sensorineural loss, reasonably good word recognition in an ear with severely impaired speech discrimination, or moderate tone decay in an ear with excessive auditory adaptation.

The problem

The problem requiring the use of masking is posed by the patient with a unilateral hearing loss or an asymmetrical bilateral loss. In an attempt

141

to reach threshold of sensitivity in the poorer ear of such a patient, the intensity of the test signal may be raised to such a level that it is transmitted across the skull and heard in the better ear before it reaches threshold level in the test ear. A number of investigators (Zwislocki, 1953; Lidén, 1954; Lidén, Nilsson, & Anderson, 1959a) have shown that a pure tone stimulus presented by air conduction to an ear with a profound hearing loss may be heard in the nontest ear when the signal intensity is 50 to 60 dB above the sensorineural sensitivity of the nontest ear. Transmission of the test stimulus across the skull to the nontest ear is referred to as *cross-over*. The intensity reduction of 50 to 60 dB in an air-conduction signal from the test ear across the skull to the nontest ear is called *interaural attenuation*. For a signal presented by bone conduction, the interaural attenuation is essentially zero. Indeed, it is possible to obtain a cross-over bone-conduction threshold response at a *better* hearing threshold level (HTL) than the actual bone-conduction sensitivity in the nontest ear (Studebaker, 1964; Sanders & Rintelmann, 1964). Thus if hearing is normal in the nontest ear, cross-over response can be obtained at the 0 dB HTL to a bone-conduction signal presented to an ear with a profound sensorineural hearing loss. Furthermore, false air-conduction thresholds at 50 to 60 dB HTL can be obtained for an ear with profound sensorineural impairment even when the nontest ear has a conductive loss of equal severity. In this case the test tone presented by air conduction has reached sufficient intensity to stimulate the nontest ear by bone-conduction.

Thus without appropriate masking, the pure tone audiogram may suggest a pure conductive hearing loss in an ear with a profound sensorineural impairment. In addition, false results may be obtained in other areas of auditory assessment, such as speech audiometry and diagnostic tests.

The solution

The solution to the problem of cross-over of the auditory stimulus is to ensure that response is from the ear being tested by eliminating the possibility of response from the nontest ear. This is accomplished by presenting a masking noise to the nontest ear at sufficient intensity to shift its sensitivity to a higher HTL, thus permitting presentation of the test signal to the test ear at higher intensities without a cross-over response from the nontest ear. The magnitude of the threshold shift in the masked ear is determined by the nature and intensity of the masking noise.

The use of a masking noise, however, introduces the possibility of a new problem. Just as the test signal may cross over to the nontest ear, so may the masking noise, presented to the nontest ear, cross over and elevate threshold in the test ear. This result is known as *overmasking*. Both clinical errors, undermasking and overmasking, may result in erroneous decisions in the audiometric assessment of a hearing disorder.

The effective application of clinical masking requires a good understanding of the answers to the following three questions:

1. When should masking be used?
2. What kind of masking noise should be used?
3. How much masking should be used?

The following sections of this chapter answer these questions through a discussion of the principles of masking based on experimental evidence.

When to mask

The answer to the question of when to mask is quite simple: Masking must be used whenever there is a possibility of the test signal being heard in the nontest ear. The possibility exists any time the test tone is presented with sufficient intensity to cross the skull and stimulate the nontest ear. Important factors in determining when to mask are

1. the intensity of the test signal,
2. auditory sensitivity in the nontest ear, and
3. interaural attenuation.

Differences in interaural attenuation for air- and bone-conduction stimuli require a different answer to the question of when to mask in air- and bone-conduction audiometry.

Air conduction

In air-conduction audiometry, masking must be used whenever the intensity of the test tone exceeds auditory sensitivity in the nontest ear by an amount greater than the expected interaural attenuation. A critical factor is that a decision of when to mask must be based on *sensorineural sensitivity* in the nontest ear and not on the air-conduction thresholds of that ear. Even when the stimulus is presented by air conduction, *cross-over occurs by bone conduction* through the skull and not by air conduction around the skull. A cross-over response will be obtained from the nontest ear whenever the air-conduction stimulus in the test ear exceeds bone-conduction thresholds in the nontest ear by about 50 dB, regardless of air-conduction thresholds in that ear. With no masking in the nontest ear, false responses to an air-conduction signal will be obtained at 50 to 60 dB HTL in an ear with a more severe hearing loss, even with air-conduction thresholds in the nontest ear at 50 to 60 dB, if bone-conduction sensitivity in that ear is normal. Thus in air-conduction testing, *interaural difference* refers to the difference between the intensity level of the test tone and bone-conduction sensitivity in the nontest ear.

Research has shown that for an air-conduction pure tone signal presented through a standard audiometer earphone, interaural attenuation ranges from 40 to about 80 dB, varying with test frequency and subject (Zwislocki, 1953; Lidén et al., 1959a). The use of a larger earphone cushion, such as the circumaural type having a larger contact area between the cushion and skull, will actually result in a decreased attenuation (Zwislocki, 1953). Because in some subjects interaural attenuation with a standard earphone may be as little as 40 dB, it seems wise to accept Studebaker's (1967) principle that whenever variability is a result of inter-subject differences, the safest course is to adopt the extreme value, in this case the smallest reported interaural attenuation. Thus the rule for when to mask in air-conduction pure tone audiometry is:

> In air conduction audiometry, the nontest ear should be masked whenever the intensity of the signal presented to the test ear exceeds bone-conduction sensitivity in the nontest ear by more than 40 dB.

Although this approach may occasionally lead to unnecessary masking, it would ensure the use of masking whenever needed.

Bone conduction

Research evidence has shown that the interaural attenuation for a pure tone stimulus presented by bone conduction is essentially zero (Feldman, 1961; Lidén et al., 1959a; Sanders & Rintelmann, 1964; Studebaker, 1964). Although some subjects show an attenuation of about 10 dB, the value varies from one subject to another and cannot be regarded as dependable. With an expectation of no interaural attenuation, some researchers have proposed that masking should always be used in bone-conduction audiometry (Glorig, 1965; O'Neill & Oyer, 1966). This approach, however, will lead to unnecessary masking in some patients. As pointed out by Studebaker (1964), whenever air- and bone-conduction thresholds are at the same HTL in the test ear without masking, the use of masking noise in the nontest ear should not affect the results.

A further factor affecting decisions regarding masking in bone-conduction audiometry is the effect of *central masking*. Central masking, probably mediated by the efferent pathways (Lidén et al., 1959b), is an elevation in the test ear threshold as a result of a masking noise in the nontest ear, even though the intensity of the masking noise is not sufficient to cross over to the test ear. Zwislocki (1953) suggested that the central masking threshold shift is on the order of approximately 5 dB. Lidén et al. (1959b) observed shifts of up to 15 dB, and Studebaker (1962), Dirks (1964), and Dirks and Malmquist (1964) found that central masking increases with increased intensity of the masking noise and may be as great as 10 to 12 dB. These findings suggest that with no masking in the nontest ear, bone-conduction thresholds may be 5 to 15 dB better than those obtained with masking, even when masking is not required to prevent cross-over of the test signal. Thus because the bone-conduction system on the audiometer usually is calibrated with normal ear data obtained with masking in the opposite ear (ANSI, S3.13-1972; ANSI, S3.26-1981), unmasked bone-conduction thresholds may underestimate sensorineural loss even without false responses from test signal cross-over. That is, as a result of the central masking effect on the normative data used to determine calibration values for bone conduction, the test ear should always show an air-bone gap if bone-conduction thresholds are obtained without masking the nontest ear. With this in mind, we can accept Studebaker's (1964) rule for when to mask in bone-conduction audiometry:

> In bone conduction audiometry, the nontest ear should be masked whenever the test ear exhibits an air-bone gap.

What kind of masking noise to use

An important decision in masking is that of what type of masking noise to use. The masking effectiveness of a noise depends not only on the intensity of the noise but also on its nature. Although the results of Wegel and Lane (1924) showed that masking can be accomplished with a pure tone, their findings indicated that a sound composed of a range of frequencies is a more effective masker. Consequently, the masking signal available on audiometers is usually some form of acoustic energy in a band of frequencies. The clinical audiometer may provide two or more different masking noises, which requires the clinician to make a choice.

Available masking noises

Over the years, three basic types of masking noise have been available for masking in pure tone audiometry: complex noise, white noise, and narrow band noise. Because the clinician may have a choice among two or more masking noises or may be limited by equipment to one of the available maskers, it is important to understand the nature of the available noises.

Complex noise. Complex noise, sometimes referred to as sawtooth noise, is a broad-band signal composed of a low-frequency fundamental plus the multiples of that fundamental. The acoustic spectrum of a typical complex noise is shown in Figure 3.1. For this particular noise, the fundamental frequency is 78 Hz, and the additional frequencies are multiples of that fundamental (156 Hz, 234 Hz, etc.). The line spectrum of Figure 3.1 demonstrates two basic problems in complex noise as a masker of pure tones. First, acoustic energy is present only at the frequencies designated by the lines and is not spread continuously across the frequency range of the noise. With energy only at discrete frequencies, it is possible for the frequency of a test pure tone to fall within three or four cycles of a frequency component of the noise, producing a "beat" or pulsing phenomenon in the ear of the listener. Lidén et al. (1959a) pointed out that the fifth harmonic of a 50-Hz fundamental will beat with a test tone of 254 Hz. A 254-Hz tone is well within the permissible variability of an audiometer test tone (ANSI, S3.6-1969).

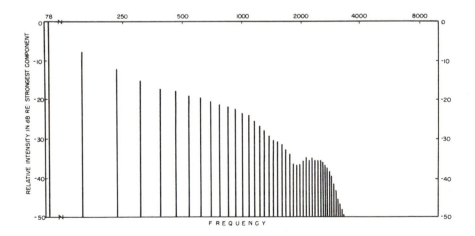

Figure 3.1. Acoustic spectrum of a sawtooth noise through a PDR-8 earphone. (From J. W. Sanders & W. F. Rintelmann, 1964, *Archives of Otolaryngology, 80*, 541–556.)

A second problem with complex noise as a masker in pure tone audiometry is the significant decrease in acoustic energy in the higher frequencies. For the noise shown in Figure 3.1, the energy present near 1000 Hz is down about 23 dB from the intensity level at 78 Hz. At 4000 Hz, the decrease in energy is greater than 50 dB. This characteristic suggests that complex noise may not be a very effective masker, at least for test tones in the middle and higher frequencies. Although the spectrum may differ somewhat from one noise generator to another, the basic limitations of the complex noise as a masker are generally characteristic of the noise. Because of these limitations, complex noise is usually no longer provided on clinical audiometers. The noise is included here because some older units still in use may include it.

White noise. White noise is a broad-band signal containing acoustic energy at all frequencies in the audible spectrum at approximately equal intensities. As shown in Figure 3.2, however, the acoustic spectrum of the noise is determined by the frequency response of the transducer. Through a TDH-39 earphone, the spectrum is essentially flat to 6000 Hz but drops off rapidly beyond that point. The acoustic spectrum of white noise is constant from one audiometer to another, provided that the same earphone is used. In contrast to complex noise, white noise is essentially equal in intensity across the frequency range to about 6000 Hz. With the newer TDH-49, 49P, 50, and 50P earphones, the spectrum is more nearly flat at 3000 and 4000 Hz by 1 or 2 dB, but the band width continues to be essentially 6000 Hz.

Narrow-band noise. Narrow-band noise is actually not a third type of noise but is rather white noise in limited bands of frequency and differs from white noise only in band width. Within the frequency band, acoustic energy is continuous and essentially equal across the band. Narrow band noise has been produced and used in the laboratory for some time (Denes & Naunton, 1952; Dirks, 1963; Egan & Hake, 1950; Jerger, Tillman, & Peterson, 1960; Koenig, 1962b; Lidén et al., 1959a; Sanders & Rintelmann, 1964; Studebaker, 1962).

For the purposes of pure tone audiometry, the narrow-band noise generator produces a separate noise band for each test frequency. For example, a 1000-Hz narrow band masker would be white noise in a limited band of frequencies with 1000 Hz at the center of the band. The acoustic spectra of narrow-band noises at three test frequencies are shown in Figure 3.3. A given noise band is described in terms of its center frequency, its band width (the span of frequencies whose intensities are no more than 3 dB below the peak component of the band), and its rejection rate (the decrease in intensity over a range of one octave on each side of the band).

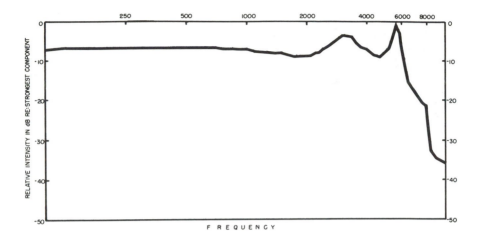

Figure 3.2. Acoustic spectrum of a broad band white noise through a TDH-39 earphone. (From J. W. Sanders & W. F. Rintelmann, 1964, *Archives of Otolaryngology, 80,* 541–556.)

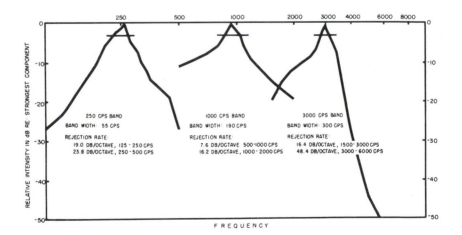

Figure 3.3. Acoustic spectra of three narrow bands of noise through a hearing aid type receiver. (From J. W. Sanders & W. F. Rintelmann, 1964, *Archives of Otolaryngology, 80,* 541–556.)

Because the latter two characteristics, band width and rejection rates, are products of the generator and the transducer used, the acoustic spectra of the noise bands may vary from one audiometer to another.

Relative masking efficiency

A critical factor in the choice of a masking noise is that of *masking efficiency*. Masking efficiency is defined as the ratio of the obtained masking to the intensity of the noise (Denes & Naunton, 1952). That is, the most efficient masking noise is the one that produces the greatest threshold shift with the least overall intensity. Thus if the three different masking noises—complex, white, and narrow band—are presented to an ear at equal overall intensity, the noise producing the greatest threshold shift could be regarded as the most efficient. Before actually measuring the threshold shift produced by each masker, let us consider the way in which masking noise affects auditory sensitivity and a method for predicting threshold shift.

The critical band concept

The *critical band concept* is a statement of masking effect relative to a band of frequencies of critical width. A thorough understanding of the concept is extremely helpful in understanding how masking noise affects auditory sensitivity. The concept developed from the early work of Fletcher and Munson (1937) and Fletcher (1940) and was elaborated in the later investigations of Hawkins and Stevens (1950) and Egan and Hake (1950). The concept is stated in two parts:

> A. In masking a pure tone with a broad band noise, the only components of the noise having a masking effect on the tone are those frequencies included in a restricted band with the test tone at its center.
> B. When the pure tone is just audible in the presence of the noise, the acoustic energy in the restricted band of frequencies is equal to the acoustic energy of the pure tone.

The width of the frequency band responsible for masking the pure tone is critical. If a band is narrowed to less than critical width without increasing intensity, the *masking effect* is decreased. If the band is widened to more than critical width, the *masking efficiency* is decreased, because the added frequencies in the band increase the overall intensity without producing a further shift in threshold. According to the first part of the critical band concept, in the masking of 1000-Hz pure tone with white noise, the only components of the noise having a masking effect are the frequencies included in a band from 968 Hz to 1032 Hz, inclusive: that is, 32 cycles

(Hz) on either side (above and below) of the 1000 Hz center frequency (see Table 3.1). The acoustic energy in the frequencies above and below that band could be removed without affecting the masking produced by the noise.

According to the second part of the critical band concept, it is the acoustic energy within the critical band of frequencies and not the overall intensity of the noise that determines the masking produced, because the overall level includes the energy in the frequencies above and below the critical band—energy that has no masking effect. In a comparison of masking efficiency for several masking noises, our concern is for the spectrum level within the critical band, often referred to as the *level per cycle*—the intensity of each individual cycle of the noise. The critical band concept can be very helpful in a comparative evaluation of noises for masking in pure tone audiometry.

Predicting masking efficiency

With the information supplied by the critical band concept, it is possible to make predictions regarding the efficiency of a masking noise. Although the concept will not hold entirely true for complex noise, given that the concept is specific to a noise of continuous and flat spectrum and complex noise is neither, we can make a general application, because the components of the noise will in effect combine their acoustic energies in masking.

According to Part 1 of the critical band concept, we can expect both complex and white noise to be inefficient to some extent, because for a given pure tone, both noises include considerable energy outside the critical band. Of the two noises, however, we should expect greater masking efficiency for white noise, because its spectrum is essentially flat; whereas in the complex noise, energy is concentrated in the lower frequencies with a rapid drop off of energy in the higher frequencies. In the masking of a pure tone in the higher frequencies with complex noise, the high intensity in the lower frequencies of the noise contributes significantly to the overall intensity of the noise but not at all to the masking of the tone.

If as stated in the critical band concept, the important factor in masking is the level per cycle within the critical band rather than the overall intensity of the noise, then narrow-band noise should show the greatest masking efficiency. If, for example, we produce each noise at a sound pressure level (SPL) of 80 dB, the level per cycle should be highest in the narrow-band noise, because the 80 dB are concentrated in a more restricted range of frequencies. This expectation can be demonstrated mathematically for white noise and narrow-band noise, because the level per cycle can be computed for a noise of continuous, flat spectrum. The level per cycle (energy in each individual cycle) is the overall intensity of the noise divided by the number of cycles in the noise band. For the white noise in our example, this would be 80 dB divided by 6000 Hz (the band width of white noise through a standard audiometer earphone). In order to carry out the computation, given that intensity in dB is a logarithm, frequency must be converted to its logarithm, and the function becomes one of subtraction.

Level per cycle = overall intensity (OA SPL) minus 10 times the logarithm of the band width (BW).

Since the logarithm of 6000 is 3.78, the formula for determining the level per cycle (LPC) of a white noise of 80 dB would be

    LPC = OA SPL − 10 log BW
    LPC = 80 − 37.8
    LPC = 42.2 dB SPL

Applying the same formula to a narrow-band noise having a band width of, let us say, 200 Hz (log of 200 is 2.3) and an overall intensity of 80 dB, the result would be

    LPC = OA SPL − 10 log BW
    LPC = 80 − 23
    LPC = 57 dB SPL

Thus for white and narrow-band noises at an overall intensity of 80 dB, the spectrum level would be 14.8 dB greater in the narrow-band noise. According to the second part of the critical band concept, we would expect the threshold shift to be 14.8 dB greater with the narrow-band noise.

Computation of the level per cycle for a narrow-band noise indicates that the narrower the band the greater the masking efficiency, as long as the band is no less than the critical width. Because the band width is determined by the characteristics of the noise generator, the efficiency of narrow-band masking may vary from one audiometer to another.

Experimental verification.   The prediction of masking efficiency with the critical band concept can be verified through the direct measurement of masked thresholds. The masking noise and the test tone are mixed in the same earphone, and hearing threshold level is determined in the presence of the masking noise. A number of investigators (Denes & Naunton, 1952; Lidén et al., 1959a; Studebaker, 1962; Sanders & Rintelmann, 1964) have carried out this kind of measurement with essentially the same results. Typical data from such a measurement are shown in Figure 3.4. The masked thresholds shown are the mean hearing threshold levels (according to the ASA, 1951, specifications) for 10 normal hearing subjects in the presence of the three masking noises at three different overall sound pressure levels. The acoustic spectra of the noises used for these measurements are those shown in Figures 3.1, 3.2, and 3.3.

The results shown in Figure 3.4 clearly support our predictions of relative masking efficiency. For a given overall intensity level, narrow-band noise showed the greatest masking efficiency. Of the two broad band noises, white noise had considerably greater masking efficiency than did the complex noise, at least in the middle and higher frequencies.

Figure 3.4 also demonstrates two additional factors of importance in clinical masking. First, for both white and narrow-band noise, masking is least effective in the lower frequencies. This is because auditory sensitivity is poorest in this frequency range, and greater intensity is required to reach hearing threshold level. Second, for both white and narrow-band noise, masking is *linear*. That is, beyond a certain minimal level, for each additional dB of noise there is an additional dB of threshold shift. This linearity is not obtained with complex noise.

Choice of masking noise.   With a verified prediction of relative masking efficiency, the question of what kind of masking noise to use has been answered. Whenever the clinician has a choice of masking noise for pure tone audiometry, narrow-band noise should be selected for its superior masking efficiency. The second choice is white noise. Although not as efficient as narrow-band noise, white noise is clearly superior to complex noise and will provide adequate masking in most cases if the output of the noise generator is sufficiently high.

How much masking?

With answers to our first two questions of when to mask and what kind of masking noise to use, we can turn to the important third question of how much masking to use. Basically, the masking noise must be sufficient to prevent a response from the nontest ear without affecting sensitivity in the test ear. The least intensity required to effect the needed threshold shift in the nontest ear has been called the *minimum effective masking level* (Lidén et al., 1959b) or the *minimum masking level* (Studebaker, 1962) and is defined as the masking level just sufficient to mask the test

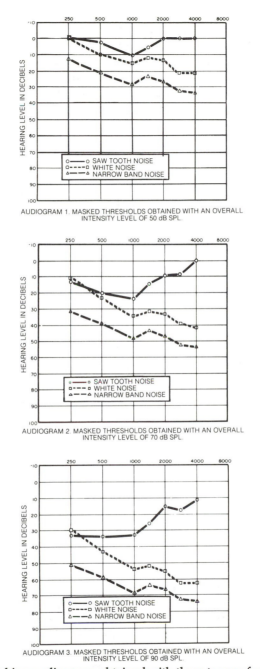

Figure 3.4. Masking audiograms obtained with three types of masking noise at three intensity levels. (From J. W. Sanders & W. F. Rintelmann, 1964, *Archives of Otolaryngology, 80,* 541–556.)

signal in the masked ear. The *maximum effective masking level* or *maximum masking level* is defined as the masking noise intensity just insufficient to mask the signal in the test ear (Studebaker, 1967). The intensity of the masking noise, then, must be at or beyond the minimum effective level without exceeding the maximum effective level. Several investigators have proposed mathematical formulas for determination of the minimum and maximum effective levels.

The formula approach

As an example of the formula approach to determining minimum and maximum effective masking levels, Lidén et al. (1959a) suggested the following for air-conduction testing:

$$M_{min} = A_t - 40 + (A_m - B_m)$$
$$M_{max} = B_t + 40, \text{ provided } M_{max} \text{ is less than D}$$

That is, the minimum masking level is equal to the air-conduction threshold in the test ear (A_t) minus the attenuation factor of 40 dB, plus the difference between the air- and bone-conduction thresholds in the masked ear (A_m and B_m). The maximum masking level is the bone-conduction threshold in the test ear (B_t) plus the attenuation factor, providing the result does not exceed the patient's discomfort level (D).

For masking in bone-conduction audiometry, the following formulas were proposed:

$$M_{min} = B_t + (A_m - B_m)$$
$$M_{max} = B_t + 40, \text{ provided } M_{max} \text{ is less than D}$$

Minimum masking level is the bone-conduction threshold in the test ear plus the difference between the air- and bone-conduction thresholds in the masked ear. The maximum level, like that for air-conduction audiometry, is the bone-conduction threshold in the test ear plus the attenuation factor of 40 dB for the masking noise, providing the maximum level does not exceed the patient's discomfort level.

Although these formulas will provide the clinician with minimum and maximum effective masking levels, the approach would be extremely cumbersome and time-consuming in clinical audiometry. The clinician would be required to carry out the arithmetic of four formulas in order to obtain air- and bone-conduction thresholds at one test frequency. Although Studebaker (1964) simplified the process somewhat by combining air- and bone-conduction testing into a single formula, he recognized the problems in the formula approach and suggested that this method, although perhaps desirable in laboratory research, is not suited to clinical audiometry.

The effective masking level approach

A direct approach to the question of how much masking to use is through the determination and use of the *effective masking level*. The effective masking level is defined as the number of dB by which the total energy in the critical band exceeds the threshold energy for a pure tone whose frequency is at the center of the band. Effective level also can be regarded as the threshold shift in dB produced in the masked ear by a given noise intensity. That is, if a masking noise shifts threshold in the masked ear from 0 dB to 30 dB hearing threshold level, the noise has produced 30 dB of effective masking, and threshold in the masked ear has been shifted to a hearing threshold level of 30 dB. Thus the effective masking level for an ear with normal sensitivity expressed in dB on the hearing threshold level scale can be regarded as the hearing level to which an ear will be shifted by a given amount of masking noise. Applying the concept of the effective masking level in this manner can greatly simplify masking procedures in audiometry.

If the numbers on the audiometer masking-noise intensity dial can be translated into effective masking levels re normal thresholds, we can predict the masked thresholds that will be produced by each setting of the dial. With this information, we can answer the question of how much masking noise to use though a direct inspection of the audiogram. If, for example, we wish to produce a minimum masking level of 10 dB in an ear with air- and bone-conduction thresholds at 0 dB HTL, we can simply turn the masking-noise intensity dial to a setting that will produce an effective masking level of 10 dB. At this masking-noise intensity, the masked air and bone threshold in the nontest ear will be at the 10 dB HTL.

The masking-noise intensity dial

In past years there has been little or no relationship between the masking effect and the numbers on the audiometer dial controlling the intensity of the masking noise. In an informal survey of eight older audiometers (portable, clinical, and research), we found that with the dial set to "60," the intensity of the masking noise (complex or white) ranged from 60 to 120 dB SPL. Obviously, on these instruments no assumptions could be made regarding the masking effect at a given setting of the dial. On the more recent audiometers, those providing narrow-band masking noise, the dial controlling the intensity of the narrow-band noise is calibrated in effective masking level re 0 dB HTL. This is possible because narrow-band masking requires a different noise band for each test frequency. Unfortunately, the dial cannot be calibrated in effective level for white noise masking, even though some audiometers providing white noise label the intensity dial "effective masking." The dial numbers may be in effective masking for one or two frequencies, but this cannot apply at all test frequencies because the sound pressure level for effective masking with white noise varies with the frequency of the test tone. It is possible, however, for the clinician to determine the relationship between dial numbers and their masking effect.

Determining effective masking level

There are two methods available to the clinician for determining effective masking levels for either white noise or narrow-band noise and relating those levels to the numbers on the masking-noise intensity dial. The first method is through computation with the critical band data.

Effective level through computation. Part 2 of the critical band concept, presented earlier, states:

> When the pure tone is just audible in the presence of the masking noise, the acoustic energy in the restricted band of frequencies (the critical band) is equal to the acoustic energy in the test tone.

From this part of the critical band concept, we can see that if the acoustic energy in a given critical band of white noise can be determined, that information can be used to predict the masking effect of the noise. As we have already seen, the spectrum level, or level per cycle, within a given band of white noise can be computed from the overall intensity of the noise and the width of the band. If we also know the width of the critical band, we can determine the acoustic energy in the critical band for a given overall intensity. The critical band widths from the data of Hawkins and Stevens (1950) are shown in Table 3.1. Each band width is reported in frequency and in 10 times the logarithm of the frequency. The total energy in a critical band is the level per cycle (energy in each individual cycle) multiplied by the number of cycles in the critical band. In the critical band having 1000 Hz as a center frequency, for example, if the level per cycle is 42.2 dB (from the example given earlier for the computation of level per cycle), and the critical band is 64 cycles in width, the total energy in the critical band would be 42.2 dB multiplied by 64 cycles. Here again, we must convert the band width to its logarithm, and the function becomes one of addition:

Energy in the critical band (CB) is equal to the level per cycle (LPC) plus 10 times the logarithm of the critical band width (CBW).

As shown earlier, the level per cycle for a given white noise, broad or narrow band, is the overall sound pressure of the noise minus 10 times the logarithm of the band width of the noise. In an earlier computation, we found that for white noise through a standard earphone at a sound pressure level of 80 dB, the level per cycle was as follows:

LPC = OA SPL − 10 log BW
LPC = 80 − 37.8
LPC = 42.2 dB SPL

Thus for white noise at an overall intensity of 80 dB and the critical band at 1000 Hz (see Table 3.1), the computation of the energy (E) in the critical band is as follows:

E in CB = LPC + 10 log CBW
E in CB = 42.2 + 18
E in CB = 60.2 dB SPL

TABLE 3.1
Critical Band Widths[a] for 11 Test Frequencies

Center Frequency Hz	Critical Band Width	
	in Hz	10 log CBW
125	70.8	18.5
250	50	17
500	50	17
750	56.2	17.5
1000	64	18
1500	79.4	19
2000	100	20
3000	158	22
4000	200	23
6000	376	25.75
8000	501	27

[a]Hawkins and Stevens (1950).

In this example, the total energy in the 1000-Hz critical band is 60.2 dB SPL. The magnitude of the difference between the energy in that critical band and the intensity necessary to reach threshold at 1000 Hz in a given ear is the effective level of the noise at that frequency in that ear. Thus, effective level, often designated as Z, can be determined as follows:

$$Z = LPC + 10 \log CBW - \text{threshold in quiet}$$

In this computation, threshold in quiet must be expressed in dB sound pressure level. According to ANSI S 3.6-1969, 0 dB HTL for the TDH-39 earphone at 1000 Hz = 7 dB SPL. Thus the effective level of white noise at a sound pressure level of 80 dB in a TDH-39 earphone in a normal ear would be:

$$Z = 42.2 + 18 - 7$$
$$Z = 53.2 \text{ dB}$$

That is, the energy in the critical band (42.2 + 18) exceeds the energy required to reach threshold in quiet (7 dB) by 53.2 dB. With an effective level of 53.2 dB, we would expect 53.2 dB of masking in a normal ear for a 1000-Hz tone. Furthermore, this masking would shift threshold to a hearing level of 53.2 dB.

Because our prediction is based entirely on computation with the critical band data, we might well ask at this point for verification. Does 80 dB of white noise actually produce a threshold shift of 53.2 dB for a 1000-Hz tone in the normal ear? The relationship between effective masking levels predicted through computation and the masking actually obtained with white noise at three different sound pressure levels in 10 normal ears is shown in Figure 3.5. Figure 3.6 reports the same data (predicted and obtained masking) for narrow band noise. In each figure, for a given overall intensity of the masking noise, one set of data points shows the masked thresholds predicted with the critical band data computations, and the second set of data reports the mean hearing threshold levels (re ASA-1951) to which the 10 normal hearers were actually shifted. Converting the measured and predicted masked thresholds to hearing threshold levels re the ANSI 53.6-1969 standard would not, of course, alter the relationship shown.

The data shown in Figures 3.5 and 3.6 verify the prediction of effective level through computation. The figures show further that if the overall intensity of the noise (white or narrow-band) is known, the hearing threshold levels to which an ear will be shifted by a given noise can be determined. This information will permit the clinician to establish the effective masking level at each test frequency for each setting of the masking-noise intensity dial.

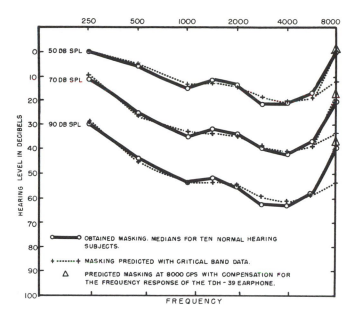

Figure 3.5. Comparison of the masking obtained with white noise at three different intensity levels for 10 normal hearing subjects and the masking predicted with the critical band data of Fletcher (1940). (From J. W. Sanders & W. F. Rintelmann, 1964, *Archives of Otolaryngology, 80,* 541–556.)

The effective masking table. For the audiometer having a masking-noise intensity dial that is not calibrated in effective masking level, the relationship between dial setting and effective masking can be established through the construction of an *effective masking table,* which should be posted at the audiometer. The first step is to measure the acoustic output of the masking noise in sound pressure level at the maximum dial setting with a sound level meter. If the clinician does not have such equipment, the measurement can be made by the people who service and calibrate the audiometer. For the maximum noise output, the level per cycle and the energy in the critical bands can be determined with the formulas given, using the critical band data from Table 3.1. Finally, the effective masking levels re audiometric zero can be determined for each test frequency by subtracting the appropriate sound pressure levels at audiometric zero (ANSI-1969) for the earphones in use from the energy in the critical bands. The resulting values are the effective levels re normal hearing at each test frequency for the maximum output of the masking noise.

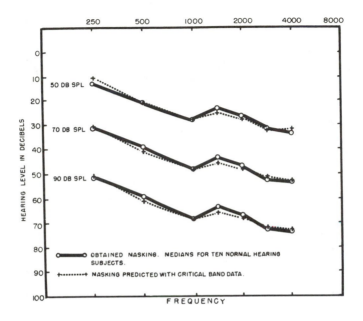

Figure 3.6. Comparison of the masking obtained with narrow bands of noise at three different intensity levels for 10 normal hearing subjects and the masking predicted with the critical band data of Fletcher (1940). (From J. W. Sanders & W. F. Rintelmann, 1964, *Archives of Otolaryngology, 80,* 541–556.)

The next step is to check the linearity of the masking-noise intensity dial. That is, does each 10-dB change on the dial bring about a 10-dB change in the intensity of the noise? On most clinical audiometers, masking-noise intensity is controlled by an attenuator that should provide satisfactory linearity. Some older instruments and most portable audiometers, however, are equipped with potentiometers that do not provide linear control. The linearity check can be made with a sound level meter, but it is done more satisfactorily with a voltmeter. If the dial departs significantly from linearity (1 or 2 dB per 10-dB step and/or a cumulative error greater than 4 or 5 dB), use the voltmeter to establish 10-dB steps and mark those on the dial. If a voltmeter is not available, this measurement can be made by the people who service the audiometer. Actually, measurement of the masking-noise intensity and a determination of masking-noise dial linearity should be part of the routine calibration of the audiometer. With linearity of the dial assured, the effective level for each dial setting can be established simply by subtracting 10 dB for each 10-dB reduction on the dial.

For example, suppose that on an audiometer equipped with white noise through a TDH-50P earphone, the maximum setting on the masking-noise intensity dial is 100 and the noise intensity at that setting is 110 dB SPL. The level per cycle of the noise would be 110 dB minus 37.8 (10 times the logarithm of 6000 Hz) or 72.2 dB. With this level per cycle and the data from Table 3.1, effective masking levels would be computed as shown for three test frequencies in Table 3.2. These are the effective levels for normal hearers and thus are the hearing levels to which an ear will be shifted with the noise-intensity dial setting of 100. These levels, *rounded off to the next lower 5-dB level*, are entered into a table of effective masking opposite the dial setting of 100. Next, for each linear setting of the masking dial, effective levels can be entered for each dial setting by subtracting 10 dB from the maximum effective levels for each 10-dB reduction on the dial. Table 3.3 illustrates the effective masking table, using the data for the three frequencies computed in Table 3.2. A table for clinical use would, of course, include effective masking levels for all test frequencies. The completed table provides for each test frequency the hearing threshold level to which a masked ear will be shifted by the masking noise at each setting of the intensity dial on a given audiometer.

Effective level by measurement. A second method for determining effective masking levels is through direct measurement with normal hearers. Although this approach is time-consuming, it will provide accurate masking data and may be necessary if any of the information for computation of effective masking levels cannot be obtained. In this method, the masking noise and the test tone are mixed in the same earphone. At several settings of the masking-noise intensity dial, thresholds are deter-

TABLE 3.2
An Illustration of the Computation of Effective Masking Levels
at Three Test Frequencies

Frequency Hz	Computation	Effective Level
250	$Z = 72.2 + 17 - 26.5^a =$	62.7
1000	$Z = 72.2 + 18 - 7.5^a =$	82.7
4000	$Z = 72.2 + 23 - 10.5 =$	84.7

[a]Audiometric zero for the TDH-50P earphone according to the ANSI standards.

TABLE 3.3
Illustration of an Effective Masking Table

Dial Setting	Effective Levels (in dB)		
	250	1000	4000
30		10	10
40		20	20
50	10	30	30
60	20	40	40
70	30	50	50
80	40	60	60
90	50	70	70
100	60	80	80

mined at each test frequency in the presence of the noise for 8 or 10 normal hearers. For each dial setting, the mean masked threshold at each frequency is the effective masking level for normal hearers and represents the hearing threshold level to which an ear will be shifted by noise at that dial setting. If the masking dial is linear, the effective masking levels for those dial settings not used for measurement can be interpolated from the obtained results, and a complete masking table can be constructed, which provides effective masking levels for each frequency at each setting of the masking noise dial. If the dial is not linear, the alternative is to mark linear points on the dial as described earlier or to measure masking in the normal ears at each dial setting.

This approach to the determination of effective masking levels assumes that the noise and test tone can be presented in the same earphone. This is not true on most one-channel audiometers. The same thing can be accomplished, however, through a simple mixing network described by Studebaker (1967) and shown in Figure 3.7. If the clinician cannot construct the network, it can be made from the diagram in a radio-television repair shop.

Effective masking and complex noise. As indicated earlier, complex noise is no longer included on clinical audiometers and has even been replaced by white noise on most portable instruments. If for whatever reason the clinician is limited to complex noise, he or she should be fully aware of its limitations. First, masking with complex noise is not linear. That is, each additional dB of noise does not necessarily produce an additional dB of masking (see Figure 3.4). Furthermore, the critical band data can-

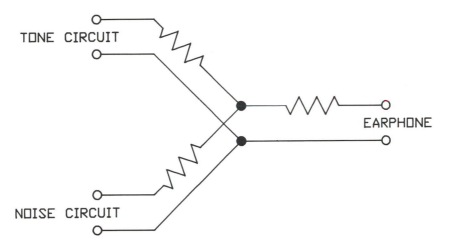

ALL RESISTORS 3.3 OHMS, 1/4 WATT

Figure 3.7. Combining network for mixing the pure tone and the masking noise into the same earphone. (From G. A. Studebaker, *Journal of Speech and Hearing Disorders*, 1967, 32, 360–371.)

not be applied to complex noise because its spectrum is neither continuous nor flat. The only approach to a determination of effective masking levels is through actual measurement with normal hearers, and that measurement must be made at each setting of the masking dial. Even with an effective masking chart, the clinician must remain aware of the possibility of a beat phenomenon between the test tone and a component of the noise.

Using effective masking levels

With a masking-noise intensity dial calibrated in effective masking level, directly or through the use of a table relating effective masking to dial setting, the clinician has an immediate indication of the hearing threshold level to which the masked ear will be shifted by each setting of the masking noise dial. To use that information appropriately, however, the clinician must be aware of several additional factors.

Effective level refers to any ear. The effective masking level has been defined as the number of dB by which the energy in the critical band exceeds the threshold energy of a pure tone whose frequency is at the center of the band. Because effective levels on the calibrated dial or in the masking table are re normal hearing (audiometric zero), they can be regarded as the hearing threshold level to which the masked ear will be shifted. This will be true for the impaired ear as well as the normal ear, provided threshold in the impaired ear is at a lower HTL than the effective level. For example, in the illustration used earlier, white noise at an overall intensity of 80 dB through a TDH-39 earphone was found to produce an effective level in the normal ear of 53.2 dB at 1000 Hz. A threshold shift of 53.2 dB in the normal ear would produce, of course, a masked hearing threshold level of 53.2 dB. If we apply that 80 dB SPL white noise to an impaired ear with HTL at, let us say, 40 dB, the threshold shift would be smaller, but the masked threshold would still be 53.2 dB HTL. Recall that the computation of effective level for a given ear requires us to subtract that ear's threshold in quiet, expressed in sound pressure level, from the total energy in the critical band. Computation of the effective masking level with white noise at an overall SPL of 80 dB for a 1000-Hz pure tone in an ear with a 40-dB hearing loss would be:

$$Z = LPC + 10 \log CBW - \text{threshold in quiet}$$
$$Z = 42.2 + 18 - 47$$
$$Z = 13.2 \text{ dB}$$

The value of 47 in the computation is the 40-dB hearing loss at 1000 Hz expressed in sound pressure level with a TDH-39 earphone (7 dB at audiometric zero plus the 40 dB HTL). The effective level, and thus the threshold shift, in this ear wold be 13.2 dB. A threshold shift of 13.2 dB from a hearing threshold level of 40 dB would result in a masked hearing threshold level of 53.2 dB, the same HTL to which the normal ear is shifted at 1000 Hz by 80 dB of white noise. Thus we can interpret effective masking levels re normal ears as the HTL to which any ear will be shifted, regardless of hearing loss in the ear, so long as the hearing loss does not exceed the effective level.

The foregoing assumes that the impaired ear will give the same linear response to white noise as will the normal ear. Although clinical experience suggests that undermasking is not a problem with the effective masking approach, there may be instances where masking an ear with sensorineural impairment produces questionable results. In such cases, the clinician should combine the effective masking level approach with the Hood technique to be described later.

Effective level is by air conduction.   In using the concept of effective masking level in clinical audiometry, it is important to recognize that the masked threshold produced by the noise is by air conduction, not bone conduction. For example, if we present masking noise at an effective level of 50 dB to an ear with air-conduction threshold at 40 dB and bone-conduction at 0 dB HTL, the air-conduction threshold in that ear will be shifted to 50 dB, but the bone-conduction threshold in that ear will be shifted to only 10 dB HTL. Increasing the effective masking level to 60 dB will shift the air threshold to 60 dB but the bone threshold to only 20 dB. The introduction of masking noise does not change the air–bone relationship in the masked ear. In an attempt to shift bone-conduction threshold in an ear with conductive impairment, effective masking is reduced by the amount of the air–bone gap. This is why in the formula approach to masking described earlier, Lidén et al. (1959a) included sub-traction of the air–bone gap in the masked ear. Given that bone-conduction sensitivity is the important concern in masking, the clinician must remain aware of the loss of effective masking due to an air–bone gap.

The occlusion effect.   The *occlusion effect*, described by Lidén et al. (1959b), Feldman (1961), Studebaker (1962), Dirks and Swindeman (1967), and others, is an improvement in bone-conduction responses in an ear covered (occluded) by an earphone. The improved responses are a result of sound pressure generated in the enclosed external auditory canal and transmitted through the middle ear. Sensitivity is not changed, but responses are obtained at a better hearing level as a result of the additional energy reaching the cochlea. Because the additional energy is transmitted through the conductive mechanism, the effect does not occur in the ear with con-ductive impairment. The effect might be as great as 25 dB (Dirks & Swindeman, 1967) but is limited to the lower frequencies, primarily 250 and 500 Hz. To overcome the occlusion effect, the minimum effective level must be increased by 30 dB when testing at these frequencies, unless the masked ear is known to have a conductive impairment.

Some illustrative cases.   The following cases are presented to illustrate the use of effective masking levels re the normal ear. Audiometric data for the cases are shown in Figure 3.8.

Case A.   An air-conduction response for a 1000-Hz tone is obtained in the right ear at 60 dB after air- and bone-conduction thresholds have been established at that frequency in the left ear at 0 dB. As we have already seen in our discussion of when to mask, the right ear response could be a result of cross-over of the test tone to the left ear, because the intensity of the tone at 60 dB exceeds bone-conduction sensitivity in the nontest ear by more than the interaural attenuation value of 40 dB. The minimum effective masking level is 10 dB. The maximum effective level is 40 dB, assuming the possibility of bone-conduction threshold in the right ear at 0 dB. If the right ear response is a result of cross-over, shift-

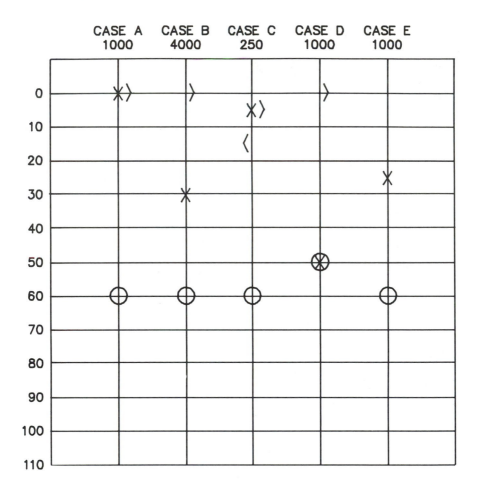

Figure 3.8. Five hypothetical cases illustrating the application of effective masking.

ing the left ear sensitivity by 10 dB should cause the right ear response to disappear. In this case, however, we can use an effective level greater than the minimum. An effective level of 40 dB would bring about a considerable shift in the left ear without danger of masking cross-over to the right ear, even if bone-conduction sensitivity in the right ear is at 0 dB. With 40 dB of effective masking in the left ear, threshold in the right ear is redetermined. If the response continues at 60 dB, we can accept it as a true threshold, because the difference between the test signal and bone-conduction sensitivity in the masked left ear is now only 20 dB, considerably less than the interaural attenuation of 40 dB. A disappearance of the right ear response with masking at a 40-dB effective level in the left ear, however, does not guarantee that the response was a result of cross-over, because it could disappear due to central masking. If, in the presence of the masking noise, the response reappears at 70 dB, this can be accepted as correct, given that the interaural difference is now only 30 dB and still not in excess of interaural attenuation. If, however, the redetermined response is at 85 dB HTL or higher (interaural difference of 45 dB or more), masking must be increased and threshold search continued until a stable response is obtained with effective level in the left ear no more than 40 dB below presentation level in the right ear. In some instances, of course, a stable response might never occur. If the actual threshold in the right ear is so poor as to be beyond the limits of audiometer output, we would eliminate response entirely with increasing levels of masking and thus demonstrate the profound nature of the hearing loss. If, however, our masking noise output is limited to an effective level no greater than 60 dB, we might continue to obtain a right ear response at 105 or 110 dB HTL that does not meet our criterion of acceptability. Under these circumstances, we would have to conclude that threshold in the right ear is at least as poor and probably poorer than the last obtained response.

Case B.   In this case, with left ear thresholds established at 30 dB by air conduction and 0 dB by bone conduction, an air-conduction response is obtained in the right ear at 60 dB HTL for a 4000-Hz tone. Here again, this right ear response must be checked with masking in the left ear, because the difference between the presentation level in the test ear and bone-conduction sensitivity in the nontest ear is 60 dB, considerably greater than the interaural attenuation of 40 dB. As in Case A, the minimum threshold shift required in the nontest ear is 10 dB. In this case, however, we cannot use an effective masking level of 10 dB, because of the air–bone gap in the nontest ear. In order to shift bone-conduction sensitivity in the left ear to 10 dB HTL, we must use an effective level of 40 dB, shifting air-conduction threshold to 40 dB and thus shifting bone-conduction threshold to 10 dB. With 40 dB of interaural attenuation for the masking noise, an effective level of 40 dB would not result in over-masking, even if bone-conduction threshold in the right ear is at 0 dB. If the right ear response continues at 60 dB with masking at an effective level of 40 dB in the left ear, it can be accepted as threshold. If it disappears, the procedure outlined for Case A must be followed until a response that meets our criterion is obtained. In this case the chances of failure to obtain an acceptable response because of insufficient masking noise output are increased by the presence of the air–bone gap in the nontest ear. It should be remembered that masking effect is decreased by an amount equal to the difference between air- and bone-conduction thresholds in the masked ear.

Case C. This case illustrates masking in bone-conduction testing with the added complication of the occlusion effect. The response in question is the unmasked bone-conduction response at 250 Hz in the right ear, with air-conduction threshold in that ear already established at 60 dB and air- and bone-conduction thresholds in the left ear at 5 dB with no air–bone gap. With no interaural attenuation expected in bone-conduction testing and with an air–bone gap in the test ear, the right ear bone-conduction response must be checked with masking in the left ear. In this case, a 10-dB threshold shift in the nontest ear is not acceptable as a minimum. With the test signal at a low frequency and no conductive component in the masked ear, we must add 30 dB of effective masking to compensate for the occlusion effect in that ear, which brings the minimum effective level to 45 dB. In this case, however, we can exceed the minimum level by 10 dB without danger of overmasking, because an effective level of 55 dB is only 40 dB above the bone-conduction response level in the test ear.

Case D. In this case, an air-conduction response is obtained at 50 dB in the right ear for a 1000- Hz tone with unmasked responses in the left ear, which indicate air-conduction threshold at 50 dB and bone-conduction threshold at 0 dB. The need for checking the right ear response with masking in the left ear is apparent. In order to overcome the air–bone gap in the left ear and bring about a shift of 10 dB in bone-conduction response, we must use an effective masking level of 60 dB. If, however, the undetermined bone-conduction sensitivity in the right ear is actually at 0 or even 5 dB, an effective level of 60 dB would be overmasking, since that noise level in the nontest ear would exceed that hypothetical bone-conduction sensitivity by more than 40 dB. If we attempt to solve the problem by establishing a bone-conduction threshold in the right ear, we face the same problem. Sufficient masking in the left ear to produce a minimum shift of 10 dB of bone-conduction response in that ear would also eliminate a true bone-conduction threshold response in the right ear, if bone-conduction threshold in that ear is actually at 0 to 10 dB. Furthermore, if we obtain an unmasked bone-conduction threshold in the right ear at 0 dB, we have no way of knowing whether 0 dB bone-conduction thresholds are correct in both ears or correct in one with cross-over response in the other. If one is due to cross-over, we have no way of telling which. Finally, the same problem exists for the air-conduction responses. The obtained response in one ear might be a result of cross-over, and as with the bone-conduction responses, we cannot tell which. This problem, described by Carhart (1960) and by Feldman (1961), and aptly labeled a "masking dilemma" by Naunton (1960), cannot be solved with standard masking procedures. The only masking solution to the problem is to increase the interaural attenuation for the masking noise by transducing the noise in an insert receiver (Zwislocki, 1953; Koenig, 1962a). Because the insert receiver results in a much smaller contact area between transducer and skull, the interaural attenuation may be increased to as much as 70 to 90 dB.

In cases like this in which masking limitations preclude an accurate assessment, an excellent procedure for determining the true nature of the hearing loss is acoustic immittance measurement. This procedure is discussed in another chapter.

Case E.   In Cases A, B, and C, we considered the amount of masking to be used when air- and bone-conduction thresholds are known for the nontest ear. This is usually not the case, however, because most clinicians complete air-conduction testing for both ears before turning to bone-conduction audiometry. In Case E, then, air-conduction responses are obtained at 60 dB in the right ear with air-conduction threshold previously established for the left ear at 25 dB. Although bone-conduction sensitivity in the left ear is unknown, it could be as low as 0 dB, and the right ear response could be a result of cross-over. In this situation the clinician has two choices. First, the right ear air response at 60 dB can be accepted temporarily and a final decision as to the need for masking made after bone-conduction testing. The second choice is to assume a bone-conduction threshold of 0 dB in the left ear and mask accordingly.

These illustrative cases certainly do not cover every problem encountered in masking in clinical audiometry. They should, however, present the principles of effective masking in a manner that will permit the clinician to reason from them to situations not included here.

The Hood technique.   As shown in several of the illustrative cases, whenever a suspect response disappears in the presence of appropriate masking, the clinician must search for the true threshold at higher hearing levels. This search may also involve increasing the effective masking level to ensure a continued nonparticipation by the nontest ear. As the intensity of the masking noise is increased, so are the chances for overmasking. An excellent procedure for ensuring sufficient masking without overmasking in the threshold search is a technique described by Hood (1960) and referred to by various terms, such as the *plateau method*, the *threshold shift method*, or the *shadowing method*. In this procedure, a questionable unmasked threshold is checked with masking in the nontest ear at the minimum effective masking level. If the response disappears, the effective masking level is increased in 10-dB steps with a redetermination of threshold at each step until a plateau of threshold response is reached—a level at which threshold response shows no further increase with increase in masking over a range of at least 20 to 30 dB of masking noise. One or more of the responses on the plateau will meet the criterion for a true threshold response. That is, the interaural difference will be 40 dB or less. The Hood technique is demonstrated with the two illustrative cases outlined in Table 3.4 and Figure 3.9.

Case 1. In this case, as shown in the figure, left ear air- and bone-conduction thresholds have been established at 0 dB. An air-conduction threshold response has been obtained in the right ear at 50 dB, although, unknown to the clinician, the actual threshold is at 80 dB. Because the unmasked response at 50 dB is a result of cross-over of the test tone to the nontest ear, masking at an effective level of 10 dB will shift bone-conduction sensitivity in the left ear to 10 dB HTL, and the cross-over response in the right ear will shift to 60 dB, as shown in the table. This response is also unacceptable, of course, because the difference between the test tone presentation level of 60 dB exceeds the masked bone-conduction threshold in the left ear by more than 40 dB. The next step is to increase the effective masking level to 20 dB. At this masking level, response in the right ear will shift to 70 dB, which is also unacceptable, because the interaural difference still exceeds 40 dB. Continuing the procedure of increasing the effective masking level in 10-dB steps with redetermination of threshold at each step will bring us to a threshold response at 80 dB. At this point, we will observe no further shifts in hearing threshold response with increase in masking level, because the response is no longer due to cross-over but rather is the true right ear

TABLE 3.4
Two Illustrative Cases of the Hood Technique

Case 1			Case 2	
Threshold Response	Effective Level		Threshold Response	Effective Level
50	0		50	0
60	10		60	10
70	20		70	20
80	30		70	30
80	40		70	40
80	50		70	50
80	60		70	60
			80	70
			90	80

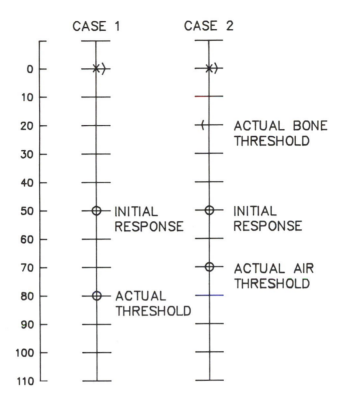

Figure 3.9. Two hypothetical cases illustrating application of the Hood technique in masking.

threshold. Further shifts in left ear threshold with masking will not affect the response.

Case 2. This case presents a somewhat different situation. Left ear thresholds have been established at 0 dB. In the right ear, air-conduction threshold response is obtained at 50 dB. This response is due to cross-over, because, again unknown to the clinician, actual threshold in the right ear is at 70 dB. Also unknown to the clinician, bone-conduction threshold in that ear is at 20 dB. With the Hood technique, we will find a response plateau in this case at 70 dB HTL in the test ear. As shown in the table, this response will remain stable over a range of effective masking levels from 20 to 60 dB. If we continue to increase the masking noise level in this case, however, we will eventually observe a further shift in threshold response. As shown in the table, at an effective level of 70 dB, threshold response will shift to 80 dB, because at this point the masking noise is more than 40 dB greater than bone-conduction sensitivity in the test ear, and overmasking has occurred. This further shift of threshold response at higher levels of masking noise should not constitute a problem, however, so long as the clinician recognizes the response plateau when it occurs. As in Case 1, responses on the plateau occurred at several effective masking levels sufficient to preclude a response from the nontest ear.

Masking in speech audiometry

With a few notable exceptions, the attention given to masking in the literature has been directed primarily toward masking in pure tone audiometry, with considerably less said about the equally important subject of masking in speech audiometry. Although both the signal and the task are different in speech audiometry, given that we are seeking recognition of spoken language rather than detection of a pure tone, the problem is the same—that is, the possibility of a false and inaccurate response as a result of cross-over of the test signal to the nontest ear. Indeed, as pointed out by Studebaker (1967), the danger is increased in word recognition testing, because the signal to the test ear is presented at suprathreshold level, increasing even further the interaural difference.

When to mask

The answer to the question of when to mask in speech audiometry is the same as that for pure tone audiometry. Masking must be used whenever the intensity of the test signal exceeds bone-conduction sensitivity for that signal by more than the expected interaural attenuation. Lidén (1954) and Lidén et al. (1959b) indicated that the interaural attenuation for speech by air conduction is 50 dB. Konkle and Berry (1983), however, present a convincing argument for an interaural attenuation of only 45 dB for threshold assessment with spondee words. They also point out that, because of differences in the nature of the tasks, interaural attenuation for word recognition tests should be regarded as 35 dB. In deciding when to mask, it must be remembered that the interaural difference must be determined as the difference between presentation level to the test ear and bone-conduction sensitivity in the nontest ear. If an air–bone gap is present in the nontest ear, bone-conduction sensitivity for speech can be taken as the pure tone average (500, 1000, and 2000 Hz) by bone conduction. If the nontest ear does not have a conductive loss, interaural difference can be based on the air-conduction pure tone average if the speech reception threshold has not been obtained. If the interaural difference is based on the pure tone average in the nontest ear, a higher effective masking level might be needed if the audiogram is irregular in configuration. In such cases, the clinician might use either the 500- and 1000-Hz average or simply the pure tone threshold at either 500 or 1000 Hz, whichever is better. Carhart (1971) reported correlation coefficients for speech reception threshold and pure tone thresholds of .90 for 500 Hz and .92 for 1000 Hz. The correlation coefficient between SRT and pure tone threshold at 2000 Hz was .78.

What kind of noise?

The question of what kind of noise to use for masking in speech audiometry is usually not a problem. Narrow bands of noise, like those used with significant advantage in pure tone audiometry, are too limited in frequency response for the relatively broad spectrum speech signal (Hirsh & Bowman, 1953; Miller, 1947; Setliff, 1971). Complex noise suffers the same deficiency it exhibits as a pure tone masker (energy concentration in the lower frequencies). On audiometers permitting speech audiometry, the clinician usually has a choice between white noise as described earlier in this chapter and *speech spectrum noise*. Speech spectrum noise is white noise filtered to a low- and middle-frequency band, simulating the long-term average spectrum of conversational speech. Because of its more limited band, speech spectrum noise is somewhat more efficient than white noise, with a masking advantage of about 8 dB (Konkle & Berry, 1983). Hawkins and Stevens (1950), Lidén (1954), and Lidén et al. (1959b) have shown that the relationship between white noise intensity level and threshold for speech is a linear function. That is, beyond a certain minimum level, each additional dB of noise produces an additional dB of shift in threshold for speech. This same linearity is found for speech spectrum noise (Konkle & Berry, 1983).

How much masking?

In deciding how much masking noise to use, the well-established one-to-one relationship between pure tone average and speech reception threshold can be used to advantage. In demonstrating the linearity of white noise masking in speech audiometry by obtaining speech thresholds in normal hearers at three different noise intensity levels, Hawkins and Stevens (1950) also found good agreement between masked thresholds for speech and masked pure tone averages. Their results are compared in Table 3.5 with masked speech reception thresholds and pure tone

TABLE 3.5
Masked Speech and Pure Tone Thresholds in Normal Hearers
Obtained With White Noise at Three Intensity Levels
Expressed in Level Per Cycle

Measures	Level Per Cycle		
	40	50	60
Average TD and TI[1]	50.9	60.4	69.8
Speech Reception Threshold[2]	49.8	59.8	69.8
Speech Reception Threshold[3]	48.4	58.4	68.3
Pure Tone Average[4]	51.0	60.8	69.7
Pure Tone Average[5]	49.2	59.0	69.0

[1]Average of threshold of detectability (TD) and threshold of intelligibility (TI) for connected discourse re threshold in quiet for the subjects tested (Hawkins & Stevens, 1950).
[2]Speech reception thresholds in dB re 22 dB SPL (Lizar et al., 1969).
[3]Speech reception thresholds in dB re 20 dB SPL (Setliff, 1971).
[4]Average masked thresholds for pure tones re thresholds in quiet for the subjects tested (Hawkins & Stevens, 1950).
[5]Average masked thresholds for pure tones re the ANSI-1969 standard (Sanders & Rintelmann, 1964).

averages from several other reports. Regarding the masked pure tone averages in the table derived from the results reported by Sanders and Rintelmann (1964), it should be pointed out that the masked thresholds obtained in their study were in hearing level according to the 1951 ASA standard; whereas the pure tone thresholds of Hawkins and Stevens (1950) were sensation levels re their subjects' thresholds in quiet. Because the thresholds in quiet were within 1 or 2 dB of the 1969 ANSI standard, the data of Sanders and Rintelmann were converted to that standard for comparison purposes here. The data in the table show excellent agreement among the studies and demonstrate the linear nature of speech masking with white noise as well as the close agreement between masked hearing for speech and for the pure tone average. This agreement permits us to determine effective masking levels for speech from those computed for pure tones.

On at least some of the newer speech audiometers, the masking-noise intensity dial is calibrated in effective masking level for speech. For those that are not, effective levels can be related to the numbers on the dial in either of two ways.

First, effective masking levels for speech can be derived from a table of effective masking for pure tones with white noise by averaging the effective levels for 500, 1000, and 2000 Hz for each dial setting. The construction of an effective masking level table for pure tones was described earlier in this chapter. Table 3.6 is a comparison of the effective masking levels for speech based on the mean effective levels computed for pure tones at 500, 1000, and 2000 Hz and the masked speech reception thresholds measured for normal hearers at three white noise intensities. The table shows an excellent agreement between the effective masking levels for speech predicted with the critical band data for pure tones and the effective levels obtained through direct measurement.

Second, effective levels can be obtained through actual measurement with a group of normal hearers. The speech signal and the masking noise are mixed into the same earphone, and speech reception thresholds are determined at three different settings of the masking dial. If the dial is linear, the average thresholds will show a linear relationship, and effective levels at other dial settings can be interpolated to complete the table. Just as with the effective masking table for pure tones, the values in the table indicate the hearing threshold levels to which the ear will be shifted with masking noise at the corresponding dial setting.

Diagnostic audiometry

Diagnostic audiometric procedures, directed toward qualitative rather than quantitative results, often present the situation in which masking is required to ensure response from the ear being tested. Although questions have been raised regarding the possibility of unusual effects when masking is used in diagnostic audiometry (Goldstein & Newman, 1985),

TABLE 3.6
Masked Thresholds for Speech Predicted With the Critical
Band Data and Masked Speech Reception Thresholds at
Three Intensity Levels Expressed in Level Per Cycle

Measures	Level Per Cycle		
	40	50	60
Pure Tone Average[1]	49.1	59.1	69.1
Speech Reception Threshold[2]	49.8	59.8	69.8
Speech Reception Threshold[3]	48.4	58.4	68.4

[1]Average masked threshold at 500, 1000, and 2000 Hz predicted with the critical band data.
[2]Speech reception thresholds in dB re 22 dB SPL (Lizar et al., 1969).
[3]Speech reception thresholds in dB re 20 dB SPL (Setliff, 1971).

there is no question that the failure to use masking will lead to erroneous results in at least some diagnostic tests. Particularly vulnerable to participation from the nontest ear are procedures such as the Carhart Tone Decay Test (Carhart, 1957; Jerger, Carhart, & Lassman, 1958) and the Performance-Intensity Tests (Jerger & Hayes, 1977; Jerger & Jerger, 1971). Tests such as these that involve presentation of the test signal at high intensity, often to an ear with unilateral sensorineural hearing loss, almost ensure a very large interaural difference with certain cross-over to the nontest ear. If tests such as these are to be used, the clinician must ensure against nontest ear response through the use of appropriate masking.

Comment

Sixteen years ago I wrote the following to introduce a chapter on clinical masking:

> Of all the clinical procedures used in auditory assessment, masking is probably the most often misused and the least understood. For many clinicians the approach to masking is a haphazard, hit-or-miss bit of guess work with no basis in any set of principles. (Sanders, 1972, p. 111)

The problem leading to the masking difficulties at that time was twofold. First, although the basic principles of accurate and effective masking were well-established through experimental research, the studies reporting those principles were published in a wide range of literature, much of which was generally unavailable to the clinician and even to many professionals and students in educational programs. Second, the masking equipment available was either inadequate or required special procedures for appropriate application. Both of those difficulties have now been overcome. Research findings have been brought together in a number of single sources that are readily available, and clinical audiometers now provide efficient masking noises calibrated in effective masking levels. Although clinical masking continues to pose challenging difficulties, the clinician now has ready access to the knowledge and equipment to solve whatever problems may arise in clinical masking.

References

American National Standards Institute. (1969). *Specifications for audiometers* (ANSI S3.6-1969). New York: Author.

American National Standards Institute. (1972). *Artificial headbone for the calibration of audiometer bone vibrators* (ANSI S3.13-1972). New York: Author.

American National Standards Institute. (1981). *Reference equivalent threshold force levels for audiometric bone vibrators* (ANSI S3.26-1981). New York: Author.

American Standards Association. (1951). *American standard specifications for audiometers for general diagnostic purposes* (ASA Z24.5-1951). New York: Author.

Carhart, R. (1957). Clinical determination of abnormal auditory adaptation. *Archives of Otolaryngology, 65,* 32–39.

Carhart, R. (1960). Assessment of sensorineural response in otosclerosis. *Archives of Otolaryngology, 71,* 141–149.

Carhart, R. (1971). Observations on relations between thresholds for pure tones and for speech. *Journal of Speech and Hearing Disorders, 36,* 476–483.

Denes, P., & Naunton, R. F. (1952). Masking in pure tone audiometry. *Proceedings of the Royal Society of Medicine, 45,* 790–794.

Dirks, D. (1963). *Factors related to reliability of bone conduction.* Unpublished doctoral dissertation, Northwestern University.

Dirks, D. (1964). Bone-conduction measurements. *Archives of Otolaryngology, 79,* 594–595.

Dirks, D., & Malmquist, C. (1964). Changes in bone-conduction thresholds produced by masking in the nontest ear. *Journal of Speech and Hearing Research, 7,* 271–278.

Dirks, D., & Swindeman, J. G. (1967). The variability of occluded and unoccluded bone-conduction thresholds. *Journal of Speech and Hearing Research, 10,* 232–249.

Egan, J. P., & Hake, H. W. (1950). On the masking pattern of a simple auditory stimulus. *Journal of the Acoustical Society of America, 22,* 622–630.

Feldman, A. S. (1961). Problems in the measurement of bone conduction. *Journal of Speech and Hearing Disorders, 26,* 39–44.

Fletcher, H. (1940). Auditory patterns. *Review of Modern Physics, 12,* 47–65.

Fletcher, H., & Munson, W. A. (1937). Relation between loudness and masking. *Journal of the Acoustical Society of America, 9,* 1–10.

Glorig, A. (1965). *Audiometry: Principles and practices.* Baltimore: Williams & Wilkins.

Goldstein, B. A., & Newman, C. W. (1985). Clinical masking. In J. Katz (Ed.), *Handbook of clinical audiology* (3rd. ed., pp. 170–201). Baltimore: Williams & Wilkins.

Hawkins, J. E., & Stevens, S. S. (1950). Masking of pure tones and of speech by white noise. *Journal of the Acoustical Society of America, 22,* 6–13.

Hirsh, I. J., & Bowman, W. D. (1953). Masking of speech by bands of noise. *Journal of the Acoustical Society of America, 25,* 1175–1180.

Hood, J. D. (1960). Principles and practices of bone conduction audiometry. *The Laryngoscope, 70,* 1211–1228.

Jerger, J., Carhart, R., & Lassman, J. (1958). Clinical observations on excessive threshold adaptation. *Archives of Otolaryngology, 99,* 409–413.

Jerger, J., & Hayes, D. (1977). Diagnostic speech audiometry. *Archives of Otolaryngology, 103,* 216–222.

Jerger, J., & Jerger, S. (1971). Diagnostic significance of PB word functions. *Archives of Otolaryngology, 93,* 573–580.

Jerger, J. F., Tillman, T. W., & Peterson, J. L. (1960). Masking by octave bands of noise in normal and impaired ears. *Journal of the Acoustical Society of America, 32,* 385–390.

Koenig, E. (1962a). On the use of hearing-aid type phones in clinical audiometry. *Acta Oto-Laryngologica, 55,* 131–143.

Koenig, E. (1962b). The use of masking noise and its limitations in clinical audiometry. *Acta Oto-Laryngologica* (Supplement 180), 1.

Konkle, D. F., & Berry, G. A. (1983). Masking in speech audiometry. In D. F. Konkle & W. F. Rintelmann (Eds.), *Principles of speech audiometry* (pp. 285–319). Baltimore: University Park Press.

Lidén, G. (1954). Speech audiometry. *Acta Oto-Laryngologica* (Supplement 114), 72–76.

Lidén, G., Nilsson, G., & Anderson, H. (1959a). Narrow-band masking with white noise. *Acta Oto-Laryngologica, 50*, 116–124.

Lidén, G., Nilsson, G., & Anderson, H. (1959b). Masking in clinical audiometry. *Acta Oto-Laryngologica, 50*, 125–136.

Lizar, D., Peck, J., Schwartz, A., & Stockdell, K. (1969). *Masking in speech audiometry*. Unpublished report, Vanderbilt University.

Miller, G. A. (1947). The masking of speech. *Psychology Bulletin, 44*, 105–129.

Naunton, R. F. (1960). A masking dilemma in bilateral conduction deafness. *Archives of Oto-Laryngology, 72*, 753–757.

O'Neill, J. J., & Oyer, H. J. (1966). *Applied audiometry*. New York: Dodd, Mead.

Sanders, J. W. (1972). Masking. In J. Katz (Ed.), *Handbook of clinical audiology*. Baltimore: Williams & Wilkins.

Sanders, J. W., & Rintelmann, W. F. (1964). Masking in audiometry: A clinical evaluation of three methods. *Archives of Oto-Laryngology, 80*, 541–556.

Setliff, W. M. (1971). *A comparison of four noises for masking speech*. Unpublished master's thesis, Vanderbilt University.

Studebaker, G. A. (1962). On masking in bone-conduction testing. *Journal of Speech and Hearing Research, 5*, 215–227.

Studebaker, G. A. (1964). Clinical masking of air- and bone-conducted stimuli. *Journal of Speech and Hearing Disorders, 29*, 23–35.

Studebaker, G. A. (1967). Clinical masking of the nontest ear. *Journal of Speech and Hearing Disorders, 32*, 360–371.

Studebaker, G. A. (1973). Auditory masking. In J. Jerger (Ed.), *Modern developments in audiology* (2nd. ed.). New York: Academic Press.

Wegel, R. L., & Lane, C. E. (1924). Auditory masking of one pure tone by another and its probable relation to dynamics of inner ear. *Physics Review, 23*, 266–285.

Zwislocki, J. (1953). Acoustic attenuation between ears. *Journal of the Acoustical Society of America, 25*, 752–759.

Zwislocki, J. (1966). Eine verbesserte vertaubungsmethode fur die audiometrie. *Translations of the Beltone Institute for Hearing Research. Acta Oto-Laryngologica, 39*, 338–356.

chapter four

Tympanometry: Basic principles and clinical applications

ROBERT H. MARGOLIS

JANET E. SHANKS

Contents

Tympanometry is the measurement of aural acoustic immittance as a function of ear canal air pressure. Since the first tympanometric recordings were reported in 1959, tympanometry has developed from an experimental procedure for estimating middle ear pressure into a routine clinical test that is useful for detecting a wide variety of middle ear pathologies. Clinical instruments, once quite limited in the choices of measurement parameters, now provide a wide range of alternatives that require the clinician to make decisions about, and understand, many physical dimensions and procedural variables. In the first section of this chapter the physical principles of tympanometry are reviewed. The second section presents a discussion of the characteristics of aural acoustic immittance instruments. The third section provides a comprehensive discussion of the clinical application of tympanometry.

Physical principles of aural acoustic immittance[1]

The middle ear is a transducer that converts acoustic energy into mechanical energy. It is so sensitive that eardrum vibrations for sounds that are near the threshold of audibility cannot be detected by the most sensitive instruments. Yet it responds with almost unmeasurable distortion to sound pressures that are a million times greater than the sound pressure at threshold. This remarkable system achieves its sensitivity and dynamic range by a delicate mechanical balance of anatomical structures that exist in an equally delicate physiological environment. It is not surprising that pathological disturbances of the middle ear produce changes in its mechanical properties. With ingenious electroacoustic devices, and an understanding of some basic physical principles, pathological changes in middle ear function can be measured, and these measurements can be exploited for diagnostic purposes.

The direct approach to the evaluation of a mechanical system is to observe the effect that a known force has on the system. By deforming the basilar membrane with a hair, von Bekesy observed its response and directly determined some of its mechanical properties. A direct approach to determining the mechanical properties of the middle ear would be to apply a known force directly to the tympanic membrane and measure its response. For clinical purposes, such a direct approach is impractical. Consequently an indirect method has been developed. By measuring the *acoustic immittance* of the air in the external auditory meatus, we can indirectly determine the properties of the middle ear. Because the acoustic characteristics of the air in the enclosed ear canal are partially determined by the middle ear, aural acoustic immittance measurements made with a probe inserted into the meatus are useful for detecting abnormal conditions of the middle ear. Proper interpretation of these indirect measurements requires a clear understanding of the interactions between the acoustic characteristics of the ear canal and the mechanical properties of the middle ear.

---

[1]See also Margolis (1981) and Van Camp, Margolis, Wilson, Creten, & Shanks (1986).

Acoustic immittance is a generic term that includes *acoustic impedance* and *acoustic admittance* and all of their components. Acoustic immittance measurement is a method for analyzing the responses of acoustic systems to sound. Other kinds of systems (e.g., mechanical and electrical systems) can be analyzed using similar techniques. Because mechanical systems are simpler and more familiar, the concept of *mechanical immittance* will be developed in this chapter, and then the same principles will be applied to acoustic systems. The immittance of a mechanical system is determined by exerting a force on the system and observing its response. In order to quantify the relationship it is necessary to understand the concept of *force*.

Force

An action that is capable of moving a body or changing the motion of a body is a force. In the international unit system (Systéme Internationale, SI)[2] the unit of force is the Newton (N). One N is the force required to change the velocity of a 1 kilogram (kg) mass by 1 meter per second (m/s) in 1 second. For example, if a 1 kg mass at rest is set in motion, thus achieving a velocity of 1 m/s in an elapsed time of 1 s, the force was 1 N.

Force can be static or dynamic. A static force is constant; it does not change with time. A dynamic force does change with time. Of course, there are an infinite variety of ways that dynamic forces can change with time. The simplest form of a dynamic force is one that changes sinusoidally, such as the one depicted in Figure 4.1. A sinusoidally changing force can be described mathematically by

$$F(t) = A \sin (2\pi ft) \tag{1}$$

where $F(t)$ is the force at any instant in time, A is the peak amplitude, f is the frequency of the sinusoidal change, and t is the time at which the measurement is made. It is convenient to express a sinusoidally changing force with one number that represents its magnitude. This is typically done by calculating the root mean square (rms) value of the sinusoidal force. That is, each instantaneous value in Figure 4.1 is squared, the squared values are averaged, and the square root of the mean is the rms force. This rms method is also used in acoustic systems to express the magnitude of a sinusoidally changing sound pressure.

Mechanical immittance

When a force is applied to an object, the object moves with a velocity that is proportional to the applied force. The relationship between the

---

[2]See Van Camp et al. (1986), for a discussion of units and unit systems.

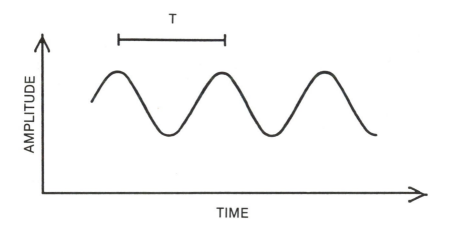

Figure 4.1. Sinusoidal waveform. The time between corresponding points on successive cycles (T) is the period.

velocity and the applied force provides the basis for quantitative analysis of the immittance characteristics of the system. That relationship can be stated in terms of a number of physical dimensions resulting in the various immittance quantities, expressed in various units of measurement.

It is important to keep in mind that *immittance* is a generic term and has no units of measurement, just as fruit has no specific color but bananas and oranges do. There are two fundamental approaches to immittance measurement: *impedance* and *admittance*.

In simple terms the *mechanical impedance* of an object is a measure of how difficult it is to move. If the same force moves one object faster than another, the first has a lower impedance than the second. Stated formally, mechanical impedance $|Z_m|$ is the ratio of the applied force F to the resulting velocity V:

$$|Z_m| = F/V \qquad (2)$$

The force may be static or dynamic. A dynamic force is usually expressed as an rms value. In a linear system, the velocity of the response to a sinusoidal force is also sinusoidal, typically expressed as an rms velocity. The frequency of the velocity waveform is identical to that of the force.

Three characteristics of a mechanical system determine its impedance: *mass, compliance,* and *friction*. Ideal mass, compliance, and friction elements are elements that possess only one of these characteristics. Ideal elements do not exist in the real world but they are useful concepts. The three types of ideal elements respond in a unique manner when acted on by a force.

When a force is applied to an ideal mass element, it moves in the direction of the applied force until another force stops it. Compliance (the opposite of stiffness) is a characteristic of a spring. When a force is applied to a spring it is compressed and it returns to its original position when the force is removed. An ideal friction element has no mass or stiffness and converts the applied mechanical force to heat until the force is dissipated or removed. The complete determination of the impedance of a mechanical system includes an analysis of the velocity of its response to an applied force and the combination of mass, compliance, and friction effects that contribute to its impedance. The impedance that results from mass elements is called *mass reactance* X_m. The impedance of spring elements is *compliant reactance* X_c. The impedance that results from friction is *resistance R*.

The admittance $|Y_m|$ of a mechanical system is the reciprocal of its impedance. That is,

$$|Y_m| = 1/|Z_m| = V/F \qquad (3)$$

Admittance is a measure of how easy it is to set the system in motion. Just as mass, stiffness, and friction contribute to the impedance of the system, each type of element contributes to its admittance. The admittance of a mass element is *mass susceptance* B_m. The admittance of a spring is *compliant susceptance* B_c. The admittance that results from friction is *conductance G*.

Acoustic immittance

Acoustic systems behave very similarly to mechanical systems, with masses, springs, and friction determining the acoustic immittance. An acoustic mass is a volume of air that moves as a unit with no compression when a force is applied to it, such as the air in an open tube. A volume of air enclosed in a rigid container is an acoustic spring. When it is compressed and released it resumes its original volume. Friction occurs as a result of collisions of molecules within the medium (air) and between the air and surrounding structures.

We can define acoustic impedance Z_a and admittance Y_a by modifying Equations 2 and 3. *Sound pressure P* is substitued for force F, and *volume velocity U* for velocity V to obtain

$$|Z_a| = P/U \qquad (4)$$

and

$$|Y_a| = U/P \qquad (5)$$

Sound pressure is the force per unit area produced by the airborne vibrations of a sound wave. Volume velocity is the volume of air that moves past an imaginary surface per unit time. Because sound is by definition dynamic, sound pressure is usually expressed as a root mean square value.

A complete description of the acoustic immittance of a system requires not only the determination of the ratios given in Equations 4 or 5, but also the relative contributions of mass, springs, and friction elements. This is done by stating the immittance in *polar* or *rectangular* notation.

When immittance is expressed in polar notation, it is stated as a ratio (P/U or U/V) and a *phase angle*. The phase angle is an expression of the time difference between the pressure and volume velocity waveforms. Just as mechanical masses, springs, and friction elements respond in unique ways to an applied force, acoustic elements respond differently to a sound pressure wave. When a sinusoidal sound is presented to an ideal acoustic mass, the sound pressure waveform *leads* the volume velocity waveform by one-fourth of a cycle ($+90°$). When the system is an ideal acoustic spring, the sound pressure waveform *lags* the volume velocity waveform by one-fourth of a cycle ($-90°$). When the acoustic system is an ideal friction element, the sound pressure and volume velocity waveforms are in phase ($0°$). The polar forms of the impedance and admittance equations are the following:

$$Z_a = P/U \underline{\angle}\ \phi_z \tag{6}$$

and

$$Y_a = U/P \underline{\angle}\ \phi_y \tag{7}$$

where ϕ_z is the phase angle of sound pressure relative to volume velocity and ϕ_y is the phase angle of volume velocity to sound pressure. For the same acoustic system, ϕ_z is equal to ϕ_y but opposite in sign. That is,

$$\phi_z = -\phi_y \tag{8}$$

When impedance is stated in rectangular notation, it is expressed in terms of its resistance and the sum of its reactance elements. Recall that the impedance phase angle ϕ_z associated with a mass element is $+90°$, and ϕ_z for a spring is $-90°$. These quantities behave as vectors that operate in opposite directions. Mass reactance always has a positive sign; compliant reactance is always negative. The *total reactance* X_t of an acoustic system is the algebraic sum of all of the mass reactances X_m and the compliant reactances X_c in the system. That is,

$$X_t = X_m + X_c \qquad (9)$$

The impedance in rectangular form is stated as

$$Z_a = R + jX_t \qquad (10)$$

Mathematically, j is equal to $\sqrt{-1}$, from complex number notation, and serves as a reminder that resistance and reactance cannot be combined by simple arithmetic because they are vectors that operate in different directions.

Similarly, acoustic admittance can be expressed in rectangular form by combining the susceptance values into a *total susceptance* B_t:

$$B_t = B_m + B_c \qquad (11)$$

The admittance is

$$Y_a = G + jB_t \qquad (12)$$

Figure 4.2 illustrates the use of vectors to express the acoustic immittance of the ear. Panel A presents an admittance vector system. On this coordinate system, compliant susceptance is represented as an arrow pointing upward (toward positive susceptance values); mass susceptance points downward (negative susceptance); and conductance points to the right. The length of each vector represents the magnitude (in acoustic mmho) of each component. The length of the resultant vector, labeled $|Y_{tm}|$, is the *admittance magnitude*, the quantity measured by most commercially available clinical acoustic immittance instruments. The angle formed by the admittance magnitude vector and the horizontal axix, ϕ_y, is the admittance phase angle. Panel B presents the impedance vectors for the same system. A mass reactance vector points upward; stiffness reactance, downward; and resistance, to the right. The values presented in these vector plots are typical of normal adult ears at 226 Hz.

From Figure 4.2 it should be apparent that the various immittance quantities are mathematically related to one another. The equations governing those relations are given in Table 4.1.

Although the immittance of a system may be equivalently stated in polar or rectangular notation, note that two numbers are always required. It has become common in aural acoustic immittance measurement to state the length of the impedance or admittance vector ($|Z_a|$ or $|Y_a|$) without the phase angle. Most clinical instruments do not provide the capability to measure the phase angle. Such an approach is an incomplete evaluation of acoustic immittance and allows the possibility that a pathological

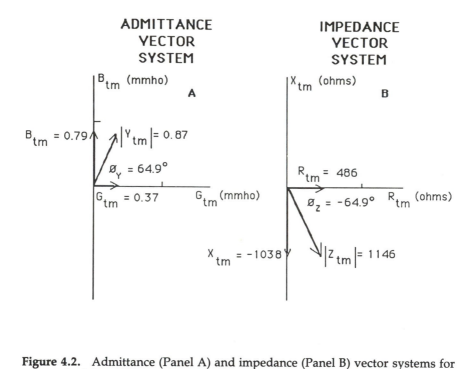

Figure 4.2. Admittance (Panel A) and impedance (Panel B) vector systems for a normal adult middle ear. Panel A shows compensated conductance (G_{tm}) and susceptance (B_{tm}) vectors and the resultant compensated admittance magnitude ($|Y_{tm}|$) vector at a normal phase angle (ϕ_y) of 64.9°. Panel B shows compensated acoustic resistance (R_{tm}) and reactance (X_{tm}) vectors and the resultant compensated impedance magnitude ($|Z_{tm}|$) vector at a normal phase angle (ϕ_z) of −64.9°.

condition may change the phase angle without changing length of the impedance or admittance vector. Cases of this nature have, in fact, been reported. Note that when the impedance or admittance vector is given without the phase angle, the magnitude $|Z_a|$ or $|Y_a|$ is placed in absolute value signs (see Equations 4 and 5) to indicate that its length, but not its direction, is known.

Frequency dependence of acoustic immittance

Acoustic resistance does not change with frequency. However, the immitances of reactive elements (acoustic springs and masses) vary with frequency. This frequency dependence is evident in the next two equations.

$$X_m = 2\pi fM \qquad (13)$$

$$X_c = \frac{-\varrho c^2}{2\pi fV} \qquad (14)$$

where ϱ is the density of the medium (usually air), and c is the velocity of sound.[3] Equation 13 expresses the relationship among mass reactance X_m, mass M, and frequency f. Note that the reactance of a mass is directly proportional to the frequency of the applied sound pressure. Equation 14 expresses the relationship among compliant reactance X_c, air volume V, and frequency. (See Lilly & Shanks, 1981, for a discussion of the constraints of this relationship.) Note that compliant reactance is inversely related to frequency. Thus changing the frequency has opposite effects on the immittance of mass and compliant elements. When a system has a combination of compliant and mass elements, as the ear does, changes in frequency may produce complex effects on the response system. In

TABLE 4.1
Immittance Equations

Defining Equations

$$Z = R + jX \qquad\qquad Y = G + jB$$

Computational Equations

$$|Z| = \sqrt{R^2 + X^2} \qquad\qquad |Y| = \sqrt{G^2 + B^2}$$

$$\phi_z = \arctan(X/R) \qquad\qquad \phi_y = \arctan(B/G)$$

Conversion Equations

$$R = \frac{G}{G^2 + B^2} \qquad\qquad G = \frac{R}{R^2 + X^2}$$

$$X = \frac{-B}{G^2 + B^2} \qquad\qquad B = \frac{-X}{R^2 + X^2}$$

$$\phi_z = -\phi_y \qquad\qquad\qquad \phi_y = -\phi_z$$

---

[3]Under standard conditions of temperature and barometric pressure, 20°C and 760 mm Hg (101386 Pa), $\varrho C^2/2\pi$ is a constant with a value of 226059. See Lilly and Shanks (1981) for a discussion.

order to gain a complete understanding of such a system, acoustic immittance measurements must be made over a wide range of frequencies.

Acoustic immittance of complex systems

Because aural acoustic immittance measurements are influenced by both the ear canal and the middle ear, it is necessary to consider how these systems interact to produce acoustic immittance measured by a probe at the lateral end of the ear canal. To understand this interaction we will consider the behavior of *series* and *parallel* systems. Figure 4.3 illustrates simple electrical systems that consist of two subsystems, Z_1 and Z_2, configured in *series* and in *parallel*. In the series system, current from the source must flow through both elements and the input impedance of the system (Z_i) is the sum of the impedances of the two subsystems:

$$Z_i = Z_1 + Z_2 \qquad (15)$$

In the parallel system, the current is divided so that some flows through Z_1 and some through Z_2 and the input impedance is given by

$$\frac{1}{Z_i} = \frac{1}{Z_1} + \frac{1}{Z_2} \qquad (16)$$

Solving for Z_i

$$Z_i = \frac{Z_1 Z_2}{Z_1 + Z_2} \qquad (17)$$

Because admittance is the reciprocal of impedance we can rewrite Equation 16 as follows:

$$Y_i = Y_1 + Y_2 \qquad (18)$$

Equations 15 and 18 reveal two simple rules regarding the immittance of series and parallel systems. The input impedance of a series system is the sum of the impedances of its components. The input admittance of a parallel system is the sum of the admittances of its components. From Equation 15 it is evident that the input impedance of a series system is greater than the impedance of any of its components. Not so obviously, but equally true, Equations 16 and 17 tell us that the input impedance of a parallel system is less than any of the component impedances. From Figure 4.3 we can infer another characteristic of parallel systems. In an

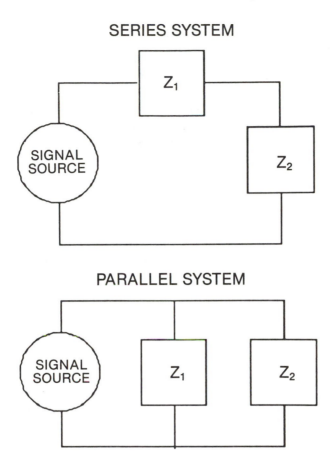

Figure 4.3. Series and parallel networks. Two impedances (Z_1 and Z_2) are configured in series (top) or parallel (bottom).

electrical parallel system, the voltages applied to parallel elements are equal. This will be true in a series system only if the impedances are equal.

Acoustic measurements made in the ear canal indicate that the ear canal space and the middle ear act as parallel acoustical elements. The impedance measured at the entrance to the ear canal is less than the impedance of the air enclosed in the ear canal. At frequencies below 1000 Hz, the sound pressure, which is analogous to electrical voltage, is equivalent at the lateral end of the ear canal and at the tympanic membrane. The ear canal and middle ear behave like the system depicted in the lower panel of Figure 4.3 where Z_1 is the impedance of the air enclosed in the ear canal and Z_2 is the impedance of the middle ear. Equation 17 can be rewritten

$$Z_i = \frac{Z_{ec}\, Z_{me}}{Z_{ec} + Z_{me}} \qquad (19)$$

where Z_i is the impedance at the plane of a probe inserted into the ear canal, Z_{ec} is the impedance of the air enclosed in the canal, and Z_{me} is the impedance of the middle ear. Because the middle ear impedance is the quantity of interest, we can solve Equation 19 for Z_{me}.

$$Z_{me} = \frac{Z_{ec}Z_i}{Z_{ec} - Z_i} \qquad (20)$$

With Equation 20 we can determine the acoustic impedance of the middle ear from the impedance measured in the ear canal (Z_i) if we know the impedance of the air enclosed in the ear canal (Z_{ec}). In the early days of clinical acoustic immittance measurement, this formula was used to estimate the middle ear impedance. Currently, commercial instruments are admittance meters. By measuring acoustic admittance rather than impedance, the simpler admittance equation can be used. Equation 15 can be rewritten

$$Y_i = Y_{ec} + Y_{me} \qquad (21)$$

Solving for Y_{me}

$$Y_{me} = Y_i - Y_{ec} \qquad (22)$$

The simpler form of Equation 22 in comparison to Equation 20 is the primary reason that clinical acoustic immittance measurements are commonly made in admittance units rather than impedance units. The relation expressed in Equations 21 and 22 indicates that the effect of ear canal volume is a simple additive constant that can be subtracted from the measured admittance to estimate the admittance of the middle ear. The correction for ear canal volume can be made by simple arithmetic by the clinician or it can be performed automatically by the instrument.

Correction for ear canal volume

Equation 22 provides a method for determining the middle ear admittance from the measured admittance at the probe tip and the admittance of the volume of air in the ear canal. One method of determining the immittance of the ear canal is to measure the volume and calculate its acoustic reactance by Equation 14. The first commercially available acoustic immittance instrument, the Zwislocki Acoustic Bridge (Zwislocki, 1963), used this method. The ear canal volume was measured by filling it with alcohol from a calibrated syringe. Although this method provides a high degree of accuracy, it is not feasible for routine clinical use. The method used instead is *tympanometry*, the measurement of aural acoustic immittance as a function of ear canal air pressure. From Equation 21 it is evident that if the middle ear admittance could be driven to zero, the measured admittance is equal to the admittance of the ear canal. Tympanometry provides a method for driving the middle ear admittance to near zero. By introducing either positive or negative air pressure into the ear canal, the middle ear is stiffened and its admittance becomes very low so that the measured admittance is a reasonable estimate of the admittance of the ear canal. Subtracting the ear canal admittance from all measured admittance values, that is, *compensation* for ear canal volume, provides estimates of the middle ear admittance Y_{me}.

Figure 4.4 presents a recording of acoustic admittance magnitude $|Y|$ as a function of ear canal air pressure—a *tympanogram*. Positive or negative ear canal air pressure decreases the measured admittance. Note that positive and negative pressure have similar, but not identical, effects. To correct for ear canal volume, the condition that best approximates $Y_{me} = 0$ should be chosen. That would be the lower of the two tail values.

Calculating static acoustic immittance

The tympanogram shown in Figure 4.4 provides acoustic admittance magnitudes ($|Y_{me}|$) over a wide range of ear canal pressures. For clinical purposes it is useful to express the acoustic immittance of the ear in one number—the *static acoustic immittance*. This value is usually taken from the peak of the tympanogram. The peak value represents the condition in which the ear canal air pressure is approximately equal to the air pressure in the middle ear. Because the middle ear pressure is a dynamically variable quantity, the peak immittance is more representative of middle ear function than the value at ambient or any other arbitrarily selected pressure. Moreover, peak admittance allows comparison of values taken under equivalent conditions—that is, with zero pressure difference on either side of the tympanic membrane. From the tympanogram in Figure 4.4, we can determine the *static admittance* as follows:

$$|Y_{me}| = |Y_{max}| - |Y_{min}| \tag{23}$$

where $|Y_{max}|$ is the peak admittance and $|Y_{min}|$ is the minimum value obtained from the lower tail value. Note that Equation 23 is identical in form to Equation 22.

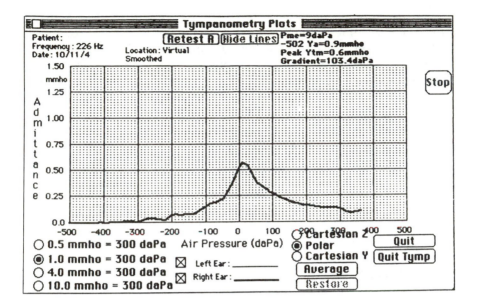

Figure 4.4. An admittance magnitude tympanogram, compensated at −400 daPa, from a normal adult ear.

Equation 23 provides a reasonable estimate of the admittance magnitude of the middle ear only when the phase angle associated with $|Y_{max}|$ and $|Y_{min}|$ are similar. With the commonly used low probe frequency (226 Hz) that condition is usually met. At higher frequencies, ear canal air pressure changes produce significant changes in phase angle, and the static immittance must be determined separately for admittance components. The MAX/MIN method (Equation 23) can be applied to the rectangular components of admittance as follows:

$$B_{me} = B_{max} - B_{min} \tag{24}$$

$$G_{me} = G_{max} - G_{min} \tag{25}$$

$|Y_{me}|$ can be calculated from its rectangular components by

$$|Y_{me}| = \sqrt{G_{me}^2 + B_{me}^2} \tag{26}$$

Instrumentation

Design principles of clinical acoustic immittance instruments

Although acoustic immittance measurements can be expressed in a variety of admittance and impedance formats, all clinical instruments are based on the same principle. A sinusoidal probe tone, most commonly 226 Hz, is presented to the sealed ear canal by a miniature loudspeaker (the driver) at a sound pressure level high enough to produce a favorable signal-to-noise ratio but below the threshold of the ipsilateral acoustic reflex (e.g., 85 dB SPL). A microphone provides a measure of the resulting sound pressure. The driver, microphone, a pressure delivery tube, and sometimes a transducer for ipsilateral acoustic reflex stimuli constitute the *probe assembly* (see Figure 4.5).

Impedance meter. Although there are no currently-produced aural acoustic impedance meters, it is important to understand the principle of impedance measurement. Figure 4.5 (middle panel) presents a block diagram of a one-component impedance meter, that is, an instrument that measures the magnitude of the impedance vector. A probe tone is presented to the driver and delivered to the ear. A microphone responds to the probe tone by changing the acoustic signal to an electrical signal, which is then filtered to reduce unwanted noise, rectified (converted to a dc voltage), and displayed on a meter, chart recorder, or video screen. The microphone voltage is proportional to the impedance at the probe tip, provided that the probe assembly is a *constant volume velocity source.* That is, volume velocity produced by the probe must be independent of the immittance characteristics of the ear. The impedance meter is a very simple device. It simply presents a volume velocity to the ear canal and measures the resulting sound pressure. The sound pressure is directly proportional to the impedance magnitude at the probe tip (Equation 4).

The impedance meter has two undesirable features. First, the probe tone sound pressure level varies from ear to ear and varies during the course of the tympanometric recording. Second, the shape of the impedance tympanogram is dependent on ear canal volume. This dependence on ear canal volume is illustrated in Figure 4.6 (top panel). Tympanograms from the same ear are shown with three hypothetical ear canal volumes (1.0, 0.5, and 0 cm³). Note the substantial effect of ear canal volume on the shape of the tympanogram.

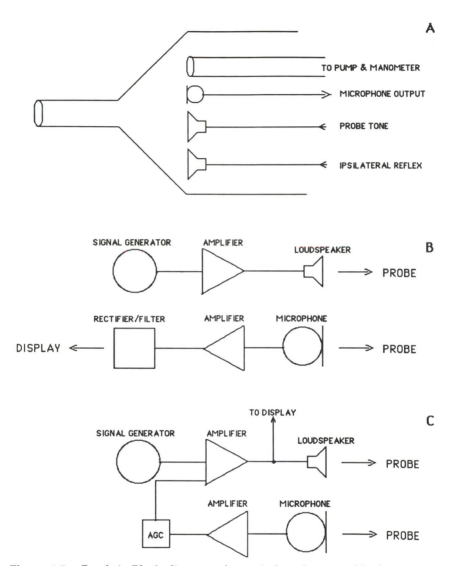

Figure 4.5. *Panel A:* Block diagram of a typical probe assembly for an aural acoustic immittance instrument. The device consists of two miniature loudspeakers to produce a probe tone and an ipsilateral acoustic reflex eliciting stimulus, a microphone to measure the probe tone sound pressure level, and a tube from a pneumatic system used to vary and measure the ear canal air pressure. *Panel B:* Block diagram of a one-component impedance meter. The loudspeaker (driver) presents the probe tone to the sealed ear canal. The microphone provides an electrical voltage that is proportional to the impedance of the "load," the ear. *Panel C:* Block diagram of an admittance meter. The probe tone is maintained at a constant sound pressure level by an AGC circuit. The voltage required to keep the probe tone sound pressure level constant is proportional to the admittance of the ear.

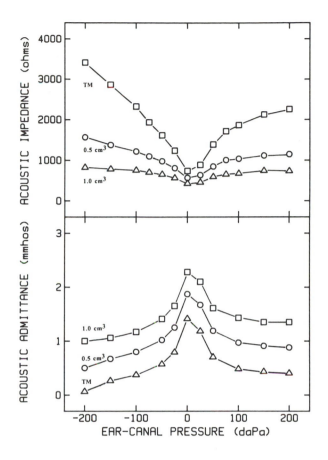

Figure 4.6. The effect of ear canal volume on uncompensated tympanograms recorded in acoustic impedance (upper panel) and in acoustic admittance (lower panel). Tympanograms are shown for ear canal volumes of 0.5cm³, 1.0 cm³, and compensated for ear canal volume (TM).

Admittance meter.   All currently-available acoustic immittance instruments measure acoustic admittance. A block diagram of an admittance meter is shown in Figure 4.5 (bottom). The admittance meter is similar to the impedance meter, but instead of measuring the sound pressure that results from a constant volume velocity probe signal, the sound pressure is kept constant with an AGC (automatic gain control) circuit. The admittance meter measures the electrical current that produces a constant ear canal sound pressure. The current required for a constant sound pressure is directly proportional to admittance magnitude at the probe tip.

Unlike impedance tympanograms, admittance magnitude tympanograms are not dependent on ear canal volume. In the lower panel of Figure 4.6 admittance tympanograms are shown with the same three assumptions of ear canal volume. Note the independence of the shape of the admittance magnitude tympanogram with volume changes.

Two-component admittance meters.   Although most commercially available instruments measure only the magnitude of acoustic admittance $|Y|$, some instruments measure both components of complex acoustic admittance. This is accomplished by measuring the phase of the probe tone in the ear canal and comparing it to the phase that occurs in calibration cavities. This phase angle measurement, along with the current needed to keep the ear canal sound pressure constant, provides the polar components of admittance (admittance magnitude and phase angle). From the polar components, the rectangular components can be calculated to produce susceptance and conductance tympanograms.

Microprocessor-based instruments.   Many of the current generation of aural acoustic immittance instruments employ dedicated microprocessors or personal computers to accomplish the processing formerly provided by analog electronic circuits. The principles of operation of these instruments are identical to those of the earlier analog devices. However, some of the components are replaced by software. The use of computers in acoustic immittance instruments provides the capabilty to calculate the values of any immittance component from admittance magnitude and phase angle. Computers also facilitate calibration of immittance instruments and provide a wider range of capabilities such as multifrequency tympanometry, automatic compensation for ear canal volume, and calculation of tympanometric variables such as static admittance and tympanometric width.

ANSI standard for acoustic immittance instruments

Although acoustic immittance measurements have been in routine clinical use since the early 1970s, a standard describing the measurement characteristics and tolerances for these instruments was not available until 1987 (ANSI, 1987). The goal of the standard is to ensure that aural acoustic immittance measurements at 226 Hz are approximately the same for an ear when measured with any instrument that meets the specifications and tolerances outlined in the standard. A secondary benefit of the standard is the promotion of uniform terminology and plotting formats. Compliance with the ANSI standard is entirely voluntary.[4]

Measurement units and terminology.   The ANSI standard recommends the use of the international units system (SI). The SI unit of air pressure, the dekapascal (daPa), replaces the unit of air pressure previously used for tympanometry (mm H_2O). The daPa and mm H_2O are related as follows:

$$1 \text{ mm } H_2O = 0.98 \text{ daPa}$$

$$1 \text{ daPa} = 1.02 \text{ mm } H_2O$$

For practical purposes, the two units can be considered to be equivalent.

Because clinical acoustic immittance measurement was widely employed for years before the existence of a standard, inconsistent and sometimes confusing terminology has been used. The standard provides the following definitions of terms, many of which have been frequently misused by manufacturers and in published reports.

Acoustic immittance refers collectively to acoustic impedance, to acoustic admittance, or to both quantities.

Acoustic compliance, the reciprocal of acoustic stiffness, is the ratio of a change in volume displacement to a change in sound pressure. This is the correct physical definition of the term and differs from the incorrect usage of "compliance" by equipment manufacturers.

Compensated static acoustic immittance is static acoustic immittance that has been compensated (or corrected) for the acoustic immittance of the ear canal. This value represents an estimate of the acoustic immittance at the lateral surface of the tympanic membrane and may be indicated by the subscript "tm." The method used for determining the acoustic immittance of the ear canal must be specified.

Peak compensated static acoustic immittance is the static acoustic immittance obtained with air pressure in the ear canal adjusted to produce a peak in the measured acoustic immittance. This value usually is obtained from a centrally located peak in the admittance tympanogram (peak Y_{tm}). This quantity is frequently referred to simply as the static admittance.

Measurement-plane tympanometry is a measurement of acoustic immittance in the measurement plane (i.e., the plane of the probe tip) and represents the combined acoustic immittance of the ear canal and the middle ear.

---

[4]See Melnick (1973) for information on the organizational structure of the American National Standards Institute.

Compensated tympanometry is a measurement of acoustic immittance that has been compensated (or corrected) for the acoustic immittance of the ear canal.

Plotting formats. Tympanometric shape is affected by the scale proportions (i.e., aspect ratio) used to plot the tympanogram. Tympanometric height and width appear to be different for identical measurements plotted on forms with different aspect ratios. The standard recommends an aspect ratio of 300 daPa to 1 acoustic mmho (or 1 cm³). Note in Figure 4.4 that a distance corresponding to 300 daPa on the abscissa is equivalent to the distance corresponding to 1 mmho on the ordinate. The standard recommends the following vertical and horizontal axis labels:

Vertical axis:
   Acoustic Admittance (10^{-8} m³/Pa × s [acoustic mmho])
Horizontal axis:
   Air Pressure (daPa) (1daPa = 1.02 mm H_2O)

Alternatively, the vertical axis label may be labeled:

   Acoustic Admittance of an Equivalent Volume of Air (cm³)
or:
   Acoustic Impedance (10^8 Pa × s/m³ [Acoustic kohm])

Because of the confusion that has existed regarding measurement units for tympanometry, the ANSI working group recommended these rather cumbersome labels for specifying tympanometric results.

Calibration. The standard describes calibration of many characteristics of acoustic immittance instruments. These are discussed in Chapter 16. Only calibration of the immittance indicator is discussed below.[5]

Acoustic immittance instruments are calibrated by comparing the instrument reading to the value expected for a known acoustic load. An enclosed volume of air is used for calibration because it approximates an ideal acoustic element for which the acoustic immittance can be determined from its volume, the probe frequency, and the atmospheric pressure (or elevation) at the test site (see Equation 14). At 20° C and an atmospheric pressure of 1.01×10^5 Pa (760 mm Hg), a 1-cm³ volume of air has an acoustic admittance magnitude of 1 acoustic mmho and an acoustic impedance magnitude of 1000 acoustic ohms at 226 Hz.

---

[5]See Lilly and Shanks (1981) and Shanks (1987) for more detailed descriptions of these procedures.

Calibration is performed by inserting the probe into the three calibration cavities that must be supplied by the manufacturer. The admittance magnitude reading is set to a value that is determined by the volume of the calibration cavity. If the probe frequency (f_p) is 226 Hz, the admittance magnitude in mmho is equal to the volume in cm^3. At higher probe frequencies, the admittance magnitude is the volume times the ratio of the probe frequency to 226. That is,

$$Y = V \frac{f_p}{226} \tag{27}$$

If calibration is not performed under standard atmospheric conditions of temperature and barometric pressure, it is extremely important to compensate for measurement conditions. As elevation increases, density and atmospheric pressure decrease and the acoustic impedance of a given volume of air also decreases. For example, at sea level and 226 Hz, a calibration cavity of 1.0 cm^3 has an admittance magnitude of 1.0 acoustic mmho and an impedance magnitude of 1000 acoustic ohms. The same calibration cavity 1 mile above sea level has an admittance magnitude of 1.22 acoustic mmho and an impedance magnitude of 818 acoustic ohms. Lilly and Shanks (1981) and Shanks (1987) provide tables to use in adjusting calibration values for elevation.

Clinical applications of tympanometry

The Vanhuyse model

The usefulness of low-frequency probe tones (i.e., 226 Hz) in detecting high-impedance middle ear pathologies such as otitis media has long been established. Similarly, the advantage of high-frequency probe tones (e.g., 678 and 800 Hz) for detecting low-impedance pathologies such as abnormalities of the tympanic membrane and ossicular chain is clear (e.g., Colletti, 1975; Funasaka, Funai, & Kumakawa, 1984; Lilly, 1984; Van Camp, Creten, Van de Heyning, Decraemer, & Vanpeperstraete, 1983; Zwislocki & Feldman, 1970). In contrast to low-frequency tympanograms, which are only single peaked or flat, high-frequency probe tones produce a wide variety of tympanometric shapes. When multipeaked tympanograms were first reported, they were thought to be indicative of tympanic membrane or ossicular chain abnormalities (Lidén, 1969). Continued experience with high-frequency tympanometry, however, revealed that multipeaked tympanograms frequently occurred in patients with no history or evidence of middle ear disease. In 1975, Vanhuyse, Creten, and Van Camp developed a model to explain the variety of tympanometric shapes that occur in both normal and abnormal ears.

Vanhuyse et al. (1975) began with some basic assumptions regarding the shapes and relative relationships between resistance and reactance tympanograms. Acoustic resistance R was assumed to be a monotonically decreasing function of ear canal pressure. Acoustic reactance X was assumed to be a symmetrical, single-peaked function. Acoustic susceptance B, conductance G, and admittance Y tympanograms were calculated from the resistance and reactance tympanograms. The model demonstrated that marked alterations in the shapes of the susceptance and conductance tympanograms result from a simple linear shift in the reactance tympanogram (Figure 4.7). Vanhuyse et al. identified four patterns of admittance tympanograms that were classified according to the number of positive and negative going peaks (*extrema*) exhibited in the susceptance and conductance tympanograms.

Type 1B1G. In Type 1B1G tympanograms, both the susceptance B and conductance G tympanograms are single peaked. This tympanometric pattern occurs when acoustic reactance X is negative (stiffness controlled) for all ear canal pressures. Furthermore, the absolute value of reactance is greater than resistance at all pressures (i.e., $|X_a| > R_a$). The corresponding admittance Y and phase angle ϕ tympanograms are also single peaked.

Type 3B1G. In Type 3B1G tympanograms, the conductance tympanogram is single peaked, but the susceptance tympanogram has a central notch due to a positive shift in the reactance tympanogram. Although reactance remains negative for all ear canal pressures, the absolute value of reactance is less than resistance near the peak and greater than resistance at extreme ear canal pressures. The central minimum in the susceptance tympanogram corresponds in presssure location to the peak reactance. The two maxima in the susceptance tympanogram occur at the pressures where the reactance and resistance tympanograms intersect. The positive susceptance maximum is higher than the negative maximum due to the asymmetry of the resistance tympanogram. When peak reactance is near zero, the admittance $|Y|$ tympanogram also may be notched.

Type 3B3G. In Type 3B3G tympanograms, the susceptance and conductance tympanograms have three extrema. This tympanometric pattern occurs when peak reactance is positive, indicating that the middle ear

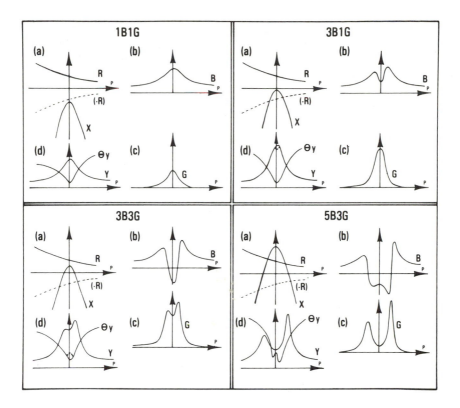

Figure 4.7. The Vanhuyse, Creten, and Van Camp (1975) model showing four patterns of admittance component tympanograms (1B1G, 3B1G, 3B3G, and 5B3G). The upper left corner of each panel shows typical acoustic resistance (R) and reactance (X) that might be obtained from a normal ear at a low-probe frequency. Also shown is the inverted resistance tympanogram ($-$R) to show the relationship between the absolute magnitudes of reactance and resistance. When the reactance and resistance do not intersect, the susceptance (B), conductance (G), admittance (Y), and phase angle (θ_y) tympanograms are single peaked (1B1G). As the reactance tympanogram shifts toward positive values, conductance, susceptance, admittance, and phase angle become double peaked, in that order. (From Osguthorpe, 1986, with permission.)

is mass controlled. A positive peak reactance value produces a negative peak susceptance value, resulting in the deeply notched susceptance tympanogram. When the central minimum of the susceptance tympanogram falls below the tail values, the ear is mass controlled. If the central minimum of a notched susceptance tympanogram is higher than the tail values, then the ear is stiffness controlled. Again, the maxima in the susceptance tympanogram occur near the points where the reactance and resistance tympanograms intersect. The maxima in the conductance tympanogram occur near the points where reactance equals zero. A notched conductance tympanogram generally occurs only in an ear that is mass controlled. The admittance tympanogram is also notched in the 3B3G pattern.

Type 5B3G. In the Type 5B3G tympanogram, the susceptance tympanogram contains five peaks and the conductance tympanogram exhibits three. The middle ear is mass controlled, and the peak reactance is greater than resistance. The maxima in the conductance tympanogram occur at the points where reactance is zero. The maximum reactance value corresponds with the central peak in the susceptance tympanogram. Again, the asymmetrical resistance tympanogram is responsible for the asymmetry in the susceptance and conductance tympanograms. This asymmetry is more evident when tympanograms are recorded in the ascending (−/+) pressure direction than in the descending (+/−) direction (Wilson, Shanks, & Kaplan, 1984).

Several studies confirmed that the Vanhuyse model accounts for a wide variety of tympanometry patterns observed in normal and abnormal ears (Creten, Vanpeperstraete, & Van Camp, 1978; Liden, Bjorkman, Nyman, & Kunov, 1977; Margolis, Osguthorpe, & Popelka, 1978; Margolis & Popelka, 1977).

Although normal 226-Hz susceptance and conductance tympanograms are always 1B1G, normal tympanograms at 678 Hz fall into all four categories. Table 4.2 shows the percentage of occurrence of each of the Vanhuyse categories among young adults for a 660-Hz (or 678-Hz) probe tone, a pump speed of 30 daPa/s and the negative to positive direction. The occurrence of multipeaked tympanograms increases for ascending (−/+) compared to descending (+/−) pressure changes (Margolis et al., 1978; Margolis, Van Camp, Wilson, & Creten, 1985; Margolis & Smith, 1977; Porter & Winston, 1973), for faster pump speeds (Creten & Van Camp, 1974), and with successive tympanometric recordings (Osguthorpe & Lam, 1981; Wilson et al., 1984). A higher rate of occurrence of multipeaked patterns suggests a shift in reactance toward positive values. These results, then, suggest that the following conditions result in higher (more positive) reactance: ascending pressure direction compared to the descending direction; faster rates of pressure change compared to slower rates; and repeated recording relative to the initial recording.

Multiple-frequency admittance tympanograms. The Vanhuyse et al. (1975) model accounts for the effect of probe frequency on tympanometric shapes. Figure 4.8 shows normal multifrequency admittance tym-

TABLE 4.2
Percentage of Occurrence of Vanhuyse Model Categories
From Normal Adult Subjects

	Category			
Study	1B1G	3B1G	3B3G	5B3G
Van Camp et al. (1983)	57	28	6	9
Wiley et al. (1987)	76	17	6	1

Note. The data were obtained from tympanograms recorded in the negative to positive direction with a pump speed of approximately 30 daPa/s and a probe frequency of 660 Hz.

panograms plotted in rectangular form (susceptance B_{tm} and conductance G_{tm}) and in polar form (admittance magnitude $|Y_{tm}|$ and phase angle ϕ_{tm}).

As probe frequency increased from 226 through 1243 Hz, the shapes of the conductance and susceptance tympanograms changed in a manner predictable from the Vanhuyse et al. model. At the lowest probe frequency, peak susceptance is about three times greater than peak conductance. This 3:1 magnitude relationship corresponds to a phase angle of 72°. The susceptance and conductance tympanograms in Figure 4.8 remain single peaked up to 678 Hz. As frequency increases, the amplitude of peak conductance and susceptance increases, but conductance increases faster until it becomes larger than susceptance at 678 Hz. As predicted by the Vanhuyse model, susceptance is the first component to notch. As frequency increases further, the notch in the susceptance tympanogram deepens and becomes negative or mass-controlled at 1017 Hz. The admittance tympanogram is the next component to notch, followed closely by notching of the conductance tympanogram. Phase angle tympanograms remain single peaked even above the resonant frequency of the middle ear.

The Vanhuyse et al. model demonstrates that the shapes of admittance component tympanograms are determined by the relationships between resistance and reactance. These amplitude relationships are depicted clearly by the plot of compensated static acoustic admittance in Figure 4.9. Each of the 10 points in the complex admittance plane were taken from the peaks of the susceptance and conductance tympanograms displayed in Figure 4.8. Conductance is represented along the x-axis and susceptance along the y-axis. A line drawn from the origin (0,0) to each

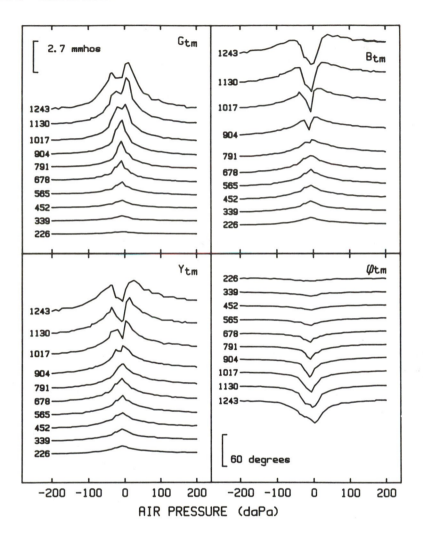

Figure 4.8. Normal, compensated conductance (G_{tm}), susceptance (B_{tm}), admittance (Y_{tm}), and phase angle (ϕ_{tm}) tympanograms for 10 probe frequencies ranging from 226 through 1243 Hz. (From Shanks, Wilson, & Palmer, 1987, with permission.)

point in the complex plane is acoustic admittance magnitude |Y|, and the angle formed between the admittance vector and the x-axis is the admittance phase angle ϕ_y. Theoretically, the admittance vector can lie anywhere between 90° and −90°. Susceptance can be either positive (stiffness controlled) or negative (mass controlled), but conductance must

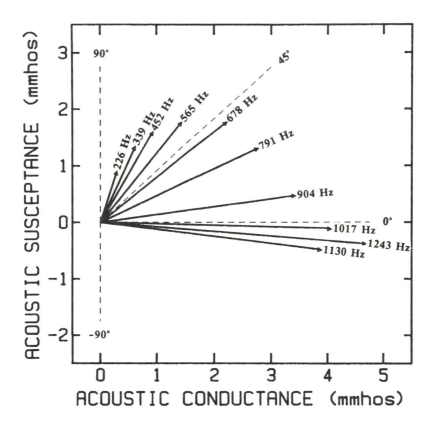

Figure 4.9. The rotation of the acoustic admittance vector, compensated for ear canal volume, over a frequency range of 226 to 1243 Hz for a normal adult ear.

always be positive. The boundaries of the vector rotation are a purely compliant (stiffness-controlled) system with the admittance vector pointing straight up (90°), or a purely mass-controlled system with the admittance vector pointing straight down (−90°). When the stiffness and mass contributions are exactly equal, at the resonant frequency of the middle ear, susceptance is 0 mmho and the admittance vector lies on the x-axis at an angle of 0°.

As probe frequency is increased from 226 to 1243 Hz, the admittance vector rotates from a phase angle of approximately 70° to about −5°. Many commercially available instruments measure only one component, admittance magnitude. This admittance measurement has been incorrectly called compliance because compliant (or stiffness) susceptance is the major contributor to admittance magnitude at low frequencies. In the example displayed for 226 Hz, susceptance is equal to 0.84 and admittance magnitude is equal of 0.88 acoustic mmho. The assumption that the admittance is a pure compliance is a reasonable approximation for normal adult ears. For abnormal adult ears, normal infant ears at 226 Hz, and for most tympanograms recorded at higher probe frequencies, the phase angle is sufficiently different from 90° that the term *compliance* is not an accurate description of the physical properties of the ear.

The Vanhuyse model predicts the following relationships between the occurrence of double-peaked tympanograms and admittance phase angle:

1. 1B1G tympanograms occur when the admittance phase angle is between 90° and 45°.

2. 3B1G tympanograms occur when the admittance phase angle is between 45° and 0°.

3. 3B3G tympanograms indicate that the admittance phase angle is between 0° and −45°.

4. 5B3G tympanograms indicate that the admittance phase angle is less than −45° and −90°.

Although there are exceptions to these relationships in normal subjects (Margolis et al., 1985), they appear to be reasonable approximations.

These same tympanometric patterns can be recorded in the presence of middle ear disease, but the frequency at which the various patterns emerge may be shifted higher or lower in comparison with normal ears. If the pathology increases stiffness, such as otosclerosis, the resonant frequency is shifted upward in frequency. Conversely, if the pathology decreases stiffness, such as ossicular discontinuity, then the resonant frequency will be shifted downward in frequency. At low frequencies such as 226 Hz, all ears whether normal or pathological are stiffness-dominated. A change in middle ear resonance does not produce a marked change in tympanometric shape. The determination of normal and abnormal results must be made on the basis of quantifiable characteristics, such as static admittance and tympanometric width. When a high-frequency probe tone is used to measure both components of complex acoustic admittance, a simple analysis of tympanometric shape may be sufficient to identify middle ear abnormalities. The clinical interpretation of tympanometric characteristics is discussed in the next section.

Clinical interpretation of tympanometric variables

Static admittance. Because tympanograms recorded with a 226-Hz probe frequency are almost always single peaked or flat, clinical interpretation is based on the height, location, and shape of the peak. The static admittance is estimated from the height of the admittance magnitude tympanogram. The standard (ANSI, 1987) refers to this quantity as the peak compensated static acoustic admittance.

Higher probe frequencies produce more complex shapes, making calculation of static admittance difficult. Interpretation of high-frequency tympanograms is facilitated by classification of shapes.

Static admittance varies with the procedural variables used to record the data. Three variables are particularly important: direction of pressure change, rate of pressure change, and method of ear canal volume compensation. These effects are summarized below.

1. Static admittance is lower for descending (positive to negative) than for ascending (negative to positive) ear canal pressure changes (Margolis & Smith, 1977; Porter & Winston, 1973; Wilson et al., 1984).

2. Static admittance is lower for slow rates of pressure change than for fast rates of pressure change (Creten & Van Camp, 1974; Ivarsson, Tjerstrom, Bylander, & Bennrup, 1983; Koebsell & Margolis, 1986; Margolis & Heller, 1987).

3. Static admittance is usually lower when ear canal volume is estimated from the positive pressure side of the tympanogram than from the negative pressure side (Shanks & Lilly, 1981).

It is important for each clinic to use normative values that were obtained with methods that are comparable to those used in the clinic. Because the effect of direction of pressure change is small at 226 Hz, it is probably reasonable to use the same norms for both pressure directions. The effect of pump speed is more significant. The static admittance obtained from preschool children with a pump speed of 200 daPa/s is about 22% higher than that obtained with a 50-daPa/s pump speed (Koebsell & Margolis, 1986). With a 400-daPa/s pump speed the static admittance is about 10% higher than at 200 daPa/s for preschool children and 8% for adults (Margolis & Heller, 1987). These differences are large enough to necessitate different norms for different pump speeds.

The method of compensation for ear canal volume also produces significant differences that necessitate different norms. Compensation at +200 daPa produces static admittance values that are consistently lower than the MAX/MIN method. Although the MAX/MIN (or −400 daPa) method produces more accurate estimates of the admittance at the tympanic membrane, screening instruments will probably continue to employ a correction at $+200$ daPa. Consequently, norms are needed for both methods.

A large-scale normative study of acoustic immittance is badly needed. Existing normative data were obtained with a variety of instruments and procedures that make compiling the data into clinical norms impossible. Table 4.3 provides some normative data based on small numbers of subjects that can be used in the interim period while we await more definitive normative studies. Clinical programs may wish to obtain their own norms.

Equivalent ear canal volume. In the presence of a flat tympanogram, an estimate of the volume of air medial to the probe can be useful in detecting eardrum perforations and evaluating the patency of a pressure-equalization (P-E) tube. Although a normal equivalent volume does not rule out the possibility of a perforation, a flat tympanogram with an abnormally large equivalent volume is evidence of a perforated eardrum or patent P-E tube.

Acoustic immittance measurements obtained with a low-probe frequency (e.g., 226 Hz) can be useful for estimating the volume of air medial to the probe (Lilly & Shanks, 1981; Lindeman & Holmquist, 1982). Tympanometric estimates of ear canal volume vary somewhat with age and sex and with the admittance component and ear canal pressure used to make the measurements.

Table 4.4 shows mean ear canal volumes and ± 2 standard deviation ranges for different patient populations and ear canal pressures. In general, females have smaller equivalent volumes than males, and children have smaller equivalent volumes than adults. The differences between males and females are small enough that separate norms are probably not necessary. Differences among age groups are more significant. The adult group data reported by Margolis and Heller (1987) show significantly larger equivalent volumes than their preschool-aged subjects. The predominantly older male subjects of Shanks (1985) had larger equivalent volumes than the younger adult groups tested by Margolis and Heller (1987) and Wiley, Oviatt, & Block (1987). Differences between equivalent volume estimates obtained at positive and negative pressures are probably not large enough to warrant separate norms (Shanks & Lilly, 1981). Equivalent volume estimates are only slightly smaller when made from susceptance versus admittance tympanograms at 226 Hz, which suggests that either is suitable for clinical use (Shanks & Lilly, 1981; Shanks, 1985; Wiley et al., 1987).

When the tympanic membrane is perforated, the volume medial to the probe is composed of the ear canal, middle ear space, antrum, and mastoid air cell system. Estimates of this volume using X-ray and fluid-

TABLE 4.3

Peak Compensated Static Acoustic Admittance (in acoustic mmho) at 226 Hz for Three Populations Obtained With Three Pump Speeds (50, 200, and 400 daPa/s) and Two Calculation Methods (MAX/MIN and +200)

Pump Speed (daPa/s):	50		200		400	
Compensation Method:	MAX/MIN	+200	MAX/MIN	+200	MAX/MIN	+200
Infants (2–4.5 months)						
Mean:	.55[4]	0.41[4]	0.45[1]	.32[1]	N/A	N/A
90% Range	0.26–0.92	0.20–0.56	0.25–0.67	0.11–0.60		
Children (3–5 years)						
Mean:	.55[2]	N/A	67[2]	.50[3]	N/A	.55[3]
90% Range	0.30–0.90		0.36–1.06	0.22–0.81		0.22–0.92
Adults						
Mean:	.85[5]	N/A	N/A	.72[3]	N/A	.78[3]
90% Range	0.56–1.36			0.27–1.38		0.32–1.46

Note. MAX/MIN values were obtained by subtracting the minimum tail value from the peak admittance. +200 values were obtained by subtracting the admittance at +200 daPa from the peak admittance. N/A = not available.

[1]Holte (1989)
[2]Koebsell & Margolis (1986)
[3]Margolis & Heller (1987)
[4]Margolis & Popelka (1975)
[5]Shanks & Wilson (1986)

TABLE 4.4

Means and ±2 Standard Deviation Ranges for Equivalent Ear Canal Volume for Various Age Groups, Sex, Admittance Component (Admittance Magnitude, Y, or Susceptance, B), and Ear Canal Pressure (in daPa) at Which Equivalent Volume Was Estimated

Study	N	Age	Sex	Component/ Pressure	Mean	±2 SD
Holte (1989)	20	3.5–4.5 mo	pooled	Y/ – 400	0.26	0.14–0.38
				Y/ + 200	0.37	0.21–0.53
Shanks (1985)	63	21–88 yr	males	B/ – 200	1.55	0.89–2.21
				Y/ – 200	1.59	0.89–2.29
Wiley, Oviatt, & Block (1987)	71	20–30 yr	pooled	B/ – 250	1.24	0.54–1.94
				B/ – 300	1.20	0.52–1.88
				B/ – 400	1.15	0.53–1.77
Margolis & Heller (1987)	47	3–6 yr	males	Y/ + 200	0.80	0.50–1.10
	45	3–6 yr	females	Y/ + 200	0.70	0.38–1.02
	49	20–62 yr	males	Y/ + 200	1.14	0.62–1.66
	38	20–62 yr	females	Y/ + 200	0.93	0.57–1.29

filling procedures in human temporal bones show large intersubject variability. Volume estimates have ranged from 2 to 22 cm³ with mean volumes ranging from 6.5 to 8.6 cm³ (Molvaer, Vallersnes, & Kringlebotn, 1978; Zwislocki, 1962). Terkildsen and Thomsen (1959) estimated volume from 220 Hz admittance tympanograms recorded from two temporal bones prior to and immediately following perforation of the tympanic membranes. Volumes estimates were 0.75 and 0.80 cm³ prior to perforation and were 4.0 and 2.6 cm³ following perforation.

It is important to note that ears with perforations and concomitant middle ear disease frequently do not produce abnormally large equivalent volume estimates (see Margolis & Shanks, 1985, Figure 23.12). Due to inflammation and/or space-occupying lesions of the middle ear, the volume in front of the probe may not be abnormally large even though the eardrum is perforated. A normal equivalent volume, then, in the presence of a flat tympanogram, does not rule out perforation of the tympanic membrane.

Tympanometry in the presence of a known perforation may be a useful indicator of the status of the middle ear and mastoid air cell systems prior to surgical intervention. Andreasson (1977) found significantly smaller volumes in patients with perforated eardrums secondary to chronic otitis media than in patients with traumatic perforations. He hypothesized that chronic middle ear disease with recurrent discharge reduces the volume by successively obstructing portions of the mastoid air cell system. This reduction in volume may be related to findings of better long-term surgical results in patients with large volumes than in those with small volumes. Holmquist (1970) and Lindeman and Holmquist (1982) concluded that the volume of the mastoid is an important factor in the long-term success of myringoplasty.

In addition to wide variations in tympanometric estimates of volume among patients with tympanic membrane perforations, variations also have been noted among their tympanometric patterns. Figure 4.10 shows three different tympanometric patterns recorded from patients with tympanic membrane perforations. The tympanograms in the left panel show the most common pattern. Susceptance and admittance magnitude at 226 Hz is high (3.6 mmho) and conductance is close to the expected value of 0 mmho for a hard-walled cavity. At 678 Hz, susceptance has increased by approximately a factor of three and conductance remained low. The tympanograms in the center panel also were recorded from a patient with a perforation, but a keratoma (cholesteatoma) filled the middle ear space and obstructed the mastoid air cell system. This decreased middle ear volume is reflected by low admittance |Y| and susceptance B at 226 Hz (approximately 1.5 cm³). In the absence of an otoscopic examination, this flat tympanometric pattern with a normal equivalent volume estimate could be confused with patterns recorded in middle ear effusion or lateral ossicular fixation. The tympanograms in the right panel were recorded from a patient with a perforation in conjunction with healthy middle ear mucosa. Susceptance and admittance measures at 226 Hz indicate a large volume (>5 cm³). At 678 Hz susceptance is off scale in the negative direction, indicating a large mass component. The complex geometry of the normal ear canal and middle ear system does not produce a pure acoustic compliance for high-frequency probe tones such as 678 Hz. This case illustrates the superiority of the low-probe frequency for estimating the volume in front of the probe.

Gradient.   A variety of measures of the sharpness of the tympanometric peak have been used to detect middle ear pathology. Brooks (1968) introduced the term *gradient* for this characteristic of the tympanogram and provided a method for its calculation. He reported that abnormal gradient was more effective for detecting middle ear effusion than static immittance or tympanometric peak pressure. Subsequent investigation supported that conclusion (Fiellau-Nikolajsen, 1983; Haughton, 1977; Paradise, Smith, & Bluestone, 1976). Two recent investigations explored

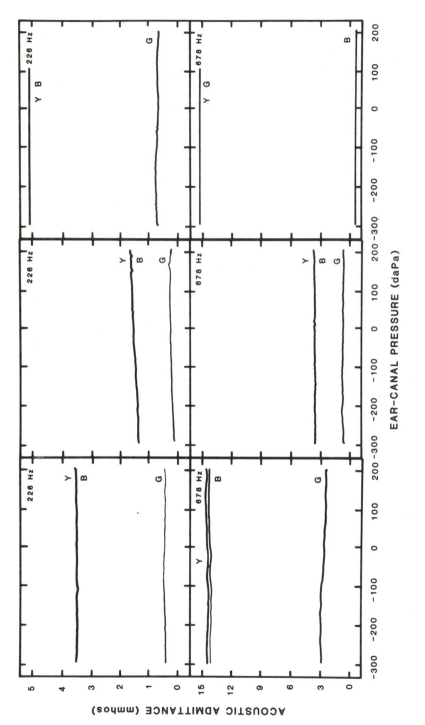

Figure 4.10. Admittance component tympanograms from three patients with tympanic membrane perforations.

the statistical properties of various gradient measures obtained from normal ears (deJonge, 1986; Koebsell & Margolis, 1986). In those studies, the measure first described by Liden and his colleagues (Liden, Harford, & Hallen, 1974; Liden, Peterson, & Bjorkman, 1970) appeared to be superior to other calculation methods. That measure, the *tympanometric width*, is illustrated in Figure 4.11. Tympanometric width is obtained by determining the pressure interval associated with a 50% reduction in admittance on either side of the peak. Some normative values for tympanometric width are presented in Table 4.5.

Ideally the tympanometric width would be calculated automatically by the acoustic immittance instrument. Several commercially-available instruments provide a gradient calculation. Caution must be observed in interpreting these measures, because manufacturers have not adopted a standard method of calculation.

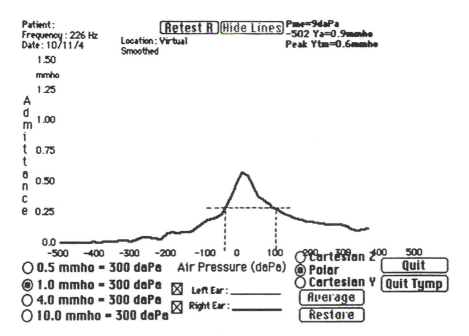

Figure 4.11. Calculation of tympanometric width from a compensated admittance magnitude tympanogram. The dashed line is placed at one-half peak compensated static admittance. In this example the tympanogram is compensated at −400 daPa. The distance along the pressure axis between points of intersection is determined. The tympanometric width is 140 daPa.

TABLE 4.5

Normative Tympanometric Width (Gradient) Data (in daPa) for Three Populations Calculated From Tympanograms Compensated by the MAX/MIN Method and by Subtracting the Admittance at +200 daPa

Ear Canal Correction	Infants		Preschool		Adults	
	MAX/MIN	+200	MAX/MIN	+200	MAX/MIN	+200
Mean	187[2]	135[2]	133[3]	100[4]	123[5]	77[4]
SD	26[2]	54[2]	42[3]	26[4]	46[5]	18[4]
90% range	150–250[2]	110–180[2]	80–200[3]	59–151[4]	60–160[1]	51–114[1]

[1]DeJonge (1986)
[2]Holte (1989)
[3]Koebsell & Margolis (1986)
[4]Margolis & Heller (1987)
[5]Shanks & Wilson (1986)

Because the tympanometric width is calculated from the peak compensated static admittance, the value is dependent on the method of ear canal volume correction. The data in Table 4.5 were obtained from studies that compensated for ear canal volume in two ways. The data from Shanks and Wilson (1986) and Koebsell and Margolis (1986) were compensated by the MAX/MIN method. Margolis and Heller (1987) used a screening instrument that automatically compensates by subtracting the admittance at +200 daPa from all tympanometric values. In a study of tympanometric width from normal subjects and patients with a variety of middle ear disorders, Koebsell, Shanks, Cone-Wesson, and Wilson (1988) demonstrated that tympanometric widths calculated from the negative side of the tympanogram were excessively variable. Calculation of tympanometric width from the peak to +200 daPa appeared to provide a more useful clinical measure.

Figure 4.12 presents two tympanograms that illustrate the clinical use of tympanometric width. The top panel illustrates a normal tympanogram from a preschool child. The shaded region indicates the upper limit of the normal range (from Margolis & Heller, 1987) positioned on the tympanogram at one-half peak admittance. The intersection of the tympanogram with the "template" indicates a normal tympanometric width. The bottom panel illustrates an abnormal tympanogram from an adult. The shaded region represents the upper limit of the normal range for adults (from Margolis & Heller, 1987). The template does not intersect the tympanogram, indicating an abnormal tympanometric width.

An abnormal gradient appears to be a strong indicator of middle ear pathology. Conditions that produce abnormal gradients, however, especially in children, are frequently transient, self-correcting conditions that do not require a medical referral. This will be discussed further in the section, *Criteria for Medical Referral*.

Tympanometric peak pressure.   The ear canal air pressure at which the peak of the tympanogram occurs is the *tympanometric peak pressure* (TPP). TPP often is used to estimate middle ear pressure. In some cases TPP provides a good estimate of the pressure behind the tympanic membrane. In others, however, TPP and the directly measured middle ear pressure are substantially different (Elner, Ingelstedt, & Ivarsson, 1971; Renvall & Holmquist, 1976). Because there is no way to know the extent of disagreement between TPP and middle ear pressure without an invasive procedure, the term tympanometric peak pressure is the appropriate term for the location of the tympanometric peak.

TPP has been widely used as a clinical measure since the advent of tympanometry. Notably, the first published report of the clinical application of tympanometry (Terkildsen & Thomsen, 1959) was subtitled "A

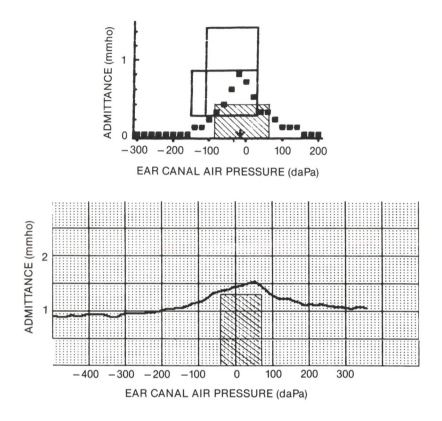

Figure 4.12. Templates used to evaluate tympanometric width. The diagonally-shaded regions represent the upper limits of the normal ranges for tympanometric width for preschool children (upper panel) and adults (lower panel). If the tympanogram intersects the template, placed at half the peak (static) admittance, the tympanometric width is within the normal range. The upper panel shows a tympanogram from a child with normal tympanometric width. The lower panel shows a tympanogram from an adult with an abnormal tympanometric width. (From ASHA, 1990, with permission.)

Method for Objective Determination of the Middle-Ear Pressure.'' Since then, TPP has been used in the classification of tympanograms (Feldman, 1976, 1977; Jerger, 1970; Liden, 1969; Paradise et al., 1976), as a pass-fail criterion in screening protocols (ASHA 1978; Harker & Van Wagoner, 1974; McCandless & Thomas, 1974), and as a diagnostic indicator for otitis media (Renvall, Liden, Jungert, & Nilsson, 1975).

The clinical use of TPP has been based primarily on the *ex vacuo* theory of middle ear function. (See Magnuson, 1983, for a review.) This theory posits that the normal middle ear is in a fluctuating state of negative pressure caused by the unidirectional diffusion of gases from the middle ear space to the mucosa and the periodic opening of the Eustachian tube. After a Eustachian tube opening, the middle ear pressure would drift from ambient pressure to a negative value that results from diffusion of gases from the air into the cells lining the middle ear cavity. This diffusion process would continue until the partial pressures of the various gases in the middle ear became equivalent to the partial pressures within the cells of the mucosa. Large negative intratympanic pressures would develop if the interval between Eustachian tube openings was long. The large negative TPPs (< -200 daPa) frequently observed in various forms of otitis media were explained on this basis.

Evidence is mounting that the foregoing description is not an accurate account of Eustachian tube physiology. It has been observed, that when the Eustachian tubes of experimental animals are chronically closed by anesthesia or ligation, negative pressures that develop are seldom more negative than -100 daPa (Cantekin, Doyle, Phillips, & Bluestone, 1980; Proud, Odoi, & Toledo, 1971). Furthermore, the small, fluctuating, negative pressures predicted to exist in normal middle ears apparently do not occur. Instead, the normal middle ear pressure, after a period of Eustachian tube closure, has been shown to be slightly positive (Hergils & Magnuson, 1985, 1987; Wiley, Oviatt, & Block, 1987) which suggests a bidirectional diffusion process, allowing gases to enter the middle ear space from the mucosa. These observations are not consistent with the *ex vacuco theory*.

Other mechanisms may account for the large negative pressures observed in patients. The ciliary action of the Eustachian tube may lower the middle ear pressure as it moves fluid through the closed tube (Hilding, 1944; Murphy, 1979). Alteration in middle ear gas composition caused by middle ear disease may also contribute to negative middle ear pressure (Cantekin et al., 1980; Yee & Cantekin, 1986). Because the diffusion of gases across a cell membrane depends on the relative concentration of gases outside and inside the cell, a change in middle ear gas composition alters the rate of diffusion, producing a greater negative pressure than would occur with normal middle ear gas composition. Another mechanism that may account for at least some large negative middle ear pressures is sniffing (Falk, 1981, 1983; Magnuson, 1981). The rush of air past an abnormally compliant Eustachian tube can produce a partial evacuation of the middle ear. Abnormally compliant Eustachian tubes may account for a substantial proportion of cases with retraction of the tympanic membrane (Magnuson, 1981; Schuknecht, 1974).

It appears, then, that negative TPP can be produced by a variety of mechanisms. In the absence of other tympanometric abnormalities, hearing loss, or medical symptoms, it is a poor indicator of middle ear effusion (Fiellau-Nikolajsen, 1983; Haughton, 1977; Paradise et al., 1976). When the tympanogram is otherwise normal, negative TPP indicates that a negative pressure exists behind the tympanic membrane, but the mechanical properties of the middle ear have not been altered. Although it may be useful to record TPP in the hearing evaluation report, it should not be used as a criterion for retest or medical referral.

Tympanometric shapes. Because much of the early work in tympanometry was done with instruments that displayed the results in relative units, qualitative analysis of tympanometric shapes, rather than quantitative analysis of tympanograms, was necessary. Several methods for classifying tympanograms according to a qualitative judgment of tympanometric shape have been employed (see Margolis & Shanks, 1984, for a review). The most commonly used system was originally proposed by Liden (1969) and modified by Jerger (1970). In that system, tympanograms were classified according to the height and location of the tympanometric peak. A normal tympanogram (Type A) has a peak that is normal in height and location. A flat tympanogram is designated Type B. A tympanogram with a negative tympanometric peak pressure is Type C. Tympanograms with a low peak or a high peak are designated Type As and Type Ad, respectively.

Other classification schemes suggested by Paradise et al. (1976) and Feldman (1977) categorized tympanograms based on peak height, tympanometric peak pressure, and shape. The Vanhuyse model provided a method of classifying tympanometric shape based on the number of peaks in the conductance and susceptance tympanograms.

Because tympanograms obtained with a low probe frequency are relatively invariant in shape, quantitative analysis of those features that are known to relate to middle ear pathology is more effective than classification of shapes. Tympanograms obtained with higher probe frequencies are more effectively evaluated by a classification of shapes for three reasons. First, static admittance and gradient are difficult to calculate due to the frequent occurrence of multiple-peaked tympanograms obtained with higher probe frequencies. Second, static admittance cannot be accurately determined from admittance magnitude tympanograms at higher frequencies where there is a significant phase shift produced by pressurizing the ear canal. Third, tympanograms obtained with higher probe frequencies are characterized by a variety of shapes that can be related to the condition of the middle ear.

In a study of patients with ossicular abnormalities and human temporal bones with experimentally produced ossicular discontinuities, Van de Heyning, Van Camp, Creten, and Vanpeperstraete (1982) determined the following simple set of rules for distinguishing normal 660-Hz multi-peaked tympanograms from abnormal ones. If any of the following conditions are met (with a 660- or 678-Hz probe tone), the tympanogram reflects a pathological condition.

1. The number of extrema exceeds five for susceptance, three for conductance, and three for admittance.

2. The outermost peaks in the conductance tympanogram do not fall between the outermost peaks in the susceptance tympanogram.

3. The pressure interval between the outermost peaks exceeds 75 daPa for tympanograms with three extrema and 100 daPa for tympanograms with five extrema.

These criteria appear to be effective for detecting the two major categories of low-impedance pathologies, eardrum abnormalities and ossicular lesions, and some high-impedance pathologies, such as otitis media in intermediate stages of development and remission.

In subsequent sections the use of tympanometric shapes obtained with high-frequency probe tones for detecting middle ear pathologies are discussed.

High-impedance pathologies

High-impedance pathologies of the middle ear are associated with the various forms of otitis media, ossicular fixation, and space-occupying lesions such as primary and invading tumors. The effects of these pathologies are complex and the degree of tympanometric abnormality is not closely related to the severity of the disease. Potentially life-threatening middle ear disease may produce subtle tympanometric abnormalities, and clinically unimportant conditions of the middle ear may produce gross irregularities in the tympanograms.

The most obvious form of high-impedance pathology is the flat tympanogram. When fluid or neoplasm occupies the normally air-filled middle ear cleft, the impedance of the middle ear is increased so that varying the ear canal air pressure has no effect on middle ear impedance and the tympanogram is flat. However, there are more moderate high-impedance conditions that represent clinically significant pathology that do not produce flat tympanograms. In some of these conditions, the tympanograms go through a stage in which, because of mass loading of the middle ear, the impedance is actually lower than normal, and a variety of multipeaked patterns occur. As the condition progresses, the tympanograms begin to flatten as the impedance becomes abnormally high.

Figure 4.13 shows a 226-Hz admittance tympanogram with a peak height (static admittance) that is just within the normal range for adults (indicated by the taller rectangle) but the tympanometric width (200 daPa)

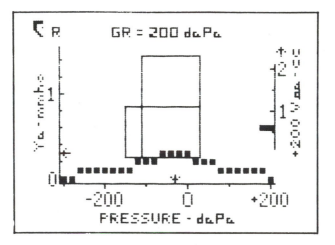

Figure 4.13. Admittance magnitude tympanogram from a patient with lateral ossicular fixation.

is abnormal. Abnormally wide tympanograms occur in certain stages of otitis media (Fiellau-Nikolajsen, 1983) and some patients with lateral ossicular fixation.

Figure 4.14 presents tympanograms from a patient with otitis media in a resolving stage. At 226 Hz, static admittance is slightly low $|Y_{tm}|$ = 0.38 mmho) and the tympanometric width is normal (TW = 105 daPa). At 678 Hz, the pattern is a very wide 3B3G, indicating a mass controlled ear, probably due to mass loading of the middle ear. The pattern is abnormal because of the broad interval between susceptance peaks.

Figure 4.15 shows tympanograms from a patient with external otitis. At 226 Hz, the tympanograms are normal in height $|Y_{tm}|$ = 0.76 mmho) and width (144 daPa). At 678 Hz, the pattern is a very wide 5B3G due to mass loading of the eardrum. Again, the pattern is abnormal because of the wide intervals between peaks.

The cases presented in Figures 4.14 and 4.15 illustrate the value of obtaining tympanograms at more than one frequency.

Figure 4.16 presents tympanograms from three patients with ossicular fixation. The tympanograms in the left panel are from a patient with lateral ossicular fixation due to adhesions involving the ossicles and tympanic membrane. The static admittance at 226 Hz is abnormally low $|Y_{tm}|$ = 0.18 mmho) and the tympanometric width is abnormally wide (226 daPa). The tympanograms in the middle and right panels are from patients with otosclerosis. The case presented in the middle panel shows a slightly low

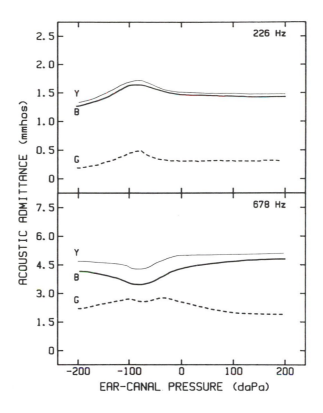

Figure 4.14. Admittance component tympanograms recorded at 226 and 678 Hz from a patient with resolving otitis media.

static admittance $|Y_{tm}|$ = 0.45 mmho) and normal tympanometric width (67 daPa) at 226 Hz. The right panel illustrates a case in which the static admittance at 226 Hz is within the normal range ($|Y_{tm}|$ = 0.70 mmho) but the tympanometric width is narrow (17 daPa). These cases demonstrate that lateral ossicular fixation is easily detected by tympanometry. Tympanograms from patients with stapedial fixation are frequently normal at 226 and 678 Hz, as they are in the middle and right panels of Figure 4.16. It may be necessary to use more than two probe frequencies to detect otosclerosis. Multifrequency tympanometry, by providing a method of estimating the resonant frequency of the middle ear, may prove to be an effective method for detecting stapedial fixation.

Although the Vanhuyse model has been primarily applied to low-impedance pathologies, it is useful for understanding high-impedance

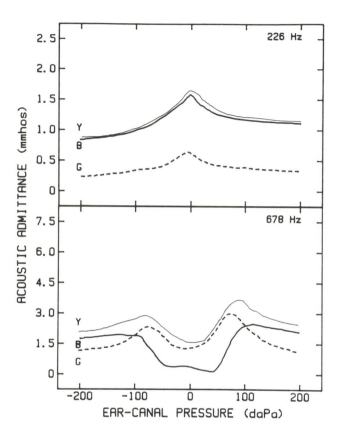

Figure 4.15. Admittance component tympanograms recorded at 226 and 678 Hz from a patient with external otitis.

pathologies as well. Van Camp, Shanks, and Margolis (1986) extended the model to account for tympanograms from patients with otitis media, lateral ossicular fixation, and otosclerosis. Figure 4.17 illustrates the assumptions made to account for tympanometric abnormalities that occur in patients with otitis media and lateral ossicular fixation. Otitis media has the effect of adding mass and resistance to the middle ear. The resistance tympanogram (R) was assumed to be normal in shape but shifted toward higher values. The reactance tympanogram was assumed to be shifted to positive values because of the mass loading of the ossicular chain. The three values (800, 1600, and 2400) indicated in Figure 4.17 represent three degrees of severity of the middle ear abnormality. These resistance and reactance tympanograms successfully predicted results from patients with otitis media (e.g., Figure 4.14).

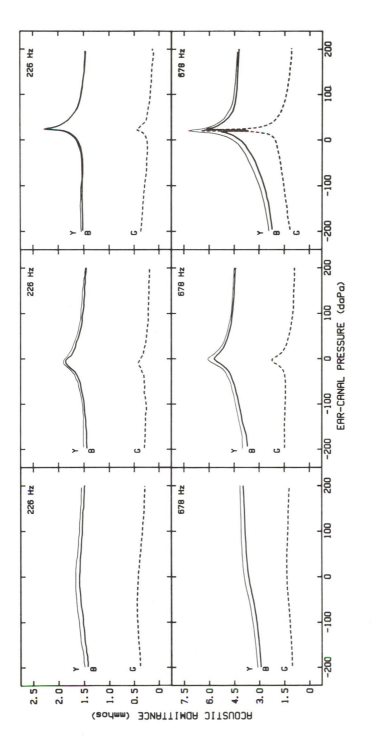

Figure 4.16. Admittance (Y), conductance (G), and susceptance (B) tympanograms recorded at 226 and 678 Hz for three patients with ossicular fixation. The tympanograms in the left panel are for a patient with lateral ossicular fixation. Those in the middle and right panels are from patients with otosclerosis.

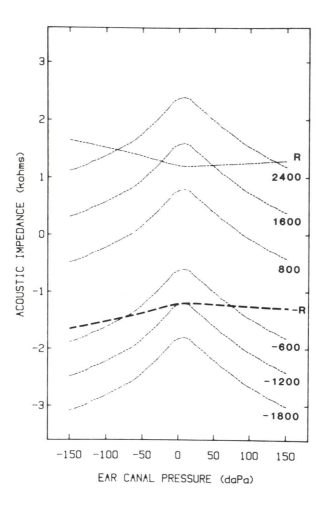

Figure 4.17. Resistance (R) and reactance tympanograms (678 Hz) for simulated cases of otitis media and lateral ossicular fixation. Otitis media shifts the reactance tympanogram toward positive values (800, 1600, 2400 acoustic ohms); lateral ossicular fixation shifts reactance toward more negative values (−600, −1200, −1800). (From Van Camp, Shanks, & Margolis, 1986, with permission.)

Lateral ossicular fixation was assumed to add stiffness to the system, shifting the reactance tympanogram toward more negative values. The three reactance tympanograms in the lower portion of Figure 4.17 (−600, −1200, −1800) represent three degrees of involvement. These resistance and reactance tympanograms appeared to account for results from lateral ossicular fixation like those shown in Figure 4.16 (left panel).

Figure 4.18 illustrates the attempt by Van Camp, Shanks, and Margolis (1986) to account for tympanometric findings in otosclerosis. Evidence from previous investigations suggested that the primary effect of stapes fixation is to add stiffness reactance to the system, leaving resistance relatively unchanged. In addition, the change in the reactance tympanogram was assumed to shift in a proportional manner. Multiplying the reactance by a constant produces a sharper tympanogram on linear coordinates. The reactance tympanograms illustrated in Figure 4.18 represent three degrees of stapes involvement. These simulations account for the shapes of tympanograms observed in otosclerotic patients (e.g., Figure 4.16 middle and right panels) reasonably well. By shifting the reactance tympanograms in a proportional manner, the admittance tympanogram becomes lower in height but the tympanometric width narrows, a finding that has been reported in otosclerosis (Ivey, 1975).

Low-impedance pathologies

Although not as common as high-impedance pathologies, low-impedance pathologies can be identified more easily because they produce an obvious alteration of tympanometric shape. These shape alterations are more evident near the resonant frequency of the middle ear than at frequencies remote from the middle ear resonance. Consequently, high-frequency probe tones such as 678 Hz are more effective than low frequencies in identifying these pathologies.

It should be noted that eardrum abnormalities that produce low-impedance tympanometric abnormalities usually are not associated with medically significant pathology and, in the absence of other evidence of ear disease, should not be regarded as a criterion for medical referral. Only when associated with other significant findings (see Table 4.6) should a medical referral be made on the basis of low-impedance tympanometric abnormality.

Figure 4.19 shows examples of 226 and 678 Hz admittance Y, susceptance B, and conductance G tympanograms recorded from two patients with tympanic membrane pathology secondary to chronic middle ear disease. The example in the left panel was recorded from a patient with a neomembrane, or monomere, resulting from a healed perforation. At 226 Hz, static admittance is high ($|Y_{tm}| = 1.76$ mmho) and tympanometric

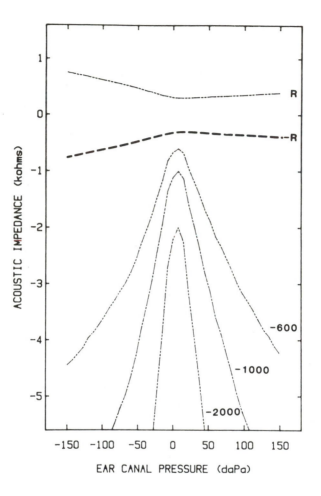

Figure 4.18. Resistance (R) and reactance tympanograms (678 Hz) for simulated cases of otosclerosis. Otosclerosis was modeled as a proportional shift of reactance toward more negative values. The reactance tympanogram was assumed to remain normal. (From Van Camp, Shanks, & Margolis, 1986, with permission.)

width (44 daPa) is narrow. At 678 Hz abnormal multipeaked patterns occurred. It is abnormal because of the excessive number of extrema (five) in the admittance magnitude |Y| tympanogram. The tympanograms in the middle panel and right panels, obtained from a patient with tympanosclerotic plaques on the tympanic membrane, were recorded with increasing ear canal pressure changes (middle panel), and decreasing ear canal pressure changes (right panel). With increasing air pressure at 226

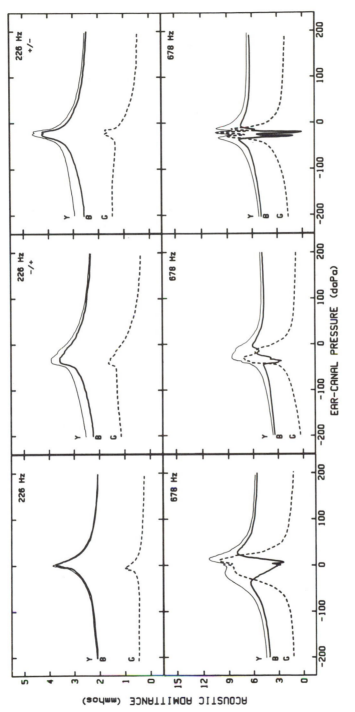

Figure 4.19. Admittance component tympanograms recorded at 226 and 678 Hz from two patients with tympanic membrane pathologies. The tympanograms in the left panel are from a patient with a neomembrane. The middle and right panels show tympanograms from a patient with tympanosclerosis, recorded with increasing pressure changes (middle panel) and with decreasing pressure changes (right panel).

Hz, static admittance and tympanometric width are within the normal ranges (1.35 mmho, 75 daPa). With decreasing air pressure, static admittance is higher ($|Y_{tm}|$ = 1.57 mmho) and tympanometric width is narrower (39 daPa). In addition, the tympanograms have three extrema, an abnormal result at 226 Hz. At 678 Hz, with increasing air pressure (middle panel) the pattern meets the requirements for normal multipeaked tympanograms, although the shapes are somewhat irregular. The decreasing pressure direction produces shapes that are abnormal because of the number of extrema in each tympanogram.

The middle and left panels of Figure 4.19 demonstrate the marked effect that the direction of pressure change can have on tympanometric shape. Notching generally is more complex or atypical for ascending pressure changes in comparsion with descending pressure. The descending direction of pressure change is recommended because it produces fewer abnormal tympanometric shapes in normal subjects (Margolis et al., 1985).

The effect of a tympanic membrane pathology on tympanometric shape emphasizes the importance of an otoscopic examination in conjunction with tympanometry. The presence of a low-impedance eardrum pathology can obscure a more medical stiffness-related pathology such as otosclerosis (Feldman, 1974). Figure 4.20 shows tympanograms recorded from a patient with a neomembrane associated with a healed perforation, in addition to surgically confirmed otosclerosis. At 226 Hz, static admittance was high ($|Y_{tm}|$ = 2.60 mmho) and tympanometric width was narrow (32 daPa). The normal 3B3G tympanogram at 678 Hz indicates a mass-controlled ear. The only tympanometric finding that was consistent with otosclerosis was the narrow width at 226 Hz. As we have seen (Figure 4.19), a narrow tympanometric width can occur in cases of tympanic membrane pathology as well. The otoscopic examination identified the neomembrane, which dominated the tympanometric pattern. A large conductive hearing loss was the only indication of a significant middle ear pathology in this patient.

Figure 4.21 shows 220- and 660-Hz tympanograms recorded from a human temporal bone with an ossicular discontinuity (from Van de Heyning et al., 1982). The static admittance at 220 Hz is normal ($|Y_{tm}|$ = 0.67 mmho). The 660-Hz tympanograms are abnormal, broad, multipeaked patterns that do not resemble any of the Vanhuyse model categories. This case is a good example of the advantage of high-frequency tympanometry for detecting low-impedance abnormalities.

Tympanometry in infants

The clinical value of tympanometry in infants under 6 months of age is controversial. Perhaps because of procedural differences among the

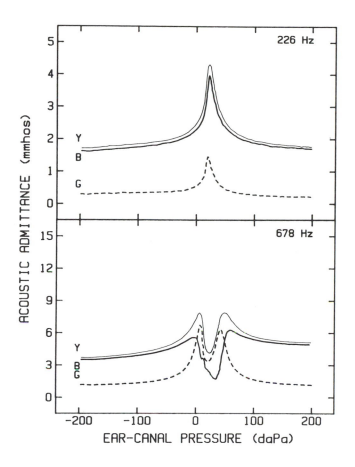

Figure 4.20. Admittance component tympanograms at 226 and 678 Hz from a patient with tympanic membrane pathology (neomembrane) and stapes fixation due to otosclerosis.

various studies, the published research in this area is inconclusive regarding normal and abnormal tympanometric characteristics in infants. Lack of a clear definition of a normal tympanogram in this population renders the studies of the clinical value of tympanometry for determining middle ear abnormalities difficult to interpret.

The earliest tympanometric recordings from infant ears were made with one-component instruments that employed a 220-Hz probe tone and expressed acoustic immittance in relative ("arbitrary") units (Bennett, 1975; Keith, 1973, 1975; Poulsen & Tos, 1978). These studies reported a frequent occurrence of double-peaked tympanograms, evidence that the

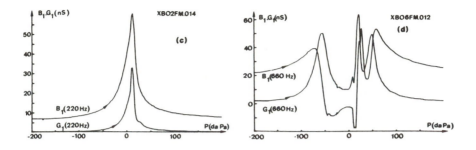

Figure 4.21. Uncompensated conductance (G_1) and susceptance (B_1) tympanograms recorded at 220 Hz (left) and 660 Hz (right) from a human temporal bone with an experimentally produced ossicular discontinuity. (From Van de Heyning, Van Camp, Creten, & Vanpeperstraete, 1982, with permission.)

neonate ear is very different from the adult ear. In retrospect, and in light of the Vanhuyse model, this result might have suggested that neonate and adult ears are sufficiently different that the rules used successfully to interpret adult tympanograms may not be appropriate for interpreting results from infants.

Some insight into the physical differences between neonate and adult ears was contributed by studies that recorded neonate tympanograms with a two-component instrument and employed more than the traditional 220- (or 226-) Hz probe frequency (Himelfarb, Popelka, & Shanon, 1979; Sprague, Wiley, & Goldstein, 1985). These results suggested that (a) unlike the adult, the neonate ear is characterized by a high resistive component at 220 Hz, (b) the impedance phase angle of the neonate ear at 220 Hz is close to 0° rather than the −70° phase angle that characterizes the adult ear, and (c) the effect of probe frequency on tympanometric shapes was not predicted by the Vanhuyse model.

Holte (1989) recorded normal, neonate tympanograms longitudinally over the first 4 months of life. Figures 4.22 and 4.23 present tympanograms from a normal neonate at 2 days and 93 days, respectively. At 2 days the 226-Hz tympanograms appear to be a 1B1G pattern. The higher conductance relative to susceptance suggests an admittance phase angle less than 45°, which would be abnormal in older children and adults. At higher probe frequencies, the conductance and susceptance tympanograms are irregular multipeaked patterns. The resistance and reactance tympanograms do not appear to be helpful in understanding the tympanometric irregularities, as they are in adult subjects with various middle ear pathologies.

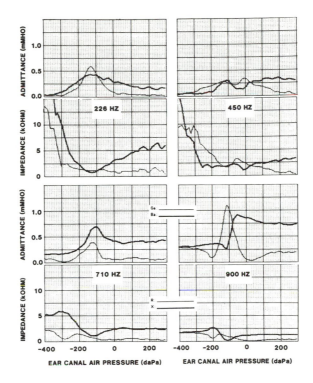

Figure 4.22.   Admittance and impedance component tympanograms from a 2-day-old infant at four probe frequencies. For each probe frequency, conductance and susceptance tympanograms are shown above and resistance and reactance tympanograms below. All tympanograms are uncompensated. (From Holte, 1989, with permission.)

The unusual characteristics of neonate tympanograms have been attributed to the incomplete development of the ear canal wall (Paradise et al., 1976; Zarnoch & Balkany, 1978). The tympanic ring of the neonate is not yet ossified. Consequently, the ear canal wall is not rigid but moves in response to ear canal air pressure changes. It is unlikely that the multipeaked neonate tympanograms at 220 Hz are due to the characteristics of the ear canal for the following reasons. First, the expected effect of a compliant ear canal wall is an increase in volume as ear canal air pressure is changed from negative to positive values, providing monotonically increasing susceptance tympanograms. This result was frequently observed in 2- to 4-month-old infants with a 660-Hz probe (Margolis, & Popelka, 1975), but not in neonates (Himelfarb et al., 1979;

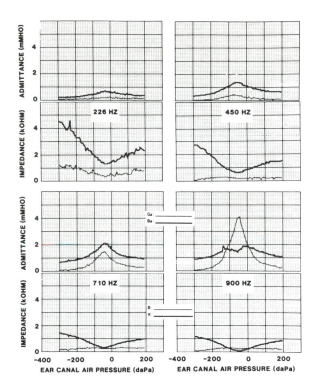

Figure 4.23. Admittance and impedance component tympanograms from a 4-month-old infant, the same subject as in Figure 4.22. (From Holte, with permission.)

Sprague et al. 1985; Holte, 1989). Second, Holte (1989) reported that there was no relationship between the occurrence of multipeaked 226-Hz tympanograms in neonates and otoscopically-observed ear canal wall mobility. It appears that the differences between neonate tympanograms and those obtained from older infants and adults cannot be completely attributable to the development of the ear canal. It is more likely that neonate tympanograms are substantially affected by the condition of the middle ear at birth. Paparella, Shea, Meyerhoff, and Goycoolea (1980) reported a significant degree of unresolved mesenchyme in the middle ears of infant temporal bones. This finding may explain the high resistive component of the impedance of the neonate ear.

Between 3 and 4 months of age, infant tympanograms become qualitatively similar to those of normal adults. Figure 4.23 presents tympanograms from a 4-month-old infant, the same ear as those in Figure

4.22. By 4 months of age, the tympanometric patterns have become consistent with the Vanhuyse model. The 226- and 450-Hz tympanograms are normal 1B1G patterns. The reactance tympanogram (shown here as uncompensated $|X|$) are symmetric patterns that progress from large negative values toward zero with increasing probe frequency. When $|X|$ becomes less than R at approximately 710 Hz, the susceptance tympanogram shows an irregularity that indicates the transition from 1B1G to 3B1G. At 900 Hz, where reactance becomes slightly positive near ambient ear canal pressure, a 5B3G pattern emerges. The effect of probe frequency in the infant tympanogram is identical to that in the adult. As frequency increases the reactance tympanogram shifts from negative to positive values with little change in resistance.

These results are consistent with those of Margolis and Popelka (1975) who reported tympanograms from 2- to 4-month-old infants. Their data suggested that by 2 to 4 months the phase angle is similar to adult ears, although reactance and resistance are about 50% higher than the adult.

Tympanometric results obtained from infants with middle ear disease are conflicting. Some investigators have reported normal tympanograms from infants with middle ear effusion, diagnosed by pneumatic otoscopy or tympanocentesis (Balkany, Berman, Simmons, & Jafek, 1978; Paradise et al., 1976; Zarnoch & Balkany, 1978). Using similar procedures, Groothuis, Sell, Wright, Thompson, and Altemeier, (1979) reported excellent agreeent between tympanometric predictions of middle ear effusion and otoscopy. In these studies tympanograms were recorded with one-component instruments with a 220-Hz probe tone and the results were recorded in "arbitrary units." It is likely that the criteria used to distinguish between normal and abnormal tympanograms differed among those studies. Using a more quantitative approach, Marchant et al. (1986) recorded acoustic susceptance tympanograms and ipsilateral acoustic reflex thresholds with a 660-Hz probe tone in infants aged 2 to 18 weeks. They reported good agreement among acoustic susceptance typanograms, ipsilateral acoustic reflex thresholds, and pneumatic otoscopy for identifying middle ear effusion.

Gradient measures have not been explored for detecting middle ear disease in infancy. It is clear that the normal gradient is age-dependent. The tympanometric widths for three age groups in Table 4.5 suggest that tympanometric width becomes narrower with age, emphasizing the need for age-dependent norms.

It is clear from quantitative studies of the neonate ear (Himelfarb et al., 1979; Holte, 1989; Sprague et al., 1985) that the tympanometric characteristics of this population are sufficiently different from the adult to deserve a unique definition of normal. To understand the physics of the infant ear, and to construct useful tests for detecting pathology, that definition should be based on an analysis similar to the Vanhuyse model. Once the rules that govern normal typanograms are developed, it may be possible to establish a set of criteria that are effective in detecting pathology. At this point, it appears that tympanograms from infants aged 4 months and older probably can be interpreted by the same rules used to interpret adult tympanograms, although normative data are badly needed for this population. The values in Tables 4.3, 4.4, and 4.5 can be used as interim norms.

Criteria for medical referral

One of the most important services that an audiologist can provide is medical referral. The outcome of the audiologic evaluation should provide the basis for determining the need for medical consultation. Because even mild middle ear pathologies usually produce significant tympanometric abnormalities, the tympanogram is a valuable source of information in the determination of the need for medical referral.

There have been many clinical studies that have attempted to determine the efficacy of tympanometry for detecting medically significant middle ear pathologies. In evaluting this research, it is important to distinguish between *measurements* and *tests*. A measurement is a procedure for assigning numbers to observations. A test is a set of rules for making a decision. Tympanometry is a measurement. It has no sensitivity or specificity. It becomes a test when we construct a set of criteria for passing or failing, for referring or not referring to a physician, or for classifying results into disease categories. A measurement is good if it accurately assigns numbers to observations. A test is good if it leads to the right decisions. Good measurements are necessary but not sufficient for good tests. For example, tympanometry provides the basis for a good test of middle ear effusion. It has not been used effectively as a test for otosclerosis. Although tympanometry can be a very good measurement of the acoustic characteristics of otosclerotic ears, the rules that have been used to classify tympanograms have not effectively distinguished between otosclerosis and normal ears. Perhaps a different set of rules would be more effective as a test for stapes fixation.

Two kinds of errors occur when a test is not perfect—false positives and misses. A false positive occurs when a normal case is erroneously classified as abnormal. A miss occurs if a pathological case is classified as normal. (See Chapter 14 for further discussion). In general, the rules that have been used to construct tests that employ tympanometry have produced a large number of false positives but not many misses. The high rate of false positives frequently results in an unacceptable high number of medical referrals of individuals who do not have medically significant pathology. Recent recognition of the high over-referral rate has resulted in a reexamination of the rules that have been used to construct tests of middle ear function. Many clinicians and investigators have concluded that tympanometry should not be used alone to determine the need for medical referral. Rather it should be part of a protocol that bases the decision on several sources of important information. The criteria for medical referral should derive from four sources: case history, visual inspection of the ear, audiometry, and tympanometry. The criteria listed in Table 4.6 and discussed below can be implemented in a screening program or in the more complete audiologic evaluation.

Case history. In the audiologic evaluation, a complete history is taken that may provide the basis for a medical referral. In a screening protocol, an abbreviated history should be obtained to acquire information necessary to determine the need for medical referral. Minimally, the history should include any recent occurrence of *otalgia* (ear pain) or *otorrhea* (ear discharge). A recent occurrence of either warrants an immediate medical referral.

Visual inspection. Although audiologists are not trained or equipped to perform diagnostic otoscopy, visual inspection of the ear should be part of every audiologic evaluation and screening. Visual inspection includes an examination of the head and neck for conditions that may portend ear disease, and otoscopic inspection of the ear canal and tympanic membrane. Conditions that warrant a medical referral include developmental defects, ear-canal abnormalities, and eardrum abnormalities. These are summarized in Table 4.6.

Audiometry. Pure tone audiometry, either threshold or screening, should be used along with tympanometry to determine the need for medical referral. The audiometric criteria used to determine the need for medical consultation may differ in various clinical programs. For most applications, the pass–fail criteria recommended in the ASHA Guidelines for Identification Audiometry (ASHA, 1985; see Table 4.6) are appropriate.

Tympanometry. Tympanometric variables recommended for use as criteria for medical referral include static admittance, equivalent ear canal volume, and tympanometric width. When values exceed appropriately selected normal ranges, these quantities provide the basis for a medical referral. A large equivalent ear canal volume, in the presence of a flat tympanogram, suggests the possibility of a perforated eardrum and requires an immediate medical referral. The other measures, static admittance and tympanometric width, should result in a medical referral only

TABLE 4.6
Criteria for Medical Referral

I. Case History
   A. Otalgia
   B. Otorrhea

II. Visual Inspection of the Ear
   A. Developmental Defects of the Head or Neck
   B. Ear Canal Abnormalities
      1. Blood or effusion
      2. Occlusion
      3. Inflammation
      4. Excessive cerumen, tumor, foreign material
   C. Eardrum Abnormalities
      1. Abnormal color
      2. Bulging eardrum
      3. Fluid line or bubbles
      4. Perforation
      5. Retraction

III. Audiometry—Air Conduction Thresholds > 20 dB HL at 1, 2, or 4 kHz

IV. Tympanometry
   A. Flat Tympanogram and Large Equivalent Ear Canal Volume
   B. Low Static Admittance on Two Successive Occurrences in a 4- to
      6-week interval
   C. Abnormally Wide Gradient on Two Successive Occurrences in a 4-
      to 6-week interval

when accompanied by another abnormality or after they are abnormal on two successive findings over a 4- to 6-week interval. Referral of all individuals with abnormal static admittance or tympanometric width, in the absence of other abnormalities, produces an unacceptably high over-referral rate.

The decision-making process for determining the need for medical referral is shown in flowchart form in Figure 4.24 (ASHA, 1990). The flow chart should not be interpreted as a protocol for the order of test administration. Rather, it indicates the logic used to determine the propriety of a medical referral based on test results.

Multiple-frequency tympanometry

Multiple-frequency tympanometry has not been fully exploited in the clinical evaluation of the ear. In patients with middle ear disease, the probe

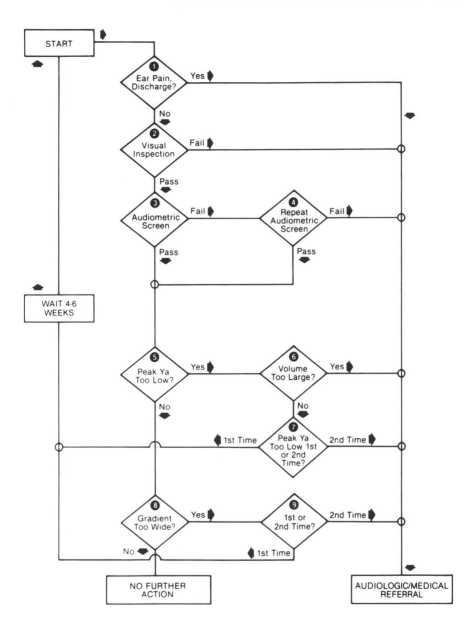

Figure 4.24. Flow chart for determining the need for audiologic or medical referral. (From ASHA, 1990, with permission.)

frequency at which the various tympanometric patterns emerge may be shifted higher or lower in comparison with normal ears. Frequently, an abnormality is most obvious when a probe frequency close to the resonant frequency of the middle ear is used (i.e. 800-1200 Hz). If the pathology increases stiffness of the middle ear, the resonant frequency is shifted upward. Conversely, if the pathology decreases stiffness or increases the mass of the middle ear transmission system, then the resonant frequency will be shifted downward. At low frequencies (e.g., 226 Hz) almost all normal and pathological ears are stiffness-dominated, and a change in middle ear resonance does not produce a marked change in tympanometric shape (see Figures 4.14, 4.15, 4.16, 4.19, 4.20, and 4.21). The determination of normal and abnormal results must be made on the basis of quanitifiable characteristics, such as static admittance and tympanometric width. When a high-frequency probe tone is used to measure both components of complex acoustic admittance, a simple analysis of tympanometric shape may be sufficient to identify middle ear abnormalities.

Colletti (1975, 1976, 1977) developed a multiple-frequency impedance procedure to identify various middle ear pathologies. He measured impedance magnitude tympanograms $|Z|$ for probe frequencies of 200 to 2000 Hz. Three distinct tympanometric patterns emerged at different frequencies (Figure 4.25). A V-shaped pattern (the inverse of admittance patterns), consistent with a stiffness-controlled middle ear, was identified for probe frequencies below 1000 Hz; a notched or W-shaped impedance pattern emerged between 650 and 1400 Hz near the resonant frequency of the middle ear; and an inverted V-shaped tympanogram was recorded above 1400 Hz, where the middle ear is mass controlled. These same three patterns were recorded in patients with middle ear pathologies, but the frequency range at which the patterns emerged was different from patients with normal middle ears. Colletti found the frequency where the W pattern first was recorded was the easiest to identify. In accordance with the Vanhuyse model, admittance and impedance magnitude tympanograms should notch near the resonant frequency of the middle ear, around 800 to 1200 Hz. The emergence of the notched pattern, therefore, provides an estimate of the resonant frequency of the middle ear. The notched pattern occurred at higher than normal frequencies in patients with otosclerosis (850 to 1650 Hz, mean = 1300 Hz), indicating an increase in resonant frequency due to an increase in stiffness reactance. Notching occurred at lower than normal frequencies in patients with ossicular discontinuity (500 to 850 Hz), indicating a decrease in stiffness reactance. The otosclerotic group showed considerable variability and overlapped the normal range. The discontinuity group showed a narrow distribution with little overlap with the other two groups.

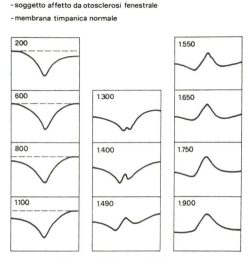

Timpanogrammi a diverse frequenze di tono sonda

- soggetto affetto da otosclerosi fenestrale
- membrana timpanica normale

From Colletti (1984)

Figure 4.25. Impedance magnitude tympanograms at probe frequencies rang-ing from 200 to 1900 Hz, from a patient with otosclerosis. (From Colletti, 1984, with permission.)

Shanks, Wilson, and Palmer (1987) found a plot comparing peak-compensated static susceptance and conductance as a function of probe tone frequency useful in describing changes in acoustic admittance as a function of probe frequency in normal and pathological ears. The static values in the upper panel of Figure 4.26 represent mean values for 10 young, normal subjects. The frequency at which conductance first became larger than susceptance was 565 Hz.

The lower portion of Figure 4.26 shows the relationship between susceptance and conductance for a patient with otosclerosis. Although the resonant frequency is not markedly different for the two graphs (the frequency at which susceptance crosses the 0 line), the frequency at which conductance becomes larger than susceptance is much higher (904 Hz). When susceptance and conductance are equal, the admittance phase angle is 45°. Figure 4.26 suggests that the probe frequency at which the admit-tance phase angle reaches 45° may be a useful method for analyzing multiple-frequency tympanograms.

Future work with multiple frequency tympanograms may allow the determination of patterns that are associated with specific pathologies. This hope is not unrealistic based on measurements by investigators such

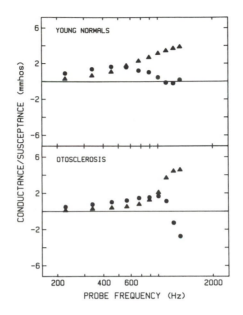

Figure 4.26. A comparison of peak compensated static acoustic susceptance (circles) and conductance (triangles) as a function of probe frequency in a group of young normal subjects (upper panel) and in a patient with otosclerosis (lower panel).

as Møller (1965), Zwislocki and Feldman (1970), and Lilly (1973). For example, in otosclerosis, acoustic reactance is decreased (i.e., more negative) and acoustic resistance is high for low frequencies and low for high frequencies in comparison with normal hearing subjects. In ossicular discontinuity, acoustic reactance is increased (more positive) and acoustic resistance is decreased in comparison with normal hearing subjects. Unique reactance and resistance values also have been reported in malleus fixation and otitis media (Wilber, 1972). The availability of clinical acoustic immittance instruments with multifrequency capability will allow further exploration of the clinical value of multiple-frequency tympanometry.

References

American National Standards Institute. (1987). *American National Standard Specifications for Instruments to Measure Aural Acoustic Impedance and Admittance (Aural Acoustic Immittance)*. (ANSI S3.39-1987). New York.

American Speech-Language-Hearing Association. (1985). *Guidelines for identification audiometry. Asha, 27*, 49–52.

Andreasson, L. (1977). Correlation of tubal function and volume of mastoid and middle ear space as related to otitis media. *Acta Oto-Laryngologica, 83*, 29–33.

ASHA Subcommittee on Impedance Measurement. (1978). Guidelines for acoustic immittance screening of middle-ear function. *Asha, 29*, 550–558.

ASHA Working Group on Acoustic Immittance Measurements. (1990). Guidelines for screening for hearing impairment and middle-ear disorders. *Asha, 32*, (Supplement 2), 17–24.

Balkany, T. J., Berman, S. A., Simmons, M. A., & Jafek, B. W. (1978). Middle ear effusion in neonates. *The Laryngoscope, 88*, 398–405.

Bennett, M. J. (1975). Acoustic impedance bridge measurements with the neonate. *British Journal of Audiology, 9*, 117–124.

Brooks, D. N. (1968). An objective method of determining fluid in the middle ear. *International Audiology, 7*, 280–286.

Cantekin, E. I., Doyle, W. J., Phillips, D. C., & Bluestone, C. D. (1980). Gas absorption in the middle ear. *Annals of Otology, Rhinology and Laryngology, 89* (Supplement 68), 71–75.

Colletti, V. (1975). Methodologic observations on tympanometry with regard to the probe-tone frequency. *Acta Oto-Laryngologica, 80*, 53–60.

Colletti, V. (1976). Tympanometry from 200 to 2000 Hz probe tone. *Audiology, 15*, 106–119.

Colletti, V. (1977). Multifrequency tympanometry. *Audiology, 16*, 278–287.

Colletti, V. (1984). *Impedenzometria.* Milano, Italy: Centro Ricerche e Studi Amplifon.

Creten, W. L., & Van Camp, K. J. (1974). Transient and quasi-static tympanometry. *Scandinavian Audiology, 3*, 39–42.

Creten, W. L., Vanpeperstraete, P. M., & Van Camp, K. J. (1978). Impedance and admittance tympanometry: I. Experimental approach. *Audiology, 17*, 97–107.

DeJonge, R. R. (1986). Normal tympanometric gradient: A comparison of three methods. *Audiology, 25*, 299–308.

Dempsey, C. (1975). Static compliance. In J. F. Jerger (Ed.), *Handbook of clinical impedance audiometry* (pp. 71–84). New York: American Electromedics.

Elner, A., Ingelstedt, S., & Ivarsson, A. (1971). The elastic properties of the tympanic membrane. *Acta Oto-Laryngologica, 72*, 397–403.

Falk, B. (1981). Negative middle ear pressure induced by sniffing: A tympanometric study in persons with healthy ears. *Journal of Laryngology and Otology, 10*, 299–305.

Falk, B. (1983). Variability of the tympanogram due to eustachian tube closing failure. *Scandinavian Audiology*, (Supplement 17), 11–17.

Feldman, A. S. (1974). Eardrum abnormality and the measurement of middle-ear function. *Archives of Otolaryngology, 99*, 211–217.

Feldman, A. S. (1976). Tympanometry: Procedures, interpretation and variables. In A. S. Feldman & L. A. Wilber (Eds.), *Acoustic impedance and admittance: The measurement of middle-ear function* (pp. 103–155). Baltimore: Williams & Wilkins.

Feldman, A. S. (1977). Diagnostic application and interpretation of tympanometry and the acoustic reflex. *Audiology, 16*, 294–306.

Feldman, R., Fria, T., Palfrey, C., & Dellecker, C. (1984). Effects of rate of air pressure change on tympanometry. *Ear and Hearing, 5*, 91–95.

Fiellau-Nikolajsen, M. (1983). Tympanometry and secretory otitis media. *Acta Oto-Laryngologica,* (Supplement 394), 1–73.

Funasaka, S., Funai, H., & Kumakawa, K. (1984). Sweep-frequency tympanometry: Its development and diagnostic value. *Audiology, 23,* 366–379.

Groothuis, J. R., Sell, S. H. W., Wright P. F., Thompson, J. M., & Altemeier, W. A. (1979). Otitis media in infancy: Tympanometric findings. *Pediatrics, 63,* 435–442.

Harker, L. A., & Van Wagoner, R. (1974). Application of impedance audiometry as a screening instrument. *Acta Oto-Laryngologica, 77,* 198–201.

Haughton, P. M. (1977). Validity of tympanometry for middle ear effusions. *Archives of Otolaryngology, 103,* 505–513.

Hergils, L., & Magnuson, B. (1985). Morning pressure in the middle ear. *Archives of Otolaryngology: Head and Neck Surgery, 111,* 86–89.

Hergils, L., & Magnuson, B. (1987). Middle-ear pressure under basal conditions. *Archives of Otolaryngology: Head and Neck Surgery, 113,* 829–832.

Hilding, A. C. (1944). Role of ciliary action in production of pulmonary atelectasis, vacuum in paranasal sinuses, and in otitis media. *Transactions of the American Academy of Ophthalmology and Otolaryngology,* 367–378.

Himelfarb. M. Z., Popelka, G. R., & Shanon, E. (1979). Tympanometry in normal neonates. *Journal of Speech and Hearing Research, 22,* 179–191.

Holmquist, J. (1970). Size of mastoid air cell system in relation to healing after myringoplasty and to eustachian tube function. *Acta Oto-Laryngologica, 69,* 89–93.

Holte, L. A. (1989). *Longitudinal tympanometry and pneumatic otoscopy in healthy newborn infants.* Unpublished doctoral dissertation, Syracuse University.

Ivarsson, A., Tjernstrom, O., Bylander, A., & Bennrup, S. (1983). High speed tympanometry and ipsilateral middle ear reflex measurements using a computerized impedance meter. *Scandinavian Audiology, 12,* 157–163.

Ivey, R. (1975). Tympanometric curves and otosclerosis. *Journal of Speech and Hearing Research, 18,* 554–558.

Jerger, J. (1970). Clinical experience with impedance audiometry. *Archives of Otolaryngology, 92,* 311–324.

Keith, R. W. (1973). Impedance audiometry with neonates. *Archives of Otolaryngology, 97,* 465–467.

Keith, R. W. (1975). Middle ear function in neonates. *Archives of Otolaryngology, 101,* 376–379.

Koebsell, K. A., & Margolis, R. H. (1986). Tympanometric gradient measured from normal preschool children. *Audiology, 25,* 149–157.

Koebsell, K. A., Shanks, J. E., Cone-Wesson, B. K., & Wilson, R. H. (1988). Tympanometric width measures in normal and pathologic ears. *Asha, 30,* 99.

Lidén, G. (1969). The scope and application of current audiometric tests. *Journal of Laryngology and Otology, 83,* 507–520.

Lidén, G., Bjorkman, G., Nyman, H., & Kunov, H. (1977). Tympanometry and acoustic impedance. *Acta Oto-Laryngologica, 83,* 140–145.

Lidén, G., Harford, E., & Hallen, O. (1974). Tympanometry for the diagnosis of ossicular disruption. *Archives of Otolaryngology, 99,* 23–29.

Lidén, G., Peterson, J., & Bjorkman, G. (1970). Tympanometry. *Archives of Otolaryngology, 92,* 248–257.

Lilly, D. J. (1973). Measurement of acoustic impedance at the tympanic membrane. In J. Jerger (Ed.), *Modern developments in audiology* (pp. 345–406). New York: Academic Press.

Lilly, D. J. (1984). Multiple frequency, multiple component tympanometry: New approaches to an old diagnostic problem. *Ear and Hearing, 5,* 300–308.

Lilly, D. J., & Shanks, J. E. (1981). Acoustic immittance of an enclosed volume of air. In G. R. Popelka (Ed.), *Hearing assessment with the acoustic reflex* (pp. 145–160). New York: Grune & Stratton.

Lindeman, P., & Holmquist, J. (1982). Volume measurement of middle ear and mastoid air cell system with impedance audiometry on patients with ear-drum perforations. *Acta Oto-Laryngologica,* (Supplement 386), 70–73.

Magnuson, B. (1981). On the origin of the high negative pressure in the middle ear space. *American Journal of Otolaryngology, 2,* 1–12.

Magnuson, B. (1983). Eustachian tube pathophysiology. *American Journal of Otolaryngology, 4,* 123–130.

Marchant, C. D., McMillan, P. M., Shurin, P. A., Johnson, C. E., Turczyk, V. A., Feinstein, J. C., & Panek, D. M. (1986). Objective diagnosis of otitis media in early infancy by tympanometry and ipsilateral acoustic reflex thresholds. *Journal of Pediatrics, 109,* 590–595.

Margolis, R. H. (1981). Fundamentals of acoustic immittance. In G. R. Popelka (Ed.), *Hearing assessment with the acoustic reflex* (pp. 117–143). New York: Grune & Stratton.

Margolis, R. H., & Heller, J. W. (1987). Screening tympanometry: Criteria for medical referral. *Audiology, 26,* 197–208.

Margolis, R. H., Osguthorpe, J. D., & Popelka, G. (1978). The effects of experimentally-produced middle ear lesions on tympanometry in cats. *Acta Oto-Laryngologica, 86,* 428–436.

Margolis, R. H., & Popelka, G. R. (1975). Static and dynamic acoustic impedance measurements in infant ears. *Journal of Speech and Hearing Research, 18,* 435–443.

Margolis, R. H., & Popelka, G. R. (1977). Interactions among tympanometric variables. *Journal of Speech and Hearing Research, 20,* 447–462.

Margolis, R. H., & Shanks, J. E. (1985). Tympanometry. In J. Katz (Ed.), *Handbook of clinical audiology* (pp. 438–475). Baltimore: Williams and Wilkins.

Margolis, R. H., & Smith, P. (1977). Tympanometric asymmetry. *Journal of Speech and Hearing Research, 20,* 437–446.

Margolis, R. H., Van Camp, K. J., Wilson, R. H., & Creten, W. L. (1985). Multifrequency tympanometry in normal ears. *Audiology, 24,* 44–53.

McCandless, G. A., & Thomas, G. K. (1974). Impedance audiometry as a screening procedure for middle ear disease. *Transactions of the American Academy of Ophthalmology and Otolaryngology,* ORL 78, 98–102.

Melnick, W. (1973). What is the American National Standards Institute? *Asha, 15,* 418–421.

Møller, A. (1965). An experimental study of the acoustic impedance of the middle ear and its transmission properties. *Acta Oto-Laryngologica, 60,* 129–149.

Molvaer, O., Vallersnes, F., & Kringlebotn, M. (1978). The size of the middle ear and the mastoid air cell. *Acta Oto-Laryngologica, 85,* 24–32.

Murphy, D. (1979). Negative pressure in the middle ear by ciliary propulsion of mucus through the Eustachian tube. *The Laryngoscope, 89,* 954–961.

Osguthorpe, J. D. (1986). Effects of tympanic membrane scars on tympanometry: A study in cats. *The Laryngoscope, 96,* 1366–1377.

Osguthorpe, J. D., & Lam, C. (1981). Methodologic aspects of tympanometry in cats. *Otolaryngology: Head and Neck Surgery, 89,* 1037–1040.

Paparella, M. M., Shea, D., Meyerhoff, W. L., & Goycoolea, M. V. (1980). Silent otitis media. *The Laryngoscope, 90,* 1089–1098.

Paradise, J. L., Smith, C. G., & Bluestone, C. D. (1976). Tympanometric detection of middle ear effusion in infants and young children. *Pediatrics, 58,* 198–210.

Poulsen, G., & Tos, M. (1978). Screening tympanometry in newborn infants and in the first six months of life. *Scandinavian Audiology, 7,* 159–166.

Porter, T., & Winston, M. (1973). Methodological aspects of admittance measurements of the middle ear. *Journal of Auditory Research, 13,* 172–177.

Proud, G. O., Odoi, H., & Toledo, P. S. (1971). Bullar pressure changes in eustachian tube dysfunction. *Annals of Otology, Rhinology, and Laryngology, 80,* 835–837.

Renvall, U., & Holmquist, J. (1976). Tympanometry revealing middle ear pathology. *Annals of Otology, Rhinology, and Laryngology, 85,* (Supplement 25), 209–215.

Renvall, U., Lidén, G., Jungert, S., & Nilsson, E. (1975). Impedance audiometry in the detection of secretory otitis media. *Scandinavian Audiology, 4,* 119–124.

Schuknecht, H. F. (1974). *Pathology of the ear.* Cambridge, MA: Harvard University Press.

Shanks, J. (1985). Tympanometric volume estimates in patients with intact and perforated eardrums. *Asha, 27,* 78.

Shanks, J. E. (1987). Aural acoustic-immittance standards. *Seminars in Hearing, 8,* 307–318.

Shanks, J. E., & Lilly, D. J. (1981). An evaluation of tympanometric estimates of ear canal volume. *Journal of Speech and Hearing Research, 24,* 557–566.

Shanks, J. E., & Wilson, R. H. (1986). Effects of direction and rate of ear-canal pressure changes on tympanometric measures. *Journal of Speech and Hearing Research, 29,* 11–19.

Shanks, J. E., Wilson, R. H., & Palmer, C. (1987). Multiple frequency tympanometry. *Asha, 29,* 131.

Sprague, B. H., Wiley, T. L., & Goldstein, R. (1985). Tympanometric and acoustic reflex studies in neonates. *Journal of Speech and Hearing Research, 28,* 265–272.

Terkildsen, K., & Thomsen, K. (1959). The influence of pressure variations on the impedance of the human ear drum: A method for objective determination of middle ear pressure. *Journal of Laryngology and Otology, 73,* 409–418.

Van Camp, K. J., Creten, W. L., Van de Heyning, P. H., Decraemer, W. F., & Vanpeperstraete, P. M. (1983). A search for the most suitable immittance components and probe-tone frequency in tympanometry. *Scandinavian Audiology, 12,* 27–34.

Van Camp, K. J., Margolis, R. H., Wilson, R. H., Creten, W. L., & Shanks, J. E. (1986). Principles of tympanometry. *Asha Monographs, 24,* 1–88.

Van Camp, K. J., Shanks, J. E., & Margolis, R. H. (1986). Simulation of pathological high impedance tympanograms. *Journal of Speech and Hearing Research, 29,* 505–514.

Van de Heyning, P. H., Van Camp, K. J., Creten, W. L., & Vanpeperstraete, P. M. (1982). Incudo-stapedial joint pathology: A tympanometric approach. *Journal of Speech and Hearing Research, 25,* 611–618.

Vanhuyse, V. J., Creten, W. L., & Van Camp, K. J. (1975). On the W-notching of tympanograms. *Scandinavian Audiology, 4,* 45–50.

Wilber, L. (1972). Use of absolute and relative impedance in defining the nature of middle ear lesions in children. In D. Rose & W. Keating (Eds.), *Impedance symposium* (pp. 109–125). Rochester, MN: Mayo Foundation.

Wiley, T. W., Oviatt, D. L., & Block, M. G. (1987). Acoustic-immittance measures in normal ears. *Journal of Speech and Hearing Research, 30,* 161–170.

Wilson, R. H., Shanks, J. E., & Kaplan, S. (1984). Tympanometric changes at 226 Hz and 678 Hz across ten trials and for two directions of ear-canal pressure change. *Journal of Speech and Hearing Research, 27,* 257–266.

Yee, A. L., & Cantekin, E. I. (1986). Effect of changes in systemic oxygen tension on middle ear gas exchange. *Annals of Otology, Rhinology and Laryngology, 95,* 369–372.

Zarnoch, J. M., & Balkany, T. J. (1978). Tympanometric screening of normal and intensive care unit newborns: Validity and reliability. In E. R. Harford, F. H. Bess, C. D. Bluestone, & J. O. Klein (Eds.), *Impedance screening for middle ear disease in children* (pp. 69–80). New York: Grune & Stratton.

Zwislocki, J. J. (1962). Analysis of the middle ear function. Part I: Input impedance. *Journal of the Acoustic Society of America, 34,* 1514–1523.

Zwislocki, J. J. (1963). An acoustic method for clinical examination of the ear. *Journal of Speech and Hearing Research, 6,* 303–314.

Zwislocki, J. J., & Feldman, A. S. (1970). Acoustic impedance of pathological ears. *Asha Monograph, 15,* 1–42.

chapter five

Acoustic-reflex measurements

RICHARD H. WILSON
ROBERT H. MARGOLIS

Contents

Introduction

The acoustically-evoked contraction of the stapedius muscle, which is called the acoustic reflex, has been the topic of considerable experimental and clinical research, beginning with the observation by Hensen (1878) that the stapedius and tensor tympani muscles in dogs contract in response to acoustic stimulation. Although debated since the work of Hensen, the function of the middle ear muscles will not be discussed in this chapter. (Borg, Counter, & Rösler, 1984 provide an excellent review of the theories of middle ear muscle function.) In this chapter, the basis and methods for the clinical application of acoustic-reflex measurements are reviewed.[1]

---

[1]See Djupesland (1976) and Wiley and Block (1984) for a review of nonacoustic-reflex measurements.

247

Lüscher made the first direct observations of the acoustic reflex in humans in 1929 (Potter, 1936). He viewed the movement of the stapedius tendon through a perforation in the tympanic membrane of a patient who had an otherwise normal middle ear. Lüscher observed the following: (a) the bilateral (consensual) nature of the acoustic reflex to monaural stimulation, (b) the frequency range of effective reflex eliciting stimuli, (c) the greater sensitivity of the reflex to complex signals in comparison to tonal signals, (d) the graded nature of the reflex, (e) the "anticipatory" characteristic of the reflex, (f) the responsiveness to certain nonacoustic stimuli, and (g) the relative independence of the muscle response to movement of the tympanic membrane.

Subsequently, several other investigators observed the acoustic reflex in patients with tympanic membrane perforations (Kobrak, 1948; Lindsay, Kobrak, & Perlman, 1936; Potter, 1936). In an attempt to develop a more widely applicable method of observation, Kobrak tried, with limited success, to induce transparency of the anesthetized tympanic membrane by coating the intact membrane with a mixture of glycerin, water, and potassium iodide. Visual observation of the acoustic reflex through the coated membrane proved to be impractical for general clinical application. Thus several early reports expressed the view that,

> The importance of the acoustic stapedius reflex for practical clinical purposes is, at present at least, very limited. Observation of the reflex can be used, however, to determine the presence of hearing in persons suspected of malingering or in children. (Lindsay et al., 1936, p. 677)

In 1946, Metz reported the development of a mechano-acoustic bridge for middle ear measurement that would eventually permit inexpensive, noninvasive recordings of the effect of the acoustic reflex on the input immittance of the middle ear. In the same report that provided the basic foundation for tympanometry, Metz (1946) also presented the first acoustic-reflex measurements that were obtained by monitoring changes in the acoustic immittance of the ear coincident with acoustic stimulation. By testing patients with a variety of otologic disorders, Metz determined the relations between acoustic-reflex thresholds and ear disease that have been only modestly refined since his pioneering efforts. The work by Metz is truly the origin of the clinical application of acoustic-reflex measurements.

The role of the tensor tympani muscle in humans was not clear to the early investigators. Hensen (1878) observed that both the stapedius and tensor tympani muscles in dogs contracted in response to acoustic stimulation, which led to the supposition that both muscles in humans must contract in response to acoustic stimulation. Kato (1913) reported, however, that only the stapedius muscle in monkeys was activated by acoustic stimulation. Metz (1946, 1952) was noncommittal as to which muscles were involved in the acoustic reflex, referring to the reflex as the intra-aural muscle reflex. Jepsen (1955), with the same "Metz" acoustic bridge, observed that patients with unilateral facial paralysis had no measurable acoustic reflex on the affected side. This evidence convinced Jepsen that only the stapedius muscle in humans was activated acoustically, and he referred to the response as the acoustic stapedius reflex. His colleague, Terkildsen, however, was unconvinced. Terkildsen (1957) reported acoustic-reflex measurements obtained manometrically, that is, by measuring air pressure changes in the ear canal. Terkildsen thought that the inward motion of the tympanic membrane and the resulting pressure decrease in the ear canal were prima facie evidence of tensor tympani contraction. Terkildsen concluded that "the existence of an acoustic reflex of the musculus tensor tympani in the human being is established" (p. 487). More recently, Brask (1978) demonstrated that the acoustic reflex produces outward, inward, or diphasic motion of the tympanic membrane. In some people there appears to be a tensor tympani reflex that is characterized by a response morphology that is different from the response morphology of a stapedius reflex. In comparison to the stapedius reflex, the tensor tympani reflex (a) is elicited at higher levels of the reflex-activator signal, (b) has a longer latency, (c) is monitored as an acoustic immittance change in the opposite direction, and (d) is associated with general body movements and the startle response (Brask, 1978; Davis, 1948; Djupesland, 1965; Salomon & Starr, 1963; Stach, Jerger, & Jenkins, 1984).

The initial clinical application of acoustic-reflex measurements was in the detection of hearing loss in difficult-to-test populations, an application that was abandoned and taken up again 35 years later (see Lindsay et al., 1936, quotation above). Metz (1946), however, had greater ambitions for the use of acoustic-reflex data. His studies of a wide variety of patients with conductive, sensorineural, and facial nerve lesions provided the basis for the use of the acoustic reflex in the differential diagnosis of auditory and neurologic disorders. His work was extended by his colleagues (Kristensen & Jepsen, 1952; Jepsen, 1953, 1955, 1963), but the routine use of acoustic-reflex measurements was not possible until a more clinically-feasible measurement method was available. Metz recognized the limitations of his mechano-acoustic bridge and anticipated the electro-acoustic devices that soon would be developed. He stated, "it would be a great advantage if it would be sufficient to connect a small apparatus (telephone) with the ear, and make the measurements on a possibly bigger apparatus placed on a table alongside the patient" (Metz, 1946, p. 233). The instrument that Metz described was developed in the same state hospital (Rigshospitalet) in Copenhagen by Terkildsen and Scott-Nielsen (1960). Their electroacoustic instrument was the prototype of the first commercially available electroacoustic immittance instrument, the Madsen ZO-61, that made routine measurements of the acoustic reflex possible. There is no question that the clinical applications of the acoustic reflex originated at Rigshospitalet in Copenhagen (Figure 5.1).

Anatomy and physiology of the acoustic reflex

Understanding the anatomy and physiology of the human acoustic reflex is severely limited by the inaccessibility of the stapedius muscle and the reflex pathways. Even in animals, the available information on the reflex pathways is incomplete. The situation is complicated further by the likelihood that substantial interspecies differences occur in the anatomy and function of the acoustic reflex. The interspecies differences that are known to exist in the acoustic tensor tympani reflex warn against assuming that the animal data accurately reflect the characteristics of the human acoustic reflex.

The Borg (1973) study of the neural pathways involved in the acoustic reflex of rabbits provides much of the available information on the acoustic-reflex arc. Borg produced brainstem lesions and measured the resultant changes in the ipsilateral and contralateral acoustic reflexes.[2] Figure 5.2 is a schematic of the neural pathways of the acoustic-reflex arc proposed by Borg. The afferent portion of the acoustic-reflex arc consists of a first order neuron in the cochlear branch of the eighth cranial nerve (CNVIII). At this stage the reflex pathways probably are undifferentiated, that is, there are no special neurons in the afferent branch of CNVIII that are devoted to the acoustic reflex. The central portion of the reflex arc consists of neurons located in the ventral cochlear nucleus (VCN) and axonal projections that are (a) primarily through the trapezoid body to the contralateral superior olivary complex (SOC), and (b) direct ipsilateral pathways to the region of the motor nucleus (MN) of the seventh cranial nerve (CNVII). From the cell bodies in the superior olivary complex, axons

---

[2]For the ipsilateral (or uncrossed) acoustic reflex, the reflex-activator signal and the probe signal are in the same ear. For the contralateral (or crossed) acoustic reflex, the reflex-activator signal and the probe signal are in opposite ears. The ear in which the probe signal is located is referred to as the "probe ear."

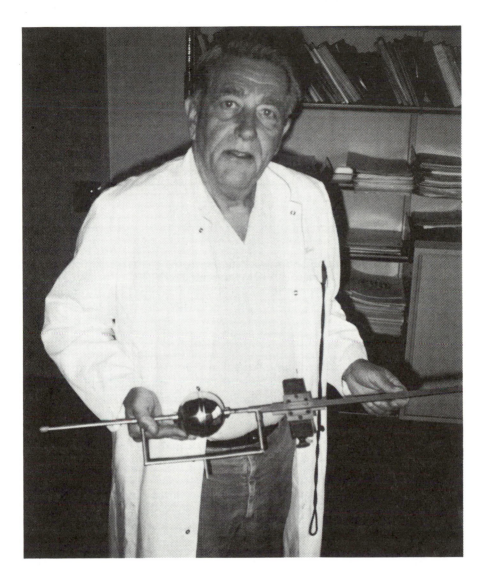

Figure 5.1.   Knut Terkildsen (1918–1984) with the Metz mechano-acoustic bridge (ca. 1980).

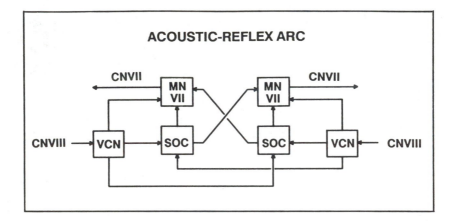

Figure 5.2.   A schematic of the acoustic-reflex arc based on the rabbit (Borg, 1973). The arc involves input through CNVIII to the ventral cochlear nucleus (VCN) from which there are neural pathways through the two superior olivary complexes (SOC) to the motor nuclei of CNVII (MN VII) and the CNVII that innervates the stapedius muscle.

project to the ipsilateral and contralateral motor nuclei of CNVII to synapse with stapedius motoneurons. The axons of the stapedius motoneurons join the trunk of CNVII, project through the internal auditory meatus, and collect into the stapedial branch of CNVII. The stapedial nerve separates from CNVII just inferior to the posterior genu (Figure 5.3) and courses anteriorly to the stapedius muscle, which is contained within a bony canal that runs roughly parallel to the facial nerve canal just inferior to the posterior genu. In addition to the "direct" pathways of the acoustic-reflex arc depicted in Figure 5.2, there may be indirect, multisynaptic pathways involving other sites in the central nervous system. For example, Borg (1973) presented evidence for a pathway involving the reticular formation. Borg and Møller (1975) suggested that the effect of central nervous system depressants on the acoustic reflex may implicate a central, multisynaptic pathway. The function of these indirect reflex pathways is unknown, but they may be involved in complex acoustic-reflex characteristics such as the "anticipatory" response, that is, the enhanced acoustic-reflex response that occurs when the reflex-activator signal is preceded by a warning signal.

The locations of the cell bodies of the efferent neurons of the acoustic-reflex arc have been studied by a number of investigators (Joseph, Guinan, Fullerton, Norris, & Kiang, 1985; Lyon, 1978, 1979; Shaw & Baker, 1983). These studies demonstrated that motoneurons of the reflex arc are located

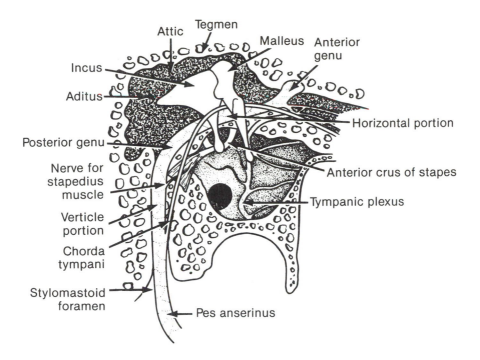

Figure 5.3.   The course of CNVII (facial nerve) through the middle ear. (From Goodhill, 1981, with permission.)

in several regions near, but not in, the motor nucleus of CNVII. Kobler, Vacher, and Guinan (1985, 1987) provide evidence from cats that motoneurons of the reflex arc are organized into regions with unique response properties. The following four types of neurons were identified: (a) contralateral units that respond only to contralateral stimuli, (b) ipsilateral units that respond only to ipsilateral stimuli, (c) "binaural and" units that respond only to binaural stimuli, and (d) "binaural or" units that respond to either ipsilateral or contralateral stimuli. These classes of motoneurons have distinctly different thresholds to acoustic stimulation (Kobler et al., 1987). In addition, there may be stapedius motoneurons that do not respond to sound (McCue & Guinan, 1983, 1988). McCue and Guinan (1988) presented evidence that these functionally distinct motoneuron groups are organized into anatomically distinct brainstem pathways. McCue and Guinan produced brainstem lesions in cats and observed the effects of the lesions on ipsilateral and contralateral acoustic reflexes. The findings suggested that the axons of the stapedial motoneurons are arranged in three distinct pathways originating from different sites in the brainstem. The three pathways are differentiated on the basis of responsiveness to stimulation of the two ears, with one pathway responsive to ipsilateral stimulation, one to contralateral stimulation, and one to stimulation of either ear. A fourth pathway may exist that is not acoustically excitable. The peripheral, efferent portion of the acoustic-reflex arc at the level of the middle ear apparently is not topographically organized in the same manner (Kobler et al., 1985). The peripheral processes of the various motoneuron groups appear to be distributed randomly within the stapedial branch of CNVII.

Because the clinical measurement of the acoustic reflex almost always is performed by measuring changes in middle ear immittance, it is important to understand the relationship between the immittance changes of the middle ear and the more direct measurement of acoustic-reflex activity. Perhaps the most direct method for measuring the acoustic reflex is the electromyographic (EMG) response that is measured directly from the stapedius muscle or tendon. Zakrisson, Borg, and Blom (1974) compared EMG responses and immittance changes produced by the acoustic reflex in patients with unilateral perforations of the tympanic membrane that allowed insertion of an electrode into the stapedial tendon. Figure 5.4 presents a sample recording. The top tracings are the integrated EMG activity, in a sense, the sum of all of the individual motor unit discharges, and an indication of the total muscle response. The middle tracings are EMG action potentials, in which each spike represents the discharge of a single motor unit. The lower panels show impedance changes in the opposite ear. Figure 5.5 shows magnitude-intensity level functions for contralateral EMG responses and for ipsilateral and contralateral impedance changes. The data, which are expressed in relative units, indicate that EMG responses and impedance changes are similarly dependent on the level of the reflex-activator signal (i.e., the stimulus used to elicit the acoustic reflex).

Recent data suggest that the differences between the ipsilateral and contralateral acoustic reflexes are greater when measured with EMG techniques than when measured with acoustic immittance procedures. In cats, Guinan and McCue (1987) observed that the EMG activity of the ipsilateral stapedius muscle was two to three times greater than the EMG activity of the contralateral stapedius muscle. In humans, the ipsilateral immittance change is only about one and one-half times greater than the contralateral immittance change (Hall, 1982).

When the stapedius muscle contracts, the stapes footplate is moved or rocked laterally from the oval window, the ossicular chain is stiffened, and the tympanic membrane is moved slightly in a direction that is dependent upon the movement of the stapes. These mechanical changes in the middle ear produce frequency-dependent changes in the sound transmis-

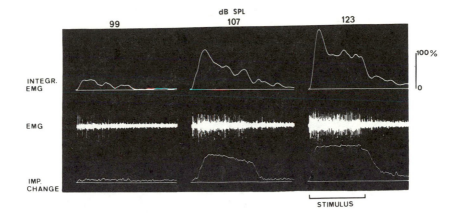

Figure 5.4. Simultaneously-recorded responses of the human stapedius muscle to a 1-s, 2000-Hz tonal stimulus. The top part of the figure depicts the integrated EMG response, a method of averaging the muscle activity. The middle part shows the raw electromyographic (EMG) response recorded from the stapedial tendon showing individual muscle action potentials. The bottom section of the figure illustrates the acoustic impedance change in the opposite ear. (From Zakrisson, Borg, & Blom, 1974, with permission.)

sion characteristics of the middle ear. As illustrated in Figure 5.6, the acoustic reflex acts as a high-pass filter on the transmission of sound through the middle ear. Stapedius contraction attenuates low-frequency signals with the maximum effect at about 600 Hz. Above 1000 Hz, there is little, if any, effect of the acoustic reflex on the sound level that reaches the inner ear (Rabinowitz, 1977). The ipsilateral acoustic reflex probably exhibits the same high-pass filter characteristic as does the contralateral reflex, but the attenuation produced by the ipsilateral reflex may be twice as large (in dB) as the attenuation produced by the contralateral reflex.

Measurement of the acoustic reflex

Measurement methods

Several methods have been used to quantify the effect of stapedial muscle contraction. The early investigators of stapedius muscle activity in response to acoustic stimulation (a) recorded the change in either EMG

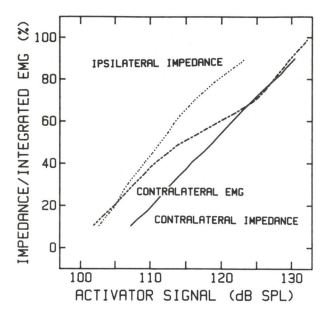

Figure 5.5. Acoustic-reflex growth functions. The dashed line shows the reflex-growth function obtained from the integrated EMG response to contralateral stimulation. The dotted and solid lines show reflex-growth functions for ipsilateral and contralateral impedance changes, respectively. (From Zakrisson, Borg, & Blom, 1974, with permission.)

activity (Perlman & Case, 1939) or tension (Lorente de Nó, 1935; Wersäll, 1958) from the stapedial muscle or tendon, (b) observed the movement of the stapedial tendon through perforations in the tympanic membrane (Lindsay et al., 1936), and (c) recorded air pressure changes in the ear canal caused by displacement of the tympanic membrane that coincided with stapedial contraction (Holst, Ingelstedt, & Örtegren, 1963; Terkildsen, 1957). When Otto Metz developed his impedance bridge and recorded acoustic-reflex responses as acoustic-immittance changes, he demonstrated that the acoustic reflex could be recorded in a clinically feasible, noninvasive manner. The method that Metz developed required the measurement of acoustic immittance during the presentation of a reflex-activator signal. In either the contralateral or ipsilateral condition, the activator signal may interact with the probe signal to produce measurement artifacts. Because the head provides isolation of the reflex-activator and probe signals in the contralateral condition, the interaction of the activator signal and the probe signal is less in the contralateral condition than

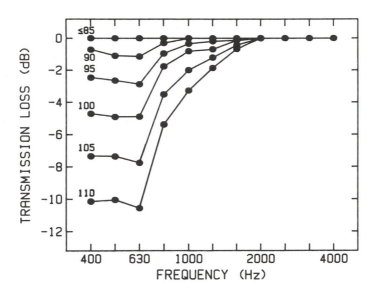

Figure 5.6. The frequency-dependent attenuation characteristics (transmission loss in dB) of the acoustic reflex from four subjects in response to 85- to 110-dB SPL reflex-activator signals. (From Rabinowitz, 1977, with permission.)

when both signals are presented to the same ear (ipsilateral). For this reason, the early clinical instruments measured only the contralateral acoustic reflex.

Two kinds of artifacts can result from interaction of the reflex-activator signal and the probe signal. Both artifacts can occur during ipsilateral or contralateral recording, but both artifacts are much more difficult to avoid in ipsilateral measurement. The *additive artifact* results from the addition of the energy in the reflex-activator signal to the energy of the probe signal. Because immittance instruments bandpass filter the probe tone, only the activator signal energy that is passed by the filter is problematic. The closer in frequency the reflex-activator signal is to the probe tone signal, the greater the likelihood is that the two signals will interact, causing an additive artifact. The additive artifact takes the form of an increase in impedance (a decrease in admittance), which can be misinterpreted as a true reflex (Margolis & Gilman, 1977; Popelka & Dubno, 1978). Because the additive artifact has no latency except for delays in the recording apparatus, it usually can be distinguished from a real acoustic reflex on the basis of latency. The *eardrum artifact* occurs primarily during ipsilateral recording with a low-frequency (226 Hz) probe tone (Kunov, 1977; Lutman

& Leis, 1980; Møller, 1978). The eardrum artifact results from a nonlinear interaction between the reflex-activator signal and the probe signal and is not related to the frequency separation between the two signals. The artifact takes the form of a decrease in impedance (increase in admittance), the opposite immittance change of a real reflex. Green and Margolis (1984) suggested that the eardrum artifact may be related to nonlinear properties of the tympanic membrane. Figure 5.7 presents a schematic representation of the additive and eardrum artifacts, a real acoustic reflex, and the simultaneous occurrence of an eardrum artifact and an acoustic reflex.

Quantification of the amplitude of the acoustic reflex

Several parameters of the acoustic reflex can be quantified with the acoustic immittance method, including threshold, temporal, and amplitude characteristics. The following discussion focuses on the measurement parameters and computations that must be considered when quantifying the amplitude of the acoustic reflex. Recall from Chapter 4 that the acoustic admittance at the probe tip (Y_a) is the complex sum of the real component of admittance, acoustic conductance (G_a), and the imaginary component of admittance, acoustic susceptance (B_a), which is expressed as

$$Y_a = G_a + jB_a \tag{1}$$

Furthermore, the acoustic admittance at the probe tip (Y_a) is the sum of the admittance of the ear canal between the probe tip and the tympanic membrane (Y_{ec}) and the admittance at the tympanic membrane (Y_{tm}) that is expressed as

$$Y_a = Y_{ec} + Y_{tm} \tag{2}$$

Although Equation 2 and the equations that follow involve the addition of vectors without regard to the phase angle, the errors encountered with a low-frequency probe tone (e.g., 226 Hz) are slight. The effect of the acoustic reflex is to produce a change in the admittance (ΔY) at the tympanic membrane. The admittance at the probe tip when the stapedius muscle is contracted (Y_r) is the sum of the admittance of the ear canal (Y_{ec}), the admittance at the tympanic membrane (Y_{tm}), and the admittance change produced by the acoustic reflex (ΔY), which is expressed as

$$Y_r = Y_{ec} + Y_{tm} + \Delta Y \tag{3}$$

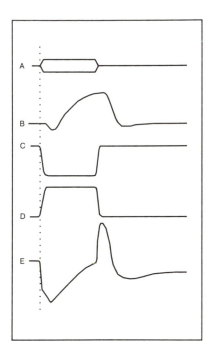

Figure 5.7. Schematic representation of (A) a reflex-activator signal, (B) an acoustic reflex measured as an impedance change, (C) an eardrum artifact, (D) an additive artifact, and (E) a simultaneously-occurring eardrum artifact and acoustic reflex. (From Green & Margolis, 1984, with permission.)

Solving Equation 3 for ΔY gives

$$\Delta Y = Y_r - (Y_{ec} + Y_{tm}) \tag{4}$$

Substituting from Equation 2, Equation 4 reduces to

$$\Delta Y = Y_r - Y_a \tag{5}$$

Because the admittance of the ear canal is a simple additive component of both Y_a (Equation 2) and Y_r (Equation 3), ΔY is not affected by ear-canal volume.

The relation between impedance change (ΔZ) and ear-canal volume is more complex than the relation between admittance change and ear-canal volume. Substituting from Equation 17 in Chapter 4, Equation 3 can be rewritten in impedance as follows:

$$Z_r = \frac{Z_{ec}(Z_{tm} + \Delta Z)}{Z_{ec} + (Z_{tm} + \Delta Z)} \tag{6}$$

ΔZ is expressed as follows:

$$\Delta Z = \frac{Z_{ec}Z_{tm} - Z_r Z_{ec} - Z_r Z_{tm}}{Z_r - Z_{ec}} \tag{7}$$

The point of this exercise is that Equations 3 and 5 express a simple relation between the admittance of the ear canal and the amplitude of the acoustic reflex (i.e., $\Delta Y_a = \Delta Y_{tm}$), whereas Equations 6 and 7 express a complex relation between the impedance of the ear canal and the amplitude of the acoustic reflex (i.e., $\Delta Z_a \neq \Delta Z_{tm}$). Although Z_{ec} must be known precisely to determine ΔZ_{tm}, Y_{ec} need not be determined to measure ΔY_{tm}.

Equations 4 and 7 produce reasonable estimates of the amplitude of the acoustic reflex only if, as was previously indicated, the admittance (or impedance) phase angle is not substantially altered by the reflex. In normal subjects >4 months of age and at a low-probe frequency (e.g., 226 Hz), only a small change in phase angle occurs when the stapedius muscle contracts. A typical acoustic reflex expressed as an admittance vector at a probe frequency of 226 Hz is depicted in the left panel of Figure 5.8. The length of the line segment from the origin to Y_{tm} is the static admittance at the tympanic membrane. The length of the line segment from the origin to Y_r is the admittance at the tympanic membrane with the stapedius muscle contracted. The difference between the lengths of the two line segments is ΔY defined in Equation 5. The actual effect of the reflex, however, is the distance from point Y_{tm} to point Y_r, which is almost exactly equivalent to ΔY because there is very little phase shift.

A typical acoustic reflex for a 678-Hz probe frequency is presented as an admittance vector in the right panel of Figure 5.8. Note that a substantial phase shift occurs when the stapedius muscle contracts. In this example, Equation 5 underestimates the admittance change produced by the reflex by 24%. To avoid underestimating the admittance change at 678 Hz, ΔY must be determined from the admittance components expressed as

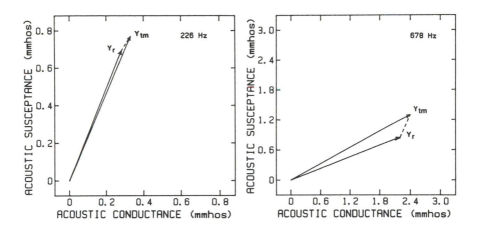

Figure 5.8. Acoustic reflex responses to a 100-dB SPL, 1000-Hz reflex-activator signal measured with two probe frequencies (226 and 678 Hz) expressed as admittance vector. Y_{tm} represents the baseline (static) admittance. Y_r is the admittance during stimulation. The reflex magnitude is represented by the dashed line between the two admittance vectors.

$$\Delta G = G_r - G_a, \text{ and} \tag{8}$$

$$\Delta B = B_r - B_a \tag{9}$$

where ΔG and ΔB are the changes in conductance and susceptance produced by the acoustic reflex, G_r and B_r are the conductance and susceptance when the stapedius is contracted, and G_a and B_a are the conductance and susceptance in the uncontracted (relaxed) state. The admittance change then is expressed as

$$\Delta Y = \sqrt{\Delta G^2 + \Delta B^2} \tag{10}$$

Equation 10 produces a better estimate of reflex magnitude than does Equation 5. To determine ΔG and ΔB, a two-component admittance meter is required. When a one-component admittance meter is used, the reflex magnitude must be determined from Equation 5. Accurate estimates of ΔY can be obtained only at low probe frequencies (e.g., 226 Hz) in normal subjects who do not exhibit a significant phase shift when the stapedius muscle contracts. That is, vectors can be added only if the vectors are identical in phase.

Several methods for quantifying the amplitude of the acoustic reflex are illustrated in Figure 5.9. The data for two subjects (S4 and S8) are

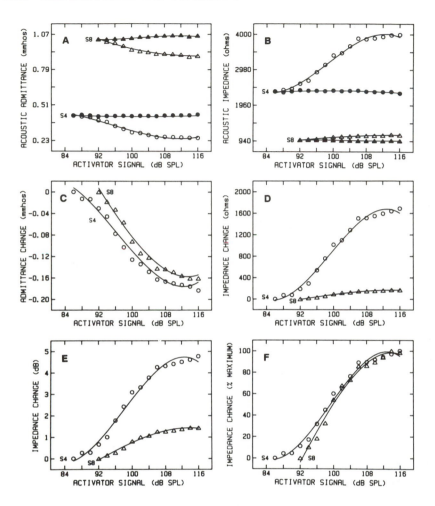

Figure 5.9. Acoustic-reflex growth functions for two subjects (S4 and S8) illustrated in various quantification units. The filled symbols represent a control baseline condition in which no reflex-activator signal was presented, and the open symbols represent the admittance magnitude during stimulation at various sound pressure levels. Panel A: Reflex-growth functions expressed as absolute acoustic admittance magnitude. Panel B: Reflex-growth functions expressed as absolute impedance magnitude. Panel C: Reflex-growth function expressed as the change in admittance between the baseline admittance and the admittance during muscle contraction shown in Panel A. Panel D: Reflex-growth functions expressed as the change in impedance between the baseline impedance and the impedance during muscle contraction shown in Panel B. Panel E: Reflex-growth functions expressed as an impedance change in decibels, which is equivalent to the change in sound pressure level of the probe tone. Panel F: Reflex-growth functions expressed as a percentage of the maximum impedance change for each subject. (Based on Figure 9, Wilson, 1981.)

based on compensated (i.e., corrected for ear-canal volume) admittance measures for a 226-Hz probe. The admittance data in acoustic mmhos (Figure 5.9, Panel A) show that the two subjects have different static admittance, evident from the different baseline values (filled symbols), but a similiar change in admittance amplitude with increases in activator signal level (open symbols). In Panel B of Figure 5.9, the reflex data are plotted in impedance (acoustic ohms). In impedance units, the static values for the two subjects (filled symbols) are different, and the reflex-growth functions (open symbols) are substantially different in slope. In the middle panels of Figure 5.9, the reflex data from the two subjects are plotted as the change in immittance between the prestimulus or baseline admittance, which is a "static" measure, and the peak values of each reflex response in admittance (Panel C) and in impedance (Panel D). Again, the reflex-growth functions for the two subjects expressed as an admittance change are similar, whereas the growth functions expressed as an impedance change are very different. In Figure 5.9, Panel E, the reflex data are expressed as the impedance change in dB (ΔdB)

$$\Delta\text{dB} = 20 \log_{10} (Z_r/Z_{tm}), \tag{11}$$

where Z_r is the impedance at the tympanic membrane during stapedial contraction and Z_{tm} is the static or baseline impedance. Note again that the reflex-growth functions are very different for the two subjects. The reflex-growth functions expressed in decibels are very similar in form to the functions expressed as an impedance change in ohms (Figure 5.9, Panel D). Because the range of the data plotted in decibels is small (≤ 5 dB), the log transformation has very little effect on the shape of the reflex-growth function. In Figure 5.9, Panel F, the reflex data are plotted as percent of the maximum impedance change. Because the largest change recorded is 100%, the two growth functions converge at the highest activator level used. When reflex magnitude is expressed in percent of maximum, the growth functions for the two subjects are very similar.

Another quantity that has been used to express the reflex magnitude is the change in the sound pressure level of the probe tone, ΔdB, that is related to the impedance of the middle ear in the following manner:

$$\Delta\text{dB} = 20 \log_{10} (Z_r/Z_a), \tag{12}$$

where Z_r is the impedance at the probe tip during stapedial contraction and Z_a is the impedance at the probe tip in the uncontracted state. Equations 11 and 12 are equivalent only in the hypothetical condition of an ear-canal volume of zero. As illustrated in Figure 5.10, however, ear-canal volume has a substantial effect on the reflex amplitudes expressed as a

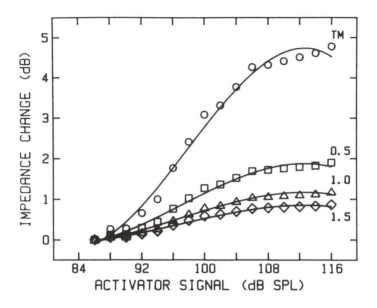

Figure 5.10.   Acoustic-reflex growth functions expressed as an impedance change (in dB) showing the effect of ear-canal volume on the amplitude of the acoustic reflex. The growth function is shown corrected to the plane of the tympanic membrane (TM), that is, an ear-canal volume of zero. The data also are presented with assumed ear-canal volumes of 0.5, 1.0, and 1.5 cm³.

change in the sound pressure level of the probe tone (Equation 12). The growth function for subject S4 (from Panel E, Figure 5.9) is replotted with four ear-canal volumes (0.5, 1.0, 1.5 cm³ and corrected to the tympanic membrane, TM, i.e., a 0-cm³ volume). The substantial effect of ear-canal volume on the amplitude of acoustic reflex plotted in acoustic impedance is obvious. The data demonstrate that comparisons between ears, or between measures obtained at different times from the same ear, cannot be compared in absolute terms when reflex magnitudes are expressed as changes in the sound pressure level of the probe tone because of the effects of variations in ear-canal volume.

Acoustic-reflex threshold

The amplitude of the acoustic reflex is dependent both on the level of the reflex-activator signal and on the characteristics of the middle ear transmission system(s). As a relative measure, the amplitude of the change in the acoustic immittance of the middle ear during contraction of the stapedius muscle is related directly to the level of the reflex-activator signal. As an absolute measure, the amplitude of the acoustic immittance of the middle ear during contraction of the stapedius muscle is related (a) directly to the level of the activator signal when measured in acoustic impedance (i.e., the higher the activator level, the higher the acoustic impedance) or (b) inversely to the activator level when measured in acoustic admittance (i.e., the higher the activator level, the lower the acoustic admittance).

Nomenclature

The relation between the level of the reflex-activator signal and the magnitude of the acoustic reflex, measured as the change in acoustic admittance, is illustrated in Figure 5.11. The top panel depicts the 1-s activator signals with increments from 80- to 110-dB HL and the acoustic reflexes elicited by the activator signals. The bottom panel of Figure 5.11 depicts the admittance change (acoustic mmhos) during contraction of the stapedius muscle. In this plot, which is an *acoustic-reflex growth function*, the *baseline admittance* data represent the acoustic admittance of the middle ear during the 100 ms prior to presentation of each reflex-activator signal (Y_{tm}) and the *peak admittance* data represent the acoustic admittance of the middle ear during the last 500 ms of each activator signal (Y_r). The acoustic admittance data (baseline, Y_{tm}, and peak, Y_r) and corresponding acoustic impedance data for the seven activator signals also are listed in Table 5.1 along with the acoustic admittance (and impedance) changes that occurred between the respective baseline and peak values.[3] Both the reflex tracings and the reflex magnitude data demonstrate that with a 226-Hz probe, the acoustic admittance of the middle ear in the reflexive state decreases as the level of the reflex-activator signal increases from 80- to 100-dB HL. Increases in the level of the activator signal above 100-dB HL do not produce continued increases in the amplitude of the reflex. Above 100-dB HL, the reflex growth function is saturated. Table 5.1 also contains the baseline (Z_{tm}), peak (Z_r), and change (ΔZ) data converted to acoustic impedance units (ohms). As the level of the activator signal

---

[3]The acoustic-admittance data in Table 5.1 are the average of 11 samples of the acoustic admittance of the middle ear during a 100-ms interval before the activator signal (Y_{tm}) and during a 500-ms interval during presentation of the activator signal (Y_r). In this manner the data were generated to three decimal points, which is beyond the measurement accuracy of instruments. To maintain simplicity, the phase angle data are omitted.

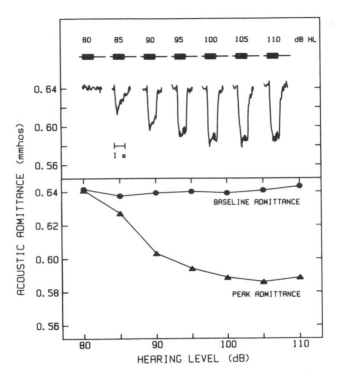

Figure 5.11. The top panel shows the acoustic-reflex responses in acoustic mmhos monitored with a 226-Hz probe and corrected for ear-canal volume. The 1-s, 1000-Hz activator signals were presented from 80- to 110-dB HL with 5-s between signal presentations. The bottom panel depicts an acoustic-reflex growth function with baseline admittance (circles) representing the acoustic admittance of the middle ear 100 ms prior to presentation of the activator signal (Y_{tm}) and peak admittance (triangles) representing the acoustic admittance during the last 500 ms of the activator signal (Y_r). (Modified from Wilson & McBride, 1978.)

increases from 80- to 100-dB HL, the Z_{tm} values fluctuate slightly around 1560 acoustic ohms, whereas the Z_r values grow consistently from 1560 acoustic ohms (no reflex at 80-dB HL) to 1698 acoustic ohms at 100-dB HL. The data expressed in acoustic ohms demonstrate that with a 226-Hz probe, the acoustic impedance of the middle ear in the reflexive state increases as the level of the reflex-activator signal increases.

With the exception of recent developments that are described in a subsequent section (Other Suprathreshold Measures of the Acoustic Reflex), the acoustic-reflex growth function is not used widely as a clinical diagnostic procedure. One point on the acoustic-reflex growth function,

TABLE 5.1

The Acoustic Admittance and Impedance Values[3] for the Acoustic Reflexes
Elicited by 1000-Hz, 80- to 110-dB HL Activator Signals.
These Are the Numeric Data (226-Hz)
For the Acoustic Reflexes Depicted in Figure 5.11

dB HL	Acoustic Admittance (mmhos)			Acoustic Impedance (ohms)		
	Y_{tm}	Y_r	ΔY	Z_{tm}	Z_r	ΔZ
80	0.642	0.641	−0.001	1558	1560	2
85	0.638	0.627	−0.011	1567	1595	28
90	0.639	0.603	−0.036	1565	1658	93
95	0.640	0.594	−0.046	1563	1684	121
100	0.639	0.589	−0.050	1565	1698	133
105	0.641	0.586	−0.055	1560	1707	147
110	0.643	0.589	−0.054	1555	1698	143

however, the *acoustic-reflex threshold*, is used extensively in the evaluation of the auditory system. The acoustic-reflex threshold is the lowest
sound pressure level or hearing level of a reflex-activator signal that elicits
a measurable immittance change that is coincident with presentation of
the activator signal. In the example given in Figure 5.11, 85-dB HL is the
lowest level at which an acoustic reflex was measured.

The level of the activator signal at which an acoustic-reflex threshold
is measured is dependent on the *sensitivity* of the measurement system.
Reflex thresholds measured with a 678-Hz probe typically are 2 to 6 dB
lower than reflex thresholds established with a 226-Hz probe (Beattie &
Leamy, 1975; Burke & Herer, 1973; Porter, 1972; Wilson & McBride, 1978).
In all probability, the difference in reflex threshold levels obtained with
the two probe frequencies is because the 678-Hz probe frequency is closer
to the lowest resonance frequency of the middle ear than is the 226-Hz
probe frequency. Reflex thresholds that are measured on a strip chart
recorder, an oscilloscope, or a computer tend to be 3 to 7 dB lower than
reflex thresholds visualized on a meter (Wilson & McBride, 1978; Wilson,
Morgan, & Dirks, 1972). Many of the currently marketed immittance
instruments feature CRT or stripchart displays that provide superior
sensitivity compared to the visual observation of a needle on a meter.

Normal reflex thresholds

There are no standards that describe procedures for the measurement of the various parameters of the acoustic reflex, including reflex threshold, or that define the normal range of levels for acoustic-reflex thresholds. Anderson and Wedenberg (1968, Figure 3) considered reflex thresholds to be abnormal if the thresholds were at levels > 90-dB HL. More recently, Jerger, Oliver, and Jenkins (1987) considered reflex thresholds to be abnormal if the reflex thresholds were > 100-dB HL. The threshold data in Table 5.2 are representative of the normative values for contralateral acoustic-reflex thresholds for adults with normal hearing. The data for the pure tone activator signals are in decibels hearing level (re: ANSI, 1969 or ISO, 1964), whereas the threshold data for the broadband noise activator signals are in decibels sound pressure level (re: 20 μPa). Several relations emerge from the data in the table. First, although there are slight variations among studies, the mean/median reflex thresholds for 250-, 500-, 1000-, 2000-, and 4000-Hz activator signals range from 80- to 90-dB HL. The Handler and Margolis (1977) and Wilson (1981) investigations reported standard deviations that can be used to define the normal range. With two standard deviations used to define the normal limits and rounding up to a 5-dB interval (the most commonly used attenuator step size), the upper limit of the normal reflex thresholds is 95-dB HL for pure tones from 250 to 2000 Hz. At 4000 Hz, the upper limit of the normal range is between 100-dB HL (Wilson, 1981) and 105-dB HL (Handler & Margolis, 1977). Second, the mean reflex threshold for the broadband noise reflex activator ranges from 70- to 75-dB SPL. Again using two standard deviations from the Wilson and Handler and Margolis studies, 90- to 95-dB SPL is the upper limit of the normal reflex threshold for broadband noise. Third, in terms of sound pressure level, the reflex threshold for the broadband noise activator is 10 to 20 dB lower than the reflex thresholds in sound pressure level[4] for 500-, 1000-, and 2000-Hz activators.

The interaural reflex threshold differences also may be useful diagnostically (Chiveralls, 1977). Contralateral reflex threshold data for the left ear and right ear of 48 young adults with normal hearing are listed in Table 5.3 (top panel) along with the absolute difference between thresholds (Wilson, Shanks, & Velde, 1981). The data, which were based on measurements made in 2-dB steps, indicate no significant difference between the reflex thresholds for the left and right ears, with an absolute difference between ears that ranged from 3.4 to 5.1 dB. The lower panel

---

[4]Using the ANSI, 1969, standard for a TDH-39 earphone, reflex thresholds for 500, 1000, and 2000 Hz are converted from hearing level to sound pressure level by adding 11.5, 7.0, and 9.0 dB, respectively, to the threshold values expressed in hearing level.

TABLE 5.2
The Mean (or Median) Contralateral, 226-Hz Acoustic-Reflex Thresholds
(dB HL re: ANSI, 1969 or ISO, 1964, for the Pure Tone Activators and dB SPL
re: 20 μPa for the Broadband Noise Activators) From Seven Studies

Study, No. of Subjects, and Statistic	Reflex-Activator Signal (Hz)					
	250	500	1000	2000	4000	Noise
Anderson & Wedenberg, 1968						
N = 200						
median	84.2	87.4	85.6	85.5	90.7	
Chiveralls, 1977						
N = 100						
median	89.8					
N = 222						
median		83.6	82.8	81.5	82.8	
Gelfand & Piper, 1981						
N = 12						
mean		81.5	82.4	83.1		76.2
SD		4.2	5.2	4.9		6.5
Handler & Margolis, 1977						
N = 17						
mean		82.5	83.0	83.0	86.5	75.0
SD		6.1	5.1	5.2	9.0	8.4
Osterhammel & Osterhammel, 1979						
N = 65						
mean		90.1	90.2	89.8	93.8	
Peterson & Lidén, 1972[a]						
N = 88						
mean	84.6	85.2	85.4	84.0	84.4	
SD	7.1	7.0	6.7	5.5	7.2	
Wilson, 1981						
N = 18						
mean	78.8	79.4	82.8	82.1	83.3	71.7
SD	6.3	4.7	4.5	4.6	5.9	8.6

[a] 800-Hz probe, ascending, amplitude measurement.

TABLE 5.3
Top Panel: The Mean Contralateral, Acoustic-Reflex Thresholds (dB HL)
for the Left and Right Ears of 48 Subjects
Bottom Panel: The Cumulative Percent of the 48 Subjects for Five 2-dB Intervals
of Absolute Reflex-Threshold Differences
(Modified from Wilson, Shanks, & Velde, 1981)

Condition	Left Ear		Right Ear		Absolute Difference	
	dB HL	SD	dB HL	SD	dB HL	SD
500 Hz	87.1	6.1	86.4	5.4	3.4	2.8
1000 Hz	86.8	5.1	86.4	6.0	3.8	2.9
2000 Hz	85.4	6.9	85.7	6.9	4.5	3.5
Noise*	77.7	9.0	77.9	10.5	5.1	4.7

	Absolute Reflex-Threshold Difference (dB)				
Condition	<2	<4	<6	<8	<10
500 Hz	25	58	75	92	98
1000 Hz	27	54	73	85	98
2000 Hz	19	42	69	83	89
Noise	15	46	69	79	83

*Broadband noise thresholds (dB SPL).

of Table 5.3 shows the cumulative percent for the absolute threshold differences between the 48 subjects for five, 2-dB intervals. For example, at 500 Hz, 58% of the subjects had acoustic-reflex thresholds that either were at the same level or were at levels <4 dB apart in the ears. The interaural acoustic-reflex thresholds differed by no more than 10 dB in 83% to 98% of the cases.

Whether or not true differences between ipsilateral and contralateral acoustic-reflex thresholds exist is uncertain. Figure 5.12 shows ipsilateral and contralateral reflex growth functions for a subject with normal hearing (Borg & Zakrisson, 1974). The data are plotted in percent of maximum impedance change. The ipsilateral growth function is steeper than the

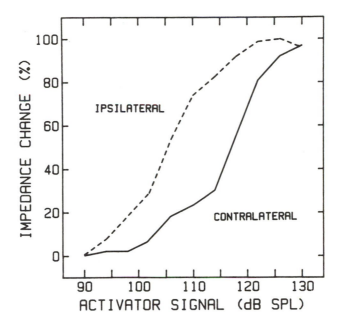

Figure 5.12. Ipsilateral (dashed line) and contralateral (solid line) acoustic-reflex growth functions expressed as a percentage of maximum impedance change. (From Borg & Zakrisson, 1974, with permission.)

contralateral function, but the two functions converge on the same point at the origin. Applying a criterion for determining the reflex threshold (e.g., 10% on the vertical axis) results in a substantial difference between the ipsilateral and contralateral reflex thresholds. If the functions converge on a point at the origin, then no true difference between the reflex thresholds exists. The available data on ipsilateral and contralateral acoustic reflexes (e.g., Møller, 1962a) suggest that ipsilateral reflex thresholds are consistently 2–14 dB lower than contralateral thresholds. It is not clear that the threshold differences are due entirely to the differences in the slopes of the reflex growth functions. It is clear, however, that the more sensitive the measurement system is, the smaller the apparent differences are between reflex thresholds for ipsilateral and contralateral activator signals.

Life span changes of the acoustic reflex

Little is known about the dynamic properties of acoustic reflexes in infants. The gross differences in middle ear characteristics between infants and adults make quantitative comparisons of acoustic-reflex magnitudes difficult. Because the reflex-threshold measurement requires only the detection of a response and not a quantification of the response, reflex thresholds are easier to compare than are other reflex characteristics that require accurate determination of the response magnitude. Still, the changes in the levels of the reflex-activator signal that result from postnatal development of the external ear are problematic in making absolute comparisons of reflex thresholds across the life span. Despite the difficulties in comparing reflex thresholds among various age groups, a general description of life span changes in acoustic-reflex thresholds is possible.

Reflex thresholds in infants. Because most commercially available aural acoustic immittance instruments offered only a low-frequency probe tone (220 or 226 Hz), early attempts to record acoustic reflexes in neonates used only one probe frequency. Although there is some disagreement on the proportion of observable responses, the early reports indicated that acoustic reflexes were not observable in most neonates (Barajas, Olaizola, Tapia, Alarcon, & Alaminos, 1981; Bennett, 1975; Keith, 1975; Keith & Bench, 1978; Stream, Stream, Walker, & Breningstall, 1978). When acoustic conductance was monitored with a two-component admittance meter, the proportion of observable neonatal acoustic reflexes was higher (88%), but reflex thresholds were substantially elevated compared to older infants and adults (Himelfarb, Shanon, Popelka, & Margolis, 1978). Sprague, Wiley, and Goldstein (1985) reported that only 50% of their neonates had observable reflexes with a 220-Hz probe tone. Inexplicably, one study (Vincent & Gerber, 1987) reported a higher proportion of observable reflexes in neonates than previous investigators have reported. Vincent and Gerber reported that 92.5% of their 2-day-old neonates had observable acoustic reflexes at 220 Hz.

Investigators who used a probe frequency higher than 226 Hz were, in general, more successful in recording acoustic reflexes from neonates (Kankkunen & Lidén, 1984; Marchant et al., 1986; McCandless & Allred, 1978; McMillan, Marchant, & Shurin, 1985; Sprague et al., 1985). Weatherby and Bennett (1980) explored most directly the effect of probe frequency on the measurement of acoustic reflexes in neonates and observed that as the probe frequency increased, the proportion of acoustic reflexes increased, and mean reflex threshold decreased. With a 600-Hz probe, 93.3% of the neonates had observable reflexes, whereas with an 800-Hz probe, 100% of the neonates had acoustic reflexes. In a subsequent investigation, Bennett and Weatherby (1982) used a 1200-Hz probe tone to measure reflex thresholds for tonal- and noise-activator signals in 4- to 8-day-old infants ($N = 28$) and reported reflex thresholds that were similar to the reflex thresholds reported for normal adults.

In summary, the extant research on acoustic-reflex thresholds in neonates suggests that the acoustic reflex is fully developed at birth and that reflex thresholds in neonates are similar to the reflex thresholds observed with adults. Several reports presented reflex thresholds that are lower than the reflex thresholds of adults (e.g., Weatherby & Bennett, 1980), but these differences may be attributable to the use of standard calibration couplers (e.g., 2-cm³ coupler) and the higher sound pressure levels that are developed in the small external ear canal of the neonate (McMillan et al., 1985). The optimal probe frequency for reflex testing in neonates appears to be above 800 Hz. The differences between ipsilateral and contralateral reflex thresholds (McMillan et al., 1985; Sprague et al., 1985) are about the same as the differences between ipsilateral and contralateral reflexes that have been reported for adults.

Reflex thresholds in aging adults.   There is some disagreement among investigators concerning acoustic-reflex thresholds in aging adults. Some studies suggest that reflex thresholds decrease with age (Jerger, Hayes, Anthony, & Mauldin, 1978; Jerger, Jerger, & Mauldin, 1972); some studies demonstrate no age-related change in the reflex threshold (Osterhammel & Osterhammel, 1979; Thompson, Sills, Recke, & Bui, 1980); some report an increase in reflex thresholds with aging (Wilson, 1981); and some report an increase in reflex thresholds for some activator signals but not other activators (Gelfand & Piper, 1981; Handler & Margolis, 1977; Silman, 1979; Silverman, Silman, & Miller, 1983). The disagreement can be attributed to the following four factors: (a) the reflex-threshold differences among age groups are small, (b) the measurement procedures used were not capable of resolving the small differences being studied, (c) the subject selection criteria were different in the various studies, and (d) the age groupings that were compared differed among studies.

    A sensitive measurement system is needed to study the effects of age on the acoustic reflex. Figure 5.13 presents reflex growth functions for two age groups (<30 years and >50 years) from Wilson (1981). The growth functions for the two age groups differ in slope, with the >50-years group (triangles) exhibiting a more gradual increase in reflex amplitude than the <30-years group (circles). In general, the growth functions converge on the same point, suggesting minimal threshold differences between the groups. In contrast, applying an absolute criterion, such as the level producing an admittance change of 0.01 mmhos, produces 3- to 11-dB threshold differences. These threshold differences result from applying a criterion change to functions that differ in slope but not in origin. Because of the slope differences in the reflex growth functions for different age groups, age-related reflex threshold differences are dependent on the criterion used to determine threshold. The reflex growth

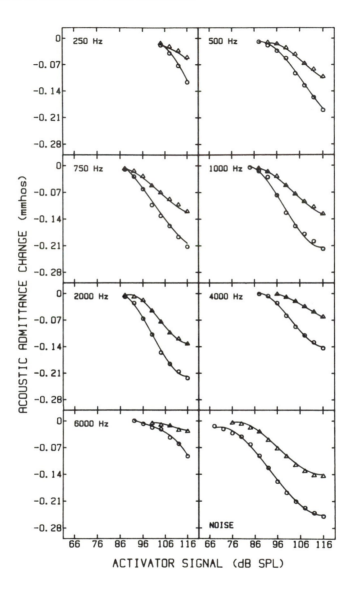

Figure 5.13. Acoustic-reflex growth functions expressed as the change in admittance magnitude at 226 Hz for two groups of subjects, aged 30 years or less (circles) and 50 years or more (triangles). (From Wilson, 1981, with permission.)

functions for tonal signals ≤2000 Hz appear to converge on the same point, suggesting that no age-related reflex threshold differences exist. With the three remaining activator signals (4000-Hz, 6000-Hz, and broadband noise), the growth functions for the two age groups converge on different origins, suggesting true reflex threshold differences for the two groups, with the >50-years group having the higher reflex thresholds.

Another complicating factor in the study of age effects is subject selection criteria, particularly regarding auditory sensitivity. Some studies selected subjects in various age groups who had "clinically normal hearing" (Gelfand & Piper, 1981; Handler & Margolis, 1977; Wilson, 1981). Other studies include subjects who had normal hearing for their age group (Osterhammel & Osterhammel, 1979). In all of the studies, sensitivity differences occurred among age groups, but the sensitivity differences were smaller in the studies that employed clinically normal subjects, as opposed to age-corrected norms. The technique of selecting clinically normal elderly subjects is useful for controlling the hearing sensitivity variable but may result in a biased control group of "supernormals," that is, a group that reflects the tail rather than the central tendency of the population represented.

With these considerations in mind, the following generalization can be drawn from studies that meet the procedural requirements of a sensitive measurement procedure. Reflex thresholds for tonal activator signals ≤2000 Hz do not change with age. Higher frequency activator signals and broadband noise produce small age-related elevations in reflex thresholds.

Abnormal reflex thresholds

An abnormality at any location in the acoustic-reflex arc can alter the characteristics of the acoustic reflex. Lesions in the afferent or input portion of the acoustic-reflex arc (viz., the middle ear, the cochlea, and CNVIII) produce either the absence of the acoustic reflex or the elevation of the acoustic-reflex threshold in the ear to which the reflex-activator signal is presented. The proportion of absent acoustic reflexes for patients with varying degrees of sensorineural hearing loss is illustrated in Figure 5.14. The percent of absent reflexes in patients with conductive hearing losses reflects the attenuation characteristics of the middle ear lesion on the reflex-activator signal. If the level of the reflex-activator signal is high enough to overcome the amount of attenuation produced by the middle ear lesion, then an acoustic reflex can be elicited in the opposite ear; the output limits of the instrumentation are the limiting factor. With a conductive hearing loss of 20 dB, 40% of the patients have no measurable acoustic reflex; with a 40-dB conductive loss, 80% of the patients have

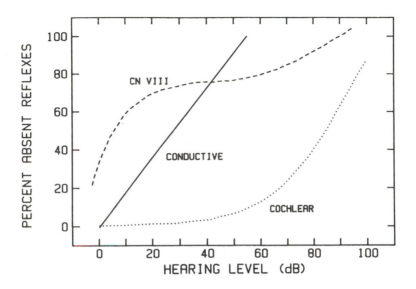

Figure 5.14. The percentage of absent acoustic reflexes in the ear to which the reflex-activator signal is presented as a function of hearing threshold sensitivity (dB HL) for patients with CNVIII hearing loss (dashed line), with conductive hearing loss (solid line), and with cochlear hearing loss (dotted line). (From Jerger, Clemis, Harford, & Alford, 1974, with permission.)

no measurable acoustic reflex (Jerger, Anthony, Jerger, & Mauldin, 1974). The acoustic reflex should be measurable with cochlear hearing losses to 40-dB HL (Jerger et al., 1972). With a 60-dB HL cochlear hearing loss, 15% of the patients do not have a measurable acoustic reflex. As the degree of cochlear hearing loss increases above 70-dB HL, the percentage of absent reflexes increases rapidly. The picture is quite different for patients with CNVIII lesions. With 0- to 10-dB HL thresholds, as many as 50% of the patients with CNVIII lesions may have no measurable acoustic reflexes (Jerger, Clemis, Harford, & Alford, 1974). As the hearing loss increases above 10-dB HL, there is a corresponding increase in the percentage of absent acoustic reflexes to 60-dB HL, at which level 80% of the patients have no measurable reflexes. Although the majority of cases in which there is no measurable acoustic reflex involve a pathological condition, a few people with apparent normal auditory systems have no measurable acoustic reflex. Jepsen (1951) reported the acoustic reflexes were not measurable in 1 of 182 subjects (<1%) who had normal auditory systems.

The relation between the degree of hearing loss and the acoustic-reflex threshold for pure tones is illustrated in the top panel of Figure 5.15. In

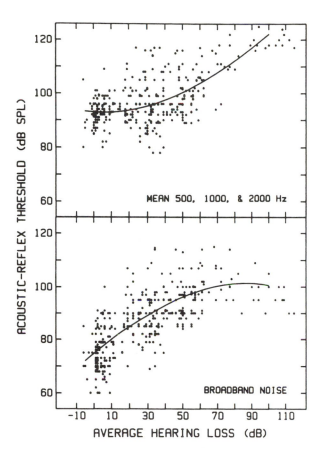

Figure 5.15. The top panel shows the mean acoustic-reflex thresholds (in dB SPL) for 500-, 1000-, and 2000-Hz activators depicted as a function of the mean hearing level (in dB HL, re: ANSI, 1969) for 355 ears at 500, 1000, and 2000 Hz. The solid line represents a best-fit, third-degree polynomial. The bottom panel shows the mean acoustic-reflex thresholds (in dB SPL) for broadband noise depicted as a function of the mean hearing level (in dB HL, re: ANSI, 1969) for 355 ears at 500, 1000, and 2000 Hz. The solid line represents a best-fit, third-degree polynomial. (From Popelka, 1981, with permission.)

the figure, the average acoustic-reflex threshold (in dB SPL) at 500, 1000, and 2000 Hz is shown as a function of the average behavioral pure tone threshold (in dB HL) at 500, 1000, and 2000 Hz. The data are based on 355 ears with cochlear hearing loss (Popelka, 1981). The reflex threshold remains at normal levels until the hearing loss exceeds 40-dB HL. As hearing loss increases above 40-dB HL, there is an almost linear increase in the level of the acoustic-reflex threshold with a slope of approximately 0.38 dB/dB. This means that for each decibel increase in hearing loss above 40-dB HL, there is an increase of 0.38 dB in the acoustic-reflex threshold. As illustrated in the bottom panel of Figure 5.15, there is a somewhat different relation between the reflex threshold for a broadband noise activator and the degree of hearing loss. As hearing loss increases to about 50-dB HL, the reflex threshold for broadband noise increases linearly with a slope of 0.4 dB/dB. As the degree of hearing loss increases above 60-dB HL, there is no corresponding increase in the level of the reflex threshold for the broadband noise activator.

When the lesion is in the efferent or output portion of the acoustic-reflex arc (viz., CNVII, the stapedius nerve, the stapedius muscle, and the middle ear), the site-of-lesion, not the degree of hearing loss, is the primary determinant of the status of the acoustic reflex in the probe ear. In patients with a suspected CNVII lesion such as Bell's palsy or a facial nerve schwannoma, absent or elevated reflex thresholds suggest that the site-of-lesion is proximal to branching of the stapedius nerve from CNVII. Normal reflex thresholds suggest the site-of-lesion is distal to branching of the stapedius nerve from CNVII. Certain neuromuscular diseases such as myasthenia gravis physiologically render the stapedius muscle unable to contract normally, thereby altering the threshold and growth characteristics of the acoustic reflexes (Blom & Zakrisson, 1974).

A middle ear abnormality in the probe ear usually precludes measurement of the acoustic reflex. In the presence of middle ear disease, the stapedius muscle may contract but the contraction is not strong enough to alter the acoustic immittance characteristics of the middle ear. An ossicular discontinuity can produce a similar effect in which the stapedius muscle contracts, but because of a disruption in the ossicular chain, the change in acoustic immittance during the reflexive state is not measurable at the tympanic membrane.

There are some middle ear disease processes, however, that do not obliterate measurement of the acoustic reflex in the probe ear. Examples of these disease processes are partial ossicular discontinuities including a fracture of the stapes crura central to insertion of the stapedius tendon (Jenkins, Morgan, & Miller, 1980), and congenital stapes anomaly (Shapiro, Canalis, Firemark, & Bahna, 1981). In these cases, the normal route of sound transmission through the middle ear is disrupted, but there is enough continuity of the middle ear system to permit monitoring of the reflex. With some otosclerotic ears, the reflex is present with the probe in the affected ear but the response is diphasic. With the diphasic pattern, transient immittance changes occur at the onset and offset of the activator signal (Flottorp & Djupesland, 1970; Terkildsen, 1964; Terkildsen, Osterhammel, & Bretlau, 1973). Finally, the audiologist must be cautious in interpreting abnormal reflex data from the probe ear. The majority of patients with abnormal reflexes in the probe ear have middle ear disorders, although, less frequently, the problem involves the stapedius muscle or CNVII.

Acoustic-reflex adaptation

During sustained activation of the acoustic reflex, the stapedius muscle begins to relax and the acoustic immittance of the middle ear mechanism begins to return to the preactivator state. Relaxation of the stapedius muscle during presentation of a reflex-activator signal is called *acoustic-reflex adaptation* (or *decay*). (For a detailed review of acoustic-reflex adaptation see Wilson, Shanks, and Lilly, 1984, and Fowler and Wilson, 1984.) In the normal auditory system, the amount and rate of reflex adaptation is directly related to the frequency of the activator signal (Djupesland, Flottorp, & Winther, 1967; Johansson, Kylin, & Langfy, 1967) and is inversely related to the level of the activator signal, especially for levels near the acoustic-reflex threshold (Dallos, 1964).

Figure 5.16 illustrates the terminology that is used to describe reflex adaptation. The top tracing in the figure is an acoustic reflex (in acoustic mmhos, left ordinate; in percent of maximum, right ordinate) elicited by a 10.2-s, 4000-Hz activator signal (bottom tracing) presented 10 dB above the acoustic-reflex threshold of a young subject with normal hearing. The letters (A–K) are used to identify the various aspects of reflex adaptation. Point B denotes the onset of the reflex-activator signal. Segment AB defines the preactivator signal baseline of middle ear activity (Y_{tm}) that corresponds to 0.79 acoustic mmhos or 0% of the maximum reflex amplitude. C is the time at which the reflex attained 10% of maximum amplitude (0.69 acoustic mmhos or 100% of maximum) that occurred at D. Point E is the time (1.6 s) at which the reflex adapted to 90% of the maximum reflex amplitude. Point F is the time (3.6 s) at which the reflex adapted to 50% of the maximum reflex amplitude. The time after onset of the activator signal at which the response adapts to 50% of maximum amplitude is called the *half-life time* and is the measure of reflex adaptation used clinically. The rate of reflex adaptation can be described as the slope of a line through the 90% (point E) and 50% (point F). Thus the slope of the adaptation function for the reflex shown in Figure 5.16 can be expressed as:

$$m = \Delta Y / \Delta t \tag{13}$$

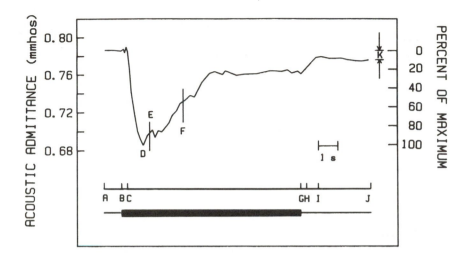

Figure 5.16. The top tracing is a reflex response (in acoustic mmhos, left ordinate; in percent of maximum, right ordinate) elicited by a 10.2-s, 4000-Hz activator signal (bottom tracing) presented 10 dB above the acoustic-reflex threshold of a young subject with normal hearing. See text for a discussion of letters A–K. (From Wilson, Shanks, & Lilly, 1984, with permission.)

in which m is the slope, ΔY is the change in acoustic mmhos that occurred between the ordinal values at 90% (0.70 acoustic mmhos) and 50% (0.74 acoustic mmhos), and Δt is the change in seconds that occurred between the abscissa values at 90% (1.6 s) and 50% (3.6 s). In this example, the rate of reflex adaptation in mmhos/second would be

$$m = -0.04 \text{ acoustic mmhos}/-2.0 \text{ s}$$
$$= 0.02 \text{ acoustic mmhos/s}$$

or the rate of reflex adaptation in percent/second would be

$$m = 40\%/-2.0 \text{ s}$$
$$= -20\%/s$$

At G in Figure 5.16 the activator signal ended, followed at H by the offset of the reflex. During segment IJ, the acoustic admittance of the middle ear approximated the preactivator signal baseline value. In the example in Figure 5.16, however, the return to the preactivator signal baseline value is not complete, with K representing the difference between the pre- (0.79 acoustic mmhos) and postactivator signal (0.78 acoustic mmhos) baselines.

This slight change in the acoustic admittance of the middle ear over 10 s to 15 s is a common occurrence that reflects the slight, but constantly changing air pressure in the middle ear (Tonndorf & Khanna, 1968; Wilson, McCullough, & Lilly, 1984; Wilson, Steckler, Jones, & Margolis, 1978). When a large pre- and poststimulus baseline acoustic immittance difference occurs, the adaptation measurement may be contaminated with the baseline shift and should be repeated.

The influence of the frequency of the reflex-activator signal on reflex adaptation is illustrated in Figure 5.17. No adaptation occurs for the 500- or 1000-Hz activator signals. With the 2000-Hz activator, adaptation to 90% of maximum is reached at 3.3 s, but adaptation to 50% is not attained over the duration of the activator signal. The reflex to the 4000-Hz activator, however, demonstrates adaptation both to 90% (1.1 s) and to 50% (2.2 s) of the maximum acoustic admittance, producing an adaptation slope of −36.4%/s. There is (a) a direct relationship between the amount and rate of reflex adaptation and the frequency of the reflex-activator signal, and (b) an inverse relationship between the frequency of the activator signal and the half-life time, that is, the higher the frequency, the shorter the half-life time of the adaptation function.

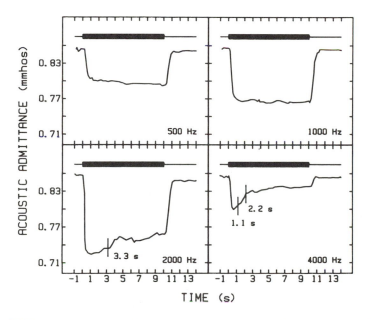

Figure 5.17. Acoustic-reflex adaptation functions elicited from a young adult with normal hearing by 500-, 1000-, 2000-, and 4000-Hz activator signals presented for 10.2 s, 10 dB above the acoustic-reflex threshold. (From Wilson, Shanks, & Lilly, 1984, with permission.)

The relation between reflex adaptation and the level of the reflex-activator signal is difficult to determine. As indicated earlier, at levels near the reflex threshold, the amount and rate of adaptation appear to be greater than at levels ≥ 10 dB above the reflex threshold (Dallos, 1964). This observation was confirmed by Djupesland et al. (1967) who observed with 250-, 500-, 1000-, 3000-, and 4000-Hz activators presented 2, 4, and 10 dB above the reflex threshold that the higher the activator level, the longer the reflex was maintained. In contrast, Wiley and Karlovich (1975) reported that as the level of a 500-Hz activator was increased from 5 to 15 dB above the reflex threshold, there was a corresponding increase in the amount of reflex adaptation; with a 4000-Hz activator, no change was noted in reflex adaptation as the level of the activator was increased. Kaplan, Gilman, and Dirks (1977) also reported that reflex adaptation at 500, 1000, 2000, 3000, and 4000 Hz was independent of the level of the activator signal (6, 12, and 18 dB above the reflex threshold). Data from three studies indicate that for activator signals less than 2000 Hz, reflex adaptation decreases as the level of the activator signal increases (Givens & Seidemann, 1979; Rosenhall, Lidén, & Nilsson, 1979; Wilson et al., 1978). For reflex-activator signals greater than 1000 Hz, there does not appear to be a systematic change in reflex adaptation as the activator level is increased (Givens & Seidemann, 1979; Wiley & Karlovich, 1975; Wilson et al., 1978). Procedural differences probably have led to different conclusions.

The clinical use of reflex adaptation was suggested by the observation that patients with CNVIII lesions exhibit a high rate of adaptation (Anderson, Barr, & Wedenberg, 1969, 1970). Abnormal reflex adaptation was defined in the original reports as a half-life time <5 s for a reflex-activator signal presented 10 dB above the reflex threshold at 500 and 1000 Hz. In contrast to the patients with CNVIII lesions, Anderson et al. reported that patients with normal hearing or with cochlear hearing loss maintained the magnitude of the acoustic reflex over the duration of the 10-s, 500- or 1000-Hz activators. Table 5.4 presents a summary of the half-life times from nine investigations of reflex adaptation on subjects with normal hearing. With minor exceptions and considering the differences in experimental protocols, there is good agreement among the results of the studies indicating the frequency-dependent nature of acoustic-reflex adaptation.

Of the original four test parameters used by Anderson et al., only the level of the reflex-activator signal (10 dB above the reflex threshold) and the half-life time measurement continue to be in common usage. The other two parameters (activator signal duration and frequency) vary from one investigation to another. Some investigators define adaptation over 10 s (Jerger, Clemis, Harford, & Alford, 1974; Olsen, Stach, & Kurdziel,

TABLE 5.4

Half-Life Times (In Seconds) for Acoustic-Reflex Adaptation in Subjects With Normal Hearing From Nine Investigations (From Wilson, Shanks, & Lilly, 1984)

| Study | Reflex-Activator Signal | | Statistic | N | Reflex-Activator Signal Frequency (Hz) | | | | | | | |
	Level	Duration (in s)			500	710	1000	1500	2000	3000	4000	6000
Anderson et al. (1969)	+10 dB[a]	10	Median	50	>10.0		>10.0		14.0		7.0	
Cartwright & Lilly (1976)	+10 dB	30–40	Mean	15	>30.0		>30.0		21.0		5.0	
Chiveralls et al. (1976)[b]	+10 dB	30	Mean	101–106	none		32.0		14.5		7.4	
			SD				6.5		5.0		2.1	
Habener & Snyder (1974)	+10 dB	10+	Mean	101–122	>10.0		>10.0		13.4		8.9	
Kaplan et al. (1977)	c	180	Model	6	240.0		158.0		25.0	13.0	7.2	
Lilly, Mekarv, & Chudnow (1983)[d]	+10 dB	120	Mean	12		78.4						
Tietze (1969)	e	180	Median	10	>100.0		>40.0	8.0	3.0	2.0	1.1	<1.0
Wilson et al. (1978)	96 dB SPL	180	Mean	7	76.6		20.8		6.2		3.5	
	104 dB SPL	180	Mean	7	141.6		41.1		16.9		4.7	
	116 dB SPL	180	Mean	7	145.3		55.9		12.5		4.4	
Wilson et al. (1984)	+10 dB	31	Mean	35	>31.0		>31.0	20.5	14.2	9.8	7.0	5.3
			SD					10.5	7.4	7.4	6.2	4.3

[a] Adaptation activator signal presented 10 dB above the acoustic-reflex threshold. [b] Includes data from Chiveralls and FitzSimons (1973). [c] Combined data for activator signals presented 6-, 12-, and 18-dB above the acoustic-reflex threshold. [d] Personal communication. [e] From the linear segment of the reflex-growth function.

1981). Other investigators define an abnormal response at either 500 or 1000 Hz. The following is a useful set of rules that can be applied to the interpretation of reflex-adaptation data (Hirsch & Anderson, 1980a, 1980b):

1. RD^{+++}, if the reflex amplitude declines ≥50% within 5 s at 500 and 1000 Hz;

2. RD^{++}, if the reflex amplitude declines ≥50% within 5 s at 1000 Hz but not at 500 Hz; and

3. RD^{+}, if the reflex amplitude declines <50% within 5 s at 500 and 1000 Hz.

RD^{+++} is a positive sign of CNVIII disease, RD^{++} is a questionable sign of CNVIII disease, and RD^{+} is not a significant sign of CNVIII disease.

Anderson et al. (1969) in the original report on reflex adaptation noted that only 1% of 600 patients with cochlear hearing loss exhibited abnormal reflex adaptation. Subsequent investigations have indicated substantially higher false-positive rates (i.e., abnormal reflex adaptation associated with cochlear hearing loss) than the 1% reported by Anderson et al. This point is illustrated by the reflex-adaptation functions shown in Figure 5.18 (Cartwright & Lilly, 1976). The data are from three groups of 15 subjects (normal hearing [squares], cochlear hearing loss from Ménière's disease [circles], and CNVIII hearing loss [triangles]) for 30-s, 500-Hz (top panel) and 1000-Hz (bottom panel) activator signals presented 10 dB above the reflex threshold. The functions in the figure illustrate that patients with cochlear hearing loss (Ménière's disease) exhibit reflex adaptation that is more than the adaptation shown by subjects with normal hearing, but less than the adaptation exhibited by patients with CNVIII lesions. Similar data from 100 ears with sensory hearing loss were reported by Olsen, Noffsinger, and Kurdziel (1975) in which abnormal reflex adaptation was demonstrated by one patient at 500 Hz and by 11 patients at 1000 Hz.

Finally, Mangham, Lindeman, and Dawson (1980) studied reflex adaptation as a function of activator level (5 to 25 dB above the reflex threshold) in patients with cochlear hearing loss and patients with CNVIII hearing loss. Mangham et al. observed that as the 500-Hz activator signal was presented at higher levels, there was a decrease in the amount of reflex adaptation for the patients with cochlear hearing loss, but there was an increase in the amount of reflex adaptation for patients with CNVIII lesions. These findings suggest that the use of multiple levels of the reflex-activator signal with reflex-adaptation measures may be useful in differentiating cochlear and CNVIII hearing losses.

Regardless of the method used clinically to define abnormal acoustic-reflex adaptation, that is, the 5-s or 10-s criteria at 500 and/or 1000 Hz, when abnormal adaptation is measured, the measurement should be

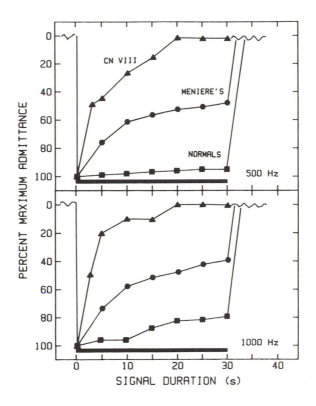

Figure 5.18. Acoustic-reflex adaptation data from three subject groups of 15 subjects each in response to 30-s, 500-Hz (top panel) and 1000-Hz (bottom panel) reflex-activator signals. (From Cartwright & Lilly, 1976, with permission.)

repeated to demonstrate reliability. Additionally, when reflex adaptation is abnormal, it may be insightful to make adaptation measurements at multiple levels above the acoustic-reflex threshold.

Other suprathreshold measures of the acoustic reflex

Throughout the 1970s, measures of the acoustic-reflex threshold and acoustic-reflex adaptation were the primary parameters of the acoustic reflex that were used routinely in the differential diagnosis of auditory disorders. Since the early 1960s, other parameters of the acoustic reflex, *viz.*, the temporal and magnitude characteristics, have been studied in animals and in young subjects with normal hearing. (Borg, 1976, provides a good review of the dynamic characteristics of the acoustic reflex.)

The animal investigations with the acoustic reflex are exemplified by the work from two laboratories. Borg (1973) reported an increase in the latency of the rabbit stapedius reflex following the creation of a lesion at the level of the trapezoid body. Mangham and Miller (1979) developed an animal model with the macaque monkey that involved the surgical implantation of balloon catheters in the left internal auditory meatus of four monkeys. To mimic the effects of a retrocochlear lesion, pressure was exerted on CNVIII by inflating the implanted balloon with saline. During the experimental procedures, acoustic-reflex measurements were made (a) with the balloon deflated, (b) during a 15- to 30-min period in which the balloon was inflated with volumes from 0.01 to 0.04 cm³, and (c) following balloon deflation. Mangham and Miller reported that measures of reflex threshold and reflex adaptation were not as sensitive to pressure on CNVIII as were measures of reflex onset latency, onset rise, and amplitude.

The temporal (latency and rise) and amplitude characteristics of the acoustic reflex in subjects with normal auditory systems have been described in numerous studies (Dallos, 1964; Gorga & Stelmachowicz, 1983; McPherson & Thompson, 1977; Møller, 1962b; Sprague, Wiley, & Block, 1981; Wilson, 1979; Wilson & McBride, 1978). Clinically, the human investigations initially concentrated on the onset latency of the acoustic reflex with the most recent focus on the amplitude characteristics of the acoustic reflex.

Acoustic-reflex latency

The latency of the acoustic reflex is the time difference, Δt, between the onset of the reflex-activator signal and the onset of the acoustic reflex. Several variables, however, compound the measurement of reflex latency. First, the commercially available electroacoustic immittance instruments have various time constants (Jerger, Oliver, & Stach, 1986; Lilly, 1984; Margolis & Gilman, 1977; Shanks, Wilson, & Jones, 1985). Second, the measurement of reflex latency is complicated by an imprecise definition of the onset of the acoustic reflex. Unlike the precise onset of an activator signal, the onset of the acoustic reflex can be monophasic or biphasic, making the reflex latency measurement difficult and arbitrary (Creten, Vanpeperstraete, Van Camp, & Doclo, 1976; Mangham, Burnett, & Lindeman, 1982, 1983; Van Camp, Vanpeperstraete, Creten, & Vanhuyse, 1975). Third, investigators use different onset landmarks to define onset of the acoustic reflex. Some investigations use the initial detectable acoustic immittance change, whereas other investigations use a percentage of the maximum immittance change, which can be 10%, 50%, or 90% (Borg, 1982; Bosatra, Russolo, & Silverman, 1984; Lilly, 1984). Fourth, the latency of the acoustic reflex is inversely related to the level of the reflex-activator signal (Dallos, 1964; Hung & Dallos, 1972; Lilly, 1964; Møller, 1958; Ruth & Niswander, 1976; Terkildsen, 1960). Fifth, the latency of the acoustic reflex covaries with the frequency and level of the activator signal. Ruth and Niswander reported that the latency was shorter for a 3000-Hz activator than for a 500-Hz activator at levels ≤104-dB SPL, whereas at activator levels >104-dB SPL, the latencies for the two frequencies were the same.

Clinically, the Clemis and Sarno (1980a, 1980b) reports typify the implementation of acoustic-reflex latency as part of the differential diagnosis. One study (1980a) included 47 subjects with normal hearing, 12 patients with Ménière's disease, 16 patients with other types of cochlear hearing loss, and 16 patients with surgically confirmed CNVIII lesions. Reflex latency, which was measured 10 dB above the reflex threshold at 1000 and 2000 Hz, was defined as the time difference between onset of the activator signal and "the first detectable increase in acoustic impedance" as measured by a commercial electroacoustic device with the output displayed on a storage oscilloscope. As shown in the histograms in Figure 5.19, the absolute latency for the normals was longer for the 2000-Hz activator (105.3 ms) than for the 1000-Hz activator (93.0 ms). The reflex latencies for both cochlear hearing loss groups (a) were about the same as the latencies measured for the normal subjects. Using the 95% confidence limit from the normal group as the normal range, 85%–95% of the patients with cochlear hearing loss were classified as normal by Clemis and Sarno. The retrocochlear group had latencies of 181.5 ms and 274.0 ms for 1000 and 2000 Hz, respectively, with no cases within the normal range. Interaural latency difference also was found to distinguish among the subject groups. The mean interaural latency difference was <25 ms for the normal subjects and the two groups with cochlear hearing loss and >90 ms for the patients with CNVIII lesions. Clemis and Sarno (1980a, 1980b), therefore, suggested that the latency of the acoustic reflex was useful in differentiating cochlear from retrocochlear disease.

In a subsequent investigation of reflex latency of four patients with confirmed CNVIII tumors, Jerger and Hayes (1983) reported that the reflex latencies for 500- to 2000-Hz activator signals presented at 100-dB SPL, which were measured on a laboratory constructed electroacoustic system, were two to nine times longer for the affected ear (mean = 184 ms; range 60 to 405 ms) than for the normal ear (mean = 40 ms; range

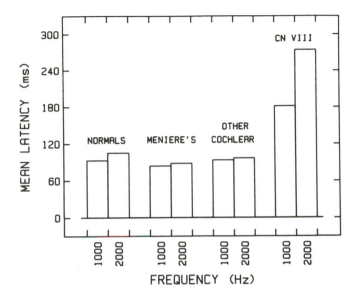

Figure 5.19. Histograms showing the mean reflex latencies (in ms) for 1000- and 2000-Hz activator signals for subjects with normal hearing (N = 47), patients with Ménière's disease (N = 12), patients with other cochlear hearing losses (N = 16), and patients with CNVIII lesions (N = 16). (Data from Clemis & Sarno, 1980a.)

30 to 45 ms).[5] Jerger and Hayes concluded that when the acoustic reflex was measurable with the activator signal presented to an ear with a CNVIII lesion, the acoustic reflex demonstrated a reduced maximum amplitude compared to the normal ear and was late with a slowly rising onset. From these observations and the measurement problems associated with the latency measurements, Jerger and Hayes suggested that suprathreshold amplitude measures of the acoustic reflex provided essentially the same diagnostic information as provided by reflex latency data, and were easier to make than were the latency measurements.

Acoustic-reflex amplitude

The magnitude or amplitude of the acoustic reflex is the difference between the immittance of the middle ear during the resting or quies-

---

[5]The latency difference between the 40-ms reported by Jerger and Hayes (1983) and the 93-ms to 105-ms latency reported by Clemis and Sarno (1980a) is attributable to different instrumentation and procedures. Jerger and Hayes did report a 78-ms latency for the normal ears when the measurements were made 10 dB above the reflex threshold.

cent state (baseline) and the immittance of the middle ear during the reflexive state (peak). During the past three decades, numerous investigations have explored the experimental parameters that affect the amplitude of the acoustic reflex, including the frequency, spectrum, level, and duration of the activator signal (Dallos, 1964; Djupesland & Zwislocki, 1971; Hung & Dallos, 1972; Metz, 1951; Møller, 1958, 1962a, 1962b; Peterson & Lidén, 1972; Silman, 1984; Wilson, 1979; Wilson & McBride, 1978). The common finding for all the investigations is the direct relation between the level of the activator signal and the amplitude of the acoustic reflex. Increases in the level of the activator signal produce increases in the amplitude of the reflex. Other observations include steeper reflex growth functions for mid-frequency activator signals than for low-frequency activators (Møller, 1961) and a hierarchy of reflex amplitudes in which binaural activator signals produce the largest reflex amplitudes, ipsilateral activator signals produce the second largest amplitudes, and contralateral activator signals produce the smallest amplitudes (Møller, 1962a). The duration of the activator signal also influences the amplitude of the acoustic reflex (Djupesland, Sundby, & Flottorp, 1973; Djupesland & Zwislocki, 1971; Jerger, Mauldin, & Lewis, 1977). As duration increases to about 500 ms, reflex amplitude increases.

Several additional characteristics of contralateral acoustic-reflex amplitude are illustrated in Figure 5.20. In the top panel of the figure are reflex growth functions for broadband noise and for 250-, 1000-, and 4000-Hz signals obtained with a 678-Hz probe and a computer-averaging technique from eight young adults with normal hearing (Wilson & McBride, 1978). The data were fit with third-degree polynomial functions, the first derivatives of which (slope functions) are illustrated in the bottom panel of Figure 5.20. The most obvious characteristic of the reflex growth functions is that increases in the level of the activator signal produce increases in the amplitude of the acoustic reflex. The growth functions are characterized by a relatively slow increase in amplitude of the reflex at low activator signal levels and at high activator levels, and by a more rapid, almost constant, increase in amplitude between the low and high activator signal levels. These two characteristics can be observed readily in "U-shaped" slope functions (mmhos/dB) in the bottom panel of Figure 5.20. The growth function for the 4000-Hz activator signal becomes asymptotic at the high signal levels, indicating that the growth function is saturated; that is, further increases in the level of the activator signal do not produce further increases in the magnitude of the acoustic reflex. These characteristics of the 4000-Hz growth function (top panel) are reflected in the 4000-Hz slope function (bottom panel) in which (a) a slow change (0 to -0.02 mmhos/dB) occurs over the first few activator levels from 88-dB SPL, (b) the maximum slope (-0.035 mmhos/dB) occurs

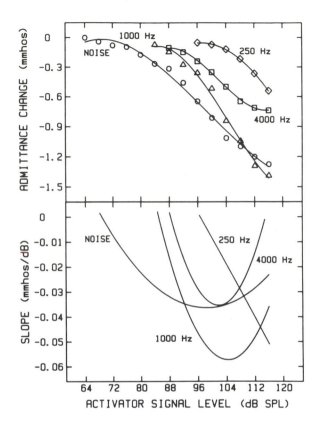

Figure 5.20. The top panel shows the mean (N = 8) reflex amplitude in admittance change (mmhos) shown as a function of the activator signal level (dB SPL). The data are modeled with best-fit, third-degree polynomials. The bottom panel shows the slope functions (mmhos/dB) calculated as the first derivatives of the polynomials used to fit the respective activator signal data. (From Wilson & McBride, 1978, with permission.)

at 102-dB SPL, and (c) the slope becomes more gradual (−0.02 to 0 mmhos/dB) at higher levels where the function begins to saturate. The dynamic range of a reflex growth function is the signal level range between reflex threshold and saturation. According to the data in Figure 5.20, the dynamic ranges are >50 dB for broadband noise, >28 dB for 1000 Hz, 23 dB for 4000 Hz, and >16 dB for 250 Hz. Three of the four dynamic ranges are "greater than" because saturation was not attained by the growth function. Finally, the status of the ear in which the measurement probe is inserted also has an influence on the amplitude of the acoustic reflex. In general, subjects with higher peak compensated static immittance exhibit larger reflex amplitudes (Lutman & Martin, 1977; Wilson, 1979, Figures 7, 8, and 9).

There are several clinical reports in the literature that indicate that patients with ear pathology have reduced reflex amplitudes. An increased rise time and a decreased magnitude of the acoustic reflex was reported as characteristic of patients with multiple sclerosis (Colletti, 1975). Silman, Gelfand, and Chun (1978) reported acoustic-reflex growth data from a case with an acoustic neuroma in the left ear. With the 500-Hz activator signal presented to the unaffected right ear, the amplitude of the reflex increased with increased activator level. With the 500-Hz activator signal presented to the affected left ear, however, the amplitude of the reflex did not increase with increases in the level of the activator signal. Ruth, Nilo, and Mravec (1978) reported that Bell's palsy patients have smaller contralateral reflex amplitudes with the measurement probe in the affected ear than with the probe in the unaffected ear. Alternatively, therefore, the reduced function of the acoustic reflex caused by the Bell's palsy, which would reduce the low-frequency attenuation characteristics of the reflex, could have permitted the 500-Hz activator signal to reach the cochlea of the affected ear at a higher than normal level, thereby increasing the amplitude of the acoustic reflex in the unaffected, contralateral ear. To clarify this issue, the Ruth et al. study must be replicated with both ipsilateral and contralateral reflex growth functions. If the alternative hypothesis were true, then the contralateral reflex amplitude would be larger than the ipsilateral amplitude, which is a relation that is reversed in the normal auditory system. Finally, data from several studies indicate that there is a decrease in the magnitude of the acoustic reflex (and growth functions) with increasing age (Thompson et al., 1980; Silman & Gelfand, 1981; Wilson, 1981).

Jerger and his colleagues (Hayes & Jerger, 1982; Jerger et al., 1987; Jerger, Oliver, Rivera, & Stach, 1986; Stach & Jerger, 1984) advocate the use of reflex amplitude measures as an indicator of auditory dysfunction. In this Jerger scheme, a probe assembly (270-Hz, 85-dB SPL probe tone) is sealed in each ear with the 500-, 1000-, or 2000-Hz activator tones (500-ms duration) presented at 110-dB SPL alternately between ears with a 1500-ms intersignal interval. The reflex to each activator signal is digitized, sorted, and averaged for the ipsilateral and the contralateral ear. Thus, four reflexes (right ipsilateral, right contralateral, left ipsilateral, and left contralateral) are obtained from 16 signal presentations. The amplitude of the reflex is the maximum decibel change (0.01 dB resolution) in the sound pressure level of the probe tone following offset of the activator signal. The reflex amplitudes for the four response modes are combined in the following ways to produce three indices of reflex amplitude:

1. Afferent Index = $(\text{Right}_{ipsi} + \text{Right}_{contra}) - (\text{Left}_{ipsi} + \text{Left}_{contra})$,
2. Efferent Index = $(\text{Right}_{ipsi} + \text{Left}_{contra}) - (\text{Left}_{ipsi} + \text{Right}_{contra})$, and
3. Central Index = $(\text{Right}_{ipsi} + \text{Left}_{ipsi}) - (\text{Right}_{contra} + \text{Left}_{contra})$,

in which Right_{ipsi} is the amplitude of the right ipsilateral acoustic reflex, Right_{contra} is the amplitude of the right contralateral acoustic reflex, Left_{ipsi} is the amplitude of the left ipsilateral acoustic reflex, and Left_{contra} is the amplitude of the left contralateral acoustic reflex. As Jerger, Oliver, Rivera, and Stach (1986), stated, "the index concept is used for two purposes: (1) to isolate the locus of reflex amplitude abnormality to (a) the probe ear, (b) the ear to which the signal is being presented, or (c) the central pathway of the crossed reflexes; and (2) to reduce the considerable inter-subject variability of individual measures of acoustic reflex amplitudes" (p. 167). The Afferent Index is sensitive to abnormalities on the input side (stimulus ear) of the acoustic-reflex arc, that is, lesions that affect the input of the reflex-activator signal, for example, cochlear and CNVIII lesions. The Efferent Index is sensitive to abnormalities on the output side (probe ear) of the acoustic-reflex arc, that is, lesions that directly affect contraction of the stapedius muscle in the probe ear, for example, CNVII and middle ear lesions. The Central Index is sensitive to abnormalities in the contralateral pathways of the acoustic-reflex arc. The reflex amplitudes from a subject with a normal auditory system are about the same for the left and right ears; therefore, the Afferent Index and the Efferent Index[6] are essentially the same or zero. Because the amplitude of the ipsilateral reflex is larger than the amplitude of the contralateral reflex, the Central Index for a subject with a normal auditory system is slightly greater than zero. As the instrumentation used by Jerger and his colleagues is unique to their facility, other clinics must establish equipment-specific norms for the three indices that are based on immittance units or the sound pressure level of the probe tone. Additionally, the approach may benefit by a method for quantifying reflex amplitude that is not sensitive to ear-canal volume (see Figure 5.10).

Detection of hearing loss from acoustic-reflex thresholds

Acoustic-reflex thresholds can provide information about hearing sensitivity (i.e., pure tone behavioral thresholds). The use of acoustic-reflex

---

[6]The Efferent Index can be influenced by a difference between ears in ear-canal volume (see Figure 5.10). With the Afferent Index and the Central Index, ear differences owing to ear-canal volume differences or peak compensated static immittance differences do not influence the indices because the characteristics of both ears are present in the expressions on either side of the minus argument.

thresholds to detect hearing loss or estimate hearing sensitivity is based on the following two relations: (a) the relation between the acoustic-reflex thresholds and the bandwidth of the reflex-activator signal, and (b) the relation between the acoustic-reflex threshold and the degree of hearing loss. In this section these two relations are described and applied to the detection of hearing loss. (Popelka, 1981, presents a thorough review of this topic.)

Lüscher (1929) was the first to point out that complex signals are more effective in eliciting the acoustic reflex than are tonal signals. The effect of bandwidth on acoustic-reflex thresholds was initially explored by Flottorp, Djupesland, and Winther (1971) and later by several other investigators (Djupesland & Zwislocki, 1973; Green & Margolis, 1983; Margolis, Dubno, & Wilson, 1980; Popelka, Karlovich, & Wiley, 1974; Popelka, Margolis, & Wiley, 1976; Schwartz & Sanders, 1976). Figure 5.21 illustrates the influence of the reflex-activator signal bandwidth on the reflex thresholds of normal subjects. Reflex thresholds remain constant as the signal bandwidth is increased to a "critical bandwidth," beyond which the reflex thresholds decrease. The bandwidth effect appears to be the same for ipsilateral and contralateral activator signals (Green & Margolis, 1983).

Thelin (1980) suggested that (a) the logarithmic bandwidth axis in Figure 5.21 does not accurately reflect the frequency representation in the auditory system, and (b) an octave scale better approximates the logarithmic frequency representation on the basilar membrane. In fact, if frequency is represented logarithmically in the auditory system as suggested by a considerable body of evidence (Zwislocki, 1965), then the log frequency axis in Figure 5.21 is not proportional to distance on the basilar membrane. Bandwidth measured in octaves, however, produces a measure that closely approximates the area of cochlear excitation (Green & Margolis, 1984). It is likely that the relatively flat portion of the acoustic-reflex threshold function in Figure 5.21 is flat because changes in the bandwidth of the reflex-activator signal in that frequency range produce very small differences in the area of excitation on the basilar membrane.

Figure 5.22 illustrates the effect of the reflex-activator signal bandwidth on acoustic-reflex thresholds plotted on an octave bandwidth axis. The effect of bandwidth on ipsilateral and contralateral acoustic-reflex thresholds are similar, that is, acoustic-reflex threshold decreases linearly with increases in activator signal bandwidth. The slope of the ipsilateral function may be slightly steeper than the slope of the contralateral function. The 5-6 dB differences in ipsilateral and contralateral acoustic-reflex thresholds may be entirely attributable to calibration differences between the two procedures (Green & Margolis, 1983). The relation illustrated in Figure 5.22 suggests a much simpler interpretation of the bandwidth effect than the "critical band" mechanism (e.g., Flottorp et al., 1971). That is,

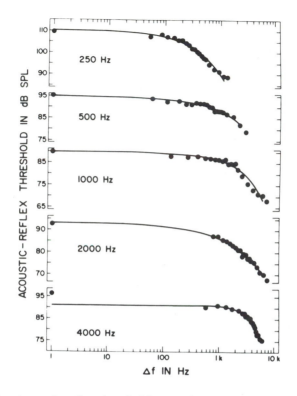

Figure 5.21. Acoustic-reflex thresholds as a function of reflex-activator signal bandwidth (Δf) in Hertz on a log-frequency axis. The activator signals were tonal complexes, logarithmically centered around the indicated frequency. The left-most data point in each function is the reflex threshold for a tonal stimulus at the indicated frequency. Each point is the mean reflex threshold for 10 normal hearing, young adult subjects. (From Popelka, Margolis, & Wiley, 1976, with permission.)

the acoustic-reflex threshold is linearly related to the area of excitation on the basilar membrane. A similar relationship has been found between loudness and signal bandwidth in octaves (Cacace & Margolis, 1985), which suggests that both loudness and acoustic-reflex threshold are linearly related to an area of excitation on the basilar membrane.

The effect of sensorineural hearing loss on acoustic-reflex thresholds was first explored by Metz, who was perplexed by the extreme variability in the relationship between sensitivity (behavioral) thresholds and acoustic-reflex thresholds. Metz (1946) stated that,

With the exception of one ear a muscle contraction can be elicited in all the ears with unilateral perception deafness or completely deaf ears from the opposite normal ears. The conditions are a little more complicated in patients with bilateral perception deafness, as a muscle contraction can be elicited in many cases, in others not, without this definitely being dependent on the magnitude of the hearing loss. However, it is impossible to elicit a muscle contraction from any of the completely deaf ears. (p. 241)

The variability in reflex thresholds from patients with sensorineural hearing loss was illustrated earlier in Figure 5.15. Reflex thresholds for tones (Figure 5.15, top panel) tend to remain unchanged for hearing losses up to about 40 dB and then increase as the degree of hearing loss increases. Acoustic-reflex thresholds for noise activator signals (Figure 5.15, bottom panel) are elevated for mild hearing losses and stabilize for more severe hearing losses. It should be pointed out, however, that most patients with severe hearing losses do not exhibit acoustic reflexes, so that the function for broadband noise in the bottom panel of Figure 5.15 probably underestimates the acoustic-reflex thresholds for severe hearing losses.

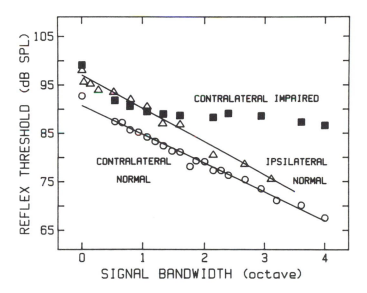

Figure 5.22. Acoustic-reflex thresholds as a function of the reflex-activator signal bandwidth (in octaves) for three subject groups. The center frequency was 2000 Hz and the left-most data point in each function is the reflex threshold for a 2000-Hz activator signal. The circles depict the contralateral reflex thresholds for normal hearing, young adult subjects from Popelka et al., 1976 (see Figure 5.21). The triangles represent ipsilateral reflex thresholds for normal hearing, young adult subjects from Green and Margolis (1983). The squares represent the mean reflex thresholds for eight subjects with noise-induced, sensorineural hearing loss. (From Popelka et al., 1976.)

The variability evident in Figure 5.15 presents a challenge to the detection of hearing loss from acoustic-reflex thresholds. A similar effect of signal bandwidth is shown in Figure 5.22. The filled, square symbols show the effect of reflex-activator signal bandwidth on acoustic-reflex thresholds for a group of patients with noise-induced sensorineural hearing loss. In comparison to the reflex thresholds from the subjects with normal hearing, the reflex thresholds from the hearing-impaired group are only slightly elevated for narrow-band activator signals but more significantly elevated for broadband activator signals.

Niemeyer and Sesterhenn (1974) were the first to use the relation between the reflex-activator signal bandwidth and the acoustic-reflex threshold to estimate the degree of hearing loss. This method for detecting hearing loss, which was dependent on the relation between the reflex thresholds for pure tone signals and noise signals, subsequently was modified by Jerger, Burney, Mauldin, and Crump (1974) and by Popelka et al. (1976). The detection methods are all based on the effect of hearing loss on the bandwidth effect in patients with sensorineural hearing loss. The various detection methods differ in the specificity of the outcome. Whereas the Niemeyer and Sesterhenn method estimates hearing loss in decibels hearing level, the Jerger et al. method classifies hearing loss into one of four severity categories. The bivariate plotting method (Figure 5.23) described by Popelka et al. (1976) is the least ambitious of the sensi-

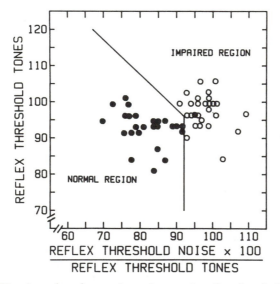

Figure 5.23. Bivariate plot of contralateral acoustic-reflex thresholds for subjects with normal hearing (filled circles) and patients with sensorineural hearing loss (open circles) exceeding 30 dB (mean at 500, 1000, and 2000 Hz). (From Margolis, Fox, Lilly, Popelka, Silman, & Trumpf, 1981, with permission.)

tivity prediction methods in that it separates subjects into two groups—normal and impaired. An evaluation of the three methods suggested that the variability illustrated in Figure 5.15 does not allow the more specific predictions of the Niemeyer and Sesterhenn method and the Jerger et al. method to be made with acceptable error rates. The bivariate plotting method, by making a gross discrimination among subjects, accomplishes that goal with acceptable false positive and hit rates (Margolis & Fox, 1977). The appropriate use of the detection procedure is as a screening device that identifies patients who need further audiologic evaluation.

Cases

This section contains cases that illustrate the use of acoustic-reflex data in the differential diagnosis of auditory disorders. Figures 5.24 through 5.33 contain simplified schematics of the acoustic-reflex arc (top panel) and pure tone audiograms[7] for the left and right ears (bottom panel). The acoustic-reflex arc is represented by the middle ear, the cochlea, CNVIII, the brainstem, CNVII, the stapedius muscle, and the middle ear. The cases that follow introduce the various threshold response patterns associated with the four acoustic-reflex conditions, namely, the left ipsilateral, right ipsilateral, left contralateral, and right contralateral. (See Jerger & Jerger, 1977, 1981, for other case studies.)

Case 1 (Figure 5.24). The acoustic-reflex arc and threshold data for a young adult subject with a normal auditory system are shown in Figure 5.24 (Case 1). As with the behavioral pure tone thresholds, the reflex thresholds are recorded on the audiogram that represents the ear to which the reflex-activator signal is presented. For example, if the activator signal is presented ipsilaterally to the right ear (probe and activator signal in the right ear), then the reflex threshold is recorded as a caret on the audiogram for the right ear. If the activator signal is presented contralaterally to the right ear (probe in the left ear and activator signal in the right ear), then the reflex threshold is recorded as a filled circle on the audiogram

---

[7]Some examples also contain pure tone, bone-conduction thresholds ([or]). For the air- or bone-conduction thresholds that required masking, the appropriate effective masking was used; to maintain clarity, however, the effective masking levels were not recorded on the audiograms. This is true for all cases except the one depicted in Figure 5.33, which is a masking dilemma. The use of only the hearing sensitivity thresholds and the acoustic-reflex thresholds given with each case is for illustrative purposes only and is not intended to preclude the other auditory tests that are involved in the differential diagnosis of auditory disorders.

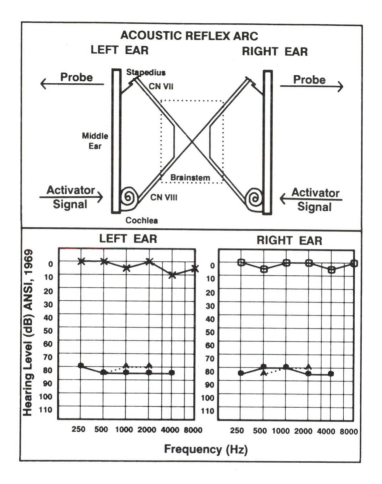

Figure 5.24. CASE 1. This case represents a young adult subject with a normal auditory system. Top panel: Schematic of the ipsilateral (uncrossed) and contralateral (crossed) auditory pathways of the acoustic-reflex arcs for the left and right ears. Bottom panel: Audiograms for the normal left and right ears on which the pure tone sensitivity thresholds are plotted along with the ipsilateral (▲) and contralateral (●) acoustic-reflex thresholds. The reflex thresholds are recorded on the audiogram for the ear to which the reflex-activator signal is presented.

for the right ear. In the cases that follow, each audiogram should have both contralateral (250-4000 Hz) and ipsilateral (500-2000 Hz) reflex thresholds recorded; an absence of the reflex symbol on the audiogram indicates that an acoustic reflex was not measurable at that activator frequency. In Case 1, the acoustic-reflex thresholds are within normal limits, that is, ≤95-dB HL for activator signals below 4000 Hz and ≤100 to 105-dB

HL for 4000 Hz. The acoustic-reflex arc for Case 1 is normal and therefore, the ipsilateral auditory pathways are depicted as the solid lines between the cochlea and stapedius muscle on the same side, and the contralateral auditory pathways are shown as the solid lines between the cochlea and stapedius muscle on opposite sides. In the cases that follow, the site-of-lesion is indicated on the schematic of the acoustic-reflex arc by a filled rectangle, and disruption of an auditory pathway(s) is indicated by a dashed line.

Case 2 (Figure 5.25). Case 2 has otosclerosis in the left ear (filled rectangle) that produced a mild, conductive hearing loss (the bone thresholds on the left ear were masked appropriately); the right ear is normal. The acoustic reflexes are absent with the probe in the left (conductive) ear and present with the probe in the right ear. Reflexes are absent probe left (impaired left ipsilateral and right contralateral reflex pathways shown by the dashed lines) because the mechanical problem in the left middle ear prevented the stapedius contraction from changing the acoustic immittance of the middle ear system. Except for 2000 Hz, the left contralateral reflex thresholds were elevated (i.e., >95-dB HL; impaired left contralateral pathway shown by the dashed line) because the left conductive component attenuated the level of the reflex-activator signal that reached the cochlea.

Case 3 (Figure 5.26). This case is identical to Case 2, except that the conductive hearing loss in the left ear of Case 3 is moderate (35- to 45-dB HL) instead of mild. The large conductive component in the left ear precludes measurement of the left contralateral acoustic reflex because the maximum output level of the reflex-activator signal does not overcome the attenuation of the activator signal produced by the conductive component.

Case 4 (Figure 5.27). Case 4 is a left cochlear hearing loss that produced a mild-to-moderate high-frequency hearing loss. The right ear is normal. All acoustic reflexes are within the normal range. Although there is a hearing loss in the left ear, reflex thresholds are ≤95-dB HL for 250 through 2000 Hz and ≤100 to 105-dB HL for 4000 Hz. The half-life times of acoustic-reflex adaptation at 500 and 1000 Hz in the left ear were normal, both being >10 s. Because the acoustic-reflex data are normal, the auditory pathways in the reflex arc are not impaired and are therefore depicted as solid lines.

Case 5 (Figure 5.28). This case has a left cochlear lesion that produced a moderate-to-profound sensorineural hearing loss. The right ear is normal. The acoustic-reflex thresholds are normal with the activator signal presented to the right ear and abnormal with the activator signal presented to the left ear. In the left ear, only the left contralateral reflexes at 250 and 500 Hz are present at elevated levels. The degree of hearing loss in

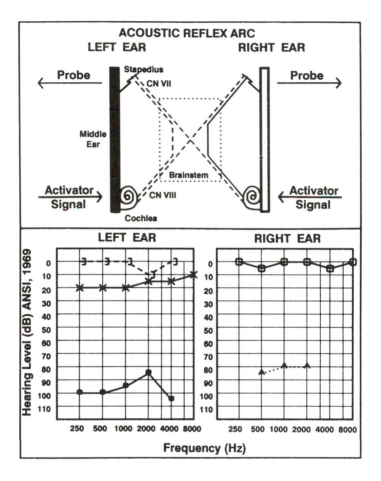

Figure 5.25. CASE 2. A left middle ear lesion (filled rectangle in the top panel) that produced a mild conductive hearing loss and no measurable acoustic reflex with the probe in the left ear (activator signal in either the left or right ears) and elevated left contralateral reflex thresholds (activator signal in the left ear, probe in the right ear). The right ipsilateral reflex thresholds are normal. The dashed lines in the schematic of the reflex arc represent the pathways that are affected by the left middle ear lesion.

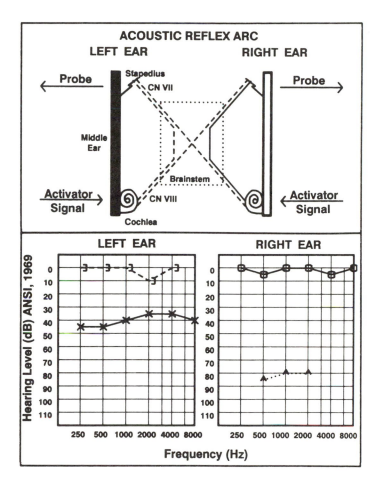

Figure 5.26. CASE 3. A left middle ear lesion (filled rectangle) that produced a moderate conductive hearing loss. No acoustic reflex was measurable with the probe in the left ear (activator signal in either the right or left ear) or with the activator signal presented to the left ear. Hearing sensitivity and the ipsilateral reflex thresholds in the right ear are normal.

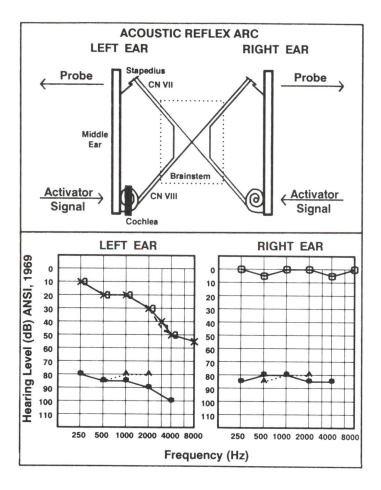

Figure 5.27. CASE 4. A left cochlear lesion that produced a mild-to-moderate high-frequency sensory (cochlear) hearing loss. The ipsilateral and contralateral reflex thresholds for the left ear are within the normal range as are the half-life times for reflex adaptation at 500 and 1000 Hz. Hearing sensitivity and the ipsilateral and contralateral reflex thresholds in the right ear are normal.

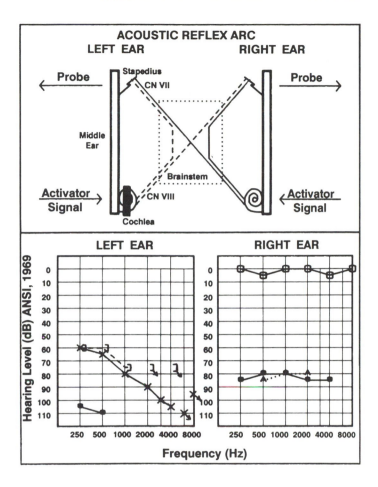

Figure 5.28. CASE 5. A left cochlear lesion that produced a moderate-to-profound sensorineural hearing loss. On the left ear, only left contralateral reflex thresholds at 250 and 500 Hz were recorded. Left ipsilateral reflexes are absent because they are beyond the output limits of the equipment. The right ipsilateral and contralateral reflex thresholds are present at normal levels.

the mid- to high-frequencies precluded the measurement (a) of the left contralateral acoustic reflexes at frequencies >500 Hz, and (b) of the left ipsilateral reflexes. Because of the high reflex threshold at 500 Hz (110-dB HL), reflex adaptation could not be measured in the left ear. These reflex findings for the left ear are reflected in the impaired ipsilateral and contralateral pathways of the acoustic-reflex arc (dashed lines). The reflex thresholds for the right ear are within normal limits. The normal right contralateral reflex thresholds (probe left) indicate a normal left middle ear, which substantiates the equality of air- and bone-conduction thresholds for the left ear.

Case 6 (Figure 5.29). In Case 6, a left CNVIII lesion produced a mild-to-moderate sensorineural hearing loss. The right ear is normal. Again, the acoustic-reflex thresholds are normal with the activator signal presented to the right ear and abnormal with the activator signal presented to the left ear. The left contralateral acoustic-reflex thresholds were present at normal levels at 250 and 500 Hz, slightly elevated at 1000 Hz, and not measurable in the higher frequencies; the left ipsilateral reflex was present only at 1000 Hz. The half-life times for reflex adaptation in the left contralateral condition were abnormal, 4 s and 1.5 s for 500 and 1000 Hz, respectively. These reflex results from the left ear are represented as the impaired pathways (dashed lines) in the acoustic-reflex arc.

Case 7 (Figure 5.30). With Case 7, a left CNVIII lesion produced a mild-to-moderate sensorineural hearing loss. The right ear is normal. The acoustic-reflex thresholds are normal with the activator signal presented to the right ear and absent with the activator signal presented to the left ear. This case is identical to Case 6 except that there are no measurable acoustic reflexes when the reflex activator is presented to the left ear, a finding that is reflected in the impaired left ipsilateral and left contralateral pathways in the reflex arc (dashed lines).

Case 8 (Figure 5.31). Case 8 illustrates a left CNVII lesion (Bell's palsy) in which the behavioral pure tone thresholds are within normal limits. The acoustic reflexes are absent with the probe in the left ear and present with the probe in the right ear. With the probe in the left ear, there were no measurable acoustic reflexes with the reflex-activator signal in the left or right ears (impaired left ipsilateral and right contralateral reflex pathways shown by the dashed lines) because the CNVII lesion inhibited innervation of the left stapedius muscle. The right ipsilateral and left contralateral reflex thresholds are within normal limits because those pathways are not involved with the left CNVII lesion.

Case 9 (Figure 5.32). This case has an intra-axial brainstem lesion that is manifested by normal behavioral pure tone thresholds. The acoustic-reflex thresholds are normal ipsilaterally and absent contralaterally. The

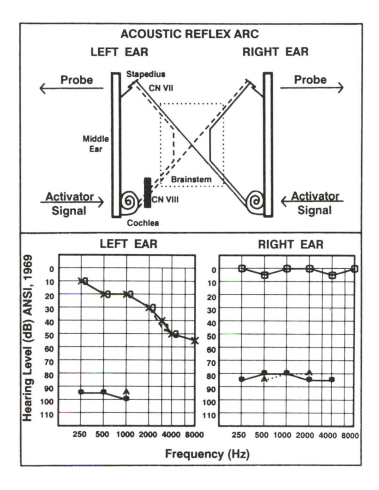

Figure 5.29. CASE 6. A left CNVIII lesion that produced a mild-to-moderate sensorineural hearing loss. Although several reflex thresholds were measurable with the activator signal presented to the left ear, abnormal reflex adaptation (6 s and 3 s for 500 Hz and 1000 Hz, respectively) was observed for the contralateral reflexes. The right ipsilateral and contralateral reflex thresholds are present at normal levels.

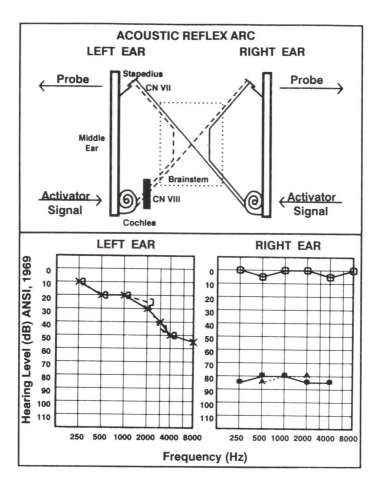

Figure 5.30. CASE 7. A left CNVIII lesion that produced a mild-to-moderate sensorineural hearing loss. No left ipsilateral or contralateral acoustic reflexes were measurable when the activator signal was presented to the left ear. The right ipsilateral and contralateral reflex thresholds are present at normal levels.

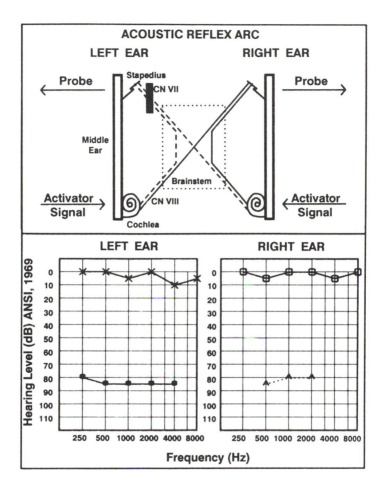

Figure 5.31.   CASE 8.   A left CNVII lesion (Bell's palsy) that produced no measurable acoustic reflexes when the probe was in the left ear (activator signal either ipsilateral left ear, or contralateral right ear). The reflexes were normal when the probe was in the right ear and the activator signal presented in either the right or left ears.

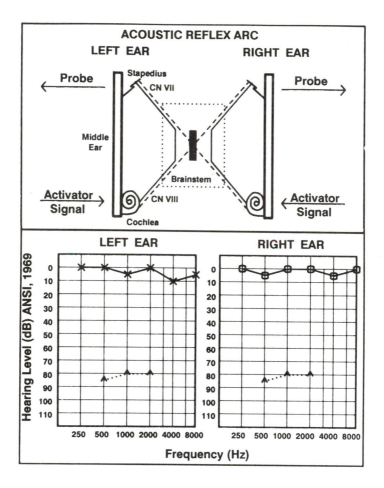

Figure 5.32. CASE 9. An intra-axial brainstem lesion that resulted in no measurable contralateral acoustic reflexes. The ipsilateral reflex thresholds in the left and right ears are present at normal levels.

left and right contralateral pathways are disrupted (dashed lines) by a lesion involving the auditory fibers that decussate.

Case 10 (Figure 5.33). Case 10 has a left ear with a moderate-to-severe sensory hearing loss, whereas the right ear has a moderate-to-severe conductive hearing loss. The unmasked bone-conduction thresholds are displayed on the left ear audiogram. Accurate masked bone-conduction thresholds could not be obtained owing to the masking dilemma. The acoustic reflexes are present only for the left ipsilateral condition. With the probe in the right ear, there were no measurable acoustic reflexes, which is consistent with the disrupted left contralateral and right ipsilateral auditory pathways. The right stapedius muscle contracted when the activator signal was presented in the left contralateral condition, but the mechanical problem in the right middle ear prevented a change in the acoustic immittance of the right middle ear. The right ipsilateral reflexes were obscured by both the attenuation of the activator signal and the mechanical problems of the right middle ear lesion. With the probe in the left ear, there were no measurable reflexes for the right contralateral condition, again because of the attenuation effects caused by the right middle ear lesion. The left ipsilateral reflexes were present at normal limits. The presence of the left ipsilateral acoustic reflexes indicates that the left middle ear functions normally, and that the hearing loss in the left ear is cochlear. One can infer that the unmasked bone-conduction thresholds originate from the right ear, which is consistent with a conductive hearing loss in the right ear.

References

American National Standards Institute. (1969). *Specifications for audiometers* (ANSI S3.6-1969). New York: Author.

Anderson, H., Barr, B., & Wedenberg, E. (1969). Intra-aural reflexes in retrocochlear lesions. In C. A. Hamberger & J. Wersäll (Eds.), *Nobel Symposium 10: Disorders of the skull base region* (pp. 48–54). Stockholm: Almqvist & Wikell.

Anderson, H., Barr, B., & Wedenberg, E. (1970). Early diagnosis of VIIIth-nerve tumours by acoustic reflex tests. *Acta Oto-Laryngologica, 262,* 232–237.

Anderson, H., & Wedenberg, E. (1968). Audiometric identification of normal hearing carriers of genes for deafness. *Acta Oto-Laryngologica, 65,* 535–554.

Barajas, J. J., Olaizola, F., Tapia, M. C., Alarcon, J. L., & Alaminos, D. (1981). Audiometric study of the neonate: Impedance audiometry. Behavioral responses and brain stem audiometry. *Audiology, 20,* 41–52.

Beattie, R. C., & Leamy, D. P. (1975). Otoadmittance: Normative values, procedural variables, and reliability. *Journal of the American Auditory Society, 1,* 21–27.

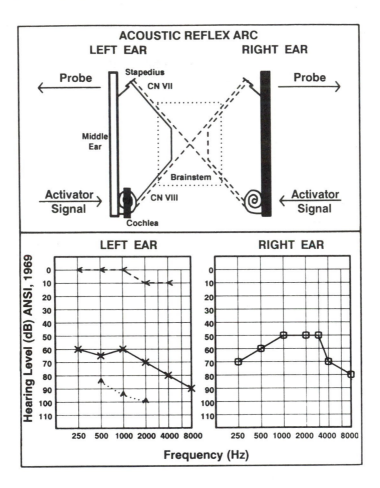

Figure 5.33. CASE 10. A left cochlear lesion that produced a moderate-to-severe sensory (cochlear) hearing loss and a right middle ear lesion that produced a moderate-to-severe conductive hearing loss. Of the acoustic-reflex measures, only the ipsilateral acoustic reflexes in the left ear were measurable.

Bennett, M. J. (1975). Acoustic impedance bridge measurement with the neonate. *British Journal of Audiology, 9*, 117–124.

Bennett, M. J., & Weatherby, L. A. (1982). Newborn acoustic reflexes to noise and pure-tone signals. *Journal of Speech and Hearing Research, 25*, 383–387.

Blom, S., & Zakrisson, J. E. (1974). The stapedius reflex in the diagnosis of myasthenia gravis. *Journal of the Neurological Sciences, 21*, 71–76.

Borg, E. (1973). On the neuronal organization of the acoustic middle ear reflex: A physiological and anatomical study. *Brain Research, 49*, 101–123.

Borg, E. (1976). Dynamic characteristics of the intra-aural muscle reflex. In A. Feldman & L. Wilber (Eds.), *Acoustic impedance and admittance: The measurement of middle ear function* (pp. 236–299). Baltimore: Williams & Wilkins.

Borg, E. (1982). Time course of the human acoustic stapedius reflex. *Scandinavian Audiology, 11*, 237–242.

Borg, E., Counter, S. A., & Rösler, G. (1984). Theories of middle-ear muscle function. In S. Silman (Ed.), *The acoustic reflex: Basic principles and clinical applications* (pp. 63–99). Orlando, FL: Academic Press.

Borg, E., & Møller, A. (1975). Effect of central depressants on the acoustic middle ear reflex in rabbit. *Acta Physiologica Scandinavica, 94*, 327–338.

Borg, E., & Zakrisson, J.-E. (1974). Stapedius reflex and monaural masking. *Acta Oto-Laryngologica, 78*, 155–161.

Bosatra, A., Russolo, M., & Silverman, C. A. (1984). Acoustic-reflex latency: State of the art. In S. Silman (Ed.), *The acoustic reflex: Basic principles and clinical applications* (pp. 301–328). Orlando, FL: Academic Press.

Brask, T. (1978). Extratympanic manometry in man. Clinical and experimental investigation of the acoustic stapedius and tensor tympani contractions in normal subjects and in patients. *Scandinavian Audiology,* (Supplement 7), 1–199.

Burke, K. S., & Herer, G. R. (1973). Impedance and admittance bridge differences in middle ear study. *Journal of Auditory Research, 13*, 251–256.

Cacace, A. T., & Margolis, R. H. (1985). On the loudness of complex stimuli and its relationship to cochlear excitation. *Journal of the Acoustical Society of America, 78*, 1568–1573.

Cartwright, D., & Lilly, D. (1976, November). *A comparison of acoustic-reflex decay patterns for patients with cochlear and VIIIth-nerve disease.* Paper presented at the American Speech-Language-Hearing Association Convention, Houston.

Chiveralls, K. (1977). Further examination of the use of the stapedius reflex in the diagnosis of acoustic neuroma. *Audiology, 16*, 331–337.

Chiveralls, K., & FitzSimons, R. (1973). Stapedial reflex action in normal subjects. *British Journal of Audiology, 7*, 105–110.

Chiveralls, K., FitzSimons, R., Beck, G., & Kernohan, H. (1976). The diagnostic significance of the stapedius reflex. *British Journal of Audiology, 10*, 122–128.

Clemis, J. D., & Sarno, C. N. (1980a). Acoustic reflex latency test in the evaluation of nontumor patients with abnormal brainstem latencies. *Annals of Otology, Rhinology, and Laryngology, 89*, 296–302.

Clemis, J. D., & Sarno, C. N. (1980b). The acoustic reflex latency test: Clinical application. *Laryngoscope, 90*, 601–611.

Colletti, V. (1975). Stapedius reflex abnormalities in multiple sclerosis. *Audiology, 14*, 63–71.

Creten, W. L., Vanpeperstraete, P. M., Van Camp, K. J., & Doclo, J. R. (1976). An experimental study on diphasic acoustic reflex patterns in normal ears. *Scandinavian Audiology, 5*, 3–10.

Dallos, P. (1964). Dynamics of the acoustic reflex: Phenomenological aspects. *Journal of the Acoustical Society of America, 36,* 2175–2183.

Davis, R. C. (1948). Motor effects of strong auditory stimuli. *Journal of Experimental Psychology, 38,* 257–275.

Djupesland, G. (1965). Electromyography of the tympanic muscles in man. *International Audiology, 4,* 34–41.

Djupesland, G. (1976). Nonacoustic reflex measurement—Procedures, interpretations and variables. In A. Feldman & L. Wilber (Eds.), *Acoustic impedance and admittance: The measurement of middle ear function* (pp. 217–235). Baltimore: Williams & Wilkins.

Djupesland, G., Flottorp, G., & Winther, F. (1967). Size and duration of acoustically elicited impedance changes in man. *Acta Oto-Laryngologica,* (Supplement 224), 220–228.

Djupesland, G., Sundby, A., & Flottorp, G. (1973). Temporal summation in the acoustic stapedius reflex mechanism. *Acta Oto-Laryngologica, 76,* 305–312.

Djupesland, G., & Zwislocki, J. J. (1971). Effect of temporal summation on the human stapedius reflex. *Acta Oto-Laryngologica, 71,* 262–265.

Djupesland, G., & Zwislocki, J. J. (1973). On the critical band in the acoustic stapedius reflex. *Journal of the Acoustical Society of America, 54,* 1157–1159.

Flottorp, G., & Djupesland, G. (1970). Diphasic impedance change and its applicability in clinical work. *Acta Oto-Laryngologica, 263,* 200–204.

Flottorp, G., Djupesland, G., & Winther, F. (1971). The acoustic stapedius reflex in relation to critical bandwidth. *Journal of the Acoustical Society of America, 49,* 457–461.

Fowler, C. G., & Wilson, R. H. (1984). Adaptation of the acoustic reflex. *Ear and Hearing, 5,* 281–288.

Gelfand, S. A., & Piper, N. (1981). Acoustic reflex thresholds in young and elderly subjects with normal hearing. *Journal of the Acoustical Society of America, 69,* 295–297.

Givens, G., & Seidemann, M. (1979). A systematic investigation of measurement parameters of acoustic-reflex adaptation. *Journal of Speech and Hearing Disorders, 44,* 534–542.

Goodhill, V. (1981). *Ear diseases, deafness, and dizziness.* New York: Harper & Row.

Gorga, M. P., & Stelmachowicz, P. G. (1983). Temporal characteristics of the acoustic reflex. *Audiology, 22,* 120–127.

Green, K. W., & Margolis, R. H. (1983). Detection of hearing loss with ipsilateral acoustic reflex thresholds. *Audiology, 22,* 471–479.

Green, K. W., & Margolis, R. H. (1984). The ipsilateral acoustic reflex. In S. Silman (Ed.), *The acoustic reflex: Basic principles and clinical applications* (pp. 276–301). Orlando, FL: Academic Press.

Guinan, J. J., & McCue, M. P. (1987). Asymmetries in the acoustic reflexes of the cat stapedius muscle. *Hearing Research, 26,* 1–10.

Habener, S. A., & Snyder, J. M. (1974). Stapedius reflex amplitude and decay in normal hearing ears. *Archives of Otolaryngology, 100,* 294–297.

Hall, J. W. (1982). Quantification of the relationship between crossed and uncrossed acoustic reflex amplitude. *Ear and Hearing, 3,* 296–300.

Handler, S. D., & Margolis, R. H. (1977). Predicting hearing loss from stapedial reflex thresholds in patients with sensorineural impairment. *Transactions of the American Academy of Ophthalmology and Otology, 84,* 425–431.

Hayes, D., & Jerger, J. (1982). Signal averaging of the acoustic reflex: Diagnostic applications of amplitude characteristics. *Scandinavian Audiology, 17* (Supplement), 31–36.

Hensen, V. (1878). Beobachtungen über die trommelfell-spanners bei hund und katze. *Archiv für Anatomie und Physiologie, Physiologische Abtheilung, 2,* 312–319.

Himelfarb, M. Z., Shanon, E., Popelka, G. R., & Margolis, R. H. (1978). Acoustic reflex evaluation in neonates. In S. E. Gerber & G. T. Mencher (Eds.), *Early diagnosis of hearing loss* (pp. 109–123). New York: Grune & Stratton.

Hirsch, A., & Anderson, H. (1980a). Elevated stapedius reflex threshold and pathologic reflex decay. *Acta Oto-Laryngologica,* (Supplement 368), 1–28.

Hirsch, A., & Anderson, H. (1980b). Audiologic test results in 96 patients with tumours affecting the eighth nerve. *Acta Oto-Laryngologica,* (Supplement 369), 1–26.

Holst, H.-E., Ingelstedt, S., & Örtegren, U. (1963). Ear drum movements following stimulation of the middle ear muscles. *Acta Oto-Laryngologica,* (Supplement 182), 140–145.

Hung, I., & Dallos, P. (1972). Study of the acoustic reflex in human beings: I. Dynamic characteristics. *Journal of the Acoustical Society of America, 52,* 1168–1180.

International Standards Organization. (1964). *Standard reference zero for the calibration of pure-tone audiometers* (ISO Recommendation R 389). New York: American National Standards Institute.

Jenkins, H. A., Morgan, D. E., & Miller, R. H. (1980). Intact acoustic reflexes in the presence of ossicular disruption. *The Laryngoscope, 90,* 267–273.

Jepsen, O. (1951). The threshold of the reflexes of the intratympanic muscles in a normal material examined by means of the impedance method. *Acta Oto-Laryngologica, 39,* 406–408.

Jepsen, O. (1953). Intratympanic muscle reflexes in psychogenic deafness. *Acta Oto-Laryngologica,* (Supplement 109), 61–69.

Jepsen, O. (1955). *Studies on the acoustic stapedius reflex in man: Measurements of the acoustic impedance of the tympanic membrane in normal individuals and in patients with peripheral facial palsy.* Unpublished doctoral dissertation. University of Aarhus, Denmark.

Jepsen, O. (1963). Middle-ear muscle reflexes in man. In J. Jerger (Ed.), *Modern developments in audiology* (pp. 193–237). New York: Academic Press.

Jerger, J., Anthony, L., Jerger, S., & Mauldin, L. (1974). Studies in impedance audiometry III. Middle ear disorders. *Archives of Otolaryngology, 99,* 165–171.

Jerger, J., Burney, P. Mauldin, L., & Crump, B. (1974). Predicting hearing loss from the acoustic reflex. *Journal of Speech and Hearing Disorders, 39,* 11–22.

Jerger, J., Clemis, J., Harford, E., & Alford, B. (1974). The acoustic reflex in eighth nerve disorders. *Archives of Otolaryngology, 99,* 409–413.

Jerger, J., & Hayes, D. (1983). Latency of the acoustic reflex in eighth-nerve tumor. *Archives of Otolaryngology, 109,* 1–5.

Jerger, J., Hayes, D., Anthony, L., & Mauldin, L. (1978). Factors influencing prediction of hearing level from the acoustic reflex. *Monographs in Contemporary Audiology, 1,* 1–20.

Jerger, J., Jerger, S., & Mauldin, L. (1972). Studies in impedance audiometry: I. Normal and sensorineural ears. *Archives of Otolaryngology, 89,* 513–523.

Jerger, J., Mauldin, L., & Lewis, N. (1977). Temporal summation of the acoustic reflex. *Audiology, 16,* 177–200.

Jerger, J., Oliver, T. A., & Jenkins, H. (1987). Suprathreshold abnormalities of the stapedius reflex in acoustic tumor: A series of case reports. *Ear and Hearing, 8,* 131–139.

Jerger, J., Oliver, T. A., Rivera, V., & Stach, B. A. (1986). Abnormalities of the acoustic reflex in multiple sclerosis. *American Journal of Otolaryngology, 7,* 163–176.

Jerger, J., Oliver, T. A., & Stach, B. (1986). Problems in the clinical measurement of acoustic reflex latency. *Scandinavian Audiology, 15,* 31–40.

Jerger, S., & Jerger, J. (1977). Diagnostic value of crossed vs. uncrossed acoustic reflexes. *Archives of Otolaryngology, 103,* 445–453.

Jerger, S., & Jerger, J. (1981). *Auditory disorders: A manual for clinical evaluation.* Boston: Little, Brown.

Johansson, B., Kylin, B., & Langfy, M. (1967). Acoustic reflex as a test of individual susceptibility to noise. *Acta Oto-Laryngologica, 64,* 256–262.

Joseph, M. P., Guinan, J. J., Jr., Fullerton, B. C., Norris, B. E., & Kiang, N. Y. S. (1985). Number and distribution of stapedius motoneurons in cats. *Journal of Comparative Neurology, 232,* 43–54.

Kankkunen, A., & Lidén, G. (1984). Ipsilateral acoustic reflex thresholds in neonates and in normal-hearing and hearing-impaired pre-school children. *Scandinavian Audiology, 13,* 139–144.

Kaplan, H., Gilman, S., & Dirks, D. D. (1977). Properties of acoustic reflex adaptation. *Annals of Otology, Rhinology and Laryngology, 86,* 348–356.

Kato, T. (1913). Zur physiologie der binnenmuskeln des ohres. *Pflüegers Archiv fuer die Gesamte Physiologie des Menschen und der Tiere, 150,* 569–625.

Keith, R. W. (1975). Middle ear function in neonates. *Archives of Otolaryngology, 101,* 376–379.

Keith, R. W., & Bench, R. J. (1978). Stapedial reflex in neonates. *Scandinavian Audiology, 7,* 187–191.

Kobler, J. B., Vacher, S. R., & Guinan, J. J., Jr. (1985). Acoustic response properties of motoneurons innervating the stapedius muscle of the cat. *Society of Neurosciences Abstracts, 11,* 288.

Kobler, J. B., Vacher, S. R., & Guinan, J. J., Jr. (1987). The recruitment order of stapedius motoneurons in the acoustic reflex varies with sound laterality. *Brain Research, 425,* 372–375.

Kobrak, H. G. (1948). Present status of objective hearing tests. *Annals of Otology, Rhinology, and Laryngology, 57,* 1018–1026.

Kristensen, H. K., & Jepsen, O. (1952). Recruitment in oto-neurological diagnostics. *Acta Oto-Laryngologica, 42,* 553–560.

Kunov, H. (1977). The 'eardrum artifact' in ipsilateral reflex measurements. *Scandinavian Audiology, 6,* 163–166.

Lilly, D. J. (1964, November). *Some properties of the acoustic reflex in man.* Paper presented at the 68th meeting of the Acoustical Society of America, Austin, Texas.

Lilly, D. J. (1984). Evaluation of the response time of acoustic-immittance instruments. In S. Silman (Ed.), *The acoustic reflex: Basic principles and clinical applications* (pp. 276–301). Orlando, FL: Academic Press.

Lindsay, J. R., Kobrak, H., & Perlman, H. B. (1936). Relation of the stapedius reflex to hearing sensation in man. *Archives of Otolaryngology, 23,* 671–687.

Lorente de Nó, R. (1935). The function of the central acoustic nuclei examined by means of the acoustic reflexes. *The Laryngoscope, 45,* 573–595.

Lüscher, E. (1929). Die funktion des musculus stapedius biem menschen. Z. *Hals-Nasen-Ohrenheilkunde, 23,* 105–132.

Lutman, M., & Leis, B. R. (1980). Ipsilateral acoustic reflex artifacts measured in cadavers. *Scandinavian Audiology, 9,* 33–39.

Lutman, M., & Martin, A. (1977). The acoustic reflex threshold for impulses. *Journal of Sound and Vibration, 51,* 97–109.

Lyon, M. J. (1978). The central location of the motor neurons to the stapedius muscle in the cat. *Brain Research, 143,* 437–444.

Lyon, M. J. (1979). Peripheral innervation of the stapedius muscle in the cat: An electron microscopic study. *Experimental Neurology, 66,* 707–720.

Mangham, C. A., Burnett, P. A., & Lindeman, R. C. (1982). Standardization of acoustic reflex latency. A study in humans and nonhuman primates. *Annals of Otology, Rhinology and Laryngology, 91,* 169–174.

Mangham, C. A., Burnett, P. A., & Lindeman, R. C. (1983). Evaluation of tensor tympani muscle dominance in the biphasic acoustic reflex. *Audiology, 22,* 105–119.

Mangham, C. A., Lindeman, R. C., & Dawson, W. (1980). Stapedius reflex quantification in acoustic tumor patients. *The Laryngoscope, 90,* 242–250.

Mangham, C. A., & Miller, J. M. (1979). A case for further quantification of the stapedius reflex. *Archives of Otolaryngology, 105,* 593–596.

Marchant, C. D., McMillan, P. M., Shurin, P. A., Johnson, C. E., Turczyk, V. A., Feinstein, J. C., & Panek, D. M. (1986). Objective diagnosis of otitis media in early infancy by tympanometry and ipsilateral acoustic reflex thresholds. *Journal of Pediatrics, 109,* 590–595.

Margolis, R. H., Dubno, J. R., & Wilson, R. H. (1980). Acoustic reflex thresholds for noise stimuli. *Journal of the Acoustical Society of America, 68,* 892–895.

Margolis, R. H., & Fox, C. M. (1977). A comparison of three methods for predicting hearing loss from acoustic reflex threshold. *Journal of Speech and Hearing Research, 20,* 241–253.

Margolis, R. H., Fox, C., Lilly, D. J., Popelka, G., Silman, S., & Trumpf, A. (1981). The bivariate plotting procedure for hearing assessment with acoustic-reflex threshold measures. In G. R. Popelka (Ed.), *Hearing assessment with the acoustic reflex* (pp. 59–84). New York: Grune & Stratton.

Margolis, R. H., & Gilman, S. (1977). Methods for measuring the temporal characteristics and filter response of electroacoustic impedance instruments. *Journal of Speech and Hearing Research, 20,* 409–414.

McCandless, G. A., & Allred, P. L. (1978). Tympanometry and emergence of the acoustic reflex in infants. In E. R. Harford, F. H. Bess, C. D. Bluestone, et al. (Eds.), *Impedance screening for middle ear disease in children* (pp. 57–67). New York: Grune & Stratton.

McCue, M. P., & Guinan, J. J., Jr. (1983). Functional segregation within the stapedius motoneuron pool. *Society of Neuroscience Abstracts, 19,* 1085.

McCue, M. P., & Guinan, J. J., Jr. (1988). Anatomical and functional segregation in the stapedius motoneuron pool of the cat. *Journal of Neurophysiology, 60,* 1160–1180.

McMillan, P. M., Marchant, C. D., & Shurin, P. A. (1985). Ipsilateral acoustic reflexes in infants. *Annals of Otology, Rhinology, and Laryngology, 94,* 145–148.

McPherson, D. L., & Thompson, D. (1977). Quantification of the threshold and latency parameters of acoustic reflex in humans. *Acta Oto-Laryngologica, 353,* 1–37.

Metz, O. (1946). The acoustic impedance measured on normal and pathological ears. *Acta Oto-Laryngologica*, (Supplement 63), 1–254.

Metz, O. (1951). Studies on the contraction of the tympanic muscles as indicated by changes in the impedance of the ear. *Acta Oto-Laryngologica*, 39, 397–405.

Metz, O. (1952). Threshold of reflex contractions of muscles of the middle ear and recruitment of loudness. *Archives of Otolaryngology*, 55, 536–543.

Møller, A. R. (1958). Intra-aural muscles contraction in man, examined by measuring acoustic impedance of the ear. *The Laryngoscope*, 68, 48–62.

Møller, A. R. (1961). Bilateral contraction of the tympanic muscles in man. *Annals of Otology, Rhinology, and Laryngology*, 70, 735–752.

Møller, A. R. (1962a). Acoustic reflex in man. *Journal of the Acoustical Society of America*, 34, 1524–1534.

Møller, A. R. (1962b). The sensitivity of contraction of the tympanic muscles in man. *Annals of Otology, Rhinology, and Laryngology*, 71, 86–95.

Møller, A. R. (1978). A comment on H. Kunov: The 'eardrum artifact' in ipsilateral reflex measurements. *Scandinavian Audiology*, 7, 61–64.

Niemeyer, W., & Sesterhenn, G. (1974). Calculating the hearing threshold from the stapedius reflex thresholds for different sound stimuli. *Audiology*, 13, 421–427.

Olsen, W. O., Noffsinger, D., & Kurdziel, S. (1975). Acoustic reflex and reflex decay. *Archives of Otolaryngology*, 101, 622–625.

Olsen, W., Stach, B., & Kurdziel, S. (1981). Acoustic reflex decay in 10 seconds and in 5 seconds for Ménière's disease patients and for VIIIth nerve tumor patients. *Ear and Hearing*, 2, 180–181.

Osterhammel, D., & Osterhammel, P. (1979). Age and sex variations for the normal stapedial reflex thresholds and tympanometric compliance values. *Scandinavian Audiology*, 8, 153–158.

Perlman, H. B., & Case, T. J. (1939). Latent period of the crossed stapedius reflex in man. *Annals of Otology, Rhinology, and Laryngology*, 48, 663–675.

Peterson, J. L., & Lidén, G. (1972). Some static characteristics of the stapedial muscle reflex. *Audiology*, 11, 97–114.

Popelka, G. R. (1981). The acoustic reflex in normal and pathologic ears. In G. R. Popelka (Ed.), *Hearing assessment with the acoustic reflex* (pp. 5–21). New York: Grune & Stratton.

Popelka, G. R., & Dubno, J. R. (1978). Comments on the acoustic-reflex response for bone-conducted signals. *Acta Oto-Laryngologica*, 86, 64–70.

Popelka, G. R., Karlovich, R., & Wiley, T. L. (1974). Acoustic reflex and critical bandwidth. *Journal of the Acoustical Society of America*, 55, 883–885.

Popelka, G. R., Margolis, R. H., & Wiley, T. L. (1976). Effect of activating signal bandwidth on acoustic-reflex thresholds. *Journal of the Acoustical Society of America*, 59, 153–159.

Porter, T. A. (1972). Normative otoadmittance values for three populations. *Journal of Auditory Research*, 12, 53–58.

Potter, A. B. (1936). Function of the stapedius muscle. *Annals of Otology, Rhinology, and Laryngology*, 45, 639–643.

Rabinowitz, W. M. (1977). *Acoustic-reflex effects on the input admittance and transfer characteristics of the human middle-ear.* Unpublished doctoral dissertation, Massachusetts Institute of Technology, Cambridge.

Rosenhall, U., Lidén, G., & Nilsson, E. (1979). Stapedius reflex decay in normal hearing subjects. *Journal of the American Auditory Society*, 4, 157–163.

Ruth, R. A., Nilo, E. R., & Mravec, J. J. (1978). Consideration of acoustic reflex magnitude (ARM) in cases of idiopathic facial paralysis. *Otolaryngology, 86,* 215–220.

Ruth, R. A., & Niswander, P. S. (1976). Acoustic reflex latency as a function of frequency and intensity of eliciting stimulus. *Journal of the American Audiology Society, 2,* 54–60.

Salomon, G., & Starr, A. (1963). Electromyography of middle ear muscles in man during motor activities. *Acta Neurologica Scandinavica, 39,* 161–168.

Schwartz, D. M., & Sanders, J. W. (1976). Critical bandwidth and sensitivity prediction in the acoustic stapedial reflex. *Journal of Speech and Hearing Disorders, 41,* 244–255.

Shanks, J. E., Wilson, R. H., & Jones, H. C. (1985). Earphone-coupling technique for measuring the temporal characteristics of aural acoustic-immittance devices. *Journal of Speech and Hearing Research, 28,* 305–308.

Shapiro, I., Canalis, R. F., Firemark, R., & Bahna, M. (1981). Ossicular discontinuity with intact acoustic reflex. *Archives of Otolaryngology, 107,* 576–578.

Shaw, M. D., & Baker, R. (1983). The locations of stapedius and tensor tympani motoneurons in the cat. *Journal of Comparative Neurology, 216,* 10–19.

Silman, S. (1979). The effects of aging on the stapedius reflex thresholds. *Journal of the Acoustical Society of America, 66,* 735–738.

Silman, S. (1984). Magnitude and growth of the acoustic reflex. In S. Silman (Ed.), *The acoustic reflex: Basic principles and clinical applications* (pp. 301–328). Orlando, FL: Academic Press.

Silman, S., & Gelfand, S. A. (1981). Effect of sensorineural hearing loss on the stapedius reflex growth function in the elderly. *Journal of the Acoustical Society of America, 69,* 1099–1106.

Silman, S., Gelfand, S. A., & Chun, T. (1978). Some observations in a case of acoustic neuroma. *Journal of Speech and Hearing Disorders, 43,* 459–466.

Silverman, C. A., Silman, S., & Miller, M. H. (1983). The acoustic reflex threshold in aging ears. *Journal of the Acoustical Society of America, 73,* 248–255.

Sprague, B. H., Wiley, T. L., & Block, M. G. (1981). Dynamics of acoustic reflex growth. *Audiology, 20,* 15–40.

Sprague, B. H., Wiley, T. L., & Goldstein, R. (1985). Tympanometric and acoustic-reflex studies in neonates. *Journal of Speech and Hearing Research, 28,* 265–272.

Stach, B., & Jerger, J. (1984). Acoustic reflex averaging. *Ear and Hearing, 5,* 289–296.

Stach, B. A., Jerger, J. F., & Jenkins, H. A. (1984). The human acoustic tensor tympani reflex. *Scandinavian Audiology, 13,* 93–99.

Stream, R. W., Stream, K. S., Walker, J. R., & Breningstall, G. (1978). Emerging characteristics of the acoustic reflex in infants. *Otolaryngology, 86,* 628–636.

Terkildsen, K. (1957). Movements of the eardrum following inter-aural muscle reflexes. *Archives of Otolaryngology, 66,* 484–488.

Terkildsen, K. (1960). The intra-aural muscle reflexes in normal persons and in workers exposed to intense industrial noise. *Acta Oto-Laryngologica, 52,* 384–396.

Terkildsen, K. (1964). Clinical application of impedance measurements with a fixed frequency technique. *International Audiology, 3,* 147–155.

Terkildsen, K., Osterhammel, P., & Bretlau, P. (1973). Acoustic middle ear muscle reflexes in patients with otosclerosis. *Archives of Otolaryngology, 98,* 152–155.

Terkildsen, K., & Scott-Nielsen, S. (1960). An electroacoustic impedance measuring bridge for clinical use. *Archives of Otolaryngology, 73,* 339–346.

Thelin, J. W. (1980). *Acoustic reflex summation in the frequency domain.* Unpublished doctoral dissertation, University of Iowa, Iowa City.

Thompson, D. J., Sills, J. A., & Recke, K. S., & Bui, D. M. (1980). Acoustic reflex growth in the aging adult. *Journal of Speech and Hearing Research, 23,* 405–418.

Tietze, G. (1969). Zum zeitverhalten des akustischen reflexes bei reizung mit dauertönen. *Archiv fuer Klinische und Experimentelle Ohren-, Nasen-, und Kehlkopfheilkunde, 193,* 43–52.

Tonndorf, J., & Khanna, S. (1968). Submicroscopic displacement amplitudes of the tympanic membrane (cat) measured by a laser interferometer. *Journal of the Acoustical Society of America, 44,* 1546–1554.

Van Camp, K. J., Vanpeperstraete, P. M., Creten, W. L., & Vanhuyse, V. J. (1975). On irregular acoustic reflex patterns. *Scandinavian Audiology, 4,* 227–232.

Vincent, V. L., & Gerber, S. E. (1987). Early development of the acoustic reflex. *Audiology, 26,* 356–362.

Weatherby, L. A., & Bennett, M. J. (1980). The neonatal acoustic reflex. *Scandinavian Audiology, 9,* 103–110.

Wersäll, R. (1958). The tympanic muscles and their reflexes. *Acta Oto-Laryngologica,* (Supplement 139), 1–112.

Wiley, T. L., & Block, M. G. (1984). Acoustic and nonacoustic reflex patterns in audiologic diagnosis. In S. Silman (Ed.), *The acoustic reflex: Basic principles and clinical applications* (pp. 387–411). Orlando, FL: Academic Press.

Wiley, T. L., & Karlovich, R. S. (1975). Acoustic reflex response to sustained signals. *Journal of Speech and Hearing Research, 18,* 148–157.

Wilson, R. H. (1979). Factors influencing the acoustic-immittance characteristics of the acoustic reflex. *Journal of Speech and Hearing Research, 22,* 480–499.

Wilson, R. H. (1981). The effects of aging on the magnitude of the acoustic reflex. *Journal of Speech and Hearing Research, 24,* 406–414.

Wilson, R. H., & McBride, L. M. (1978). Threshold and growth of the acoustic reflex. *Journal of the Acoustical Society of America, 63,* 147–154.

Wilson, R. H., McCullough, J. K., & Lilly, D. J. (1984). Acoustic-reflex adaptation: Variability in subjects with normal hearing. *Journal of Speech and Hearing Research, 27,* 586–595.

Wilson, R. H., Morgan, D. E., & Dirks, D. D. (1972, October). *Relationships between the acoustic reflex and the loudness discomfort level.* Paper presented at the meeting of the 11th International Congress of Audiology, Budapest, Hungary.

Wilson, R. H., Shanks, J. E., & Lilly, D. J. (1984). Acoustic-reflex adaptation. In S. Silman (Ed.), *The acoustic reflex: Basic principles and clinical applications* (pp. 329–387). Orlando, FL: Academic Press.

Wilson, R. H., Shanks, J. E., & Velde, T. M. (1981). Aural acoustic-immittance measurements: Inter-aural differences. *Journal of Speech and Hearing Research, 46,* 413–421.

Wilson, R. H., Steckler, J. F., Jones, H. C., & Margolis, R. H. (1978). Adaptation of the acoustic reflex. *Journal of the Acoustical Society of America, 64,* 782–791.

Zakrisson, J.-E., Borg, E., & Blom, S. (1974). The acoustic impedance change as a measure of stapedius muscle activity in man. *Acta Oto-Laryngologica, 78,* 357–364.

Zwislocki, J. J. (1965). Analysis of some auditory characteristics. In R. D. Luce, R. B. Bush, & E. Galenter (Eds.), *Handbook of mathematical psychology* (Vol. 3, pp. 1–97). New York: Wiley.

Acknowledgments.   We extend our appreciation to Cynthia G. Fowler and Janet E. Shanks for their comments on the various drafts of this manuscript. Carol Zizz contributed to the project in several ways. Portions of this project were funded by the Rehabilitation Research and Development Service and by the Medical Research Service of the Veterans Health Services and Research Administration.

chapter six

Auditory evoked potentials: Basic aspects

JOHN D. DURRANT

KENNETH E. WOLF

Contents

Introduction

Noninvasive electrophysiology and the measurement of evoked sensory potentials have assumed increasing importance in clinical audiology.

Thanks to modern technology, the necessary instrumentation has become cost-effective, and auditory evoked potential (AEP) evaluations have become a part of the services offered routinely by audiologists, whether in private practice or in university/hospital centers. The AEP is a computer-extracted electric response of the auditory nerve and brain that lasts several hundred milliseconds or longer (Figure 6.1).

Its earliest components, the short latency responses, are reflected in the electrocochleogram (ECochGm) and the auditory brainstem response (ABR). These responses are now the most popular clinically, both for purposes of otoneurologic evaluation and estimating hearing sensitivity, but the various later components also are clinically useful. For example, responses in the 10- to 50-ms epoch, known as the middle latency responses (MLRs), are recorded with minor procedural changes from recordings of the short latency potentials and can be particularly useful for obtaining near-threshold information for low-frequency stimuli. The late/long latency evoked potentials have histories of clinical application exceeding all of the above-mentioned responses (see Reneau & Hnatiow, 1975). The late responses also can provide the basis for determining reasonably good estimates of hearing thresholds. They also have been of keen interest with regard to the extent to which they reflect perceptual attributes of sound, the issue of interhemispheric differences, and even cognition.

It is beyond the scope of a textbook chapter to do justice to any single component of the AEP, let alone the entire response, considering the

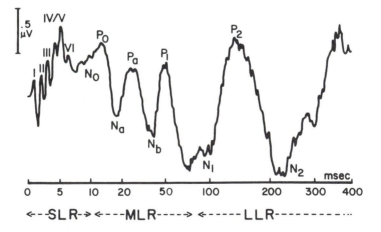

Figure 6.1. Auditory evoked potential: time windows of short- (SLR), middle- (MLR), and long- (LLR) latency responses (logarithmic time base). (Based on a figure from Michelini, Arslan, Prosser, & Pedrielli, 1982, from ASHA, 1988, with permission.)

intense interest evoked potentials have created and the resulting volu-
minous literature in all areas. In this book, various (particularly clinical)
issues thus have been presented in other chapters (i.e., Chapters 7 and
8), with an overview of the basic aspects of AEP measurement provided
here. Emphasis in this chapter is on the short latency responses, although
overviews of the middle and longer latency potentials are provided. In
brief, this chapter is intended to serve as an introduction to AEP measurement, to the major components of the AEP, and to the fundamentals of
AEP measurement and clinical applications.

Rudiments of instrumentation for AEP measurement

Electrical interface to the subject

The nervous system is constantly active and generating electrical potentials. These electrical events may be conducted to the body's surface
where, with suitable methods and instrumentation, they may be recorded.
These potentials are minute (e.g., microvolts or less, where 1 microvolt
= 1/1,000,000 volt), and they are buried in a background of electrical noise,
making them difficult to detect or measure. Additionally, the skin is electrically insulative, particularly the corneum stratum (the outermost layer).
There also is a fundamental difference between bioelectricity (ion-
mediated current) and physical electricity (electron-mediated current).
Therefore, applying an electrode (i.e., a metal conductor) to the skin, constitutes a barrier over which there can be no net charge transfer. Such
an interface thus opposes current flow and can be characterized by its
impedance (Geddes, 1972).

Electrode impedance is a product of the electrode characteristics (i.e.,
surface area and material), the tissue to which it is interfaced (e.g., skin,
muscle, etc.), and anything in between (e.g., oil, dirt, fluid, etc.). Silver,
gold, and platinum have relatively low impedances and are widely used
in clinical electrophysiology. Additionally, silver is useful because it can
be plated with salt, forming a silver-silver-chloride (Ag-AgCl) electrode.
This further lowers impedance and forms a reversible or nonpolarized
electrode, making it possible to record very low-frequency potentials (i.e.,
approaching dc). Impedance also is lowest when the electrode makes
direct contact with body fluids, for example, just under the skin's surface. This can be accomplished with needle electrodes, but this approach
is unattractive for clinical work. Good electrical contact, however, can

be obtained by cleansing the skin thoroughly and applying an electrolyte gel, paste, or cream. The latter improves conductivity of the dead skin layer, gives contact stability, and effectively increases the electrode-surface area. Various methods for obtaining low-electrode impedances may be found in electroencephalography texts (e.g., Binnie, Rowan, & Gutter, 1982). Interelectrode impedances, that is, the impedances between each possible pair of electrodes, should be measured routinely and, as a rule, should not exceed 5 kohms. Most important, the interelectrode impedance should be balanced between electrode pairs in order to optimize common-mode rejection of noise (see the Amplification section below).

Signal processing

The desired signal, the AEP, is buried in a background of physical and biological electrical noise. The noise background can be reduced substantially via computer-based time ensemble averaging, thereby improving the signal-to-noise ratio (SNR). The recorded signal and noise are continuous functions in time that must be sampled in discrete pieces, as illustrated in Figure 6.2, Panel A. This is accomplished through analog-to-digital (A-D) conversion, wherein the amplitude of the signal (over a given interval of time) is translated into a binary value for computations by the computer.

The more points that can be sampled in the waveform, the more accuracy with which it can be represented in the computer's memory (Figure 6.2, Panel B). The sampling rate of the A-D conversion process thus determines the temporal resolution of the waveform (i.e., the number of data points per cycle). There also is a limit to the resolution of the signal's amplitude. Amplitude resolution depends on the numeric precision of the A-D converter, that is, the number of bits representing full scale. Manufactured evoked response test equipment typically provides temporal resolution of at least 40 microseconds per data point and 8 to 12 bit resolution of amplitude (1/256 to 1/4096). With amplitude resolution in the thousands of microvolts and recorded signals in the microvolt or submicrovolt range, the recorded potentials must be amplified prior to signal averaging, as discussed below.

The basis for the noise reduction is that any signal not time-locked with the stimulus is likely to be cancelled over time. Synchronous signals will be preserved. The improvement in the SNR is proportional to the square root of the number (N) of samples that are averaged (Picton & Hink, 1974). For example, increasing N by a factor of 4 will increase the SNR by a factor of 2. The recording of reproducible AEPs typically requires Ns of hundreds (longer latency potentials) to thousands (shorter latency potentials).

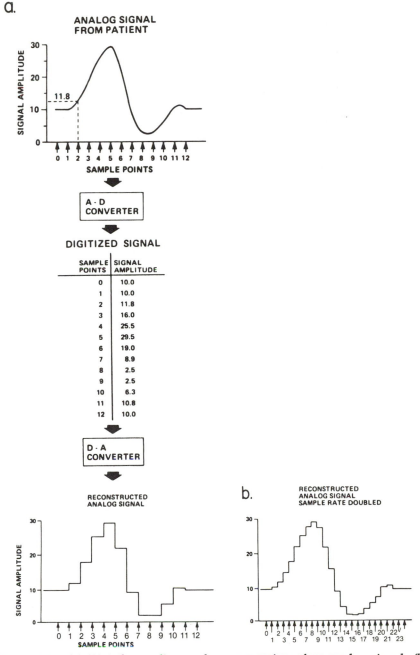

Figure 6.2. (a) Digital sampling and reconstruction of an analog signal. (b) Reconstructed signal sampled at twice the rate as in (a). (Adapted from Coats, 1983, with permission.)

Amplification

The objective of amplification is twofold. The first is to magnify the recorded signal (which contains both the AEP and background noise) to bring it within the range of amplitude resolution of the A-D converter. The second purpose is to optimize the voltage sampling for the desired potential while, as much as possible, rejecting unwanted signals. This is possible by differential recording, that is, using an amplifier with a balanced input. The differential amplifier thus amplifies the difference in voltage sampled by its two inputs. Consequently, one input is negative and inverts the signal, whereas the other is positive and is noninverting. A connection also is made between the subject and the electrical ground, that is, the chasis of the amplifier. Signals/noise common to the two inputs will tend to be cancelled, with complete cancellation occurring when the common-mode signal/noise is of equal amplitude and phase at the two inputs. For AEP measurement, the three electrodes required (connected to the inverting and noninverting inputs and ground) generally are placed on the head. Most myogenic artifacts and extraneous electrical noises will appear at the two electrode sites with nearly equal amplitudes and phases, and an improvement of SNR will be realized via common-mode rejection. Signals not common to the two inputs (which still is likely to be more background noise than AEP) will be amplified, as desired. The required gain depends on the AEP being sought, but typically ranges from 10,000 (for the longest latency potentials) to 500,000 (for the shortest latency potentials).

Filtering and other methods of noise and artifact rejection

Much background noise actually can be removed via filtering, because the noise generally has a much broader spectrum than the desired AEP component. This can be done before and/or after signal averaging, but some prefiltering usually is desirable. High-pass filtering is used to eliminate very low-frequency and direct-current (dc) potentials to minimize baseline drift and other artifacts. Low-pass filtering is used to reject signals of frequencies beyond the sampling limits of the A-D conversion process as well as high-frequency noise. In general, the better the SNR is before averaging, the more efficient the averaging process will be. However, analog filtering introduces phase shifts that become increasingly severe as the filter cutoff frequencies are approached and the filter may ring and otherwise color the response by its own characteristics. Because different AEP components have different spectra, they will not be affected in the same manner by a given filter. Therefore, analog filtering using extremely narrow bandwidths and/or steep filter skirts generally is avoided.

Digital filtering, on the other hand, can provide precise filtering without the above-mentioned artifacts (Boston & Ainslie, 1980; Domico & Kavanagh, 1986). This is accomplished computationally, that is, by the computer after signal averaging. Most currently available instruments use a combination of analog (pre-) filtering and digital (post-hoc) filtering, that is, bandpass filtering at the amplifier stage with, at least, low-pass digital filtering available to effect smoothing.

Even with analog prefiltering, it is not unlikely that a noise artifact will occur during the sampling epoch that may not be cancelled by averaging within a practical time period of signal averaging. For example, an incidental swallow can create a large electromyogenic artifact; such incidental events never may be averaged out completely. Such artifacts often are much greater in magnitude than the desired potential, so they usually can be detected and excluded on the basis of their amplitude. Most commercially available test systems provide control of the permissible amplitude limits or automatically reject overscale signals. In the case of the latter, control of the maximal permissible amplitude is tied to the gain setting. Amplitude artifact rejection typically involves the detection of any instant of overscale voltage, generally within the sampling epoch or a specified portion thereof; any time an artifact occurs, the entire sweep is excluded from the average. It is important to recognize that there is a cost in efficiency of data collection, and amplitude artifact rejection is most effective in eliminating samples containing incidental voltage spikes in otherwise quiet recordings. It is not a very effective means of dealing with overall noisy subjects, and its usage does not diminish the need for careful electrode application, cooperation of the subject (if the individual is not sedated), and appropriate filtering.

The tremendous amplification required for recording AEPs makes the recordings susceptible to the pickup of extraneous electrical noises via electrostatic and/or electromagnetic coupling. These include 60-Hz noise from electric (especially fluorescent) lights and other electrical devices and wiring, radiation from power transformers and electrical machinery, and stimulus artifact radiation from the earphone. Sixty-cycle noise (and harmonics and related artifacts thereof) generally is substantially reduced by the signal averaging process itself, if the sampling epoch is not synchronized with the noise. The phase of the noise will vary randomly within the sampling epoch and (largely) be cancelled. Nevertheless, various precautions are worthwhile for optimal noise reduction, such as proper shielding of equipment and, perhaps, for the subject (i.e., using a shielded test suite). Proper grounding also is important for minimizing 60-Hz artifact via ground loops (Pfeiffer, 1974), as well as ensuring proper electrical safety for patient and examiner (Binnie et al., 1982). It is also helpful to dress the electrode leads close to the subject's body, braiding and/or shielding excess leads, and making the leads as short as practical. Stimulus artifact can be minimized by electromagnetically shielding the earphone (Elberling & Solomon, 1973). Another way to minimize contamination of the desired response with stimulus artifacts was described by Sohmer and Pratt (1976), wherein a tube is used to couple the earphone to the subject's ear, that is, an acoustic delay line. This may now be accomplished through the use of tubal insert earphones (Clemis, Ballad, & Killion, 1986). Some evoked response test instruments also permit the zeroing of samples over a specified interval, for instance, the first 1 ms, which may be used to blank out the stimulus artifact without interfering much with the acquisition of the desired response. Lastly, the use of alternating stimulus polarity (see below) can be used to minimize stimulus artifact via phase cancellation.

Sound stimulation

Spectral and temporal factors.   As a general rule, the more concise the stimulus, temporally, the better synchronized the neural discharges elicited and the more robust the evoked potentials. The click, a sound obtained by applying a dc pulse to an earphone, loudspeaker, or bone vibrator, provides an excellent stimulus for eliciting AEPs. Its brief duration minimizes stimulus artifact while providing a broad spectrum stimulus (Figure 6.3, Panel a.2); the result is the excitation of many nerve fibers with excellent synchronization. Earphones, however, do not perfectly reproduce the spectrum of a dc pulse (Figure 6.3, Panel a.2), and the auditory system itself filters the stimulus. Therefore, frequency limits are imposed upon click stimulation (Durrant, 1983).

Frequency specificity (at least to some extent) can be obtained via sinusoidal pulses (tone pips or bursts) or bandpass-filtered clicks (e.g., ringing a filter with a dc pulse). Such stimuli are transients, so they have continuous (Figure 6.3, Panel b) rather than discrete spectra, as in the case of pure tones. The energy in their spectra is concentrated around a central frequency (Figure 6.3, Panel b), and the use of sinusoidal pulses has been shown to produce even short latency potentials whose latencies vary as a function of frequency (for a given intensity), reflecting somewhat the traveling-wave propagation time in the cochlea (Naunton & Zerlin, 1976). Further details of such relationships for other AEPs are discussed in sections that follow.

There also are various temporal parameters associated with stimulation, which in turn affect the spectrum of the stimulus. However, they also may have effects more or less specific to the temporal parameter,

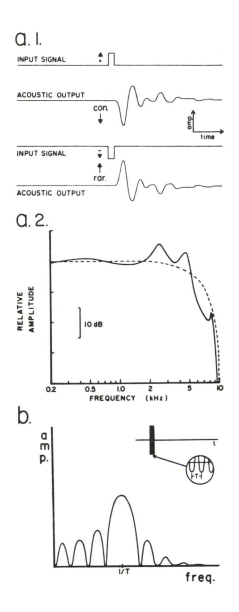

Figure 6.3.   Panel a.1: Acoustic output of an earphone (Telephonics TDH 39) in response to direct current pulses (input signal), producing clicks (acoustic output), of condensation (con.) or rarefaction (rar.) polarities. Panel a.2: Spectrum of the click (solid line) versus the electrical pulse (dashed line). (From Durrant, 1983, with permission.) Panel b: Spectrum of a brief tone burst. (From ASHA, 1988, with permission.)

such as plateau duration, rise-fall duration, and the gating function by which the amplitude envelope of the sinusoid is shaped (e.g., rectangular, cosine, etc.). The AEPs are relatively insensitive to plateau duration of the stimulus since they are largely onset responses. Rise-fall duration, however, is influential. In general, the longer the rise time, the less the amplitude and the longer the latency of the evoked potential will be (see below). Stimulus repetition rate is another important parameter. The repetition rate of the stimulus must be slow enough to avoid adaptation but high enough for efficient data collection (particularly important in testing newborns/infants; see Chapter 8). Typical rates range from 1/s or less to 50/s or more, depending on AEP component of interest and/or purpose of the AEP evaluation.

Stimulus calibration.   As with other audiometric procedures, evoked response evaluation requires calibration of the test stimulus. The intensity of the click stimulus frequently is reported in terms of dB above the behavioral threshold of a group of normal listeners and referred to as nHL. Regretfully, there currently are no hearing level standards for clicks and other brief transients. Existing audiometric calibration procedures are not applicable; sound level meters typically used for audiometric calibration require long duration signals for accurate measurement. A popular method of physical calibration of evoked potential test equipment is to determine the peak-equivalent sound pressure level (peSPL). This measurement is obtained by using an oscilloscope to match the amplitude of a sine wave with the peak amplitude of the click stimulus. The long duration pure tone can then be measured on a sound level meter. The behavioral threshold of the click has been found to be approximately 30 dB peSPL (Stapells, Picton, & Smith, 1982). Cann and Knott (1979) also described a method of determining the starting phase of the acoustic signal relative to the polarity or starting phase of the signal driving the transducer.

When determining hearing levels, the psychophysical method for threshold measurement and number and rate of stimulus presentations are important factors. The integrity of the hearing of the normative group sample must be affirmed. For more in-depth discussions of these and other aspects of stimulus calibration (e.g., choice and effect of pulse duration for click stimulation), the reader is referred to Durrant (1983) and Gorga, Abbas, and Worthington (1985).

Electrocochleography

The recording of stimulus-related potentials from the cochlea and eighth nerve is called electrocochleography (ECochG), and the record of the recorded potentials is the electrocochleogram (ECochGm). The ECochGm consists of several potentials (Figure 6.4): the cochlear microphonic (CM) and the summating potential (SP), which are generated by the hair cells (i.e., prior to excitation of the auditory nerve), and the whole-nerve action potential (AP), which is the compound action potential of the eighth nerve. The CM has much the same waveform as the stimulus. For example, a sinusoidal voltage is recorded in response to a pure tone burst. However, the CM often is observed to be asymmetrical about the zero axis, due to the presence of the summating potential. The SP can be isolated via low-pass filtering or phase cancellation of the CM (Dallos, 1973; Coats, 1981). Depending on the combination of stimulus parameters and recording site and method, the SP may be of either positive or negative polarity. When elicited by a transient stimulus such as a click, the SP appears as a transient deflection upon which the AP is superimposed and forms a shoulder on the leading edge of the AP waveform, as shown in Figure 6.4 (Coats, 1981). However, in the click-evoked ECochGm obtained via noninvasive ECochG in humans, the N1 component of the AP is the most salient feature (Coats, 1974). (For a more extensive overview of these potentials, see Durrant & Lovrinic, 1984.)

Recording methods and parameters

There are two general recording techniques available for noninvasive ECochG, extratympanic (Berlin, Cullen, Ellis, Lousteau, Yarbrough, & Lyons, 1974; Ruth, Lambert, & Ferraro, 1989; Stypulkowski & Staller, 1987) and ear canal (Coats, 1974; Durrant, 1977, 1986). The method of Cullen and his associates involved the use of a silver wire electrode wrapped in a saline-soaked cotton pledget, placed against the tympanic membrane. Interest in this method recently has been rekindled by a new electrode designed by Stypulkowski, which uses a very flexible silastic tube to hold the wire and a foam-rubber electrolyte-impregnated tip. (The tube also can be used for sound delivery.) In contrast, Coats's (1974) design and similar ones (e.g., Durrant, 1977, 1986) employ a light, springy "clip" to hold a small electrode against the canal wall near (but not touching) the eardrum. These types of electrode assemblies generally are tolerated well by subjects, even while they wear earphones. They are capable of providing recordings of the AP traceable to or close to the perceptual limits of the stimulus (Figure 6.5). However, there is a considerable amount of variability in extratympanic or ear canal ECoChG (Durrant, 1986), which may lead to much less successful recordings in some subjects, although this appears to be less of a problem with the Stypulkowski design (Stypulkowski & Staller, 1987).

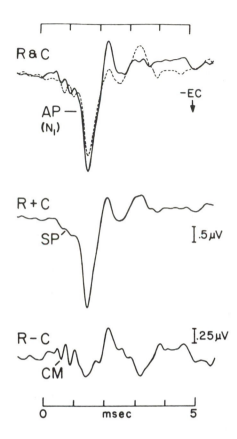

Figure 6.4. Component potentials of the (human) electrocochleogram recorded from the ear canal using condensation (C) and rarefaction (R) clicks: action potential (AP), cochlear microphonic (CM), summating potential (SP). The CM and SP can be selectively enhanced by manipulating the R and C responses, as indicated. Ear-canal negative (−EC) potentials are plotted as downward deflections. (Based on a figure by Coats, 1981, from ASHA, with permission.)

Other ear canal electrode designs have been described wherein the electrode is placed much less deep in the ear canal (e.g., Yanz & Dodds, 1985; Whitaker, 1986). There also now are earplug-type ear canal electrodes available commercially (Nicolet tiptrodes), which replace the tips and are used with the drivers of tubal insert earphones. Such shallow ear canal electrodes compare favorably in performance with electrodes of the Coats type, when the latter is placed laterally in the ear canal (Ferraro, Murphy, & Ruth, 1986). These more recent designs have substantially reduced the inherent impedance problem of ear canal electrodes.

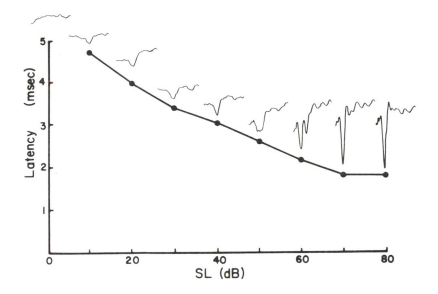

Figure 6.5. AP latency-intensity function and corresponding ECochG tracing (recorded via an ear canal electrode). (From ASHA, 1988, with permission.)

Still, as demonstrated by Coats (1974), a price is paid in that the farther out in the canal the recording is made, the smaller the recorded potential.

Differential recording, again, requires two electrode leads besides ground. The second electrode (sometimes referred to as the reference) is usually a disk EEG-type recording electrode, and its site is no less important than that of the ear canal electrode. At first glance, the ipsilateral earlobe or mastoid might seem most appropriate, but these are not inactive sites (see the section on ABRs). Preferable sites are the nasion or contralateral earlobe/mastoid, which are relatively inactive for the ECochGm. Durrant (1977; also see Durrant, 1986) also suggested recording between the ear canal and the vertex or forehead to provide simultaneous pickup of the eighth nerve and brainstem components (Figure 6.6).

Stimulus variables

The AP, like all compound nerve potentials, grows in proportion to the strength of the stimulus, but equally remarkable is the concomitant decrease in its latency. Latency is the time interval between stimulus onset and onset or peak of the response. Because the latency of the occurrence

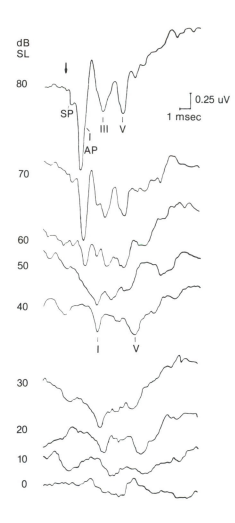

Figure 6.6. Combined ECochGm and ABR recording at different sensation levels of the click stimulus, obtained by differential recording between the forehead at hairline (inverted input) and the ear canal (noninverted input). Using this montage and configuration of inputs to the recording amplitude, both ear canal negative and forehead/vertex positive potentials are plotted as downward deflections. (From Durrant, 1986, with permission.)

of the peak of the AP (i.e., N1) is easier to measure, it is the preferred measure, at least for clinical purposes. The typical graph of AP (peak) latency versus stimulus level is shown in Figure 6.5; in general such graphs are called latency-intensity functions. The basis of this phenomenon is evident from the recordings presented in Figure 6.7

wherein broad-band and derived narrow-band click-elicited APs are shown. These data show that the high-level response reflects more basalward (i.e., high-frequency) contributions of eighth nerve fibers in the cochlea, whereas the contributions from lower frequency regions tend to cancel one another (Eggermont, 1976a). The latencies and broader waveforms of low-level responses (Figure 6.7, Panel a) correspond more to responses generated by lower frequency bands, namely around 2 kHz (Figure 6.7, Panel b), which is consistent with the greater sensitivity of the 2-kHz region near threshold. The latency-intensity shift largely reflects the time required for the traveling wave to propagate between the corresponding places along the basilar membrane.

Nonpathologic variables

As noted earlier, considerable variability between subjects often is observed in the amplitude of the ECochG. This, however, appears to be inherent to the pickup of the AP at extracochlear sites and not necessarily to the method of recording. For instance, transtympanic recordings from the promontory using needle electrodes produce on the order of 10 times larger signals than do extratympanic/ear canal recordings but can yield a range of AP amplitudes as much as 20:1 (e.g., see data of Eggermont, 1976b). This range exceeds the range of amplitudes recorded with non-invasive methods (Durrant, 1986). The main difficulty with the extra-tympanic methods, compared to the transtympanic, is a matter of SNR, that is, the more remote the site of recording, the poorer is the SNR. This is because the signal, the AP, gets smaller while the noise remains essen-tially constant. In contrast to amplitude, the variability of latency is much less and is relatively independent of recording technique (Durrant, 1986). In general, standard deviations are typically less than 0.2 ms for the AP recorded from normal hearing subjects.

Pathologic variables and clinical applications of ECochG

The primary categories of clinical utility for AEP evaluations are in otoneurologic/differential diagnostics and hearing threshold estimation. Noninvasive ECochG has not proven too valuable for threshold estima-tion and is not considered as reliable as transtympanic ECochG (Probst, 1983). In differential diagnoses most clinical interest in ECochG has been directed toward the identification, assessment, and monitoring of Ménière's disease or hydrops. Advances in this area stem largely from the work of Coats (1981, 1986; see also Ferraro, Arenberg, & Hassanein, 1985; and Staller, 1986); these advances follow observations of Eggermont

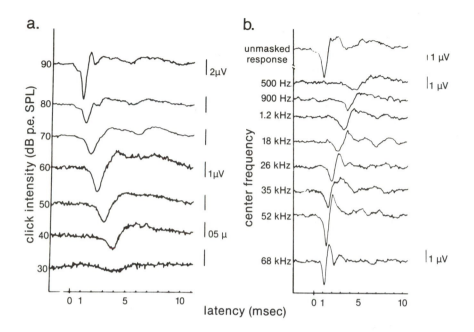

Figure 6.7. Panel a: Wide-band click-evoked APs (from Eggermont, Odenthal, Schmidt, & Spoor, 1974, with permission). Panel b: Derived narrow-band responses with click stimulus presented at 90 dB peSPL (from Eggermont, 1976a, with permission). Both sets of recordings are from the promontory via a trans-tympanic electrode.

(1976b) and Gibson, Moffat, and Ramsden (1977). Namely, many patients with Ménière's disease demonstrate enhanced SPs, as illustrated in Figure 6.8. Such enhancement of the SP is rarely, if ever, seen in cases of retrocochlear lesions and is seen infrequently in other cochlear disorders.

The major application of noninvasive ECoChG to differential diagnostic testing, otherwise, is the facilitation of the ABR evaluation, that is, to improve detection and definition of the AP and, thereby, provide information important to the interpretation of the ABR (discussed below). As illustrated in Figure 6.9, cochlear and more peripheral pathologies can be reflected clearly in the latency-intensity functions of the AP. Latency shifts of the AP will be, for the most part, echoed by the latency-intensity functions of the later waves of the AEP, especially the ABR (Davis, 1976). Additionally, as shown previously in Figures 6.5 and 6.6, ECochG can provide measurable APs at levels approaching the perceptual limits of the stimulus. Thus measurable APs can be obtained

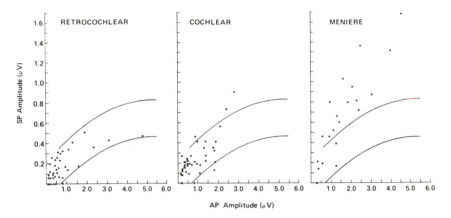

Figure 6.8. Scatter plots of SP versus AP amplitudes for three groups of pathologic ears. The curves represent best-fit estimates of ± 2 SD for responses obtained from normal ears. Recordings from ear canal. (From Coats, 1981, with permission.)

in cases with peripheral hearing losses (Stypulkowski & Staller, 1987) for whom even high levels of stimulation will lead, at most, to relatively low sensation levels of stimulation. Consequently, the contribution of peripheral components to observed prolongations of later waves of the AEP can be more critically assessed when supplemented by ECochG techniques (Ferraro & Ferguson, 1989).

Measurement of auditory brainstem evoked potentials

Shown in Figure 6.10 is the typical ABR, as obtained in a normal hearing and neurologically intact subject, using moderately high levels of click stimulation and recording between vertex and the ipsilateral earlobe/ mastoid with surface (disc) electrodes. This ostensibly yields the same short latency AEP as reported by Jewett, Romano, and Williston (1970). From another perspective, this is simply another method of noninvasive ECochG. Indeed, using this recording montage, but connecting the earlobe lead to the noninverting input of the differential amplifier (i.e., rather than the vertex lead, as in Figure 6.10), Sohmer and Feinmesser (1967) earlier described a potential that proved to contain not only the AP, but up to seven component waves (see peak labels in Figure 6.10 in parentheses; Sohmer, Feinmesser, & Szabo, 1974). Of course, the peaks

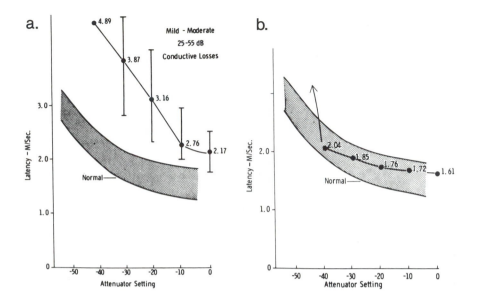

Figure 6.9. AP latency-intensity functions for group of patients with mild-to-moderate conductive (Panel a) and sloping sensorineural hearing loss (Panel b). (Data from recordings from surface of the eardrum; adapted from Berlin, Cullen, Ellis, Lousteau, Yarbrough, & Lyons, 1974, with permission.)

of their recorded response were negative rather than positive, as in Figure 6.10, but it was Jewett and Williston's (1971) polarity convention and peak labeling scheme that subsequently prevailed as the most widely accepted representation of the ABR. Far more important than the vertex positive-versus-negative convention was the revelation that what Sohmer and Jewett had recorded independently were potentials containing both eighth nerve and brainstem potentials (Jewett, 1970). Therefore, (Jewett) Wave I of the auditory *brainstem* potential actually arises from the auditory nerve (Sohmer et al., 1974; Buchwald & Huang, 1975) and is none other than the N1 component of the AP. Furthermore, Wave II of the human ABR now is attributed predominantly to the eighth nerve (Møller & Jannetta, 1982). Only the waves beyond II (or N2) appear to arise from brainstem level generators per se. Consequently, Waves I, II, and III arise from structures ipsilateral to the side of stimulation, whereas later waves may come from structures that receive ipsilateral, contralateral, or bilateral inputs from the auditory periphery (Achor & Starr, 1980a, 1980b; Buchwald & Huang, 1975; Møller, Jannetta, Bennett, & Møller, 1981; Wada & Starr, 1983a, 1983b, 1983c).

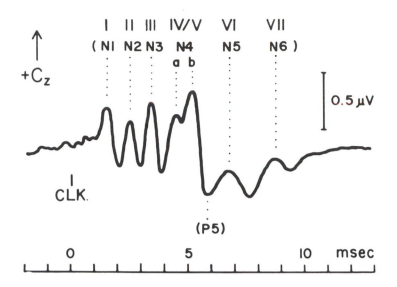

Figure 6.10. Auditory brainstem response. Onset of click (CLK) stimulus and vertex positive deflection (+Cz) as indicated. (From ASHA, 1988, with permission.)

Frequently measured parameters of the ABR waveform are illustrated in Figure 6.11. The amplitude measures commonly used are peak-to-peak, that is, the voltage difference between the designated positive peak and the subsequent negative peak/trough. Although avoiding the difficulty of determining the true baseline of the potential, this parameter may compound effectively amplitude measures of potentials actually arising from separate generators (Hughes, Fino, & Hart, 1985; Wada & Starr, 1983a, 1983b, 1983c). Relative amplitude measures also have been employed, namely the ratio of the Wave V to Wave I amplitudes. However, by far the most extensively used measures for clinical purposes are those of latency. As defined earlier, the (absolute) latency is the time difference between the onset of the stimulus to the peak of the wave (Figure 6.10). Relative latency measures also are of keen interest and are referred to as interwave latencies or interpeak intervals, namely the differences between absolute latencies of two peaks (e.g., I-V). By convention, the ABR evaluation favors the vertex-positive peaks of the waveform, but this may not be entirely justified from the perspective of assessment of all generators (Hughes et al., 1985) and/or the fact that the negative peaks can provide useful alternative measures (e.g., if residual noise has obscured a positive peak).

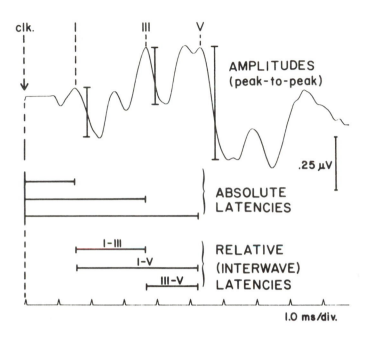

Figure 6.11. Fundamental measures of amplitude and latency of the ABR. (From ASHA, 1988, with permission.)

Stimulus parameters

Intensity. The effects of (click) stimulus level and typical latency-intensity functions of major components of the ABR are shown in Figure 6.12. Naturally, the amplitude of the response diminishes with decreasing intensity, but more notable is the tendency for the earliest waves to disappear in the noise floor of the recording. Otherwise, the latency-intensity functions of the brainstem components roughly parallel those of Wave I, that is, the AP (N1). The basis for the latency-intensity shift, again, is attributed primarily to the basalward spread of excitation with increasing intensity. This has been demonstrated for the ABR by Don and Eggermont (1978), as illustrated in Figure 6.13.

Spectrum. The fact that the abrupt onset and broad spectrum of a click synchronizes and excites a broad population of neuronal discharges also makes the click a very effective stimulus for the ABR, indeed for most AEPs. The click also can provide general high-frequency threshold information (Don, Eggermont, & Brackmann, 1979), although brief tone bursts

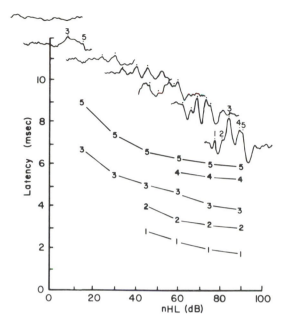

Figure 6.12. ABR latency-intensity functions and corresponding waveforms. (From ASHA, 1988, with permission.)

and similar transients and related methods are essential for more frequency-specific information (Stapells, Picton, Perez-Abalo, Read, & Smith, 1985). Again, stimulus frequency specificity is not compatible with stimulus brevity, so there is a spread of energy around the central frequency and, with increasing stimulus intensity, a basalward spread of excitation (Folsom, 1984). Low-frequency sinusoidal pulses also have, effectively, longer rise times than high-frequency, which adds to the propagation delay in the cochlea, causing longer ABR latencies. There also is a concommitant reduction of synchrony so that low-frequency stimuli are not nearly as reliable as high-frequency stimuli for eliciting the ABR. Still, the ABR can be evoked by stimuli with spectral lobes centered at frequencies of 500 Hz or lower (Stapells & Picton, 1981; Suzuki, Hirai, & Horiuchi, 1977). With the use of such stimuli, Wave V may be tracked down to the limits of visual detection of the response, with observed stimulus levels within 10 dB of behavioral thresholds at corresponding audiometric frequencies, at least down to 500 Hz (Suzuki & Yamane, 1982).

The ABR is relatively insensitive to the stimulus duration (Gorga, Beauchaine, Reiland, Worthington, & Javel, 1984) but quite dependent

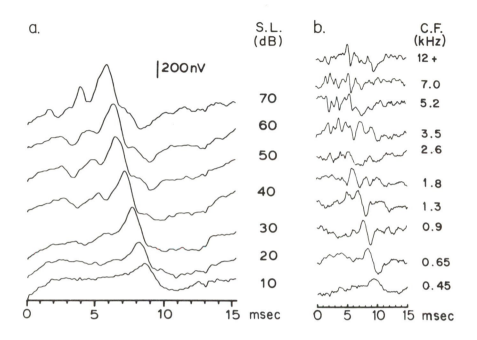

Figure 6.13. Panel a: Broad-band click-elicited ABRs. (From Don, Eggermont, & Brackmann, 1979, with permission.) Panel b: Derived narrow-band responses. (Adapted from Don & Eggermont, 1978, with permission.)

on the rise-fall times (Kodera, Marsh, Suzuki, & Suzuki, 1983). The more gradual the rise-fall time is, the lower the amplitude and the longer the latencies of the waves will be, with Wave V being the least sensitive to this stimulus parameter (Hecox, Squires, & Galambos, 1976). The gating function itself also is important; it is what mainly determines the spectrum. Various functions are available to minimize spectral splatter (Harris, 1978; Nuttall, 1981), although stop-band masking may be added to further ensure frequency specificity (Picton, Ouellette, Hamel, & Smith, 1979; Stapells et al., 1985). Another method for obtaining frequency-specific information, albeit more time-consuming, is the "subtractive" masking method originally described by Teas, Eldredge, and Davis (1962). It is this method that was used by Don et al. (1979) to derive the narrow-band ABRs shown in Figure 6.13, Panel b (as well as the narrow-band APs shown previously in Figure 6.7 [Eggermont, 1976]).

Polarity.   Although not affecting the spectrum of the stimulus and imperceptible to the listener, polarity or starting phase of the stimulus often affects the detailed morphology of the ABR waveform. For example, condensation and rarefaction clicks frequently are observed to differentially affect the amplitudes, latencies, and/or resolution of some peaks of the ABR (Figure 6.14), although these effects are variable across subjects (i.e., opposite or negligible effects) and latency differences usually amount to no more than 0.1–0.2 ms in normal subjects. However, a sloping high-frequency hearing loss can lead to more dramatic effects of stimulus polarity (Coats & Martin, 1977). These effects depend largely on the low-frequency components of the stimulus (Fowler & Swanson, 1986), because the auditory neurons are most capable of preserving phase information for low-frequency stimuli. (See also Moller, 1986; and Salt & Thornton, 1983.) Use of alternating stimulus polarity offers the advantage of canceling stimulus artifact. It may be preferable, however, to avoid muddling the polarity effects (and the distortion of the waveform that can result) and separately collect responses to each phase. With many of the commercially available test units, these responses can be combined later in the computer memory to derive the alternating polarity response if desired and/or if necessary.

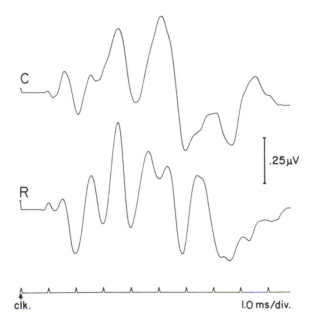

Figure 6.14. Effects of click polarity on the ABR: C—condensation, R—rarefaction. (From ASHA, 1988, with permission.)

Repetition rate of stimuli.   Because signal averaging requires many repetitions of the stimulus, the efficiency of data collection is directly dependent on repetition rate. However, due to adaptation, the ABR is sensitive to stimulus repetition rate (Fowler & Noffsinger, 1983; Picton, Stapells, & Campbell, 1981), as shown by Figure 6.15. As stimulus rate is increased, the latencies of the waves are prolonged and amplitudes are decreased. Rates of 10/s or less are necessary for maximal definition of all the waves, although rates up to 20/s may be used with little compromise. Rates of 30/s or higher may be used if only Wave V definition is essential. Such high stimulus rates are particularly attractive for deriving thresholds in newborns and difficult-to-test subjects wherein time is of the essence. High stimulus rates also are used by some clinicians as a way of stressing the system and, perhaps, exaggerating an otherwise marginal abnormality in the response, that is, by adapting the system. However, high repetition rates may not involve adaptation alone and results obtained must be interpreted accordingly (Durrant, 1986).

Masking

There is still considerable debate as to whether or not masking is ever needed for ABR testing. First, at least for clicks, there appears to be greater transcranial attenuation than encountered in pure tone audiometry (Finitzo-Hieber, Hecox, & Cone, 1979). Additional transcranial attenuation can be realized through the use of recently developed insert earphones (Clemis et al., 1986). Second, in terms of determining the possibility of retrocochlear pathology, a response to crossover stimuli would be so delayed that it might raise as much suspicion as an absent response. Nevertheless, in the audiologic-oriented evaluation, much the same consideration for masking must be given as in behavioral audiometry.

Monaural versus binaural stimulation

Binaural stimulation greatly enhances the amplitude of the response. Were the central pathways conveying right- and left-eared information totally separately, it might be expected that the binaurally-stimulated ABR would be twice as large as the monaurally-elicited response. As illustrated by Figure 6.16, the binaural ABR does approach the sum of the monaural ABRs, but not quite (Dobie & Norton, 1980). The difference between the binaural and summed monaural ABRs yields the binaural interaction potential (Dobie & Berlin, 1979; Dobie & Nornton, 1980). This potential is most prominent in the Wave V-VII time frame and is attributed to neurons that are shared by the left and right brainstem auditory pathways. Perhaps because the binaural interaction potential is small and intimately

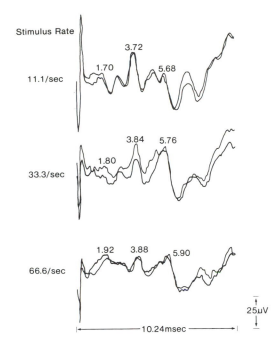

Figure 6.15. Effect of click repetition rate on the ABR. (From ASHA, 1988, with permission.)

depends on the nuances of the morphology of the monaural ABRs, its clinical utility has yet to be established (Fowler & Swanson, in submission).

Recording methods and parameters

Because the generators of the ABR are located at appreciable distances from the recording electrodes, small variations in electrode placement are not critical (Martin & Moore, 1978). An electrode in the vicinity of an imaginary line drawn between vertex and mid-forehead at the hairline picks up the primary brainstem waves as positive potentials relative to ground, and this zone provides optimal pickup of the brainstem potentials (van Olphen, Rodenburg, & Verway, 1978; Beattie, Beguwala, Mills, & Boyd, 1986). However, the area of the earlobe or mastoid, although providing optimal pickup of the eighth nerve response (via surface recording methods), is not totally inactive for the brainstem potentials (Terkildsen, Osterhammel, & Huis int Veld, 1974). Still, recording between vertex/

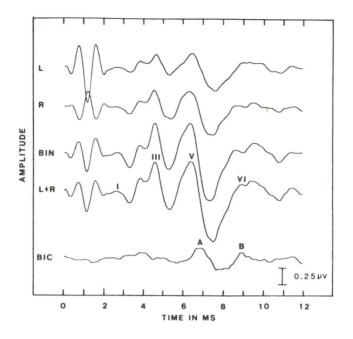

Figure 6.16. Binaural (BIN) versus monaural ABRs (L + R) and the derivation (i.e., BIN − [L + R]) of the binaural interaction component (BIC, demarked by Peaks A and B). (From ASHA, 1988, with permission.)

forehead to earlobe/mastoid is the most widely used recording montage because it does provide pickup of eighth nerve and brainstem components simultaneously and is inherently less noisy than recordings between vertex and a noncephalic reference.

Two- or multichannel recordings also have gained popularity for clinical purposes, most commonly using the ipsilateral and contralateral recording montages. The vertex/forehead inputs are tied together and leads from each earlobe/mastoid are connected to a separate channel. As shown in Figure 6.17, Wave I is attenuated/negligible in the contralateral recording, and there are waveform differences between the ABRs recorded via the two channels. These differences are largely attributable to the difference in "view" of the generators provided by the two channels (Durrant, Boston, & Martin, in press). Analyses of three-dimensional voltage space (bearing in mind that the head is a solid conductor), have shown that each ABR wave has an associated voltage plane of particular orientation (Williston, Jewett, & Martin, 1981; Pratt, Martin, Bleich, Kaminer, & Har'El, 1987). Consequently, as one moves about the head and alters

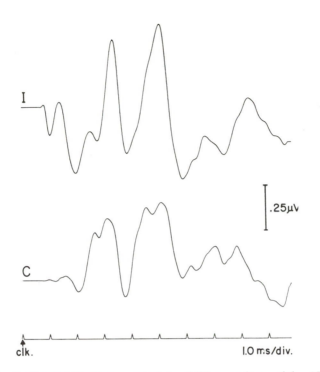

Figure 6.17. Ipsilateral (I) versus contralateral (C) recordings of the ABR. (From ASHA, 1988, with permission.)

the axis of orientation of the bipolar electrode pair (like turning the "rabbit ears" type of indoor television antenna), more-or-less different wave morphologies should be observed. Consequently, both amplitude and latency differences will be observed (e.g., see Creel, Garber, King, & Witkop, 1980; Stockard, Stockard, & Sharbrough, 1978). As illustrated in Figure 6.17, the second channel may resolve the peaks of the IV/V complex better, thereby ensuring the proper labeling of the Wave V peak (although they typically do not have identical latencies). Corroboration of the interpretation of the ipsilaterally recorded ABR perhaps represents the broadest clinical usage of two-channel recordings currently, although multichannel recordings may enhance the detection of pathology, per se (e.g., see Hashimoto, Ishiyama, & Tozuka, 1979; Hammond & Yiannikas, 1987).

Because the amplitudes of its component waves fall in the submicrovolt range and the background noise is in the tens of microvolts, the ABR usually requires amplifier gains of 100,000 to 500,000 and Ns of 500 to 2000, or more. Again, some analog prefiltering is helpful in improving the SNR, even with signal averaging. The normal ABR elicited by high-intensity stimuli are composed of frequencies between 50 and 1000 Hz (Kevanishvili & Aphonchenko, 1979), with a shift toward lower frequency content at low stimulus levels (Elberling, 1979). Nevertheless, current practices deemphasize the low-frequency content, because much emphasis is placed on the peak latencies. The peaks themselves represent relatively high-frequency features of the ABR. Therefore, typical band-passes used clinically in analog prefiltering are 100–3000 Hz (6 dB/oct roll-offs). In signal averaging, sampling epochs of 10 to 15 ms are typical. However, a lower low-frequency cutoff and epochs of 20 ms are desirable when recording responses to low-frequency stimuli (Suzuki & Horiuchi, 1977).

Nonpathologic variables

Beside stimulus parameters, there are various nonpathologic or subject variables that are worth considering in order to fully appreciate the clinical utility, limitations, and interpretation of the ABR evaluation. First, the widespread popularity of ABR measurement for clinical purposes is owed partly to the fact that the ABR is relatively unaffected by changes in subject state, including natural and sedated sleep (Amadeo & Shagass, 1973) and attention (Picton & Hillyard, 1974). Sedation often is required for the ABR evaluations in young children and other uncooperative subjects in order to obtain acceptable background noise and adequate time to collect data, although newborns usually are testable under natural sleep conditions (Fria, 1980). In some cases and for other purposes (e.g., intra-operative monitoring) examination of patients under anesthesia may be required. Anesthesias also do not alter the latencies or amplitudes of the potentials unless the core temperature of the body is lowered below 33° C or if the anesthetics are inherently depressive to the brainstem. A reduction in core temperature prolongs the latency of the ABR (Stockard, Sharbrough, & Tinker, 1978).

Substantial maturational changes occur in the ABR during early life, both in terms of waveform morphology (Figure 6.18, Panel a) and latencies (Figure 6.18, Panel b; Cevette, 1984; Fria, 1980; Salamy, Fenn, & Bronshvag, 1979; Salamy & McKean, 1976; Starr, Amlie, Martin, & Sanders, 1977). This necessitates the use of age-adjusted norms for the interpretation of ABR evaluations in premature infants and newborns. Failure to account for the maturation variable also can lead to substantial errors in hearing level estimation (Klein, 1984).

The early maturational changes are ostensibly complete within 2 years (chronological age). Throughout childhood the ABR changes little, until adolescence when males begin to develop slightly longer latencies than

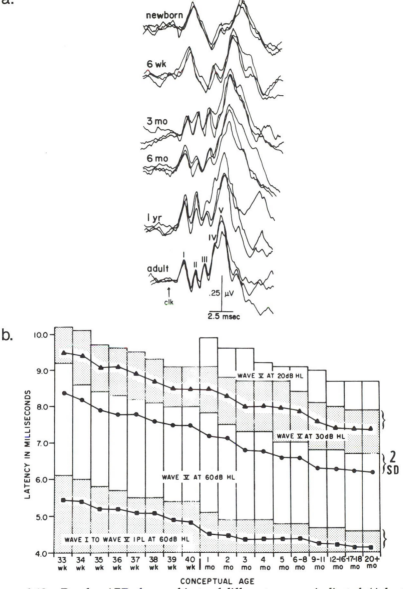

Figure 6.18.   Panel a: ABRs from subjects of different ages, as indicated. (Adapted from Salamy & McKean, 1976, with permission.) Panel b: ABR Wave V latencies and I–V interpeak latencies at indicated nHLs versus conceptual age. Conceptual ages in months (mo) are actually 44 weeks (wk) plus the indicated number of months. Horizontal bars above each data point demark latencies that are 2 SDs above the means (N = 580 newborns). (Adapted from Cevette, 1984, with permission.)

do females. By adulthood the gender difference amounts to approximately 0.2 ms in absolute Wave V latency, on average (Rowe, 1978; Jerger & Hall, 1980). Separate norms thus are preferred for the most critical interpretation of the ABR in males versus females. As adults age, latencies of all the waves may again increase, especially over the age of 50. Age-related changes may be potentiated by the presence of hearing loss, although it may be that ABRs recorded in older subjects are simply more variable (Jerger & Hall, 1980). Nevertheless, separate norms may be desirable for older subjects.

Pathologic variables

Peripheral hearing loss.   It should be evident from the latency-intensity function (refer to Figures 6.12 and 6.13) that whenever the level of the stimulus is either directly or effectively reduced, the latency, if not the waveform, of the ABR will be affected. The impact on the ABR, as manifested by latency-intensity functions, are much the same as demonstrated earlier for the AP (see Figure 6.9), but are worth repeating and elaborating here. Because conductive hearing losses cause sound energy to be attenuated, the latency-intensity function is shifted along the intensity axis by essentially the amount of the conductive hearing loss (Figure 6.19). The I-V interpeak interval is altered little (Mendelson, Salamy, Lenoir, & McKean, 1979; see also review by Fria, 1980), but the waves prior to Wave V may be lost at low levels and impede this measurement (see Figure 6.25). However, the shift of the latency-intensity function may not be parallel if the loss involved has a sloping configuration (Gorga, Reiland, & Beauchaine, 1985).

Cochlear hearing losses effectively reduce the sensation level and also cause shifts in the latency-intensity function. However, the results are more complex in the cases of cochlear than in conductive hearing losses. The overall effect is dependent on the severity and configuration of the loss (Bauch & Olsen, 1986) and the frequency composition of the stimulus. For otoneurologic-oriented evaluations, the click is the most widely used; thus the discussion, for the moment, will focus on this stimulus. Low-frequency hearing losses, in general, have little or no effect on the click-elicited ABR (Rosenhamer, Lindstrom, & Lundborg, 1981). With high-frequency hearing loss, essentially normal ABRs also are recordable if it is possible to stimulate at approximately 20 dB or more above the pure tone threshold at 4000 Hz and the degree of loss in the vicinity of 4000 Hz is no worse than mild to moderate in severity (Selters & Brackmann, 1977; Rosenhamer et al., 1981). Latency-intensity functions in such cases converge upon the normative functions at high stimulus levels, as

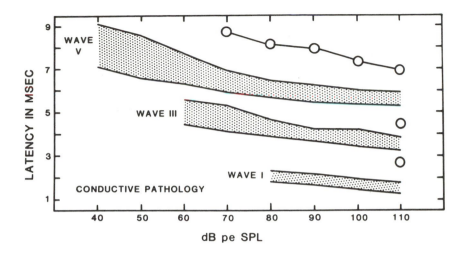

Figure 6.19. Example of the effects of conductive pathology on latencies of ABR Waves I, III, V. Stippled area represents ±2 SDs of latencies for normal hearing subjects. (From ASHA, 1988, with permission.)

illustrated by Figure 6.20. (This particular case demonstrated a fairly flat hearing loss of moderate degree.) Precipitously sloping high-frequency losses of moderate or worse severity, however, cause increased latencies (Coats & Martin, 1977; Gorga, Reiland, & Beauchaine, 1985; Gorga, Worthington, Reiland, Beauchaine, & Goldgar, 1985). Although a converging pattern in the latency-intensity function may still be evident, at high stimulus levels the latencies are less likely to fall within normal ranges. The ABR waveform also is likely to be degraded, with the detection of the earlier waves being most vulnerable. In such cases, the dominant tonotopical region along the basilar membrane being stimulated is presumably more apicalward than in the normal ear (i.e., the stimulus at the cochlear level is effectively low-pass filtered), so there is an additional propagation delay in the cochlea.

It thus is essential to account for peripheral hearing loss in the interpretation of the ABR. It should be noted that the impact of high-frequency hearing loss is not necessarily the same for all ABR waves; consequently, the interpeak intervals may be altered (Coats & Martin, 1977; Fowler & Noffsinger, 1983; Keith & Greville, 1987). The determination of the interpeak interval is given high priority clinically, because it provides some of the most compelling information by which it is possible to differentiate between cochlear or more peripheral pathologies and retrocochlear lesions (see below). The compromising of the definition of the earlier

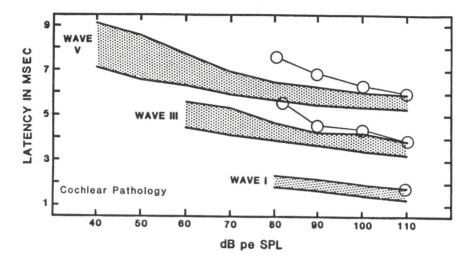

Figure 6.20. Example of the effects of cochlear pathology on latencies of ABR Waves I, III, V. Stippled area represents ±2 SDs of latencies for normal hearing subjects. (From ASHA, 1988, with permission.)

waves can be circumvented through the use of noninvasive ECochG to enhance Wave I, as mentioned earlier. Still, much interest exists in the prospect of somehow correcting absolute latencies for hearing loss. Various corrections for Wave V latency have been suggested to take into account degree of peripheral loss (e.g., see Selters & Brackmann, 1977).

Retrocochlear pathology.   It is beyond the scope of this chapter to delve extensively into the effects of the various known retrocochlear pathologies; this topic is taken up in Chapter 7. Suffice it to say at this juncture that any pathology that effectively blocks the conduction of action potentials, causes dysynchrony of neural discharges, reduces the available neuronal pool, and/or alters the orientation of the generators will lead to abnormalities in the ABR latency and/or waveform. Only the more straightforward type of retrocochlear lesion will be illustrated here, that of a tumor affecting the eighth nerve (Figure 6.21). It is well established that such a lesion, if not so severe as to greatly disrupt cochlear blood supply, will cause abnormalities in the ABR for waves following Wave I (Starr & Achor, 1975). However, the points to be made here are that what is being sampled via the ABR evaluation is not etiology but functional impact of the lesion, and there is no precise coupling between a given etiology and ABR waveform abnormalities (Figure 6.21). Furthermore, various pathologies may cause similar patterns of findings if they affect the same function

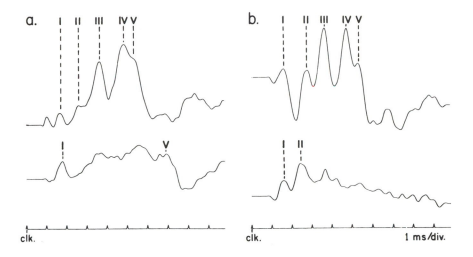

Figure 6.21. ABRs recorded from patients with surgically confirmed acoustic tumors: Panel a—neuroma, Panel b—meningioma in the cerebellopontine angle. Upper trace: normal ear response; lower trace: pathological ear response. (From ASHA, 1988, with permission.)

and level of the system. For example, a focus of multiple sclerosis in the cochlear nucleus with root entry involvement can mimic a tumor in the cerebellar pontine angle (Furman, Durrant, & Hirsch, 1989). Vasocompression of the eighth nerve can have similar effects. Thus it is important to use and interpret the ABR evaluation for what it is, a neurologic screening test, albeit a powerful test for such purposes.

The actual detection of an abnormality and arriving at an interpretation suggesting the presence of retrocochlear pathology depends on the criteria for normalcy of the ABR and the parameters used. There are no firmly established rules determining which of the various parameters are best suited to this task. Each parameter has its strengths and weaknesses, and most clinicians tend to use a multiparameter approach. Like multiple tests, however, it should be kept in mind that not all ABR measures are independent from one another, which can influence the sensitivity and specificity of any given test strategy (Turner, Frazer, & Shepard, 1984; Turner & Nielsen, 1984; Turner, Shepard, & Frazer, 1984; see also Chapter 13).

The weakest measure of the ABR for diagnostic purposes tends to be amplitude, again due to its high variability (Thornton, 1975). The use of relative amplitudes, particularly the ratio between Wave V (or IV/V) and Wave I has been suggested as an alternative (Starr & Achor, 1975), but in practice the V:I ratio does not improve precision of measurement beyond that of the absolute measures (Durrant, 1986). Still, the consistent observation of a relatively small Wave V, compared to Wave I, warrants follow-up.

Certainly, the most basic approach to ABR evaluation is that based on the absolute latencies. This, however, tends to be the approach most subject to interpretational error due to the influence of the various non-pathological and pathological variables noted above. Some of these variables are circumvented by reliance on interpeak intervals. Prolongation of these intervals is presumed to reflect increased time required for peripheral nerve and/or central propagation of nerve impulses (Starr & Achor, 1975) and is strongly suggestive of retrocochlear pathology (see Figure 6.21, Panel a). Therefore, lesion of the eighth nerve generally leads to prolongation of the I-III interval and lesions of the brainstem to III-V prolongation, although the more peripheral lesions may lead to too much desynchrony of the brainstem waves for the former to be seen clearly (Figure 6.21). It also may take the entire I-V interval for the effects of the more peripheral lesion to lead to a significant deviation from the norm. The limitation of interpretation based on interpeak intervals is the vulnerability of the ABR to the effects of peripheral hearing loss—the inadequate definition of the earlier waves.

In the neurologically intact, normal hearing subject, the ABRs recorded with each ear of stimulation differ only slightly (Starr & Achor, 1975), that is, 0.2 ms or less in most cases. This provides the basis for a sensitive test of abnormality, because the subject is his or her own control. Interaural latency comparisons are applied primarily to absolute Wave-V latencies (Selters & Brackmann, 1977; Clemis & McGee, 1979) but also can be applied to interpeak intervals. Here, too, hearing loss, particularly unilateral/asymmetrical types, can create a substantial interpretational obstacle but may be circumvented if interpeak measures are available.

The most clear-cut reflection of pathology, when observed, is the absence of waves (Figure 6.21). As a general rule, the absence of waves prior to V, although being a confounding variable for interpretation, tends to occur due to nonpathologic and (peripheral) pathologic factors, whereas the absence of waves after Wave I strongly suggests pathology of the auditory nerve and/or lower brainstem auditory pathways. Similarly, absence of waves following III is suggestive of pathology affecting the pontine level, presumably at or above the superior olivary complex. Even here, the rules are not rigorous, and the functional nature of the test must be kept in mind. Thus if an eighth nerve tumor or vasocompression, for instance, restricts or cuts off the cochlear blood supply, then an intact Wave I is not likely. Lastly, the presence/absence of the ABR waves, and normality of the ABR waveform itself, is inherently a subjective matter, and this interpretation too can be biased by the various variables discussed above.

Middle latency auditory evoked potentials

The middle latency potentials receive their name simply because of where they fall in the time domain following stimulus onset, namely, after the ABR or early potentials and before the cortical or late components. These potentials typically occur in the time window of about 10 ms to 100 ms. Literature prior to the early 1970s referred to these AEPs as the early response, a reference that shifted to the ABR after the initial reports of Jewett, Sohmer, and their respective associates, as discussed earlier in this chapter.

The middle latency potentials have been studied for more than 30 years (Geisler, Frishkopf, & Rosenblith, 1958). The first account described an evoked potential within 100 ms that was detectable near the subject's threshold; thus the response was believed to be cortical in origin. Since that initial report, interest in the middle latency potentials has waxed and waned. This time zone of the AEP often has been involved in deep controversy, contributing to the declining investigative interest during the period of rising interest in the ABR, but the middle latency potentials now are receiving renewed research and clinical interest (Musiek, Geurkink, Weider, & Donnelly, 1984; Jerger & Jerger, 1985).

The following AEPs have been referred to as or associated with the time zone of middle latency AEPs, although they are of arguably different origins.

SN10 potential

The slow negative wave (SN10), occurring about 10 ms following stimulus onset, was described by Davis and Hirsh (1979). This is a large vertex-negative response, obtained using low-frequency tone bursts, and occurs at the end of the ABR. The SN10 appears to be greatly dependent on filter parameters and requires the high-pass filter cutoff to be reduced to as low as 10–40 Hz. Some investigators have questioned the reliability of the SN10 for assessing low-frequency hearing sensitivity in children (Hawes & Greenberg, 1981; Weber, 1987), which originally commanded much of the attention in this potential (Davis & Hirsh, 1979). Thus the

SN10 has neither received the interest nor the acceptability afforded to some of the other AEPs.

Middle latency response (MLR)

The MLR has received the most attention of the middle latency AEPs, and, perhaps by default, the most controversy. It consists of a series of waves between 10 and 100 ms, the first of which is a positive peak identified as Po. Subsequent peaks are labeled P (positive) and N (negative) with alphabetically increasing subscripts (see Figure 6.1). Pa, occurring at about 30 ms, is typically the most robust and is the primary peak of interest, much as Wave V is in the ABR (Mendel & Wolf, 1983). Much of the MLR research was initiated by the work of Goldstein and Mendel and their colleagues, with interest focused on estimation of hearing sensitivity, particularly for low-frequency hearing (Thornton, Mendel, & Anderson, 1977; McFarland, Vivion, & Goldstein, 1977). Recent reports, however, suggest that the MLR may be useful in the assessment of the integrity of the central auditory nervous system as well (Harker & Backoff, 1981; Musiek et al., 1984; Vedder, Barrs, & Fifer, 1988).

Although the original report on the MLR by Geisler and his associates (1958) was followed by others (e.g., Lowell, 1961), the enthusiasm was soon cooled when the neurogenic origin of the MLR was challenged by Bickford, Jacobson, and Cody (1964). They suggested that the response actually is generated in the muscles of the head and neck. The controversy continued until Harker, Hosick, Voots, and Mendel (1977) reported the observation of MLRs elicited by moderate- (and low-) level stimuli from a subject under drug-induced paralysis, demonstrating that the MLR is not myogenic (see Mendel, 1977; and Musiek et al., 1984). Nevertheless, recordings of the MLR can be contaminated by what indeed is a sound-evoked myogenic response—the postauricular muscle response. (Another contaminant is electrical, 60-Hz noise.) The clinical value and audiometric utility of the MLR, however, has not been established on the basis of the origin of the MLR, but rather on the demonstrated absence or presence of a response to specific stimuli (Frye-Osier, 1983). Still, the controversy persisted long enough to discourage growth in MLR research.

The controversy surrounding the MLR has shifted in the 1980s from origin(s) to effects of filtering. Many of the earlier MLR studies used narrow filter bandwidths and steep filter skirts (McFarland, Vivion, Wolf, & Goldstein, 1975; McRandle, Smith, & Goldstein, 1974; Mendel, Adkinson, & Harker, 1977) in recording from adults and children. Of course, such filtering, when implemented via analog devices, induces a phase shift and distorts the MLR. This prompted the recommendation for the use of either wide-band analog filtering or zero-phase-shift digital filtering (Scherg, 1982). Others, however, have reported that MLRs were not easily identified in infants and children when using wide-band filters with shallow slopes (Sprague & Thornton, 1982; Susuki, Hirabayashi, & Kobayashi, 1983). Notably absent were the later peaks, Pb and Pc, but Suzuki and his co-workers did observe Pa in the vast majority of the children tested. These observations were ostensibly the same as those from earlier studies of Wolf and Goldstein (1978, 1980). They reported that the MLR recorded from neonates to low-level tonal stimuli is poorly organized beyond Pb but that the earliest components are present and easily identified.

Despite the debate over filtering, there is excellent agreement between MLR threshold and voluntary behavioral threshold data, and it would not be surprising that the ideal filter characteristics for reliable and valid threshold estimation may not be the same as those required to maximize waveform morphology at suprathreshold levels. This dichotomy is not unique to the MLR and also pervades clinical applications of the ABR. Nor has there been solidarity in the representation of the ABR waveform (and the underlying methods of measurement). Fria (1980) compared ABRs from three classic studies, namely Jewett and Williston's (1971), Sohmer and Feinmesser's (1973), and Starr and Achor's (1975). The representative ABRs from these studies were different morphologically but all represented equally valid ABRs. Still, it was the relatively narrow-band ABR, as recorded by Starr and Achor, that became clinically acceptable. Similarly the distortion imposed by filtering has made the MLR easier to identify and use clinically (Musiek et al., 1984). Several authors agree that the questions related to filtering need to be explored further but that the MLR is a clinically useful AEP for assessing low-frequency hearing sensitivity and evaluating the integrity of the central auditory nervous system (Jerger & Jerger, 1985; Kileny & Shea, 1986; Mendel & Wolf, 1983; Weber, 1987; see also Chapters 7 and 8).

Steady-state (40-Hz) potential

A different procedure for obtaining an MLR was proposed by Galambos, Makeig, and Talmachoff (1981). Stimuli are presented at repetition rates of 40/s, hence the name, 40-Hz Event Related Potential (ERP) or Steady State Evoked Potential (SSEP; Weber, 1987). The resulting morphology of the response is sinusoidal, with about a 25-ms period of four cycles over a 100-ms epoch (Figure 6.22). The 40-Hz ERP is larger than the traditional MLR, although Wave Pa of the MLR is equally detectable to the 40-Hz ERP at near-threshold levels (Brown & Shallop, 1982). Furthermore, although the amplitude of the 40-Hz ERP is larger than the MLR under click stimulation, the amplitude advantage disappears when 500-Hz tone

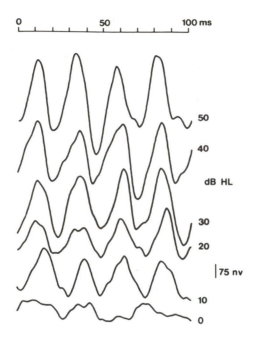

Figure 6.22. 40-Hz ERPs from a normal subject, elicited by 500-Hz tone bursts presented at hearing levels indicated. (From Brown & Shallop, 1982, with permission.)

bursts are used (Kileny & Shea, 1986). Both responses, therefore, are equally viable for threshold estimation in adults. However, the 40-Hz ERP does appear to be sensitive to patient state and may be too unstable for clinical application in infants and children (Kileny, 1983) or for use with patients in natural or drug-induced sleep (Brown & Shallop, 1982).

Recording parameters for MLR measurement

The remainder of this section is devoted to the MLR per se. The MLR may be recorded successfully with most commercial evoked potential equipment on the market today. Many of the recording parameters are similar to those used to record the ABR, with appropriate changes in time window and filter settings. Electrodes are placed typically at the vertex and the earlobe or mastoid ipsilateral to the ear stimulated, and it is this montage that yields the largest MLR. The contralateral earlobe or mastoid, or the forehead usually serves as the ground site. The MLR may be recorded ipsilateral or contralateral to the ear of stimulation without substantially affecting the MLR in adults (Peters & Mendel, 1974), but only the ipsilaterally recorded MLR is reliably demonstrable in the neonate (Wolf & Goldstein, 1978, 1980). The contralaterally recorded MLR begins to mirror the ipsilateral MLR by 28 weeks of age, attaining or approximating adult symmetry sometime around the first year of life (Reed, Hirsch, & Goldstein, 1980).

The MLR is of sufficient amplitude that fewer samples per average are needed compared to the ABR. The MLR may be present with as few as 256 samples (McFarland et al., 1975); however, 512 to 1,024 samples per average are more typically needed for acceptably reproducible responses (Mendel & Wolf, 1983).

Despite a great deal of discussion about filtering in the literature, filter settings have not been standardized (i.e., no more so than they have for any of the other AEPs). Typical filter settings range from 20 to 30 Hz for the low-frequency cutoff to 100 to 250 Hz for the high-frequency cutoff. However, bandpasses as wide as 5–1500 Hz may be used with the advantage of somewhat preserving the ABR (Ozdamar & Kraus, 1983; Kavanagh, Harker, & Tyler, 1984; Kavanagh & Domico, 1987). Given the lower frequency characteristic of the MLR, the sampling epochs used may be as wide as 100 ms, but 50–75 ms may be adequate for most applications (Mendel & Wolf, 1983).

MLR measures

The basic measures of the MLR are similar to other AEPs and include assessment of waveform morphology, latencies of peaks, and amplitude measures. The characteristic MLR has a series of peaks designated Po, Na, Pa, Nb (Figure 6.23, Panel A; Goldstein & Rodman, 1967). Some researchers have included later peaks in the MLR, labeled Pb through Nd (e.g., Vivion, Wolf, Goldstein, Hirsch, & McFarland, 1979; Wolf & Goldstein, 1978, 1980), whereas others appear to favor labeling only the positive peaks (Musiek & Geurkink, 1981). Latency measures usually are limited to absolute latency only, but interpeak latency measures and interaural latency differences can be obtained easily, if desired. Peak-to-peak measures are the most common of the amplitude measures; amplitudes of MLRs usually range from about 0.5 to 2.0 microvolts.

Stimulus parameters

The MLR amplitude increases and latency decreases as the stimulus intensity increases (Goldstein & Rodman, 1967; Zerlin & Naunton, 1974), thus following the same trends established by other AEPs described earlier

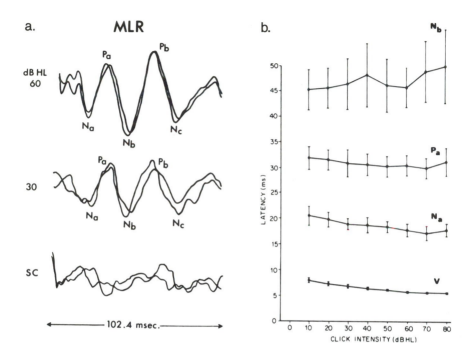

Figure 6.23. (a) Test–retest tracings of MLRs obtained at indicated stimulus levels (SC: silent/nonstimulus control). (From Mendel & Wolf, 1983, with permission.) (b) Latency-intensity functions of MLR component waves and Wave V of the ABR, for comparison. Data points are means and vertical bars are standard deviations for a group of normal listeners. (From Ozdamar & Kraus, 1983, with permission.)

in this chapter (Figure 6.23, Panel B). The MLR can be detected at or near the behavioral threshold in adults (McFarland et al., 1977; Thornton et al., 1977) and infants (Mendel et al., 1977; Wolf & Goldstein, 1978, 1980). Threshold estimations with click stimuli have been reported to be equally sensitive to those based on measurements of the ABR (Frye-Osier, Goldstein, Hirsch, & Weber, 1982; Musiek & Geurkink, 1981).

It is well established that MLRs can be elicited by tone bursts (Zerlin, Mowry, & Naunton, 1971). The amplitude and latency of the MLR has been found to decrease as stimulus frequency increases (McFarland, Vivion, & Goldstein, 1977; Thornton et al., 1977), and this trend is even more dramatic in neonatal subjects (Frye-Osier & Hirsch, 1980; Wolf & Goldstein, 1980). Thus frequency-specific threshold information can be obtained using the MLR, and it currently is considered to be one of the best electrophysiologic procedures for estimating low-frequency hearing sensitivity (Kileny & Shea, 1986; Mendel, 1980; Mendel & Wolf, 1983; Musiek & Geurkink, 1981).

MLRs usually are elicited using fairly low repetition rates. However, stimulus rates as rapid as 16 per second can be used without affecting MLR latency or amplitude (McFarland et al., 1975). Most studies have used rates less than 10 per second, with 9.1 to 9.6 per second being common (Mendel & Wolf, 1983).

Nonpathologic variables

MLRs have been reported to be stable under a variety of subject states. Mendel and his colleagues reported a number of studies in the 1970s that showed the MLR could be recorded reliably in different stages of natural and drug-induced sleep. Peak latencies were unaffected by sleep state; however, there were amplitude decreases with deep stages of sleep (Mendel, 1977). Such stability made the MLR a promising tool for estimating hearing sensitivity in difficult-to-test populations.

The MLR is present in neonates and infants and has been reported to be detectable when elicited by tone bursts at or near adult behavioral thresholds (Frye-Osier & Hirsch, 1980; McRandle et al., 1974; Mendel et al., 1977; Wolf & Goldstein, 1978, 1980). These reports, however, have been challenged recently (Kraus, Smith, Reed, Stein, & Cartee, 1985; Okitsu, 1984; Suzuki, Hirai, & Horiuchi, 1981; Suzuki et al., 1983).

There currently is a dearth of information on the effects of aging on the MLR. Because age effects have been found for both the short latency and long latency AEPs, such effects on the MLR would not be surprising, if not expected.

Pathologic variables and clinical applications

Audiometric-like applications were suggested above. Indeed, clinical application of the MLR has been concentrated heavily on the estimation of hearing sensitivity. MLRs have been obtained with tone bursts at or near threshold in a group of subjects with known conductive, sensorineural, or mixed hearing losses (McFarland, Vivion, & Goldstein, 1977). The tone burst-elicited MLR also has been shown to have potential for use in the evaluation of pseudohypacusics and the determination of organic hearing loss (Musiek & Donnelly, 1983; Musiek et al., 1984).

In contrast, there is much less information available on the use of the MLR to assess the central auditory nervous system, but the literature in this area is showing signs of growth. Robinson and Rudge (1977, 1978) reported that 12% of their patients with multiple sclerosis had abnormal MLRs with normal ABRs. MLRs also have been reported to be useful in the evaluation of patients suspected of having acoustic tumors, not in the detection of the tumors, but in predicting their size or estimating the low- and mid-frequency hearing sensitivity of these patients (Harker & Backoff, 1981; Musiek & Donnelly, 1983; Wolf, Pulec, Hodell, & Millen, 1979). Recent reports have described the clinical value of the MLR in the detection of cortical lesions (Jerger & Jerger, 1985; Kraus, Ozdamar, Hier, & Stein, 1982; Musiek & Donnelly, 1983; Musiek et al., 1984). MLRs were abnormal, whereas ABRs and pure tone audiometry were within normal limits in patients with cortical lesions. In such cases, brainstem dysfunction must either be ruled out or accounted for (Musiek et al., 1984).

The MLR, therefore, has been suggested to be a viable clinical tool in the assessment of the peripheral and central auditory systems. Still, more clinical research and clinical experience in a variety of centers is needed in order to expand the knowledge base regarding the clinical utility of the MLR.

Long latency potentials

It has been known for over a half century that auditory and other sensory stimulation can evoke a response in the electrical brain wave (e.g., a detectable change in the ongoing EEG; Davis, 1939). Of course, evoked potential methodology has progressed greatly since the earliest days of manual superposition of raw EEG tracings and the computer-based methods of today. The long latency potentials reflect long-lasting reactions of the cortex to sound, starting over 50 ms after the onset of stimulation (see Figure 6.1). This section focuses on the long latency response (LLR), comprising component potentials known as P1, N1, P2, and N2 (with particular emphasis on the N1-P2 complex).

The LLR occupies the time window of approximately 50 to 250 ms. Even later potentials may be identified, such as P300 and the contingent negative variation (CNV). The P300, commonly referred to as the cognitive potential, is discussed in Chapter 7, and treatment of the CNV is simply beyond the practical limits of this chapter. These responses, especially the CNV, have received little audiologic-oriented interest. However, all the long latency potentials have possible audiologic application. In fact, the LLR was studied and used extensively in audiologic, as well as neurologic and other, applications well in advance of the advent of the ABR evaluation. Perusal of the literature suggests that there may well have been unwarranted abandonment of the LLR in audiology, or at least acute withdrawal of academic/professional nourishment. (See also

Chapter 8.) In any event, the LLR is a hearty and relatively easy-to-record potential with which the audiologist should be familiar. Reneau and Hnatiow (1975) have comprehensively reviewed much of the literature up to the mid-1970s, which has provided an in-depth overview of the various characteristics of the LLR. The following is a brief summary thereof. The reader also is referred to overviews by Davis, (1976), Goldstein (1973), Picton, Woods, Baribeau-Braun, and Healey (1977), and Polich and Starr (1983).

Basic LLR recording parameters and measures

The methods already described for the measurement of short and middle latency potentials generally are applicable to the LLR. However, the relatively low-frequency characteristic of LLRs requires a lower bandpass in analog prefiltering (e.g., 1–100 Hz, if only the N1-P2 complex is of interest). The best methods for measuring the LLR are recording differentially between the vertex and the earlobe/mastoid (contralateral or both tied together) or between vertex and a noncephalic reference. Unlike ABR recordings, in recording the LLR the electrodes, in principle, can be placed physically near the generators. However, the amplitude of the LLR actually decreases laterally from the vertex, that is, over the temporal region, where it may even reverse polarity (Goff, 1978; Peronnet & Giard, 1981; Picton, Woods, Stuss, & Campbell, 1976; Vaughan & Ritter, 1970). This presumably is due to the location of much of the auditory cortex on the superior surface of the temporal gyrus, lying in the Sylvian fissure. Despite their small size, the responses recorded over the temporal region may show asymmetries reflecting regional damage or even asymmetries related to side of stimulation/dominance in the normal subject (Cacace, Dowman, & Wolpaw, 1988; Peronnet & Michel, 1977; Wolpaw & Pendry, 1977).

As seen in Figure 6.1, the amplitude of the (vertex recorded) LLR is in the microvolt range, and N1-P2 can reach 10s of microvolts at moderate to high levels of stimulation. Therefore, amplifier gain need be no more than 50,000 (as a rule), and reasonably stable responses are obtainable with Ns of 100 or less, depending on recording parameters and stimulus characteristics.

Stimulus variables

The LLR is elicited readily by various stimuli, including clicks, brief or long-lasting tone bursts, other transient stimuli, intensity increments in otherwise steady-state stimuli, transient frequency modulations of a steady carrier, and speech (Reneau & Hnatiow, 1975). Thus the LLR is at least as sensitive to changes in the stimulus as to stimulus onset. For example, Durrant (1987a) demonstrated LLRs stimulated by a frequency-modulated eight-tone carrier whose component tones are spaced every other critical band and alternatingly modulated across one-critical-band intervals. Additionally, with the ability to use relatively long rise/fall times and durations (see below), relatively narrow-band stimuli are usable to achieve excellent frequency specificity.

The frequency of the stimulus appears to affect the amplitude of the LLR only slightly, at least within audiometric frequencies. Some researchers (e.g., Antinoro, Skinner, & Jones, 1969) have reported a tendency toward decreased amplitude with increasing frequency (all other parameters being equal). Intensity naturally influences the LLR, as reflected in the input-output function and the now-familiar latency-intensity function (Figure 6.24). However, the latency-intensity shift of the LLR tends to be confined to relatively low sound levels, namely those below 50 dB HL, and is most dramatic near threshold (Picton et al., 1977). More attention actually has been given to the input-output function of the LLR with particular attention to its possible relation to the loudness power function. Some researchers have suggested the input-output function to be representable as a power function but with an exponent smaller than that of the loudness function (Butler, Keidel, & Spreng, 1969; Davis, Bowers, & Hirsh, 1968). Others suggest an input-output function that approaches a straight line when LLR amplitude is plotted against stimulus level, although this tends to occur only over the lower hearing level range (see Figure 6.24; Antinoro, Skinner, & Jones, 1969; Durrant, 1987b; Picton et al., 1977). At higher levels there is a trend toward saturation of output.

Temporal aspects of stimulation also are important. Repetition rate has a similar effect on the LLR as it does on the shorter latency potentials. Amplitude decreases with increasing rate, with maximal amplitudes being observed at rates of 0.1/s or less (Picton et al., 1977). However, rates of 0.5 to 1.0/s provide a good compromise between response amplitude and efficiency of data collection. Duration and rise/fall times of stimuli can influence the LLR, but the effects of duration, per se, are not straightforward. This perhaps reflects the interaction between on- and off-effects of stimulation (Reneau & Hnatiow, 1975). Generally, an increase in rise time leads to an amplitude decrease and latency increase in the LLR (Ruhm & Jansen, 1969; Skinner & Antinoro, 1971). However, compared to the ABR and MLR, relatively long rise times (e.g., 10 ms or longer) may be employed quite effectively in the elicitation of the LLR, with the advantage that spectral splattering is greatly reduced. Therefore, frequency specificity of stimulation of the LLR is not nearly the problem that it is in the elicitation of the ECochGm, ABR, or even the MLR. In short,

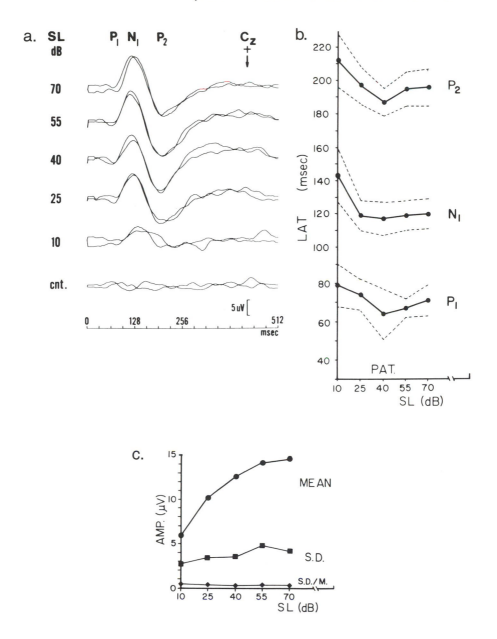

Figure 6.24. Test–retest tracings of LLRs (a) obtained at indicated stimulus levels (cnt: nonstimulus controls). Latency-intensity (b) and input-output functions (c) of LLR component waves. Data points are mean values. Standard deviations are indicated by dashed lines in Panel b and plotted directly in Panel c. (Adapted from Durrant, 1987b, with permission.)

with the LLR, audiometric-like stimulation can be closely approximated, if not replicated.

Nonpathologic variables

Other major nonpathologic variables of the LLR are those of maturation and level of arousal. As with the earlier potentials, the most significant developmental changes occur in early maturation (Davis & Onishi, 1969). LLRs tend to be smaller and have longer latencies in young children, with adult-like responses appearing within the first decade of life (Beagley & Kellogg, 1969; Price & Goldstein, 1966; Skinner & Antinoro, 1969; Suzuki & Origuchi, 1969). LLRs have been recorded successfully in very young, premature, and even fetal infants (Davis & Onishi, 1969; Engel & Young, 1969; Sakabe, Arayama, & Suzuki, 1969).

Recordings in young children are best achieved under sleep (Suzuki & Taguchi, 1968), although the LLR varies substantially from one stage of sleep to the next. With deeper stages of sleep, both amplitudes and latencies of the LLR component potentials increase (Skinner & Antinoro, 1969), although there is some question as to the integrity of the classically defined peaks in the deeper sleep stages (i.e., are they in fact the same or different potentials? Cody, Klass, & Bickford, 1967). Various sedatives also have been used in LLR recordings (including, for example, chloral hydrate; Skinner & Antinoro, 1969) with little or no substantive differences from natural sleep (Reneau & Hnatiow, 1975).

Less dramatic, but no less significant, are the effects of attentional state (Picton & Hillyard, 1974). Thus whether the subject is attending to the stimulus can influence the LLR. Consequently, the subject must be maintained at a constant level of arousal and attentional state to achieve the most consistent results. Even voluntary motor function as minor as thumb movement (performed in a task related to the stimulus event) can influence the LLR (Tapia, Cohen, & Starr, 1987). Additionally, short-term habituation of the LLR occurs with repetitive stimulation, wherein amplitude decreases exponentially, recovering spontaneously upon interruption/change of stimulation (Ohman & Lader, 1977). It is doubtlessly these variables and the associated complexities of the behavior of the LLR that have subdued interest in the LLR in the audiologic arena (coupled with the emergence of and rising interest in the shorter latency potentials).

Pathologic variables and clinical applications

The LLR can be affected by peripheral pathology. These effects are much as reflected in behavioral audiologic measures, including the manifestation of such phenomena as loudness recruitment (Cody, Griffing, &

Taylor, 1968; Shimizu, 1968). Indeed, loudness balance and LLR balance functions have been demonstrated that are quite similar (Knight & Beagley, 1969). The effects of retrocochlear lesions depend on level of lesion. Lesions at lower levels of the auditory system (e.g., eighth nerve tumor) yield mixed results (Shimizu, 1968; Townsend & Cody, 1970). Cortical lesions, of course, can affect the LLR, but the effects depend on site(s), extent, and nature of the lesion. Lesions of or in the immediate vicinity of the auditory cortex are expected to have the most profound effects on the LLR, but the effects of temporal lobe lesions (including bilateral involvement of primary auditory cortex) are not entirely predictable (Knight, Hillyard, Woods, & Neville, 1980; Woods, Clayworth, Knight, Simpson, & Naeser, 1987; Woods, Knight, & Neville, 1984). Not surprisingly then, diffuse/spotty cortical or subcortical lesions, such as multiple sclerosis, may have negligible effects on the LLR, at least when stimulated and recorded conventionally (Paty, Deliac, Gioux, & Franqui-Zannettacci, 1981; Durrant, Eidelman, Rossman, & Boston, 1988). Although there has not been great interest developed in the LLR for clinical assessment of cortical lesions (compared to, say, the pattern-reversal visual evoked potential), the advent of mapping of cortical potentials may help to renew clinical interest. Mapping, as currently practiced, is the use of multiple channels of recording together with computer graphics to generate a color-coded display that can reveal lesioned areas (e.g., see Duffy, 1985; Baran, Long, Musiek, & Ommaya, 1988).

As noted earlier, the LLR has a long history of interest in the audiometric arena (Reneau & Hnatiow, 1975). Although there has been in the past (Rose, Keating, Hedgecock, Schreurs, & Miller, 1971; Rose, Keating, Hedgecock, Miller, & Schreurs, 1972) and there continues to be reservations about the routine use of electric response audiometry (Polich & Starr, 1983), the LLR can provide the basis for obtaining an objective audiogram that often approximates the behavioral audiogram within 10 to 20 dB in adults and children (Hyde, Alberti, Matsumoto, & Li, 1986; Reneau & Hnatiow, 1975). However, thresholds in young children may be slightly, but systematically, overestimated (McCandless, 1967). The LLR has also been used successfully with mentally and other multiply handicapped subjects (Rose & Rittmanic, 1968), yielding acceptable intertest agreement with the behavioral audiogram with relatively minor compromises of results compared to those of normal subjects (Nodar & Graham, 1968).

In the present authors' opinion, the strength of the LLR actually may lie in the assessment of pseudohypacusis, for which electric response audiometry appears to provide valid results (McCandless & Lentz, 1968). Findings from an exemplary case are shown in Figure 6.25. This individual had a long-standing asymmetrical bilateral impairment with essentially

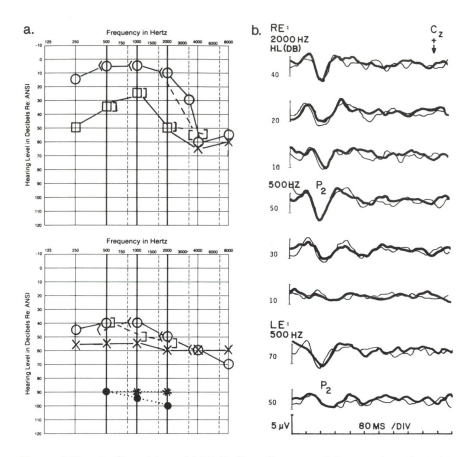

Figure 6.25. Audiometric and LLR findings for a pseudohypacusic patient. (a) Previous audiogram (top) and audiogram in question plus acoustic reflex thresholds (bottom). (b) LLRs obtained in AEP evaluation for right ear (RE) and left ear (LE), using tone bursts of indicated frequency and hearing levels.

normal low-frequency hearing in the better ear. One day, he appeared in his otologist's office, distressed over a perceived decrease in his hearing—including in his better ear. These complaints were corroborated by audiological assessment (Figure 6.25), which, in turn, was corroborated by tests performed by a second audiologist. Results on the Doerfler-Stewart test tended to support the patient's reported symptoms. Upon evaluation of the LLR, however, the sensitivity of the better ear was found to be unchanged, essentially, in reference to previous audiograms. Also, the results of the LLR evaluation were consistent with the 500-Hz (elevated) threshold demonstrated previously for the poorer ear. Thus a nonorganic component to this patient's hearing loss was demonstrated. Recognizing the value of the LLR in the assessment of pseudohypacusis, LLR evaluations have long been used in Canada as an adjunct to the hearing assessment of compensation cases for occupational hearing loss (Hyde et al., 1986). (For further discussion of pseudohypacusis, see Chapter 12.)

It is tempting to suggest that the LLR is underused in audiologic, and perhaps even otoneurologic, applications today (see also Chapters 7 and 8). In "objective" testing of the suspected functional case the authors believe that, not only is LLR evaluation worthy of consideration, it may be preferable to tests of the shorter latency potentials. The latter generally require very relaxed and/or sedated subjects to yield good threshold estimates and require great care in stimulus generation, if pure-tone-like threshold information is paramount. The LLR, on the other hand, can be readily recorded from awake/alert subjects, are very robust responses, and readily provide frequency-specific information.

Conclusion

Advances in technology and auditory evoked potential measurement have placed a powerful diagnostic instrument at the audiologist's fingertips, thus providing information about all levels of the auditory system. Volumes of scientific data now exist concerning the various components of the auditory evoked potential, and still more on clinical applications. Yet, the literature in the area continues to proliferate. Therefore, one need only ask, "What is it that I am trying to learn about the auditory system?" and then choose the appropriate AEP component(s) and corresponding recording and stimulus parameters to obtain the desired response. This is not to say that auditory evoked potential measurement is any more of a panacea today than it (misguidedly) was thought to be previously. Nor is AEP measurement a replacement for other methods. It must be applied judiciously with a full appreciation for its weaknesses, as well as its strengths. With knowledge, skill, and experience, however, AEP measurement can be used effectively to enhance differential diagnosis, monitor the status of the auditory system, and/or provide reliable estimates of hearing sensitivity in the absence of valid behavioral threshold data.

Acknowledgments

This chapter was developed in large part from a semifinal draft of *The Short Latency Auditory Evoked Potentials*, a tutorial document developed by the Working Group on Auditory Evoked Potential Measurement of the American Speech-Language-Hearing Association, on which the authors served (JDD, Chair). Therefore, we wish to acknowledge the efforts and contributions of members of the Committee on Audiologic Evaluation and peer reviewers, too numerous to mention, and especially, those of our fellow working group members, Drs. Cynthia Fowler, John Ferraro, Richard Folsom, and Bruce Weber. We dedicate this chapter to them.

References

Achor, L. J., & Starr, A. (1980a). Auditory brain stem responses in the cat I: Intracranial and extracranial recordings. *Electroencephalography and Clinical Neurophysiology, 48,* 154–173.

Achor, L. J., & Starr, A. (1980b). Auditory brain stem responses in the cat II: Effects of lesions. *Electroencephalography and Clinical Neurophysiology, 48,* 174–190.

Amadeo, M., & Shagass, C. (1973). Brief latency click-evoked potentials during waking and sleep in man. *Psychophysiology, 10,* 244–250.

Antinoro, F., Skinner, P. H., & Jones, J. J. (1969). Relation between sound intensity and amplitude of the AER as a function of stimulus frequency. *Journal of the Acoustical Society of America, 46,* 1433–1436.

American Speech-Language-Hearing Association. (1988). *The short latency auditory evoked potentials.* Rockville, MD: Author.

Baran, J. A., Long, R. R., Musiek, F. E., & Ommaya, A. (1988). Topographic mapping of brain electrical activity in the assessment of central auditory nervous system pathology. *American Journal of Otology, 9*(Supplement), 72–76.

Bauch, C. D., & Olsen, W. O. (1986). The effect of 2000–4000Hz hearing sensitivity on ABR results. *Ear and Hearing, 7,* 314–317.

Beagley, H. A., & Kellogg, S. E. (1969). A comparison of evoked response and subjective auditory thresholds. *International Audiology, 8,* 345–353.

Beattie, R. C., Beguwala, F. E., Mills, D. M., & Boyd, R. L. (1986). Latency and amplitude effects of electrode placement on the early auditory evoked response. *Journal of Speech and Hearing Disorders, 51,* 63–70.

Berlin, C. I., Cullen, J. K., Ellis, M. S., Lousteau, R. J., Yarbrough, W. M., & Lyons, G. D. (1974). Clinical application of recording human VIIIth nerve action potentials from the tympanic membrane. *Transactions of the American Academy of Ophthalmology and Otolaryngology, 78,* 401–410.

Bickford, R. G., Jacobson, J. L., & Cody, D. T. R. (1964). Nature of average evoked potentials to sound and other stimuli in man. *Annals of the New York Academy of Science, 112,* 204–223.

Binnie, C. D., Rowan, A. J., & Gutter, T. (1982). *A manual of electroencephalographic technology.* Cambridge, MA: Cambridge University Press.

Boston, J. R., & Ainslie, P. J. (1980). Effects of analog and digital filtering on brain stem auditory evoked potentials. *Electroencephalography and Clinical Neurophysiology, 48,* 361–364.

Brown, D. D., & Shallop, J. K. (1982). A clinically useful 500 Hz evoked response. *Nicolet Potentials, 1,* 9–12.

Buchwald, J. S., & Huang, C. M. (1975). Far-field acoustic response: Origins in the cat. *Science, 89,* 382–384.

Butler, R. A., Keidel, W. D., & Spreng, M. (1969). An investigation of the human cortical evoked potential under conditions of monaural and binaural stimulation. *Acta Oto-Laryngologica, 68,* 317–326.

Cacace, A. T., Dowman, R., & Wolpaw, J. R. (1988). T complex hemispheric asymmetries: Effects of stimulus intensity. *Hearing Research, 34,* 225–232.

Cann, J., & Knott, J. (1979). Polarity of acoustic click stimuli for eliciting brainstem auditory evoked responses: A proposed standard. *American Journal of Electroencephalography and Technology, 19,* 125–132.

Cevette, M. J. (1984). Auditory brainstem response testing in the intensive care unit. *Seminars in Hearing, 5,* 57–68.

Clemis, J. D., Ballad, W. J., & Killion, M. C. (1986). Clinical use of an insert earphone. *Annals of Otology, Rhinology and Laryngology, 95,* 520–524.

Clemis, J. D., & McGee, T. (1979). Brainstem electric response audiometry in the differential diagnosis of acoustic tumors. *Laryngoscope, 89,* 31–42.

Coats, A. C. (1974). On electrocochleographic electrode design. *Journal of the Acoustical Society of America, 56,* 708–711.

Coats, A. C. (1981). The summating potential and Ménière's disease. *Archives of Otolaryngology, 107,* 199–208.

Coats, A. C. (1983). Instrumentation. In E. J. Moore (Ed.), *Bases of auditory brainstem evoked responses* (pp. 197–220). New York: Grune & Stratton.

Coats, A. C. (1986). Electrocochleography: Recording techniques and clinical applications. *Seminars in Hearing (Electrocochleography), 7,* 247–266.

Coats, A. C., & Martin, J. L. (1977). Human auditory nerve action potentials and brainstem evoked responses. *Archives of Otolaryngology, 103,* 605–622.

Cody, D. T. R., Griffing, T., & Taylor, W. F. (1968). Assessment of the newer tests of auditory function. *Annals of Otology, Rhinology and Laryngology, 77,* 686–705.

Cody, D. T. R., Klass, D. W., & Bickford, R. G. (1967). Cortical audiometry: An objective method of evaluating auditory function in awake and sleeping man. *TransAmerican Academy of Ophthalmology and Otology, 19,* 81–91.

Creel, D., Garber, S. R., King, R. A., & Witkop, C. J., Jr. (1980). Auditory brainstem anomalies in human albinos. *Science, 209,* 1253–1255.

Cullen, J. K., Jr., Ellis, M. S., Berlin, C. I., & Lousteau, R. J. (1972). Human acoustic nerve action potential recordings from the tympanic membrane without anesthesia. *Acta Oto-Laryngologica, 74,* 15–22.

Dallos, P. (1973). *The auditory periphery.* New York: Academic Press.

Davis, H. (1976). Principles of electric response audiometry. *Annals of Otology, Rhinology and Otolaryngology, 85* (Supplement 28), 1–96.

Davis, H., Bowers, C., & Hirsh, S. K. (1968). Relations of the human vertex potential to acoustic input: Loudness and masking. *Journal of the Acoustical Society of America, 43,* 431–438.

Davis, H., & Hirsh, S. K. (1979). A slow brainstem response for low-frequency audiometry. *Audiology, 18,* 445–461.

Davis, H., & Onishi, S. (1969). Maturation of auditory evoked potentials. *International Audiology, 8,* 24–33.

Davis, P. A. (1939). The electrical response of the human brain to auditory stimuli. *American Journal of Physiology, 126,* 475–476.

Dobie, R. A., & Berlin, C. I. (1979). Binaural interaction in brainstem-evoked responses. *Archives of Otolaryngology, 105,* 391–398.

Dobie, R. A., & Norton, S. J. (1980). Binaural interaction in human auditory evoked potentials. *Electroencephalography and Clinical Neurophysiology, 49,* 303–313.

Domico, W. D., & Kavanagh, K. T. (1986). Analog and zero phase-shift digital filtering of the auditory brainstem response waveform. *Ear and Hearing, 7,* 377–382.

Don, M., & Eggermont, J. J. (1978). Analysis of the click-evoked brainstem potentials in man using high-pass noise masking. *Journal of the Acoustical Society of America, 63,* 1084–1092.

Don, M., Eggermont, J. J., & Brackmann, D. E. (1979). Reconstruction of the audiogram using brain-stem responses and high-pass noise masking. *Annals of Otology, Rhinology and Laryngology, 88* (Supplement 57), 1–20.

Duffy, F. H. (1985). The beam method for neurophysiological diagnosis. *Annals of the New York Academy of Sciences, 457,* 19–34.

Durrant, J. D. (1977). Study of a combined noninvasive-ECochG and BSER recording technique. *Journal of the Acoustical Society of America, 62,* S87.

Durrant, J. D. (1983). Fundamentals of sound generation. In E. J. Moore (Ed.), *Bases of auditory brain-stem evoked responses* (pp. 15–49). New York: Grune & Stratton.

Durrant, J. D. (1986). Combined ECochG-ABR versus conventional ABR recordings. *Seminars in Hearing (Electrocochleography), 7,* 289–305.

Durrant, J. D. (1987a). Pattern-reversal auditory evoked potential. *Electroencephalography and Clinical Neurophysiology, 68,* 157–160.

Durrant, J. D. (1987b). Auditory-evoked potential to pattern-reversal stimulation. *Audiology, 26,* 123–132.

Durrant, J. D., Boston, J. R., & Martin, W. H. (in press). Correlation study of two-channel recordings of the brain-stem auditory evoked potentials. *Ear and Hearing.*

Durrant, J. D., Eidelman, B. H., Rossman, R. N., & Boston, J. R. (1988). Preliminary study of pattern-reversal AEPs in multiple sclerosis cases. *Asha, 30,* 174.

Durrant, J. D., & Lovrinic, J. H. (1984). *Bases of hearing science* (2nd ed.). Baltimore: Williams & Wilkins.

Eggermont, J. J. (1976a). Analysis of compound action potential responses to tone bursts in the human and guinea pig cochlea. *Journal of the Acoustical Society of America, 60,* 1132–1139.

Eggermont, J. J. (1976b). Electrocochleography. In W. D. Keidel & W. D. Neff (Eds.), *Handbook of sensory physiology. Vol. V/3: Auditory system—clinical and special topics* (pp. 625–705). Berlin: Springer-Verlag.

Eggermont, J. J., Odenthal, D. W., Schmidt, P. H., & Spoor, A. (1974). Electrocochleography: Basic principles and clinical application. *Acta Oto-Laryngologica* (Supplement 316), 1–84.

Elberling, C. (1979). Auditory electrophysiology: Spectral analysis of cochlear and brainstem evoked potentials. *Scandinavian Audiology, 8,* 57–64.

Elberling, C., & Solomon, G. (1973). Cochlear microphonics recorded from the ear canal in man. *Acta Oto-Laryngologica, 75,* 489–495.

Engel, R., & Young, N. (1969). Calibrated pure tone audiograms in normal neonates based on evoked electroencephalographic responses. *Neuropediatrics, 1,* 149–160.

Ferraro, J. A., Arenberg, I. K., & Hassanein, R. S. (1985). Electrocochleography and symptoms of inner ear dysfunction. *Archives of Otolaryngology, 111,* 71–74.

Ferraro, J. A., & Ferguson, R. (1989). Tympanic ECochG and conventional ABR: A combined approach for the identification of wave I and the I-V interwave interval. *Ear and Hearing, 10,* 161–166.

Ferraro, J. A., Murphy, G. B., & Ruth, R. A. (1986). A comparative study of primary electrodes used in extratympanic electrocochleography. *Seminars in Hearing, 7,* 279–287.

Finitzo-Hieber, T., Hecox, K., & Cone, B. (1979). Brainstem auditory evoked potentials in patients with congenital atresia. *Laryngoscope, 89,* 1151–1158.

Folsom, R. C. (1984). Frequency specificity of human auditory brainstem responses as revealed by pure-tone masking profiles. *Journal of the Acoustical Society of America, 66,* 919–924.

Fowler, C. G., & Noffsinger, D. (1983). The effects of stimulus repetition rate and frequency on the auditory brainstem response in normal, cochlear-impaired, and VIII nerve/brainstem-impaired subjects. *Journal of Speech and Hearing Research, 26,* 560–567.

Fowler, C. G., & Swanson, M. R. (in submission). *Binaural and monaural phasic differences in the auditory brainstem response.*

Fria, T. J. (1980). The auditory brainstem response: Background and clinical applications. *Monographs in Contemporary Audiology, 2,* 1–44.

Frye-Osier, H. A. (1983). *Simultaneous early- and middle-components of the averaged electroencephalic response elicited from neonates by narrow-spectrum signals.* Unpublished doctoral dissertation, University of Wisconsin–Madison.

Frye-Osier, H. A., Goldstein, R., Hirsch, J. E., & Weber, K. (1982). Early and middle AER components to clicks as response indices for neonatal hearing screening. *Annals of Otolology, Rhinology and Laryngology, 91,* 272–276.

Frye-Osier, H. A., & Hirsch, J. E. (1980). *Normal middle component AERs to narrow-spectrum stimuli: A clinical tool.* Paper presented at the annual convention of the American Speech-Language-Hearing Association, Detroit.

Furman, J. M. R., Durrant, J. D., & Hirsch, W. L. (1989). Eighth nerve signs in a case of multiple sclerosis. *American Journal of Otolaryngology, 10,* 376–381.

Galambos, R., Makeig, S., & Talmachoff, P. J. (1981). A 40-hz auditory potential recorded from the human scalp. *Proceedings of the National Academy of Science, 78,* 2643–2647.

Geddes, L. A. (1972). *Electrodes and the measurement of bioelectric events.* New York: Wiley-Interscience.

Geisler, C., Frishkopf, L., & Rosenblith, W. (1958). Extracranial responses to acoustic clicks in man. *Science, 128,* 1210–1211.

Gibson, W. P. R., Moffat, D. A., & Ramsden, R. T. (1977). Clinical electrocochleography in the diagnosis and management of Meniere's disorder. *Audiology, 16,* 389–401.

Goff, W. (1978). The scalp distribution of auditory evoked potentials. In R. F. Naunton & C. Fernandez (Eds.), *Evoked electrical activity in the auditory nervous system* (pp. 505–524). New York: Academic Press.

Goldstein, R. (1973). Electroencephalic audiometry. In J. Jerger (Ed.), *Modern developments in audiology* (2nd ed., pp. 407–435).

Goldstein, R., & Rodman, L. (1967). Early components of averaged evoked responses to rapidly repeated auditory stimuli. *Journal of Speech and Hearing Research, 10,* 697–705.

Gorga, M. P., Abbas, P. J., & Worthington, D. W. (1985). Stimulus calibration in ABR measurements. In J. T. Jacobson, (Ed.), *The auditory brainstem response* (pp. 49–62). San Diego: College-Hill.

Gorga, M. P., Beauchaine, K. A., Reiland, J. K., Worthington, D. W., & Javel, E. (1984). The effects of stimulus duration on ABR and behavioral thresholds. *Journal of the Acoustical Society of America, 76,* 616–619.

Gorga, M. P., Reiland, J. K., & Beauchaine, K. A. (1985). Auditory brainstem responses in a case of high-frequency conductive hearing loss. *Journal of Speech and Hearing Disorders, 50,* 346–350.

Gorga, M. P., Worthington, D. W., Reiland, J. K., Beauchaine, K. A., & Goldgar, D. E. (1985). Some comparisons between auditory brainstem response thresholds, latencies, and the pure-tone audiogram. *Ear and Hearing, 6,* 105–112.

Hammond, S. R., & Yiannikas, C. (1987). The relevance of contralateral recordings and patient disability to assessment of brain-stem auditory evoked potential abnormalities in multiple sclerosis. *Archives of Neurology, 44,* 382–387.

Harker, L., & Backoff, P. (1981). Middle latency electric auditory responses in patients with acoustic neuroma. *Otolaryngology and Head and Neck Surgery, 89,* 131–136.

Harker, L., Hosick, E. C., Voots, R. J., & Mendel, M. I. (1977). Influence of succinylcholine on middle components auditory evoked potentials. *Archives of Otolaryngology, 103,* 133–137.

Harris, F. J. (1978). On the use of windows for harmonious analysis with the discrete Fourier Transform. *Proceedings of the IEEE, 66,* 51–83.

Hashimoto, I., Ishiyama, Y., & Tozuka, G. (1979). Bilaterally recorded brain stem auditory evoked responses. Their asymmetric abnormalities and lesions of the brain stem. *Archives of Neurology, 36,* 161–167.

Hawes, M. D., & Greenberg, H. J. (1981). Slow brain stem responses (SN10) to tone pips in normally hearing newborns and adults. *Audiology, 20,* 113–122.

Hecox, K., Squires, N., & Galambos, R. (1976). Brainstem auditory evoked responses in man. I. Effect of stimulus rise-fall time and duration. *Journal of the Acoustical Society of America, 60,* 1187–1192.

Hughes, J. R., Fino, J. J., & Hart, L. A. (1985). The significance of the negativities in the brainstem auditory evoked potential (BAEP). *International Journal of Neuroscience, 28,* 111–118.

Hyde, M., Matsumoto, N., Alberti, P., & Li, Y. (1986). Auditory evoked potentials in audiometric assessment of compensation and medicolegal patients. *Annals of Otology, Rhinology and Laryngology, 95,* 514–519.

Jerger, J., & Hall, J. (1980). Effects of age and sex on auditory brainstem response. *Archives of Otolaryngology, 106,* 387–391.

Jerger, S., & Jerger, J. (1985). Audiologic applications of early, middle and late auditory evoked potentials. *Hearing Journal, 38,* 31–36.

Jewett, D. L. (1970). Volume-conducted potentials in response to auditory stimuli as detected by averaging in the cat. *Electroencephalography and Clinical Neurophysiology, 28,* 609–618.

Jewett, D. L., Romano, M. N., & Williston, J. S. (1970). Human auditory evoked potentials: Possible brain-stem components detected on the scalp. *Science, 167,* 1517–1518.

Jewett, D. L., & Williston, J. S. (1971). Auditory-evoked far fields averaged from the scalp of humans. *Brain, 94,* 681–696.

Kavanagh, K. T., & Domico, W. (1987). High pass digital and analog filtering of the middle latency response. *Ear and Hearing, 8,* 101–109.

Kavanagh, K. T., Harker, L. A., & Tyler, R. S. (1984). Auditory brainstem and middle latency responses: I. Effects of response filtering and waveform identification; II. Threshold responses to a 500-Hz tone pip. *Annals of Otology, Rhinology and Laryngology, 93* (Supplement 108), 1–12.

Keith, W. J., & Greville, K. A. (1987). Effects of audiometric configuration on the auditory brain stem response. *Ear and Hearing, 8,* 49–55.

Kevanishvili, Z., & Aphonchenko, V. (1979). Frequency composition of brainstem auditory evoked potentials. *Scandinavian Audiology, 8,* 51–55.

Kileny, P. (1983). Auditory evoked middle latency responses: Current issues. *Seminars in Hearing, 4,* 403–413.

Kileny, P., & Shea, S. L. (1986). Middle-latency and 40 Hz auditory evoked responses in normal-hearing subjects: Click and 500-Hz thresholds. *Journal of Speech and Hearing Research, 29,* 20–28.

Klein, A. J. (1984). Frequency and age-dependent auditory evoked thresholds in infants. *Hearing Research, 16,* 291–297.

Knight, J. J., & Beagley, H. A. (1969). Auditory evoked response and loudness function. *International Audiology, 8,* 382–386.

Knight, R. T., Hillyard, S. A., Woods, D. L., & Neville, H. J. (1980). The effects of frontal and temporal-parietal lesions on the auditory evoked potential in man. *Electroencephalography and Clinical Neurophysiology, 50,* 112–124.

Kodera, K., Marsh, R. R., Suzuki, M., & Suzuki, J. (1983). Portions of tone pips contributing to frequency-selective auditory brainstem responses. *Audiology, 22,* 209–218.

Kraus, N., Ozdamar, O., Hier, D., & Stein, L. (1982). Auditory middle latency responses (MLRs) in patients with cortical lesions. *Electroencephalography and Clinical Neurophysiology, 45,* 275–287.

Kraus, N., Smith, D. I., Reed, N. L., Stein, L. K., & Cartee, C. L. (1985). Auditory middle latency responses in children: Effects of age and diagnostic category. *Electroencephalography and Clinical Neurophysiology, 62,* 343–351.

Lowell, E. (1961). Measurement of auditory threshold with a special purpose analog computer. *Journal of Speech and Hearing Research, 4,* 105–112.

Martin, M. E., & Moore, E. J. (1978). Scalp distribution of early (0 to 10 msec) auditory evoked responses. *Archives of Otolaryngology, 103,* 326–328.

McCandless, G. A. (1967). Clinical application of evoked response audiometry. *Journal of Speech and Hearing Research, 10,* 468–478.

McCandless, G. A., & Lentz, W. E. (1968). Amplitude and latency characteristics of the auditory evoked response at low sensation levels. *Journal of Auditory Research, 8,* 273–282.

McFarland, W. H., Vivion, M. D., & Goldstein, R. (1977). Middle components of the AER to tone-pips in normal-hearing and hearing-impaired subjects. *Journal of Speech and Hearing Research, 20,* 781–798.

McFarland, W. H., Vivion, M. C., Wolf, K. E., & Goldstein, R. (1975). Reexamination of effects of stimulus rate and number on the middle components of the averaged electroencephalic response. *Audiology, 14,* 456–465.

McRandle, C. C., Smith, M. A., & Goldstein, R. (1974). Early averaged electroencephalic responses to clicks in neonates. *Annals of Otology, Rhinology and Laryngology, 83,* 695–702.

Mendel, M. I. (1977). Electroencephalic tests of hearing. In S. E. Gerber (Ed.), *Audiometry in infancy* (pp. 174–181). New York: Grune & Stratton.

Mendel, M. I. (1980). Clinical use of primary cortical responses. *Audiology, 19,* 1–15.

Mendel, M. I., Adkinson, C. D., & Harker, L. A. (1977). Middle components of the auditory evoked potentials in infants. *Annals of Otology, Rhinology and Laryngology, 86,* 293–299.

Mendel, M. I., & Wolf, K. E. (1983). Clinical applications of the middle latency responses. *Audiology: A Journal for Continuing Education, 8,* 141–155.

Mendelson, T., Salamy, A., Lenoir, M., & McKean, C. (1979). Brainstem evoked potential findings in children with otitis media. *Electroencephalography and Clinical Neurophysiology, 105,* 17–20.

Michelini, S., Arslan, E., Prosser, S., & Pedrielli, F. (1982). Logarithmic display of auditory evoked potentials. *Journal of Biomedical Engineering, 4,* 62–64.

Møller, A. R. (1986). Effect of click spectrum and polarity on round window N1N2 response in the rat. *Audiology, 25,* 29–43.

Møller, A. R., & Jannetta, P. J. (1982). Comparison between intracranially recorded potentials from the human auditory nerve and scalp recording auditory brainstem responses (ABR). *Scandinavian Audiology, 11,* 33–40.

Møller, A. R., Jannetta, P. J., Bennett, M., & Møller, M. B. (1981). Intracranially recorded responses from the human auditory nerve: New insights into the origin of brainstem evoked potentials (BSEP). *Electroencephalography and Clinical Neurophysiology, 52,* 18–27.

Musiek, F., & Donnelly, K. (1983). Clinical applications of the auditory middle latency responses: An overview. *Seminars in Hearing, 4,* 391–401.

Musiek, F., & Geurkink, N. (1981). Auditory brainstem and middle latency evoked response sensitivity near threshold. *Annals of Otology, Rhinology and Laryngology, 90,* 236–240.

Musiek, F., Geurkink, N., Weider, D., & Donnelly, K. (1984). Past, present, and future applications of the auditory middle latency response. *The Laryngoscope, 94,* 1545–1552.

Naunton, R. F., & Zerlin, S. S. (1976). Basis and some diagnostic implications of electrocochleography. *The Laryngoscope, 86,* 475–482.

Nodar, R. H., & Graham, J. T. (1968). An investigation of auditory evoked responses of mentally retarded adults during sleep. *Electroencephalography and Clinical Neurophysiology, 25,* 73–76.

Nuttall, A. H. (1981). Some windows with very good sidelobe behavior. *IEEE Transactions on Acoustics, Speech, and Signal Processing, 29,* 84–91.

Ohman, A., & Lader, M. (1977). Short-term changes of the human auditory evoked potentials during repetitive stimulation. In J. E. Desmedt (Ed.), *Auditory evoked potentials in man. Psychopharmacology correlates of EPs. Progress in clinical neurophysiology* (Vol. 2, pp. 93–118). Basel, Switzerland: Karger.

Okitsu, T. (1984). Middle components of the auditory evoked response in young children. *Scandinavian Audiology, 13,* 83–86.

Ozdamar, O., & Kraus, N. (1983). Auditory middle-latency responses in humans. *Audiology, 22,* 34–59.

Paty, J., Deliac, P., Gioux, M., & Franqui-Zannettacci, M. (1981). An approach to diagnosis of multiple sclerosis with cerebral evoked potentials (visual, auditory, somatosensory). In C. Barber (Ed.), *Evoked potentials* (pp. 593–603). Baltimore: University Park Press.

Peronnet, F., & Giard, M-H. (1981). Inter-hemispheric and inter-aural differences in the human auditory evoked potential. In C. Barber (Ed.), *Evoked potentials* (pp. 317-324). Baltimore: University Park Press.

Peronnet, F., & Michel, F. (1977). The asymmetry of the auditory evoked potentials in normal man and in patients with brain lesions. In J. E. Desmedt (Ed.), *Auditory evoked potentials in man: Psychopharmacology correlates of evoked potentials* (pp. 130-141). Basel, Switzerland: Karger.

Peters, J. F., & Mendel, M. I. (1974). Early components of the averaged electroencephalic response to monaural and binaural stimulation. *Audiology, 13,* 195-204.

Pfeiffer, R. R. (1974). Consideration of the acoustic stimulus. In W. D. Keidel & W. D. Neff (Eds.), *Handbook of sensory physiology. Vol. V/1: Auditory system—Anatomy and physiology (ear)* (pp. 9-38). Berlin: Springer-Verlag.

Picton, T., Woods, D., Stuss, D., & Campbell, K. (1976). *Methodology and meaning of human evoked-potential scalp distribution studies.* Paper presented at the International Congress on Event-Related Slow Potentials of the Brain, Hendersonville, North Carolina.

Picton, T. W., & Hillyard, S. A. (1974). Human auditory evoked potentials. II: Effects of attention. *Electroencephalography and Clinical Neurophysiology, 36,* 191-199.

Picton, T. W., & Hink, R. F. (1974). Evoked potentials: How? What? and Why? *American Journal of EEG Technology, 14,* 9-44.

Picton, T. W., Ouellette, J., Hamel, G., & Smith, A. D. (1979). Brainstem evoked potentials to tonepips in notched noise. *Journal of Otolaryngology, 8,* 289-314.

Picton, T. W., Stapells, D. R., & Campbell, K. B. (1981). Auditory evoked potentials from the human cochlea and brainstem. *Journal of Otolaryngology, 10* (Supplement 9), 1-41.

Picton, T. W., Woods, D. L., Baribeau-Braun, J., & Healey, T. M. G. (1977). Evoked potential audiometry. *Journal of Otolaryngology, 6,* 90-118.

Polich, J. M., & Starr, A. (1983). Middle-, late-, and long-latency auditory evoked potentials. In E. J. Moore (Ed.), *Bases of auditory brain-stem evoked responses* (pp. 345-361). New York: Grune & Stratton.

Pratt, H., Martin, W. H., Bleich, N., Kaminer, M., & Har'El, Z. (1987). Application of the three-channel Lissajous trajectory of auditory brainstem-evoked potentials to the question of generators. *Audiology, 26,* 188-196.

Price, L. L., & Goldstein, R. (1966). Averaged evoked responses for measuring auditory sensitivity in children. *Journal of Speech and Hearing Disorders, 31,* 248-256.

Probst, R. (1983). Electrocochleography: Using extratympanic or transtympanic methods? ORL—*Journal of Otorhinolaryngology and Related Specialties, 45,* 322-329.

Reed, N., Hirsch, J. E., & Goldstein, R. (1980). Maturation of early and middle components AERs in infants. *Journal of the American Speech-Language-Hearing Association, 22,* 769-770.

Reneau, J. P., & Hnatiow, G. Z. (1975). *Evoked response audiometry: A topical and historical review.* Baltimore: University Park Press.

Robinson, K., & Rudge, P. (1977). Abnormalities of the auditory evoked potentials in patients with multiple sclerosis. *Brain, 100,* 19-40.

Robinson, K., & Rudge, P. (F1978). The use of the auditory evoked potential in the diagnosis of multiple sclerosis. *Journal of Neurological Sciences, 45,* 235-244.

Rose, D. E., Keating, L. W., Hedgecock, L. D., Miller, K. E., & Schreurs, K. K. (1972). A comparison of evoked response audiometry and routine clinical audiometry. *Audiology, 11*, 238–243.

Rose, D. E., Keating, L. W., Hedgecock, L. D., Schreurs, K. K., & Miller, K. E. J. (1971). Aspects of acoustically evoked responses-interjudge and intrajudge reliability. *Archives of Otolaryngology, 94*, 347–351.

Rose, D. E., & Rittmanic, P. A. (1968). Evoked response tests with mentally retarded. *Archives of Otolaryngology, 88*, 495–498.

Rosenhamer, H. J., Lindstrom, B., & Lundborg, T. (1981). On the use of click-evoked electric brainstem responses in audiological diagnosis. III. Latencies in cochlear hearing loss. *Scandinavian Audiology, 10*, 3–11.

Rowe, M. J. (1978). Normal variability of the brainstem auditory evoked response in young and old adult subjects. *Electroencephalography and Clinical Neurophysiology, 44*, 459–470.

Ruhm, H. B., & Jansen, J. W. (1969). Rate of stimulus change and the evoked response: Signal rise time. *Journal of Auditory Research, 9*, 211–216.

Ruth, R. A., Lambert, P. R., & Ferraro, J. A. (in press). Electrocochleography: Methods and clinical applications. *American Journal of Otology, 9* (Supplement), 1–11.

Sakabe, N., Arayama, T., & Suzuki, T. (1969). Human fetal evoked response to acoustic stimulation. *Acta Oto-Laryngologica* (Supplement 252), 29–36.

Salamy, A., Fenn, E., & Bronshvag, M. (1979). Ontogenesis of human auditory brainstem evoked potential amplitude. *Developmental Psychology, 12*, 519–526.

Salamy, A., & McKean, C. M. (1976). Postnatal development of human brainstem potentials during the first year of life. *Electroencephalography and Clinical Neurophysiology, 40*, 418–426.

Salt, A. N., & Thornton, A. R. (1983). The effects of stimulus rise-time and polarity on the auditory brainstem responses. *Scandinavian Audiology, 13*, 119–127.

Scherg, M. (1982). Distortions of the middle latency auditory response produced by analog filtering. *Scandinavian Audiology, 11*, 57–60.

Selters, W. A., & Brackmann, D. E. (1977). Acoustic tumor detection with brain stem electric response audiometry. *Archives of Otolaryngology, 103*, 181–187.

Shimizu, H. (1968). Evoked response in eighth nerve lesions. *The Laryngoscope, 78*, 2140–2152.

Skinner, P., & Antinoro, F. (1969). Auditory evoked responses in normal hearing adults and children before and during sedation. *Journal of Speech and Hearing Research, 12*, 394–401.

Skinner, P., & Antinoro, F. (1971). The effect of signal rise time and duration on the early components of the auditory evoked cortical response. *Journal of Speech and Hearing Research, 14*, 552–558.

Sohmer, H., & Feinmesser, M. (1967). Cochlear action potentials recorded from the external ear in man. *Annals of Otology, Rhinology and Laryngology, 76*, 427–435.

Sohmer, H., & Feinmesser, M. (1973). Routine use of electrocochleography (cochlear audiometry) on human subjects. *Audiology, 12*, 167–173.

Sohmer, H., Feinmesser, M., & Szabo, G. (1974). Electrocochleographic (auditory nerve and brain-stem auditory nuclei) responses to sound stimuli in patients with brain damage. *Electroencephalography and Clinical Neurophysiology, 37*, 663–669.

Sohmer, H., Gafni, M., & Chisin, R. (1978). Auditory nerve and brainstem responses: Comparison in awake and unconscious subjects. *Archives in Neurology, 35,* 228–230.

Sohmer, H., & Pratt, H. (1976). Recording of the cochlear microphonic potential with surface electrodes. *Electroencephalography and Clinical Neurophysiology, 40,* 253–260.

Sprague, B. H., & Thornton, A. R. (1982, November). *Clinical utility and limitations of middle-latency auditory-evoked potentials.* Paper presented at the annual convention of the American Speech-Language-Hearing Association, Toronto.

Staller, S. (1986). Electrocochleography in the diagnosis and management of Ménière's disease. *Seminars in Hearing (Electrocochleography) 7,* 267–277.

Stapells, D. R., & Picton, T. W. (1981). Technical aspects of brainstem evoked potential audiometry using tones. *Ear and Hearing, 2,* 20–29.

Stapells, D. R., Picton, T. W., Perez-Abalo, M., Read, D., & Smith, A. (1985). Frequency specificity in evoked potential audiometry. In J. T. Jacobson (Ed.), *The auditory brainstem response* (pp. 147–177). San Diego: College-Hill.

Stapells, D. R., Picton, T. W., & Smith, A. D. (1982). Normal hearing thresholds for clicks. *Journal of the Acoustical Society of America, 72,* 74–79.

Starr, A., & Achor, L. J. (1975). Auditory brainstem responses in neurological disease. *Archives of Neurology, 32,* 761–768.

Starr, A., Amlie, R. N., Martin, W. H., & Sanders, S. (1977). Development of auditory function in newborn infants revealed by auditory brainstem potentials. *Pediatrics, 60,* 831–839.

Stockard, J. J., Sharbrough, F. W., & Tinker, J. A. (1978). Effects of hypothermia on the human brainstem auditory response. *Annals of Neurology, 3,* 368–370.

Stockard, J. J., Stockard, J. E., & Sharbrough, F. W. (1978). Nonpathologic factors influencing brainstem auditory evoked potentials. *American Journal of Electroencephalogram Technology, 18,* 177–209.

Stypulkowski, P. H., & Staller, S. J. (1987). Clinical evaluation of a new ECochG recording electrode. *Ear and Hearing, 8,* 304–310.

Suzuki, J. I., & Yamane, H. (1982). The choice of stimulus in the auditory brainstem response test for neurological and audiological examinations. *Annals of the New York Academy of Sciences, 388,* 731–736.

Suzuki, T., Hirabayashi, M., & Kobayashi, K. (1983). Auditory middle responses in young children. *British Journal of Audiology, 17,* 5–9.

Suzuki, T., Hirai, Y., & Horiuchi, K. (1977). Auditory brainstem responses to pure tone stimuli. *Scandinavian Audiology, 6,* 51–56.

Suzuki, T., Hirai, Y., & Horiuchi, K. (1981). Simultaneous recording of early and middle components of auditory electric response. *Ear and Hearing, 2,* 276–278.

Suzuki, T., & Horiuchi, K. (1977). Effect of high-pass filter on auditory brainstem responses to tone pips. *Scandinavian Audiology, 6,* 123–126.

Suzuki, T., & Origuchi, K. (1969). Averaged evoked response audiometry (ERA) in young children during sleep. *Acta Oto-Laryngologica* (Supplement 252), 19–28.

Suzuki, T., & Taguchi, K. (1968). Cerebral evoked response to auditory stimuli in young children during sleep. *Annals of Otology, Rhinology and Laryngology, 77,* 102–110.

Tapia, M. C., Cohen, L. G., & Starr, A. (1987). Attenuation of auditory-evoked potentials during voluntary movement in man. *Audiology, 26,* 369–373.

Teas, D. C., Eldredge, D. H., & Davis, H. (1962). Cochlear responses to acoustic transients and interpretation of the whole nerve action potentials. *Journal of the Acoustical Society of America, 34,* 1438–1459.

Terkildsen, K., Osterhammel, P., & Huis int Veld, F. (1974). Far field electrocochleography, electrode positions. *Scandinavian Audiology, 3,* 123–129.

Thornton, A., Mendel, M. I., & Anderson, C. (1977). Effects of stimulus frequency and intensity on the middle components of the averaged electroencephalic response. *Journal of Speech and Hearing Research, 20,* 81–94.

Thornton, A. R. D. (1975). Statistical properties of surface-recorded electrocochleographic responses. *Scandinavian Audiology, 4,* 91–102.

Townsend, G. L., & Cody, D. T. R. (1970). Vertex response: Influence of lesions in the auditory system. *The Laryngoscope, 80,* 979–999.

Turner, R. G., Frazer, G. J., & Shepard, N. T. (1984). Formulating and evaluating audiological test protocols. *Ear and Hearing, 5,* 321–330.

Turner, R. G., & Nielsen, D. W. (1984). Application of clinical decision analysis to audiological tests. *Ear and Hearing, 5,* 125–133.

Turner, R. G., Shepard, N. T., & Frazer, G. J. (1984). Clinical performance of audiological and related diagnostic tests. *Ear and Hearing, 5,* 187–194.

Van Olphen, A. F., Rodenburg, M., & Verway, C. (1978). Distribution of brain stem responses to acoustic stimuli over the human scalp. *Audiology, 17,* 511–578.

Vaughan, H. G., Jr., & Ritter, W. (1970). The sources of auditory evoked response recorded from the human scalp. *Electroencephalography and Clinical Neurophysiology, 28,* 360–367.

Vedder, J. S., Barrs, D. M., & Fifer, R. C. (1988). The use of middle latency response in diagnosis of cortical deafness. *Otolaryngology and Head and Neck Surgery, 98,* 333–337.

Vivion, M. C., Wolf, K. E., Goldstein, R., Hirsch, J. E., & McFarland, W. H. (1979). Toward objective analysis for electroencephalic audiometry. *Journal of Speech and Hearing Research, 22,* 88–102.

Wada, S.-I., & Starr, A. (1983a). Generation of auditory brain stem responses (ABRs). I. Effects of injection of a local anesthetic (procaine HCL) into the trapezoid body of guinea pigs and cat. *Electroencephalography and Clinical Neurophysiology, 56,* 326–339.

Wada, S.-I., & Starr, A. (1983b). Generation of auditory brainstem responses (ABRs). II. Effects of surgical section of the trapezoid body on the ABR in guinea pigs and cat. *Electroencephalography and Clinical Neurophysiology, 56,* 340–351.

Wada, S.-I., & Starr, A. (1983c). Generation of the auditory brainstem responses (ABRs). III. Effects of lesions of the superior olive, lateral lemniscus and inferior colliculus on the ABR in guinea pig. *Electroencephalography and Clinical Neurophysiology, 56,* 352–366.

Weber, B. A. (1987). Assessing low frequency hearing using auditory evoked potentials. *Ear and Hearing, 8*(4 Supplement), 49S–54S.

Whitaker, S. R. (1986). Sequential electrocochleography and auditory dehydration testing in patients with Ménière's disease. *Seminars in Hearing (Electrocochleography), 7,* 329–336.

Williston, J. S., Jewett, D. L., & Martin, W. H. (1981). Planar curve analysis of three-channel auditory brainstem responses: A preliminary report. *Brain Research, 223,* 181–184.

Wolf, K. E., & Goldstein, R. (1978). Middle component averaged electroencephalic responses to tonal stimuli from normal neonates. *Archives of Otolaryngology, 104,* 508–513.

Wolf, K. E., & Goldstein, R. (1980). Middle component AERs from neonates to low-level tonal stimuli. *Journal of Speech and Hearing Research, 23,* 185–201.

Wolf, K. E., Pulec, J. L., Hodell, S. F., & Millen, S. J. (1979). *Auditory brainstem and middle latency responses from acoustic tumor patients.* Paper presented at the annual convention of the American Speech-Language-Hearing Association, Atlanta.

Wolpaw, J. R., & Pendry, J. K. (1977). Hemispheric differences in the auditory evoked response. *Electroencephalography and Clinical Neurophysiology, 43,* 99–102.

Woods, D. L., Clayworth, C. C., Knight, R. T., Simpson, G. V., & Naeser, M. A. (1987). Generators of middle- and long-latency auditory evoked potentials: Implications from studies of patients with bitemporal lesions. *Electroencephalography and Clinical Neurophysiology, 68,* 132–148.

Woods, D. L., Knight, R. T., & Neville, H. J. (1984). Bitemporal lesions dissociate auditory evoked potentials and perception. *Electroencephalography and Clinical Neurophysiology, 57,* 208–220.

Yanz, J. L., & Dodds, H. J. (1985). An ear-canal electrode for the measurement of the human auditory brainstem response. *Ear and Hearing, 6,* 98–104.

Zerlin, S., & Naunton, R. F. (1974). Early and late averaged electroencephalic responses at low sensation levels. *Audiology, 13,* 366–378.

Zerlin, S., Mowry, H. J., & Naunton, R. F. (1971). Effect of frequency and intensity on early components of the evoked cortical response. *Asha, 13,* 556.

chapter seven

Auditory evoked responses in site-of-lesion assessment

FRANK E. MUSIEK

Contents

Introduction

This chapter focuses on four categories of auditory evoked responses (AER) relative to their use in site-of-lesion determination. Electrocochleography is reviewed briefly with regard to its use in the diagnosis of endolymphatic hydrops. Major emphasis is placed on the auditory brainstem response (ABR), which commonly is used to define lesions of the eighth nerve and pons and to differentiate them from cochlear pathology. The middle latency response (MLR) and late auditory evoked response (LAER) are the other electrophysiologic measures to be reviewed. These middle and late responses, though beginning to receive much interest in site-of-lesion research, are not yet as reliable or refined as the ABR. These "later" auditory responses (or potentials) are used to assess a more difficult and

383

complex region, the cerebrum, which cannot be evaluated by the ABR. The scope of this chapter cannot permit a presentation of all the uses of AER. As a result, some valuable applications and discussions are omitted. What is presented will be referenced in a manner to provide a basis for further reading.

Electrocochleography (ECochG)

Interest in ECochG has been revived for three possible clinical applications: the diagnosis and monitoring of endolymphatic hydrops (Coats, 1981), the enhancement of Wave I amplitude for ABR interpretation (Coats, 1986), and for intraoperative purposes. Currently, there are three recording techniques for ECochG: (a) transtympanic, where the electrode penetrates the tympanic membrane to contact the promontory (Eggermont, 1976); (b) extratympanic, where the electrode is placed in the ear canal (Durrant, 1986); and (c) tympanic, where the electrode is placed on the tympanic membrane (Cullen, Ellis, & Berlin, 1972; Stypulkowski & Staller, 1987).

The transtympanic method, widely used in Europe, results in the largest and most readable recordings of the summating potential (SP) and action potential (AP). In the United States, however, its invasive nature has made it less popular than the other two approaches.

Comparing SP-AP amplitudes has been the basis for the prediction of endolymphatic hydrops, with a relatively large SP indicating presence of the disorder. It must be realized, however, that the SP-AP comparison procedure has only moderate sensitivity/specificity for detecting hydrops. (See Chapter 14 by Turner for a discussion of sensitivity/specificity.) In Staller's (1986) review of the literature, hydrops was correctly classified in 57% to 68% of the patients using ECochG. There are a number of factors that have served to impede sensitivity and use of ECochG for hydrops detection. For example, the SP-AP ratio is quite variable even in normal hearing subjects, especially if the absolute amplitude of the AP is small (Chatrian, Wirch, Edwards, Turella, Kaufman & Snyder, 1985; Staller, 1986). Also, Ménière's patients with either minimal or severe high-frequency hearing loss yield poor hit rates using ECochG for categorization (Coats, 1986). The highly variable diagnostic criteria often used for characterizing an hydropic condition may be a factor affecting ECochG accuracy in predicting Ménière's disease. Even when the disease is properly categorized, symptoms may fluctuate, a situation that many claim can be monitored by ECochG recordings over time (Ferraro, Arenberg, & Hassanein, 1985; Staller, 1986; Whitaker, 1986).

These factors, as well as variable effects of intensity (Chatrian et al., 1985), electrode type (Ferraro, Murphy, & Ruth, 1986), and waveform morphology relative to electrode placement in the ear canal (Coats, 1986), make ECochG a procedure to be used and interpreted with caution in defining endolymphatic hydrops.

ECochG could prove to be a valuable contribution in obtaining an otherwise unmeasurable Wave I for ABR interwave measures. Clearly, the transtympanic ECochG provides for an improved Wave I recording, and in a very high percentage of cases with hearing loss Wave I can be obtained. For tympanic membrane electrodes Ferraro and Ferguson (1989) reported recording a Wave I in eight hearing impaired subjects who by standard ABR recordings did not have a Wave I. Though the findings are not as convincing as with the tympanic membrane electrode, the foam type, extratympanic electrode may also help in obtaining a Wave I in some patients with an absent Wave I by conventional ABR (Musiek and Baran, in press). Along a similar line, Ruth, Mills, and Jane (1986) discussed the benefits of using extratympanic electrodes for recording the ABR in patients requiring intraoperative monitoring of certain auditory structures at risk for iatrogenic damage. In many cases of intraoperative monitoring, there is high-frequency hearing loss or during surgery the middle ear may fill with blood causing a conductive loss. In both of these situations Wave I becomes more difficult to obtain by conventional ABR. However, with a canal electrode chances of obtaining a Wave I is improved. ECochG also can provide information as to the status of the cochlea during surgery but it is not a good measure of neural integrity.

Though ECochG procedures appear to be potentially helpful in hydrops, enhancing Wave I, and for certain aspects of intraoperative monitoring, its universal clinical value is still uncertain. More research of the clinical efficacy ECochG is needed to determine its contribution to audiology and otology.

The auditory brainstem response

Since the first publications on site-of-lesion information (Robinson & Rudge, 1975a; Starr & Achor, 1975), the ABR has become the audiologic test of choice for evaluating neurological lesions of the eighth nerve and brainstem. The ABR continues to be such a powerful diagnostic procedure that it has taken a considerable period of time to realize the extent of its uses. Throughout this chapter the strengths and weaknesses of ABR are discussed. One of the primary considerations in the application of ABR relates to its generator sites.

Generator sites and ABR interpretation

Wave V is generated by the lateral lemniscus and more caudal auditory neuron tracts (Møller & Møller, 1985), which means that the more rostral parts of the (auditory) brainstem, including the inferior colliculus (midbrain) and medial geniculate bodies (caudal thalamus), are minimally or not involved in the generation of the first five ABR waves. Lesions limited to the midbrain and/or thalamus should not affect the ABR. Clinical cases, as well as animal data, have been reported to support this concept (Jerger, Neely, & Jerger, 1980; Musiek, 1986a; Wada & Starr, 1983). In most cases, however, lesions are seldom isolated to just the rostral brainstem in that they often affect the pons, which in turn results in ABR abnormality. The fact that the generator sites of ABR are limited to the pons and more caudal structures is important for clinical interpretation and test selection in evaluating brainstem disorders.

Patient selection for ABRs

ABR is a powerful tool for detecting eighth nerve and brainstem lesions. Careful judgment must be used in selecting appropriate patients for ABR testing. Failure to refer patients for ABR testing is perhaps the weakest link in diagnostic audiology, that is, once a patient is referred for ABR testing, the chance of detecting the presence of an eighth nerve or brainstem lesion is good. It is the patient not referred that is of concern.

It is important to realize that pure tone thresholds are not always a good indicator of an acoustic nerve or brainstem lesion. It has been well documented that some patients with various types of posterior fossa lesions, including acoustic neuromas, have very good hearing sensitivity for pure tones (Jerger & Jordan, 1980; Musiek, Kibbe-Michal, Geurkink, Josey, & Glasscock, 1986). Retrocochlear involvement, therefore, is not always anchored to peripheral hearing deficit.

As shown in a recent study (Musiek, Kibbe-Michal, et al., 1986) the patient's symptoms (otologic, neurologic, and auditory) may, in some cases, be better indicators of neuro-auditory involvement than are pure tone thresholds. It is well known that most brainstem lesions and lesions of the more rostral auditory system have little if any affect on pure tone sensitivity and routine speech recognition measures (Jerger & Jordan, 1980). These patients should have ABR testing and should not be overlooked because of normal or symmetrical pure tone audiograms. It should also be remembered that, though rare, some patients with fluctuating hearing and or low-frequency sensorineural loss, or sudden hearing loss could have an eighth nerve or brainstem involvement (often multiple sclerosis). Patients with these auditory findings and the appropriate constellation of symptoms, or lack of a definite diagnosis, deserve ABR work-ups.

Normal radiologic findings should not necessarily preclude doing ABR testing. Radiologic procedures reflect anatomy and not function; ABR is a functional test and may yield abnormalities not observed on radiologic exams (Josey, Glasscock, & Musiek, 1988).

On the other hand, some patients are not good candidates for ABR testing. This is not to say they should not be tested, but that the potential for ambiguous results should be clearly understood by the examiner and referring clinician. Patients with severe hearing loss, especially in the high frequencies, and tense, nervous individuals or patients with neuromotor problems (because of excessive muscle artifact) often are difficult to test.

It is difficult to provide general guidelines for patient selection for ABR, as each patient should be evaluated individually. However, thoughtful judgment should be given in deciding when to use ABR testing, because patient selection can influence the cost-benefit ratio of this procedure.

Sensitivity and specificity

Studies in which extensive analyses of published data on ABR have been conducted indicate that ABR has excellent sensitivity and specificity for appropriate categorization of cochlear and eighth nerve lesions (see Chapter 14 by Turner; Jerger, 1983; Musiek, Mueller, Kibbe, & Rackliffe, 1983; Turner & Nielsen, 1984). It is common to note sensitivity in excess of 90% for acoustic tumor detection using ABR, yet the false-positive rate for patients with cochlear impairment is relatively low (Table 7.1). These sensitivity-specificity data are relevant only for cochlear pathology versus eighth nerve tumors. It is doubtful if the ABR would be as diagnostically efficient for various brainstem lesions (Musiek, 1986b).

Although the ABR has good sensitivity-specificity in separating cochlear from eighth nerve lesions, there are certain populations that can provide diagnostic problems, and if these patients make up a major portion of a clinician's practice, sensitivity and specificity will suffer. Patients for whom the early ABR waves cannot be obtained and who have a delayed absolute latency for Wave V are difficult to evaluate. These patients are often elderly and have severe hearing loss at the high frequencies. Jerger (1983) has shown that when the PTA2 (the average of 1000, 2000, and 4000 Hz) exceeds 65 dB HL, the ABR (using a 90 dB nHL click) may become

TABLE 7.1
Some Major Studies Indicating the Sensitivity of ABR for
Confirmed Acoustic Tumors and False-Positive Rate as Tested
on Various Cochlear Lesions

Study	Hit Rate	No. Subjects	False-Positive Rate
Selters and Brackmann (1979)	92.7%	94	8%* (n = 266)
Clemis and McGee (1979)	92.0%	29	33% (n = 115)
Glasscock et al. (1979)	98.0%	49	7%* (n = 399)
Harker (1980)	94.6%	36	9% (n = 111)
Eggermont et al. (1980)	95.0%	36	
Terkildsen et al. (1981)	96.0%	56	9% (n = 71)
Bauch et al. (1982)	96.0%	26	25% (n = 229)
	χ = 94.9	326	15.2 (n = 1,091)

*Approximated. Table has been adapted from Musiek and Gollegly (1985).

difficult to interpret. Hyde (1985) has shown that the degree of 4000-Hz hearing loss and the age of the patient can affect the latency of Wave V in a nonlinear fashion. The nonlinearity seems to begin between 50 and 60 years of age and when the threshold at 4000 Hz exceeds 65 dB HL. Musiek, Kibbe-Michal, and Josey (1987) showed that ABRs remain relatively sensitive and specific if the patient's age is 65 years or less and if pure tone thresholds do not exceed 65, 70, and 75 dB HL at 1000, 2000, and 4000 Hz, respectively. This applies only when using an 80 to 90 dB nHL click as the stimulus. The specific effects of cochlear hearing loss on various ABR indices will be discussed later.

The sensitivity of ABR to brainstem lesions is not as high as for acoustic tumors, although much depends on the type of brainstem lesion. Almost all patients with pontine gliomas have demonstrated abnormal ABRs, though most reports (e.g., Chiappa, 1983) are limited to a few cases. House and Brackmann (1979) reported that 15 of 20 patients (75%) with a variety of extra-axial tumors of the low pons (cerebellopontine angle [CPA] area) had abnormal ABRs. In a recent study that analyzed ABRs from 23 patients with a variety of brainstem lesions, 17 demonstrated abnormal ABRs (Musiek, 1986b). The wide variety and nature of the many disorders of the brainstem make the ABR evaluation of these lesions more challenging than that of acoustic tumors. In addition, it is extremely difficult to acquire patients with various brainstem anomalies that can be tested validly by ABR. This is an area of ABR clinical application that requires better quantification.

Multiple sclerosis (MS) often is considered a brainstem disease, but this is not always the case (Rubens, Froehling, Slater, & Anderson, 1985). This disease affects the white matter and can include any of the anatomical areas of the brain containing myelin. In many cases of MS the auditory tracts of the brainstem may not be involved; this disease cannot be classified as exclusively a brainstem disorder unless neurologic and radiologic evaluations clearly indicate this is so. For this reason and several others which will be discussed later, ABR sensitivity to MS varies dramatically, though, on the average, it is about 60% (Chiappa, 1983; Jerger, Oliver, Chmiel, & Rivera 1986; Musiek, Gollegly, Kibbe-Michal, & Reeves, 1989).

Little data exist about the specificity of ABR in discriminating eighth nerve from brainstem lesions. Antonelli, Bellotto, and Grandori (1987) reported that eighth nerve and brainstem lesions can be correctly categorized a high proportion of the time by ABR, but a number of indices must be analyzed (i.e., interwave intervals, wave presence–absence). Though the ability of ABR to discriminate between eighth nerve and brainstem lesions is debatable, certain ABR patterns of abnormality are consistent with brainstem involvement. For example, an absent Wave V, with all other waves present and normal, is highly indicative and specific to brainstem involvement, as is an extended III-V interval. On the other hand, a I-III extension could represent an acoustic tumor or brainstem lesion. Also, because many acoustic tumors affect the brainstem and many brainstem lesions affect the auditory nerve, there can be overlap in the kind of ABR results observed in these two sites of lesion. However, this type of situation compromises the specificity of ABR for distinguishing eighth nerve from brainstem lesions.

ABR indices in site-of-lesion determination

There are a variety of ABR measurements that can be used clinically (Musiek, 1982; Musiek & Gollegly, 1985). These measurements are not of equal value diagnostically, but each has certain clinical situations for which it may be best suited. Indices of latency, waveform morphology, and amplitude ratio, as well as the effects of repetition rate and intensity level are discussed with reference to cochlear, eighth nerve, and brainstem involvement.

Latency indices in cochlear involvement. The focus here is on three latency measures: absolute, interwave interval (IWI), and interaural latency difference (ILD). In cochlear lesions, the absolute latency of Waves I, III, and V often depends on the degree of hearing loss at the mid to high frequencies (1000, 2000, 3000, and 4000 Hz), with the higher frequencies being more critical. For example, Bauch and Olsen (1986a) found that in cochlear pathology, more abnormal ABRs were noted when 3000-Hz hearing was depressed compared with 2000 or 4000 Hz, although a number of other reports suggest that 4000 Hz is a key frequency (Rosenhamer, 1981; Selters & Brackmann, 1977). The spectral energy of the stimulus also plays a critical role. Generally, the lower the frequency of the peak energy of the stimulus, the greater the delay in ABR latencies. The same stimulus (such as a rectangular electric wave) passed through different tranducers can result in acoustic events with different spectral components and different ABR results (Weber, Seitz, & McCutcheon, 1981).

It has been shown that as the hearing sensitivity at the high frequencies decreases, the absolute ABR wave latencies increase (Coats & Martin, 1977; Galambos & Hecox, 1978; Hyde, 1985; Rosenhamer, 1981). This latency delay is related to the time required for the traveling wave to reach an area of the cochlear partition that is sufficiently intact to allow a response (Don & Eggermont, 1978). Though the increase in absolute latency generally does correlate with increased high-frequency hearing loss, the variability that surrounds this trend is considerable (Rosenhamer, 1981).

Absolute latencies are normal in many cases of high-frequency cochlear hearing loss. If the stimulus is presented at a sufficient sensation level (SL), the cochlear-involved ear behaves similarly to a normal ear with regard to absolute latency. However, often a sufficient SL cannot be obtained at certain frequencies, and only a portion of the click's energy is effective (Gorga, Reiland, & Beauchaine, 1985). Therefore, one would expect a latency delay.

Some patients with cochlear hearing loss appear to have a much steeper Wave V intensity function than do normal hearing persons (Galambos & Hecox, 1978; Gorga, Worthington, Reiland, Beauchaine, & Goldgar, 1985; Hyde, 1985; Rosenhamer, 1981). The configuration of the pure tone hearing loss may be important in determining the shape of the latency-intensity function (Coats & Martin, 1977); flat cochlear losses, such as seen in Ménière's disease, seem to have shallower slopes for their intensity-latency function and result in less latency shift than do high-frequency losses (Gorga, Worthington, et al., 1985; Møller & Blegvad, 1976). In many cases of flat hearing loss, all intensity levels in which an ABR is present are within normal latency range, but there is great variability for this finding (Gorga, Reiland, et al., 1985; Hyde, 1985). Steep intensity-latency slopes and normal ABR at low SLs have been considered an indication of recruitment in cochlear-damaged ears (Galambos &

Hecox, 1978), though a recent report provides evidence against this concept (Gorga, Reiland, et al., 1985).

If high-frequency hearing loss does cause a delay in the absolute latency of Wave V, and the earlier waves cannot be observed, how can a clinician be sure that this increased latency is not reflecting an eighth nerve tumor effect? The answer to this still remains a major challenge to ABR interpretation. Certain formulas have been used to offset or account for absolute latency delays of sloping high-frequency cochlear losses (Jerger & Mauldin, 1978; Selters & Brackmann, 1977), and though these may be of value in some cases, they are not in others.

A formula proposed by Prosser and Arslan (1987) incorporates Wave V absolute latency of the pathological ear, the sensation level (re: 2-4 kHz pure tone threshold) at which a 90 dB nHL click is presented, and the latency of Wave V from a normal intensity function. Based on these factors, Prosser and Arslan properly categorized all patients with retro-cochlear involvement. Certainly, the preliminary data look appealing, but further evaluation is needed. Absolute latency measures, because of the variable effects of cochlear hearing loss, may be risky to use as the sole ABR index in site-of-lesion determination. It also has been shown that age and degree of high-frequency hearing loss both result in delays of Wave V (Eberling & Parbo, 1987; Hyde, 1985), and if these two factors can be controlled to some degree, separation between cochlear and eighth nerve lesions, based on absolute latency, can be improved (Eberling & Parbo, 1987; Musiek, Kibbe-Michal, & Josey, 1987).

Cochlear hearing loss is also a factor in the use of the ILD. Because the ILD is the comparison of absolute latencies of Wave V (Selters & Brackmann, 1977) or Wave III (Møller & Møller, 1983), much of the afore-mentioned discussion pertaining to the effects of cochlear hearing loss is applicable for this index. When the cochlear hearing loss is symmetrical, the ILD is most valuable; when there is asymmetry between ears, ILD interpretation is more difficult (Rosenhamer, 1981). Bauch and Olsen (1989) reported that as the difference in hearing threshold between ears for frequencies 2, 3, and 4 kHz increased, so did the ILD. A significant portion of the patients with asymmetrical and cochlear hearing loss yielded abnormal ILDs (Table 7.2). These investigators also demonstrated that as the hearing of the better ear became worse, more patients had ILDs that exceeded the criteria for abnormality. Hyde (1981) noted a 14% false-positive rate for patients with hearing loss (presumed cochlear) when a criteria of 0.2 ms ILD was used. Even in cases of symmetrical cochlear hearing loss, some patients have ILDs exceeding 0.3 ms (Musiek & Johnson, 1987).

There have been attempts to offset the effect of cochlear loss on the ILD. One strategy is to allow a 0.1-ms latency adjustment for every 10

TABLE 7.2
Percentage of Patients With Asymmetric Cochlear Hearing Loss
That Exceed Various Interaural Latency Difference (ILD) Criteria

Difference Between Ears	> .2 (ILD)	> .3 (ILD)	> .4 (ILD)
0–19 dB (n = 105)	13%	8%	7%
20–39 dB (n = 43)	28%	19%	9%
40–59 dB (n = 52)	42%	40%	28%
≥ 60 dB (n = 12)	82%	82%	82%

Adapted from Bauch and Olsen (1986), with permission.

dB of hearing loss at 4000 Hz greater than 50 dB HL (Selters & Brackmann, 1977; 1979). Another strategy is to use any ILD greater than 0.3 ms as a retrocochlear indicator, but if hearing loss is 65 dB HL or greater, 0.4 ms should be the criteria for abnormality (Clemis & McGee, 1979). These "adjustments" are useful for some patients but have definite limitations and, at times, may even confuse ABR interpretation. For example, in some patients, when a correction factor is applied, the "good" ear may end up with an abnormal latency delay relative to the ear suspected of neural involvement.

Most clinicians would agree that IWIs, unlike absolute latencies or ILDs, are minimally affected by cochlear hearing loss (Chiappa, 1983; Eggermont, Don, & Brackmann, 1980; Rosenhamer, 1981). Coats and Martin (1977) claimed that the I-V interval may actually decrease as a function of high-frequency hearing loss. Eberling and Parbo (1987) reported that this trend is more prominent in men than in women. However, Keith and Greville (1987) reported that the I-V interval is extended in notched type cochlear hearing losses, a trend that has not been reported before. Nonetheless, the IWI, when it can be obtained, is clearly the ABR measure least affected by cochlear hearing loss and is therefore a powerful indicator of eighth nerve or brainstem dysfunction.

Latency indices in eighth nerve and brainstem involvement. Because the absolute latency measure is affected by both cochlear and retrocochlear involvement, it has limitations in discriminating these lesion sites. However, group data clearly show that the absolute latency of Wave V is significantly greater for eighth nerve tumors than for cochlear lesions (Musiek, Kibbe-Michal, et al., 1987; Prosser & Arslan, 1987). However, on an individual basis, such as required in the clinic, the differentiation of cochlear and eighth nerve involvement can be most difficult when hearing loss is present.

Absolute latencies perhaps could be made more differential if criteria were established for various degrees of hearing loss or by using Prosser and Arslan's approach mentioned earlier. Currently, this measure simply cannot provide the specificity or sensitivity of the IWI or ILD.

The ILD has excellent sensitivity and specificity for the detection of eighth nerve tumors (Table 7.3 and Figure 7.1). Practically all published studies show better than 90% hit rates and relatively low false-positive rates (Bauch, Rose, & Harner, 1982; Clemis & McGee, 1979; Hyde, 1981; Musiek, Josey, & Glasscock, 1986b; Selters & Brackmann, 1979; Terkildsen, Osterhammel, & Thomsen, 1981). The ILD criteria for abnormality assumed ranges from >0.2 to >0.4 ms (Bauch et al., 1982; Bauch & Olsen, 1989; Selters & Brackmann, 1977). Perhaps the most commonly recommended ILD criterion for retrocochlear involvement is >0.3 ms (Clemis & McGee, 1979; Hyde, 1981; Musiek, Josey, & Glasscock, 1986b; Terkildsen et al., 1981; Thomsen, Terkildsen, & Osterhammel, 1978). These criteria, as mentioned earlier, may be adjusted to offset the effects of cochlear hearing loss.

Though there have been numerous reports on ILDs in patients with acoustic neuromas, few data are available for this measure in patients with brainstem lesions. This lack of data prompted a recent study at our center (Musiek, Johnson, Gollegly, Josey, & Glasscock, 1989). Our findings in patients with brainstem lesions showed the ILD to be much less sensitive for this group than in patients with acoustic tumors (Table 7.3). This probably occurs because brainstem lesions can affect both ipsilateral and contralateral auditory tracts. Therefore, ABRs from each ear may be delayed,

TABLE 7.3
Interaural Latency Difference (ILD) Data for Eighth Nerve (VIIIn) Tumors and Brainstem (BS) Lesions with Bilaterally Symmetrical Hearing

ILD	VIIIn (n = 16)	BS (n = 16)
> .2 ms	16 (100%)	10 (63%)
> .3 ms	16 (100%)	9 (56%)
> .4 ms	16 (100%)	8 (50%)

Note. All above patients had bilaterally symmetrical hearing (within 10dB 500–4000 Hz).

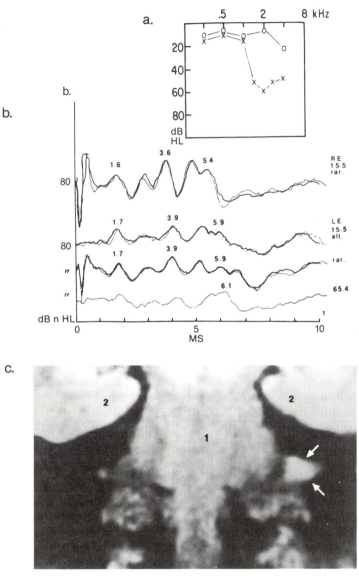

Figure 7.1.   Audiogram (a), ABR (b), and MRI (c) of a 48-year-old woman with a 2-year history of hearing difficulty in the left ear. No tinnitus or balance problems were noted. Neurological exam was normal. This patient had a very small (0.5 cm) acoustic neuroma on the left side. The ABR shows an unusual morphology in the area of Wave V for a rarefaction click. This was not as evident with an alternating click, or at a high rep rate. The ILD was the primary abnormality in this case. The MRI shows the tumor (arrows) at the most medial aspect of the internal auditory meatus where the auditory nerve emerges to connect to caudal and posterior-lateral aspect of the pons (1). The cerebellar hemispheres are also evident (2).

but not necessarily one more significantly than the other. Because most acoustic tumors are unilateral and affect generators ipsilateral to the side with the lesion, latency differences between ears are likely to occur.

The IWI, when the necessary waves can be obtained, is probably the most powerful diagnostic index for eighth nerve and brainstem lesions. In acoustic neuromas the I-III interval is the one most often extended (Eggermont et al., 1980; Møller & Møller, 1983; Musiek, Josey, & Glasscock, 1986b), although the III-V can also be affected by these tumors (Musiek, Josey, & Glasscock, 1986b). It also must be realized that an extended I-III does not always result in an extended I-V interval; all IWIs (I-III, III-V, and I-V) must be considered when they are measurable (Musiek, Josey, & Glasscock, 1986b). This may slightly increase the false-positive rate for nontumor patients but is clinically worthwhile, as it should reduce the number of false-negatives.

Though there is considerable overlap of IWI effects in eighth nerve and brainstem lesions, there are some group trends that may help separate these lesion sites. Antonelli et al. (1987) and others (Chiappa, 1983; Lynn & Verma, 1985; Starr & Hamilton, 1976) have shown that the earlier wave intervals (I-II and I-III) are affected more by eighth nerve lesions, whereas the later intervals (III-V) are affected more by brainstem involvement. In some cases the IWIs have been able to differentiate lesions of the upper pons and midbrain from the lower pons (Antonelli et al., 1987; Gilroy, Lynn, Ristow, & Pellerin, 1977; Hashimoto, Ishiyama, & Tozuka, 1979), but this type of interpretation must still be viewed as tenuous. Because many brainstem lesions have secondary effects (edema, vascular insufficiency, etc.), Waves III and V have multiple generators, and the brainstem is so compact and neurally complex that defining the precise locus of brainstem involvement is often beyond ABR capability. It should be kept in mind, however, that identifying the presence of a lesion regardless of its site in the brainstem is what is critical. Radiologic procedures can be used to identify the specific location of the lesion.

Waveform morphology (wave presence–absence). Poorly formed waveforms can at times provide clinical information about abnormality, but these judgments are most difficult to make and may be a result of a number of nonpathological factors (e.g., poor electrodes; muscle or electrical artifact). Therefore, this discussion focuses on wave absence, as it is a more reliable and interpretable finding with regard to its effect on ABR waveform morphology.

If cochlear involvement is severe enough, it will preclude obtaining any ABR waves. Reproducible ABRs often are not observed in cases of severe-to-profound high-frequency hearing loss. Therefore, when ABR waves are absent, it does not necessarily mean an eighth nerve tumor exists, but it cannot be ruled out.

In cochlear impairment (especially high-frequency hearing loss), the early waves (I and III) tend to be absent more often than Wave V (Fowler & Noffsinger, 1983; Musiek, Kibbe-Michal, et al., 1987; Selters & Brackmann, 1977). As with normal hearing individuals, Wave V is the most robust wave in patients with cochlear hearing loss.

Total absence of the main ABR waves (I, III, and V) occurs in a significant portion of patients with eighth nerve tumors. Several investigators have indicated that nearly one-half of the patients with acoustic tumors have totally absent ABRs (Bauch, Olsen, & Harner, 1983; Selters & Brackmann, 1977, 1979). Other reports show the incidence of ABR absence in acoustic tumors to be about 30% (Harker, 1980; Musiek et al., 1986a; Rosenhall, 1981), whereas in a few instances it has reportedly been less than 20% (Clemis & McGee, 1979; Terkildsen et al., 1981). In almost one-half of the cases of acoustic neuromas Wave I is absent, making it difficult to use various IWI measures (Figure 7.2). This remains one of several major shortcomings and challenges of the diagnostic ABR. As mentioned earlier, the development of a noninvasive, clinically feasible ear canal or tympanic membrane electrode for electrocochleography may solve this dilemma by providing a means for a more reliable measurement of Wave I (Stypulkowski & Staller, 1987).

An eighth nerve or brainstem lesion is a strong possibility in clinical situations where Wave I is present and the later waves (III and V) are

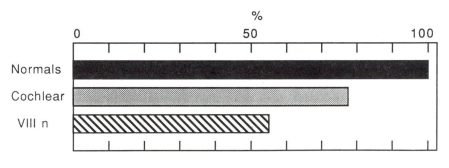

Wave I Presence

Figure 7.2. The presence of Wave I by percentage, in normal ears (N = 50), ears with cochlear hearing loss (N = 70), and ears with eighth nerve tumors (N = 61). The normal and cochlear ears were selected at random from clinical files, whereas the eighth nerve data were based on previously published work (Musiek, Josey, & Glasscock, 1986).

absent (Antonelli et al., 1987; Terkildsen et al., 1981). This occurs most often when there is good peripheral hearing (House & Brackmann, 1979; Musiek & Gollegly, 1985). When Wave V is absent, and Waves I and III are present, there is a high probability that only the brainstem is involved (Antonelli et al., 1987; Starr & Achor, 1975; Stockard et al., 1977, 1980). Antonelli et al. (1987) reported a high incidence ($\geq 90\%$) of Wave I presence and a relatively low occurrence of Wave V presence with low brainstem ($\approx 50\%$) and high brainstem (15%) lesions.

Repetition rate. The comparison of high- and low-repetition rate ABRs is done to enhance the probability of detecting an eighth nerve or brainstem abnormality (Figure 7.3). In pathological neural conditions (e.g., tumors and demyelinization), the refractory period of the nerve is increased (Tasaki, 1954) and high repetition rates would presumably serve to stress the nerve fiber(s) more than at low rates. A high stimulation rate would result in a nerve fiber firing before it totally recovers (from previous discharge), which results in decreased nerve conduction velocity (Tasaki, 1954), and hence a longer latency evoked potential. Because not all fibers in the system may be equally affected by pathology, a group of nerve fibers may have a variety of latencies, so that the compound potential becomes asynchronous (Campbell & Abbas, 1987) and a poor waveform results.

From a clinical perspective, there is evidence that cochlear pathology does not result in any greater latency shift of Wave V at high rates than that which results in a normal auditory system (Debruyne, 1986; Fowler & Noffsinger, 1983; Gerling & Finitzo-Hieber, 1983). In cochlear hearing loss it is important that the morphology of Wave V is reasonably good before using a high repetition rate. A poor Wave V at a low repetition rate may disappear at a high rate and not indicate a central nervous system (CNS) problem. The criteria for determining an abnormal amount of shift in comparing low and high rates has not been well-documented. For adults, Hecox (1980) suggested using 0.006 ms, multiplied by the difference between high and low repetition rates, plus 0.4 ms. Musiek and Gollegly (1985) used a 0.1-ms shift for every 10 clicks per second increase, plus a variance factor of 0.2 ms. Wave V latency shifts greater than those permitted by these formulas may indicate CNS involvement.

There have been a variety of reports where a high-rate ABR has resulted in an abnormal shift or poor waveform morphology in patients with eighth nerve or brainstem lesions (Campbell & Abbas, 1987; Gerling & Finitzo-Hieber, 1983; Paludetti, Maurizi, & Ottaviani, 1983; Weber & Fujikawa, 1977; Yagi & Kaga, 1979).

Abnormal findings also have been noted in patients with multiple sclerosis (MS; Antonelli, Bellotto, Bertazzolli, Busnelli, Castro, Felisati,

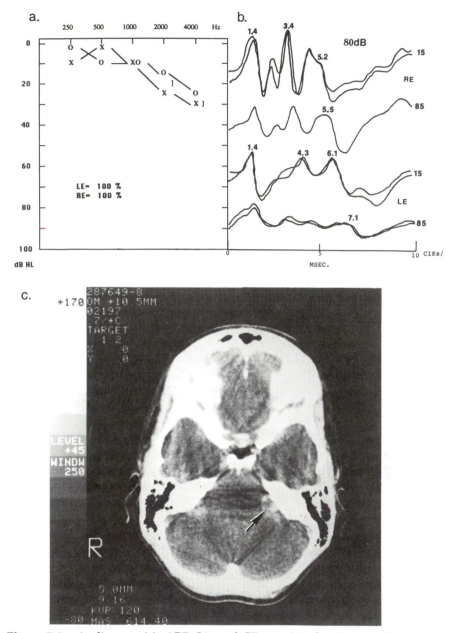

Figure 7.3. Audiogram (a), ABR (b), and CT scan (c) of a 34-year-old woman who complained of tinnitus, fluctuating hearing, and a blocked sensation in the left ear, present for about 6 months. There was no complaint of any type of balance disorder. An acoustic tumor slightly more than 1 cm in size was confirmed at surgery. The ABR from the left ear reveals an abnormal I-III, ILD and high rep rate shift.

& Romagnoli, 1986; Robinson & Rudge, 1977; Stockard & Rossiter, 1977). Despite these reports, high rates often do not enhance ABR sensitivity to CNS involvement (Campbell & Abbas, 1987; Chiappa, 1983). It does seem evident that increased rates may be of help in defining CNS involvement on an individual basis. This, coupled with the fact that there is little time and effort involved in doing a high-rate ABR, make it a viable clinical procedure.

Amplitude ratio.   In animal experiments in which specific brainstem lesions have been made, ABR amplitudes are generally affected more than latencies (Wada & Starr, 1983). Although ABR wave amplitudes are sensitive to neural lesions, clinical application of this measurement has not met with much success, primarily because of great intra- and intersubject variability. An alternative to absolute amplitude measures is the V-I amplitude ratio. This measure has less variability but still must be used with caution (Chiappa, 1983; Rowe, 1981), and a variety of recording and stimulus parameters must be controlled (Musiek, Kibbe, Rackliffe, & Weider, 1984). Normative data from a number of studies indicate Wave V to be consistently larger than Wave I, which is the basis for clinical use of amplitude ratios (Chiappa, Gladstone, & Young, 1979; Musiek, Kibbe, et al., 1984; Rowe, 1978). A study at our center (Musiek, Kibbe, et al., 1984) showed that 44% of the patients with retrocochlear pathology, 0% of the patients with cochlear lesions, and 8% of the patients with normal hearing demonstrated abnormal amplitude ratios (Figure 7.4). Intensity, rate, filtering, click polarity, and electrode montage were kept constant. Wave I and Wave V absolute amplitudes also had to replicate within 20% to be used in this study. Other reports have shown the V-I amplitude ratio to be of value in detecting neurological involvement (Rosenhall, Hedner, & Bjorkman, 1981; Stockard & Rossiter, 1977). It has also been observed that in some patients with brainstem involvement Waves I or II become larger than normal, affecting the V-I amplitude ratio (Musiek, Weider, & Mueller, 1983; Starr & Achor, 1975). Factors such as stimulus intensity and rate, filtering, electrode position, and the type of averager used can affect amplitude measures (Chiappa, 1983; Musiek, Kibbe, et al., 1984; Rowe, 1978, 1981). With this in mind, investigators should collect their own norms and establish their own criteria for the V-I amplitude ratio.

Intensity function.   ABRs conducted at more than one intensity, especially when hearing is normal, can be of value in site-of-lesion assessment. In situations in which it is difficult to discern Wave V, a drop in intensity will often reduce the amplitude of other waves and Wave V will be relatively more prominent (Starr & Achor, 1975). Also, a lower intensity may help in detecting or enhancing abnormality in the ABR waveform (Figure 7.5). In our clinic, intensities of 60 and 80 dB nHL are used for site-of-lesion testing. As shown, neurologic lesions can affect the ABR threshold estimate, but the quantification and factors surrounding this effect await further research. Nonetheless, this concept is an important one in ABR threshold testing of neurologically involved patients.

ABR indices in perspective

Not all of the ABR indices mentioned are of equal diagnostic value. In certain situations some indices cannot be employed and the clinician must use whatever is available. The latency measures, especially the IWI and ILD, are overall the most valid and reliable diagnostic ABR measures. The other indices must be used with more caution, as they probably do not have the validity and reliability of the latency measures. Clinical situations do occur, however, in which the "softer" indices can be highly predictive. For example, an absent Wave V with Waves I and III present strongly suggests brainstem involvement. Another strong indicator of neurologic involvement would be a normal waveform at a low rate and an absent response at a high rate. The value of a given ABR index must be assessed on an individual basis, with consideration given to the validity, reliability, time required, and utility of the data.

Laterality aspects of ABR

One of the intriguing and diagnostically informative aspects of ABR is its laterality effect. In small unilateral acoustic tumors the ABR abnormality is ipsilateral to the side of the lesion with essentially no effect on the opposite ear. However, if the acoustic tumor is large, an ABR obtained from the opposite ear can also be affected (Møller & Møller, 1983; Musiek & Kibbe, 1986; Nodar & Kinney, 1980; Rosenhall et al., 1981; Shannon, Gold, & Himmelfarb, 1981; Zapulla, Greenblatt, & Karmel, 1982). This finding indicates that the brainstem has been displaced, compressed, or in some way functionally compromised (Musiek & Kibbe, 1986; Nodar & Kinney, 1980; Rosenhall et al., 1981; Zapulla et al., 1982). It appears that this contralateral effect from a large tumor often modifies the ABR components in a particular way. Musiek and Kibbe (1986) found that in 11 of 15 patients with large acoustic neuromas, the ABR from the opposite ear demonstrated normal Waves I and III and abnormally delayed or absent Waves IV and V. If the acoustic tumor is large enough (>2 cm), bilaterally abnormal ABRs can result (Hall, 1983).

In brainstem lesions the ABR abnormalities are most often ipsilateral to the side of the lesion (Chiappa, 1983; Musiek & Geurkink, 1982; Oh,

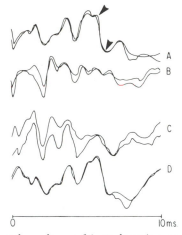

Figure 7.4. ABR tracings from four subjects focusing on the V-I amplitude ratio. Tracing A is from a normal adult; B is from a patient with multiple sclerosis; C is from a patient with a pontine lesion; and D is from a patient with Ménière's disease. Note the difference in the V-I amplitude ratio when comparing the patients with brainstem involvement with normal and cochlear involved subjects. (From Musiek et al., 1984, with the publisher's permission.)

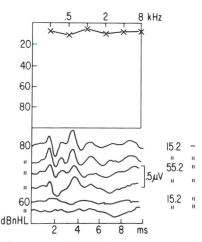

Figure 7.5. Left ear audiogram and ABR from a young adult patient who suffered a left, lateral pontine contusion. At 80 dB n HL, Waves I, II and III are normal; however, the IV-V "complex" is of low amplitude. This is even more noticeable at a high rep rate (55.2 clicks per second). The most striking abnormality is noticed at 60 dB n HL, where there is no ABR with normal pure tone thresholds for that ear. In this case the intensity function has enhanced the abnormality. This illustrates that in a patient with neurological involvement ABR may not be an accurate predictor of hearing threshold, an important consideration in testing neurologically-involved infants by ABR for hearing sensitivity. In this patient the ABR was entirely normal for the right ear. (From Musiek & Geurkink, 1982, with the publisher's permission.)

Kuba, Soyer, Choi, Bonikowski, & Vitek, 1981). Bilaterally abnormal ABRs are also noted in brainstem involvement, even if the lesion involves only one side of the brainstem. This finding is related to the compactness and numerous decussating auditory fibers in the brainstem (Chiappa, 1983; Oh et al., 1981). Midline lesions of the brainstem, especially of the low pons, often can result in bilateral ABR abnormalities (Musiek, 1986b).

At the midline in the caudal pons a heavy neural network of crossing fibers exist; therefore, it is highly probable that ipsilateral and contralateral brainstem fiber tracts are affected. This may also be the reason that a high percentage of intra-axial lesions yield abnormal ABR results, as intra-axial lesions are more midline than extra-axial lesions (Musiek & Baran, 1986). It is of special interest that contralateral ABR abnormality is seldom observed exclusively in brainstem involvement (Brown, Chiappa, & Brooks, 1981; Chiappa, 1983; Musiek & Geurkink, 1982; Oh et al., 1981). (See Table 7.4.)

These ABR laterality findings not only provide important clinical correlations but also provocative notions as to underlying neuroanatomy and generator sites for the ABR (Chiappa, 1983; Musiek, 1986b; Musiek & Kibbe, 1986).

ABR correlates to selected pathologies

There is an ever-growing list of neuro-auditory disorders for which ABR results can be abnormal (Rowe, 1981). Some of the more common and/or significant pathologies that occur are mass lesions, both intra- and extra-axial, as well as degenerative and vascular disorders.

Mass lesions (extra-axial). The extra-axial tumor originates outside but close to the brainstem, generally growing in a manner that directly affects

TABLE 7.4
ABR Laterality Findings in Brainstem Lesions

Investigator	Patients With Abnormal ABRs	Ipsilateral Abnormality Only	Bilateral Abnormality Only	Contralateral Abnormality Only
Oh et al. (1981)	8	7	1*	0
Musiek (1986)	10	6	4*	0

*Ipsilateral auditory brainstem response (ABR) was more abnormal in all cases.

the brainstem. The most common posterior fossa tumor (the general region in which CPA and brainstem tumors occur), is the acoustic schwannoma, for which ABR is an excellent diagnostic tool, as mentioned earlier. Meningiomas are the next most common extra-axial posterior fossa tumor (Huertas & Haymaker, 1969). Additional extra-axial tumors include fifth and seventh nerve neuromas and various tumors of the cerebellum. ABR sensitivity for these latter groups of tumors is not as good as for acoustic tumors (House & Brackmann, 1979; Rowe, 1981; Stockard et al., 1977) and is probably poorest for the cerebellar tumors (Stockard et al., 1977). It should be remembered, however, that most of these studies of ABR results on extra-axial brainstem tumors, other than acoustic neuromas, have small numbers of patients, and further study of these populations is needed.

Mass lesions (intra-axial). Intra-axial mass lesions, most commonly gliomas, arise from within the brainstem. ABRs were abnormal in 90%–100% of all brainstem gliomas reviewed, although no studies had a large series of patients (Brown et al., 1981; Hashimoto et al., 1979; Nodar, Hahn, & Levine, 1980; Starr & Hamilton, 1976; Stockard, Stockard, & Sharbrough, 1980). As mentioned earlier, these lesions (especially those in the pons) are often positioned so that the diffuse crossing auditory tracts of the brainstem are compromised (Musiek & Baran, 1986). This results in an abnormal ABR a high percentage of the time.

Degenerative lesions. MS is the most common degenerative disorder for which ABR is employed. The percentage of MS patients with abnormal ABRs ranges from under 50% to nearly 100% (Chiappa, Jarrison, Brooks, & Young, 1980; Grenman, Lang, Panelius, Salmivally, Laine, & Rintamaki, 1984; Stockard et al., 1977), with the average about 60% (Jerger et al., 1986). This great variability in ABR sensitivity reflects the nature of the disease (it may or may not affect the auditory tracts of the auditory nerve, brainstem, and cortex), the different classifications of MS (definite, probable, possible), varying degrees of peripheral hearing loss, differing ABR pass–fail criteria, and various methodological approaches (Verma & Lynn, 1985; Keith & Jacobson, 1985; Musiek et al., 1989; Noffsinger, Olsen, Carhart, Hart, & Sahgal, 1972).

In reviewing ABR results from various reports it appears that MS can provide practically every kind of ABR abnormality (Chiappa et al., 1980; Chiappa, 1983; Jerger et al., 1986; Keith & Jacobson, 1985; Musiek et al., 1989; Robinson & Rudge, 1977). Perhaps the most common ABR trends—if there are any—may be an extension of the III-V interval and the absence or degradation of the later waves (Chiappa et al., 1980; Stockard & Rossiter, 1977). These trends are grossly consistent with ABR results in brainstem involvement and are generally different from findings in acoustic tumors (refer to earlier discussion on latency and waveform morphology), though in some cases MS can mimic acoustic neuroma findings on ABR.

Patients with MS may have hearing loss as one of their initial symptoms, with or without deficits on the pure tone audiogram (Figure 7.6). These symptoms often are overlooked by both the patient and the clinician, as attention is focused more on acute visual or motor symptoms (Musiek et al., 1989).

Another degenerative neurologic disorder with strong correlates to ABR is Charcot-Marie-Tooth (CMT) syndrome. CMT syndrome, an inherited disorder, classically causes slow, chronic degeneration of peripheral nerves, resulting in distal muscle atrophy of the feet and/or hands (Cruse, Conomy, & Wilbourne et al., 1977). There also is evidence that CMT syndrome affects hearing (Cruse et al., 1977; Musiek, Weider, & Mueller, 1982). All ABR findings reported for patients with CMT syndrome have been abnormal, including no response in one individual with relatively good peripheral hearing (Figure 7.7), and an extended I-III interval in several others (Satya-Murti & Cacace, 1982).

Olivopontocerebellar degeneration (OPCD) involves specific atrophy of the (pontine) olives, pons and cerebellum, with occasional involvement of the spinal cord and ventricular system. The age of onset varies from adolescence to the sixth decade, and it has a strong genetic characteristic (Lynn, Cullis, & Gilroy, 1983). ABR results combined from four studies showed abnormality in 18 of 37 patients with OPCD (Lynn et al., 1983; Nuwer, Perlman, Packwood, & Pieter-Kark, 1983; Pederson & Trojaborg, 1981; Satya-Murti, Cacace, & Hanson, 1980). The most extensive ABR study (involving 20 patients) was conducted by Lynn et al. (1983), who showed most abnormal ABRs to be bilateral (10 of 11 patients), with a variety of latency and morphological abnormalities affecting both early and late waves.

There are a number of ABR reports on other CNS degenerative diseases, such as Friedreich's ataxia, Parkinson's disease, and the various leukodystrophies (see Chiappa, 1983; Rowe, 1981, for review); however, the small numbers of patients and the diversity of these disorders make it difficult to describe general ABR findings.

Vascular disorders. ABR abnormalities in brainstem strokes have been shown, in combining results from six major studies, to occur in 82% of the patients (Table 7.5). Transient ischemia of the brainstem, however, does not generally reveal a high incidence of ABR abnormality (Chiappa, 1983).

A vascular entity with relatively new ABR correlations is the vascular loop (Møller, Møller, & Jannetta, 1982). A loop or bulge, usually in the

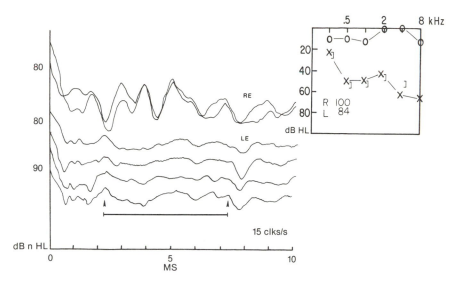

Figure 7.6. Audiogram and ABR from a 42-year-old woman whose initial symptoms were sudden hearing loss and tinnitus for the left ear, followed (within the same week) by mild unsteadiness. Left facial numbness and tingling occurred about 2 months later. The subsequent diagnosis was multiple sclerosis. The ABR is normal for the right ear. The left ear shows an extended I-V interval (5 ms) and the ILD is abnormal.

anterior inferior cerebellar artery (AICA) at the CPA region, can result in pressure on the low brainstem and/or on the seventh and eighth cranial nerves. Symptoms related to vascular loop syndrome can be facial spasm, dizziness, and hearing loss (Møller et al., 1982). The ABR IWIs are significantly affected, with the I-III being the most commonly prolonged interval (Møller & Møller, 1985). Surgical intervention can ameliorate patients' symptoms and improve their ABR results (Møller et al., 1982).

Aneurysm of the brainstem, a rare and serious condition, cannot only result in various vascular disturbances of other vessels of the brainstem but may also mimic a mass lesion (Musiek, Geurkink, & Spiegel, 1987). A basilar artery aneurysm in the low pons often is initially diagnosed as a CPA tumor, though in at least one well-documented case the ABR was slightly different than the classic ABR findings in tumor cases (Musiek et al., 1987). (See Figure 7.8).

It must be kept in mind that the main blood supply for the brainstem is the basilar artery, which is located on the ventral surface of the brainstem, whereas most of the auditory tract is on the dorsal-lateral surface (Musiek & Baran, 1986). Secondary and tertiary branches leading

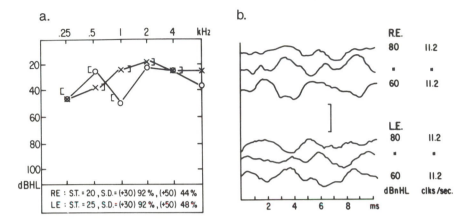

Figure 7.7. Audiogram (a) and ABR (b) from a 54-year-old patient with Charcot-Marie-Tooth (CMT) disease (see text). This patient had extreme difficulty hearing when using a telephone and whenever there was background noise. These complaints brought her to our medical center, where the subsequent diagnosis of CMT disease was made. The ABR shows essentially unreadable waveforms despite relatively good hearing sensitivity at the high frequencies. Speech discrimination scores revealed roll-over bilaterally (AD = right ear; AS = left ear; ST = spondee threshold; SD = speech discrimination; calibration marker is 0.5 microvolts). (From Musiek et al., 1982, with publisher's permission.)

to the dorsal-lateral areas of the pons would probably have to be compromised in order to adversely affect the ABR.

In summary, there is no question that ABR has greatly enhanced our ability to make accurate site-of-lesion determinations. It has changed the approach to site-of-lesion evaluation and is being used by increasing numbers of clinicians in a variety of disciplines.

Clearly, ABR has excellent sensitivity for detecting acoustic tumors and can differentiate these lesions from those of the peripheral end organ. It appears that the ABR is generally more sensitive to acoustic neuromas than are various lesions of the brainstem, though its sensitivity varies across different kinds of brainstem lesions. ABR may be of little value in detecting abnormality confined to the rostral most brainstem (midbrain, thalamus), as recent research indicates that the first five waves originate in the eighth nerve and pons (Møller & Møller, 1985).

There are a variety of indices that can be used with ABR in site-of-lesion testing. The ILD and IWI are probably the most robust and dependable measures; however, in the appropriate situation, rate and

TABLE 7.5
Auditory Brainstem Response (ABR) Results in Brainstem Stroke

Study	n	Abnormal ABR	Normal ABR	Sensitivity (in %)
Hashimoto et al. (1979)	15	15	0	100
Green and McLeod (1979)	4	4	0	100
Kjaer (1980)	15	13	2	87
Brown et al. (1981) (taken from Chiappa, 1983)	13	9	4	69
Oh et al. (1981)	7	6	1	86
Rogazoni et al. (1982)	11	6	5	55
TOTAL	65	53	12	(Avg.) = 82

intensity functions as well as V-I amplitude ratios and absolute latencies can be of value.

The one major difficulty surrounding ABR in site-of-lesion testing is when Wave I cannot be obtained. This situation often compromises the clinician's interpretation, but certain ECochG applications may help resolve this problem.

Middle latency response (MLR) in site-of-lesion testing

The MLR occurs after the ABR and within a time frame of 100 ms, poststimulus. It is composed of a number of negative and positive waves (Figure 7.9), which are generally larger than the ABR Wave V. More normative information on the MLR can be found in Chapter 6. In site-of-lesion evaluation, attention is focused on the Pa and Na waves because of their consistent presence in human and animal studies.

MLR does not appear to have the sensitivity to higher level auditory lesions that ABR has to eighth nerve or pontine lesions, although MLR

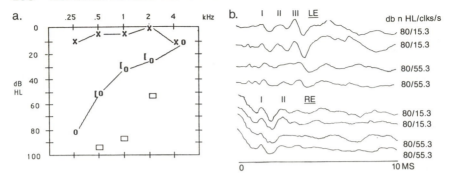

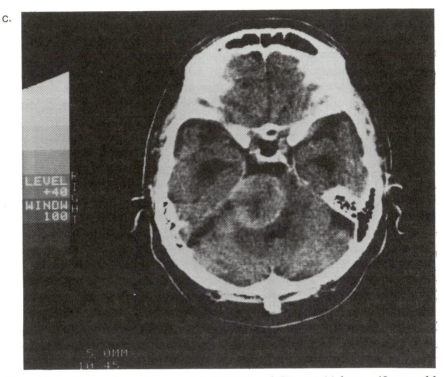

Figure 7.8. Pure tone audiogram (a) ABR (b) and CT scan (c) from a 48-year-old man with a large (4–5 cm), right-sided basilar artery aneurysm at the low anterior-lateral region of the pons. The audiogram reflects a discrepancy between ascending (indicated by the squares) and descending thresholds. The ABR shows only Waves I and II (which are of normal latencies) on the involved side. The ABR from the nonaffected ear revealed normal early waves (I, II, and III) but an absent or highly distorted IV-V complex. The right ear ABR indicates the auditory nerve to be functioning, but with dysfunction commencing at the level of the cochlear nucleus. The ABR from the left ear indicates compression and/or displacement of the brainstem (affecting the later waves) from the right-sided lesion, similar to what is often observed in large acoustic neuromas (see text). (From Musiek et al., 1987, with the publisher's permission.)

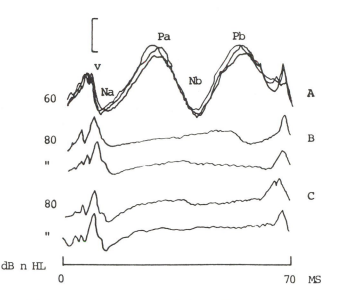

Figure 7.9. MLR from a normal, young adult (A). The next two tracings (B) are for right ear stimulation recorded at electrode positions T-3 and T-4, whereas the following two traces (C) are from the same electrode positions but are for left ear stimulation. The B and C traces are MLRs from a young adult with bilateral temporal lobe epilepsy. The ABR for both subjects can be seen at the left. The total absence of an MLR is consistent (in this case) with bilateral auditory cortex involvement. The stimulus was a click presented at a rate of 15 per second and filtering was 30–1500 Hz. The calibration marker at the top left equals 0.4 microvolts.

can be used to assess the integrity of the auditory system rostral to the pons. Another MLR advantage is that tone pips can be used at practically any frequency, increasing the opportunity to find a frequency of bilaterally similar sensitivity for interaural comparisons in patients with hearing loss. This is not to say that tone pips cannot be used with ABR, but that they are more easily accommodated with MLR.

If the MLR is to be used in detecting neurologic disorders, consideration must be given to filtering effects. As mentioned in earlier chapters, narrow filtering bands with sharp roll-offs may distort the MLR and lead the clinician to make incorrect judgments (Hall & Mackey-Hargadine, 1984; Kileny, 1983). Employing a wide filter band (i.e., 20-1500 Hz) with a gradual roll-off (6-12 dB/octave) is an important recommendation to follow.

Another advantage of using broadband filtering is that the ABR and MLR can be recorded simultaneously (Kraus, Ozdamar, Hier, & Stein,

1982). This can be a valuable procedure if the clinician is unsure if the brainstem or cortex is involved at the site of the lesion. In essence, with one set of recordings, integrity of the eighth nerve, brainstem and (auditory) cerebrum can be grossly checked.

In assessing cerebral lesions, especially in cases of unilateral damage, it is necessary to place the electrodes over each hemisphere (i.e., T-3, T-4, C-3, C-4, C-5, C-6) to best depict the problem (Kraus et al., 1982). Often the electrode that is closest to the lesion will provide the best indication of abnormality (Kileny, 1985; Kraus et al., 1982; Musiek, Geurkink, Weider, & Donnelly, 1984). Comparisons of responses from each hemi-sphere and ear can be valuable indices in determining unilateral abnor-mality, because there is little intrasubject variability in normal hearing subjects (Kileny, Paccioretti, & Wilson, 1987). However, for absolute amplitude measures (Pa Wave), intersubject variability in normal hear-ing subjects is relatively high (Kraus et al., 1982) and therefore is not a good differential measure. Absence of an MLR in patients 10 years of age or older with good peripheral hearing is a strong indication of higher auditory level dysfunction (Kileny et al., 1987; Musiek et al., 1984). How-ever, in younger, normal children, the MLR may be absent or delayed due to maturational effects (Kraus, Smith, Reed, Stein, & Cartee, 1985; Musiek, Geurkink et al., 1984).

Lesion effects—eighth nerve

Several investigators have reported increased latency of MLR waves for acoustic tumors (Harker & Backoff, 1981; Terkildsen, et al., 1981). Harker and Backoff (1981) reported that MLRs are present in a high percentage (97%) of acoustic neuroma patients but that there was not a high sensi-tivity (24% false-negative rate) to small lesions of this type. They point out that the MLR may provide some insight as to the size of the acoustic tumor, because, contrary to small tumors, large lesions often do affect the MLR. Though the MLR does have some interesting correlates to acoustic tumors, it is not as valuable as the ABR for evaluating this type of lesion.

Cerebral lesions

Based on its proposed generator sites, which include thalamic areas and the auditory cortex (Picton, Hillyard, Krausz, & Galambos, 1974), the MLR should be of greatest value in evaluating cerebral lesions. The published reports on MLR and lesions of the cerebrum can be divided into patients with unilateral lesions and those with bilateral lesions. Kraus et al. (1982) reported on 22 patients with one hemisphere involved and 2 patients with bilateral lesions. The temporal lobe was involved in the majority of these patients. In approximately 50% of these patients the MLR was normal. These investigators showed that the MLR abnormalities were most evident when recorded from the electrode over the damaged hemisphere and when the lesion was at or near the primary auditory cortex. Kileny et al. (1987) showed a significant reduction in the Na-Pa amplitudes from the affected hemisphere when compared with the normal hemisphere in nine patients with unilateral damage. These authors also showed significantly reduced Na-Pa amplitudes for patients with temporal lobe involvement compared with patients with cerebral lesions outside the temporal lobe.

Bilateral temporal lobe lesions often result in complete (central) deafness (Graham, Greenwood, & Lecky, 1980), and the MLR has often been applied in these patients (Woods, Clayworth, Knight, Simpson, & Naeser, 1987). Most bitemporal lobe lesions result in absent or abnormal MLRs (Graham et al., 1980; Ho, Kileny, Paccioretti, & McLean, 1987; Ozdamar, Kraus, & Curry, 1982; Rosati, Bastiani, Paolino, Prosser, Arslan, & Artioli, 1982; Woods et al., 1987; see Figure 7.9). However, some patients with bitemporal lobe lesions have recorded normal MLRs (Parving, Solomon, Eberling, Larsen, & Lassen, 1980; Woods et al., 1987). These latter results could be due to a number of factors, such as the extent of the lesion, its precise location with regard to how much of the auditory cortex is involved, and the duration of the lesion. Many factors such as these cannot be determined in detail with the present technology, making it difficult to evaluate the worth of the procedure. It is hoped that more data on MLR correlations to brain lesions may provide some answers to the many complex questions surrounding higher auditory processing.

Late auditory evoked responses (LAERs)

LAERs discussed in this section are the N1, P2, and P3 wave components (see Chapter 6, and Figure 7.10). The N1 and P2 waves are responses to externally generated (acoustic) events and are commonly termed *exogenous potentials*. These potentials can be obtained with the subject "passively" listening to the stimulus. The P3 (P-300) is a response to an internally-generated event (attention, recognition, categorization, etc.) brought about by cognitively processing acoustic stimuli; that is, the subject must manipulate the stimuli in a cognitive manner (Squires & Hecox, 1983).

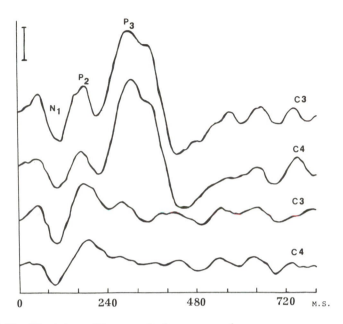

Figure 7.10. The late auditory evoked responses from a young, normal adult. The top two traces include the P-300 (endogenous) or P3 wave obtained by using a traditional oddball paradigm with 1000- and 2000-Hz tones. The bottom traces show only the exogenous, late responses (N1, P2) obtained employing a 1000-Hz tone. All responses were obtained from a right ear stimulus with the electrode recording sites shown at the extreme right of each tracing. The calibration marker at the left top equals 4.88 microvolts.

Like the MLR, the LAERs are attractive means for the evaluation of cortical and subcortical functions. LAERs are relatively easy to obtain, are present in nearly 100% of the normal population, are large in amplitude, and can be obtained with a variety of acoustic stimuli. On the other hand, LAERs can be variable and are affected by sleep, sedation, and various drugs (Goldstein, 1973). Though the specific generators of the late responses are not known, they are probably generated within the cerebrum (Vaughn & Ritter, 1970, and see Chapter 6).

A variety of acoustic stimuli (e.g. clicks, tones, phonemes, or even short words) can be used to evoke the late responses (Haaland, 1974; Squires & Hecox, 1983). The use of speech as a stimulus could prove most valuable in assessing various types of brain-damaged patients. Interestingly, however, one of the first site-of-lesion studies using LAERs was done on acoustic neuromas (Shimizu, 1968), which showed both N1 and P2 latencies increased and amplitudes decreased for the ear with the acoustic tumor, relative to the normal ear. Further research in this area was not pursued; instead, LAER was applied to cerebral lesions. Similar to the MLR, unilateral cerebral lesions can best be evaluated by electrodes positioned over each hemisphere (Peronnet & Michel, 1977). They showed reduced or absent N1 and P2 responses from electrodes placed over or near the damaged brain region, whereas electrodes placed over normal areas of the brain yielded normal responses. LAERs often demonstrate reduced amplitudes from the hemisphere with the lesion (Figure 7.11). Reports on late potentials and brain lesions subsequent to Peronnet and Michel's have revealed similar findings (Musiek, 1986b; Scherg & von Cramon, 1986).

Knight, Hillyard, Woods, and Neville (1980) reported significant N1 amplitude reduction for patients with temporal-parietal lesions, compared with normal hearing persons and with patients with frontal lobe involvement. In bilateral temporal lobe lesions, investigators and clinicians have turned to the LAER to provide insight into (auditory) cortical function, primarily because many of these patients present with cortical deafness. In a number of reports of patients with bitemporal lesions, the LAER has been essentially absent (Graham et al., 1980; Jerger, Weikers, Sharbrough, & Jerger, 1969; Michel, Peronnet, & Schott, 1980; Woods et al., 1987). Other reports on bitemporal lesions have shown decreased amplitudes and/or delayed N1-P2 waves (Albert, Sparks, Stockert, & Sax, 1972; Goldstein, Brown, & Hollander, 1975; Miceli, 1982; Rosati et al., 1982). Normal LAERs in bitemporal lesions have also been reported (Woods et al., 1987) but to a lesser degree than abnormal results. In analyzing the data in the review by Woods et al. (1987), and including two patients of our own, we found that 19 of 26 patients with bitemporal lesions had abnormal N1 and P2 responses. Of these 19 patients with abnormal findings, 12 had absent responses, whereas the others demonstrated amplitude, latency, or waveform abnormalities. Scherg and von Cramon (1986) reported good sensitivity of the LAER to various auditory cortex lesions. They commented that this increased sensitivity is related to obtaining potentials from tangential and radial dipoles, which can better measure the various spatial projections of auditory cortex activity.

The P3 is obtained by having the subject listen to two different sounds, such as 1000- and 2000-Hz tones. One group of tones (1000 Hz) occurs a high proportion of time (80%–85%), and are termed the *frequent* stimuli, whereas the other tones (2000 Hz) are termed the *rare* stimuli, occurring only 15%–20% of the time in a given trial. The subject is asked to attend to and count the number of rare tones while ignoring the frequent stimuli. The responses to the rare tones are averaged separately from the responses to the frequent tones. The focusing of attention (and other related, subtle cognitive events) on the rare tones results in P3 wave generation,

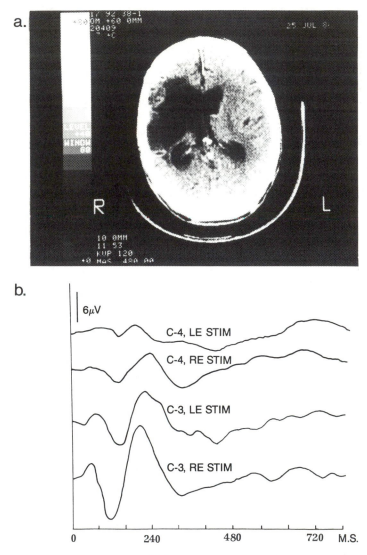

Figure 7.11. The CT scan (a) and late exogenous (b) auditory evoked responses (N1, P2) from a patient in his mid-fifties who suffered a right hemisphere stroke, resulting in much parietal and temporal lobe damage, several years prior to this evaluation. A talented musician prior to the stroke, this patient lost much of his musical skills and appreciation after the vascular accident. The evoked responses show markedly reduced amplitudes recorded from the right hemisphere (C-4) compared with the left hemisphere (C-3). Also, the ear contralateral to the damaged hemisphere yielded smaller amplitudes compared with the ipsilateral ear. The stimulus was a 1000-Hz tone presented at a rate of about 1 per second. This patient had essentially normal pure tone thresholds bilaterally. (Taken in part from Musiek, 1986b, with the publisher's permission.)

whereas the frequent tones are responsible for the N1 and P2 responses. By using this procedure, termed the *oddball* paradigm, N1, P2, and P3 responses can be obtained.

The P3 has not been highly utilized in defining focal brain lesions. However, a recent report revealed that P3 waves are absent in normal hearing, nondemented subjects with deep (subcortical) brain lesions (infarcts or tumors; Musiek, Gollegly, Verkest, & Kibbe-Michal, 1987). The most common application of the auditory P3 has been in the studies of aging, dementia, and disorders of attention. It has been well-documented that the P3 latency changes with age (Goodin, Squires, & Starr, 1978; Polich, Howard, & Starr, 1985). Though there is high variability (Kileny & Kripal, 1987), P3 decreases in latency into the teenage years, then begins to increase in latency at about the third decade (Goodin et al., 1978; Polich et al., 1985).

A number of studies have shown markedly increased P3 latencies in patients with various types of dementia (Canter, Hallett, & Growdon, 1982; Goodin et al., 1978; Squires & Hecox, 1983). Because of these findings, evaluation of patients with dementia has become one of the most common clinical uses of the P3 response.

The P3 responses also may prove helpful in monitoring the recovery of patients who have suffered head injuries (Figure 7.12) Levin (1985), in defining attention disorders in children (Loiselle, Stamm, Maitinsky, & Whipple, 1980), and in depicting auditory-language processing deficits post stroke (Squires & Hecox, 1983).

It must be remembered, however, that most P3 studies on various populations with CNS disorders are preliminary, with interesting but often perplexing results. Though the P3 has promise in diagnostic application, considerable research must be done on a variety of clinical populations before the P3 response can become a useful and dependable clinical tool.

Topographic brain mapping (TBM)

TBM provides a measure of electrical activity over different areas of the brain. This electrical activity is acquired from EEG and evoked potential measurements. The TBM EEG displays electrical activity in delta, theta, alpha, and beta frequency bands, whereas the evoked potential displays indicate changes in electrical activity related to sensory stimulation of an appropriate type. Though the EEG part of the TBM is critical to the optimal use of the procedure (Finitzo & Pool, 1987), the focus here is on the (auditory) evoked potential segment of the procedure.

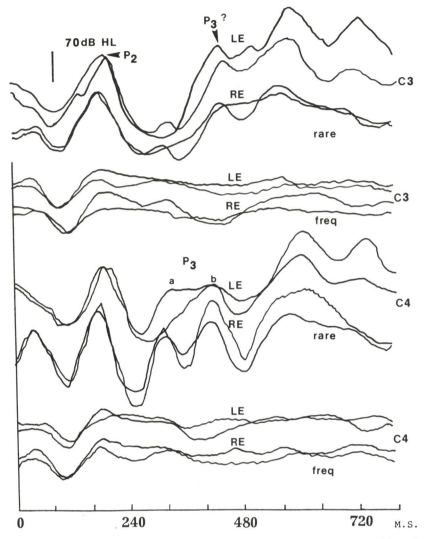

Figure 7.12. The P3, N1, and P2 evoked responses from a 39-year-old patient who suffered a closed head injury in an automobile accident. Although he attempted to return to work, he was unable to do his job, as he often became confused, had trouble following directions, and could not perform complex tasks. The "rare" traces recorded from the C-3 electrode site (left parietal area) show what may be the P3 (arrow), which is delayed to a latency of almost 450 ms for both left and right ear stimulations. Also, the amplitude of P3 is decreased relative to the P2 wave. The C-4 tracing of the P3 is closer to normal, although its amplitude may still be decreased and the waveform is not highly replicable. The C-4 tracing has a bifid P3 often termed 3a and 3b. This patient had normal peripheral hearing bilaterally. A traditional oddball paradigm was used to obtain the P3 response, with 1000- and 2000-Hz tones presented at a rate of about 1 per second. The calibration marker equals 4 microvolts (upper left).

TBM evoked potentials start with a classical evoked response procedure, but these potentials are recorded simultaneously from multiple electrode sites (usually 18–24) over the head. This provides topographical information about the evoked response. The various evoked responses can be obtained at multiple electrode sites and interpreted in the traditional manner, or further analysis can take place.

The TBM procedure can assess the evoked response at each electrode site every 4 ms for a 512-ms poststimulus analysis time period, producing 128 images. These 128 different images represent the varying characteristics of the evoked response over time (i.e., temporal displays of AER activity; Finitzo & Pool, 1987). Each image is played in rapid succession, which results in an image of continuous activity. This can be analyzed for high and low activity areas over the brain and can be color coded, which yields the map of activity (Finitzo & Pool, 1987).

The activity levels of certain brain areas can be compared with normal data to yield a significance probability map to help define abnormalities (Duffy, Bartels, & Burchfiel, 1981).

TBM is currently an experimental tool, and its clinical applications are certainly in their infancy. Interesting and provocative findings have been reported in patients with dyslexia (Duffy, Denckla, Bartels, & Sandini, 1980), dementia (Duffy, Albert, & McAnulty, 1984), spasmodic dysphonia (Finitzo, Freeman, Chapman, & Watson, 1987), brain tumors (Duffy et al., 1981), and strokes involving the middle cerebral artery (Pool, Finitzo, Tzong-Hong, Rogers, & Pickett, 1989).

In summarizing the information on the middle and late auditory evoked responses, there are several prominent notions. There is a definite need for electrophysiologic procedures that can evaluate the most rostral portions of the auditory system. These tests could complement the ABR and various central psychophysical tests to allow assessment of the complete auditory system. Currently, however, MLRs and LAERs do not appear to have the sensitivity or reliability of ABR or even the better central behavioral tests in site-of-lesion evaluation. It is difficult to determine the value of MLRs and LAERs in assessing cerebral involvement because so few studies have been reported using these procedures. More studies that correlate specific, well-defined lesions of the cerebrum with MLR, LAER, or TBM results would advance our knowledge of the late and middle potentials. In reviewing the studies that are available on MLRs and LAERs, it appears that abnormalities are observed when the auditory cortex and/or its association areas are compromised. This may or may not be true for the P3 response.

Multiple electrode recordings can also have an advantage in depicting cerebral abnormality with MLRs and LAERs (Kraus et al., 1982; Peronnet & Michel, 1977). Furthermore, the use of radial and tangential dipoles in the LAER evaluation of cerebral lesions could be of value, and research in this area should continue (Scherg & von Cramon, 1986).

Speech stimuli also can be employed with the LAERs. Using the P3 oddball paradigm, procedures could be designed to mimic various behavioral tests such as dichotic listening and auditory discrimination tasks. This could permit measurements of electrophysiological and psychophysical responses at the same time.

Further analysis of MLR, LAER, and TBM procedures is needed to allow their optimal clinical use. The informational value of these evoked responses has not been fully explored as it has been for the ABR, which provides distinct diagnostic information. It is also with the ABR that the greatest number of evaluations and greatest amount of clinical experience have been obtained. Not until there is a similar amount of clinical and basic research experience with the middle and late responses will their true overall value be assessed and appreciated.

Acknowledgments

Thanks to Mike Gorga, PhD, and Roger Ruth, PhD, for their review of an earlier draft of this chapter, and to Alice Witterschein and Cathy Coffin for their help with the preparation of this manuscript.

References

Albert, M. Sparks, R., Stockert, T., & Sax, D. (1972). A case study of auditory agnosia, linguistic, and nonlinguistic processing. *Cortex, 8,* 427–443.

Antonelli, A., Bellotto, R., Bertazzolli, M., Busnelli, G., Castro, M., Felisati, G., & Romagnoli, N. (1986). Auditory brainstem response test battery for multiple sclerosis patients: Evaluation of test findings and assessment of diagnostic criteria. *Audiology, 25,* 227–238.

Antonelli, A., Bellotto, R., & Grandori, F. (1987). Audiologic diagnosis of central versus eighth nerve and cochlear auditory impairment. *Audiology, 26,* 209–226.

Bauch, C., & Olsen, W. (1986). The effect of 2000-4000 Hz hearing sensitivity on ABR. *Ear and Hearing, 7,* 314–317.

Bauch, C., & Olsen, W. (1989). Wave V interaural latency differences as a function of asymmetry in 2000-4000 Hz hearing sensitivity. *American Journal of Otology, 10,* 389–392.

Bauch, C., Olsen, W., & Harner, S. (1983). Auditory brainstem response and acoustic reflex test: Results for patients with and without tumor matched for hearing loss. *Archives of Otolaryngology Head Neck Surgery, 109,* 522–525.

Bauch, C., Rose, D., & Harner, S. (1982). Auditory brainstem response results from 255 patients with suspected retrocochlear involvement. *Ear and Hearing, 3,* 83–86.

Brown, R., Chiappa, K., & Brooks, A. (1981). Brainstem auditory evoked responses in 22 patients with intrinsic brainstem lesions: Implications for clinical interpretations. *Electroencephalography and Clinical Neurophysiology, 51,* 38.

Campbell, K., & Abbas, P. (1987). The effect of stimulus repetition rate on the auditory brainstem response in tumor and nontumor patients. *Journal of Speech and Hearing Research, 30,* 494–502.

Canter, N., Hallett, M., & Growdon, J. (1982). Lecithin does not affect EEG spectroanalysis or P-300 in Alzheimer's disease. *Neurology, 32,* 1262–1266.

Chatrian, G., Wirch, A., Edwards, K., Turella, G., Kaufman, M., & Snyder, J. (1985). Cochlear summating potential to broadband clicks detected from the human auditory meatus. *Ear and Hearing, 6,* 130–137.

Chiappa, K. (1983). *Evoked potentials in clinical medicine* (pp. 125–128, 165–177). New York: Raven Press.

Chiappa, K., Gladstone, K., & Young, R. (1979). Brainstem auditory evoked responses: Studies of waveform variations in 50 normal human subjects. *Archives of Neurology, 36,* 81–87.

Chiappa, K., Jarrison, J., Brooks, E., & Young, R. (1980). Brainstem auditory evoked responses in 200 patients with multiple sclerosis. *Annals of Neurology, 7,* 135–143.

Clemis, J., & McGee, T. (1979). Brainstem electric response audiometry and the differential diagnosis of acoustic tumors. *The Laryngoscope, 89,* 31–42.

Coats, A. (1981). The summating potential and Ménière's disease: I. Summating potential amplitude in Ménière and Non-Ménière ears. *Archives of Otolaryngology, 107,* 199–208.

Coats, A. (1986). Electrocochleography: Recording techniques and clinical applications. *Seminars in Hearing, 7,* 247–264.

Coats, A., & Martin, J., (1977). Human auditory nerve action potentials and brainstem evoked responses. *Archives of Otolaryngology, 12,* 506–622.

Cruse, R., Conomy, J., & Wilbourne, A., et al. (1977). Hereditary hypertrophic neuropathy combining features of tic douloureux, Charcot-Marie-Tooth disease and deafness. *Cleveland Clinic Quarterly, 44,* 107–111.

Cullen, J., Ellis, M., & Berlin, C. (1972). Human acoustic nerve action potential recordings from the tympanic membrane without anesthesia. *Acta Oto Laryngologica (Stockholm), 74,* 15–22.

Debruyne, F. (1986). Influence of age and hearing loss on the latency shifts of the auditory brainstem response as a result of increased stimulation rate. *Audiology, 25,* 101–106.

Don, M., & Eggermont, J. (1978). Analysis of the click-evoked brainstem potentials in man using high-pass noise masking. *Journal of the Acoustic Society of America, 63,* 1084–1092.

Duffy, F., Albert, M., & McAnulty, G. (1984). Brain electrical activity in patients with presenile and senile dementia of the Alzheimer's type. *Annals of Neurology, 16,* 439–448.

Duffy, F., Bartels, P., & Burchfiel, J. (1981). Significance of probability mapping: An aide to the topographic analysis of brain electrical activity. *Electroencephalography and Clinical Neurophysiology, 51,* 455–462.

Duffy, F., Denckla, M., Bartels, P., & Sandini, G. (1980). Dyslexia: Regional differences in brain electrical activity by topographic mapping. *Annals of Neurology, 7,* 412–420.

Durrant, J. (1986). Observations on combined noninvasive electrocochleography and auditory brainstem response recording. *Seminars in Hearing, 7,* 289–303.

Eberling, C., & Parbo, J. (1987). Reference data for ABRs in retrocochlear diagnosis. *Scandinavian Audiology, 16,* 49–55.

Eggermont, J. (1976). Summating potentials in electrocochleography: Relation to hearing disorders. In R. Ruben, C. Elberling, & G. Salomon (Eds.), *Electrocochleography* (pp. 67–87). Baltimore, MD: University Park Press.

Eggermont, J., Don, M., & Brackmann, D. (1980). Electrocochleography and auditory brainstem electric responses in patients with pontine angle tumors. *Annals of Otology, Rhinology and Laryngology, 89,* 1–19.

Ferraro, J., Arenberg, I., & Hassanein, R. (1985). Electrocochleography and symptoms of inner ear dysfunction. *Archives of Otolaryngology, 111,* 71–74.

Ferraro, J., & Ferguson, R. (1989). Tympanic ECochG and conventional ABR: A combined approach for the identification of Wave I and the I-V interwave interval. *Ear and Hearing, 10,* 161–166.

Ferraro, J., Murphy, G., & Ruth, R. (1986). A comparative study of primary electrodes used in extratympanic electrocochleography. *Seminars in Hearing, 7,* 279–285.

Finitzo, T., Freeman, F., Chapman, S., & Watson, B. (1987). Windows on the CNS in vocal controlled disorders. *Asha, 29,* 201.

Finitzo, T., & Pool, K. (1987). Brain electrical activity mapping: A future for audiologists or simply a future conflict? *Asha, 29,* 21–25.

Fowler, C., & Noffsinger, D. (1983). Effects of stimulus repetition rate and frequency on the auditory brainstem response in normal, cochlear-impaired, and VIII nerve/brainstem-impaired subjects. *Journal of Speech and Hearing Research, 26,* 560–567.

Galambos, R., & Hecox, K. (1978). Clinical applications of the auditory brainstem response. *Otolaryngology Clinics of North America, 11,* 709–722.

Gerling, I., & Finitzo-Hieber, T. (1983). Auditory brainstem response with high stimulus rates in normal and patient populations. *Annals of Otology, Rhinology and Laryngology, 92,* 119–123.

Gilroy, J., Lynn, G., Ristow, G., & Pellerin, R. (1977). Auditory evoked brainstem potentials in a case of "locked-in" syndrome. *Archives of Neurology, 34,* 492–495.

Goldstein, R. (1973). Electroencephalic audiometry. In J. Jerger (Ed.), *Modern developments in audiology* (pp. 407–433). New York: Academic Press.

Goldstein, M., Brown, M., & Hollander, J. (1975). Auditory agnosia and cortical deafness: Analysis of a case with a three-year follow-up. *Brain Language, 2,* 324–332.

Goodin, D., Squires, K., Starr, A., (1978). Long latency event-related components of the auditory evoked potential. *Brain, 101,* 635–648.

Gorga, M., Reiland, J., & Beauchaine, K. (1985). Auditory brainstem responses in a case of high frequency conductive hearing loss. *Journal of Speech and Hearing Disorders, 50,* 346–350.

Gorga, M., Worthington, D., Reiland, J., Beauchaine, K., & Goldgar, D. (1985). Some comparisons between auditory brainstem response thresholds, latencies, and the pure tone audiogram. *Ear and Hearing, 6,* 105–112.

Graham, J., Greenwood, R., & Lecky, B. (1980). Cortical deafness: A case report and review of the literature. *Journal of Neurological Science, 48*, 35–49.

Grenman, R., Lang, H., Panelius, M., Salmivally, A., Laine, H., & Rintamaki, J. (1984). Stapedius reflex in brainstem auditory evoked responses in multiple sclerosis patients. *Scandinavian Audiology, 13*, 109–113.

Haaland, K. (1974). The effect of dichotic, monaural, and diotic verbal stimuli on auditory evoked potentials. *Neuropsychologia, 12*, 339–345.

Hall, J. (1983). Auditory brainstem response audiometry. In J. Jerger (Ed.), *Hearing disorders in adults: Current trends* (pp. 3–56). San Diego, CA: College Hill Press.

Hall, J., & Mackey-Hargadine, J. (1984). Auditory evoked responses in severe head injury. *Seminars in Hearing, 5*, 313–336.

Harker, L. (1980, August). *ABR in cases of acoustic tumors.* Paper presented at the Symposium on Auditory Evoked Response in Otology and Audiology, Cambridge, MA.

Harker, L., & Backoff, P. (1981). Middle latency electric auditory response in patients with acoustic neuroma. *Otolaryngology and Head and Neck Surgery, 89*, 131–136.

Hashimoto, I., Ishiyama, Y., & Tozuka, G. (1979). Bilateral recorded brainstem auditory evoked responses: Their asymmetric abnormality in lesions of the brainstem. *Archives of Neurology, 36*, 161–167.

Hecox, K. (1980, August). *ABR and brainstem involvement.* Paper presented at the Symposium on Auditory Evoked Response in Otology and Audiology, Cambridge, MA.

Ho, K., Kileny, P., Paccioretti, D., & McLean, D. (1987). Neurologic, audiologic, and eletrophysiologic sequelae of bilateral temporal lobe lesions. *Archives of Neurology, 44*, 982–987.

House, J., & Brackmann, D. (1979). Brainstem audiometry in neurologic diagnosis. *Archives of Otolaryngology, 105*, 305–309.

Huertas, J., & Haymaker, W. (1969). Localization of lesions involving the statoacoustic nerve. In W. Haymaker (Ed.), *Bing's localization in neurological disase* (15th ed., pp. 186–216). St. Louis, MO: C. V. Mosby.

Hyde, M. (1981). The auditory brainstem response in neuro-otology: Perspectives and problems. *American Journal of Otology, 10*, 117–125.

Hyde, M. (1985). Effect of cochlear lesions on the ABR. In J. Jacobson (Ed.), *The auditory brainstem response* (pp. 133–146). San Diego, CA: College Hill Press.

Jerger, S. (1983). Decision matrix and information theory analysis in the evaluation of neuroaudiologic tests. *Seminars in Hearing, 4*, 121–132.

Jerger J., & Jordan, C. (1980). Normal audiometric findings. *American Journal of Otology, 1*, 157–159.

Jerger, J., & Mauldin, L. (1978). Prediction of sensorineural hearing level from the brainstem evoked response. *Archives of Otolaryngology, 103*, 181–187.

Jerger, J., Neely, J., & Jerger, S. (1980). Speech, impedance, and auditory brainstem response audiometry in brainstem tumors. *Archives of Otolaryngology, 106*, 218–223.

Jerger, J., Oliver, T., Chmiel, R., & Rivera, V. (1986). Patterns of auditory abnormality in multiple sclerosis. *Audiology, 25*, 193–209.

Jerger, J., Weikers, F., Sharbrough, W., & Jerger, S. (1969). Bilateral lesions of the temporal lobe: A case study. *Acta Oto-Laryngology* (Supplement 258), 1–51.

Josey, A., Glasscock, M., & Musiek, F. (1988). Correlation of ABR and medical imaging in patients with cerebellopontine angle tumors. *American Journal of Otology, 9*(Supplement), 12–16.

Keith R., & Jacobson, J. (1985). Physiological responses in multiple sclerosis and other demyelinating diseases. In J. Jacobson (Ed.), *The auditory brainstem response* (pp. 219–236). San Diego, CA: College Hill Press.

Keith, W., & Greville, K. (1987). Effects of audiometric configuration on the auditory brainstem response. *Ear and Hearing, 8*, 49–55.

Kileny, P. (1983). Auditory evoked middle latency responses: Current issues. *Seminars in Hearing, 4*, 403–413.

Kileny, P. (1985). Middle latency (MLR) and late vertex auditory evoked responses (LVAER) in central auditory dysfunction. In M. Pinheiro & F. Musiek (Eds.), *Assessment of central auditory dysfunction: Foundations and clinical correlates* (pp. 87–102). Baltimore, MD: Williams & Wilkins.

Kileny, P., & Kripal, J. (1987). Test–retest variability of auditory event-related potentials. *Ear and Hearing, 8*, 110–114.

Kileny, P., Paccioretti, D., & Wilson, A. (1987). Effect of cortical lesions on middle latency auditory evoked responses (MLR). *Electroencephalography and Clinical Neurophysiology, 66*, 108–120.

Knight, R., Hillyard, S., Woods, D., & Neville, H. (1980). The effects of frontal and temporal-parietal lesions on the auditory evoked potential in man. *Electroencephalography and Clinical Neurophysiology, 50*, 112–124.

Kraus, N., Ozdamar, O., Hier, D., & Stein, L. (1982). Auditory middle latency responses (MLRs) in patients with cortical lesions. *Electroencephalography and Clinical Neurophysiology, 54*, 275–287.

Kraus, N., Smith, D., Reed, N., Stein, L., & Cartee, C. (1985). Auditory middle latency responses in children: Effects of age and diagnostic category. *Electroencephalography and Clinical Neurophysiology, 62*, 343–351.

Levin, H. (1985). Neurobehavioral recovery. In D. Becker & J. Povlishock (Eds.), *Central nervous system trauma status report* (pp. 281–300). Bethesda, MD: Neurological and Communicative Disorders in Stroke, National Institute of Health.

Loiselle, D., Stamm, J., Maitinsky, S., & Whipple, S. (1980). Evoked potential and behavioral signs of auditory dysfunctions in hyperactive boys. *Psychophysiology, 17*, 193–201.

Lynn, G., Cullis, P., & Gilroy, J. (1983). Olivopontocerebellar degeneration: Effects on auditory brainstem responses. *Seminars in Hearing, 4*, 375–383.

Lynn, G., & Verma, N. (1985). ABR and upper brainstem lesions. In J. Jacobsen (Ed.), *The auditory brainstem response* (pp. 203–218). San Diego, CA: College Hill Press.

Miceli, G. (1982). The processing of speech sounds in a patient with cortical auditory disorder. *Neuropsychologia, 20*, 5–20.

Michel, F., Peronnet, F., & Schott, B. (1980). A case of cortical deafness: Clinical and electrophysiological data. *Brain Language, 10*, 367–377.

Møller, K., & Blegvad, B. (1976). Brainstem response in patients with sensorineural hearing loss. Monaural vs. binaural stimulation. The signification of the audiogram configuration. *Scandinavian Audiology, 5*, 115–120.

Møller, M., & Moller, A. (1983). Brainstem auditory evoked potentials in patients with cerebellopontine angle tumors. *Annals of Otology, Rhinology and Laryngology, 92*, 645–650.

Møller, M., & Møller, A. (1985). Auditory brainstem evoked responses (ABR) in diagnosis of eighth nerve and brainstem lesions. In M. Pinheiro & F. Musiek (Eds.), *Assessment of central auditory dysfunction: Foundations and clinical correlates* (pp. 43–65). Baltimore, MD: Williams & Wilkins.

Møller, M., Møller, A., & Jannetta, P. (1982). BSER in patients with hemifacial spasm. *The Laryngoscope, 92*, 848–852.

Musiek, F. (1982). ABR in eighth nerve and brainstem disorders. *American Journal of Otology, 3*, 243–248.

Musiek, F. (1986a, October). *ABR and psychophysical tests in brainstem lesions.* Paper presented at the International Congress of Brainstem Evoked Potentials, New York.

Musiek, F. (1986b). Neuroanatomy, neurophysiology, and central auditory assessment: Part II. The cerebrum. *Ear and Hearing, 7*, 283–293.

Musiek, F., & Baran, J. (in press). *Canal electrode electrocochleography in patients with absent Wave I ABRs.*

Musiek, F., & Baran, J. (1986). Neuroanatomy, neurophysiology, and central auditory assessment: Part I. Brainstem. *Ear and Hearing, 7*, 207–219,

Musiek, F., & Geurkink, N. (1982). Auditory brainstem response (ABR) and central auditory test (CAT) findings for patients with brainstem lesions: A preliminary report. *The Laryngoscope, 92*, 891–900.

Musiek, F., Geurkink, N., & Spiegel, P. (1987). Audiologic and other clinical findings in a case of basilar artery aneurysm. *Archives of Otolaryngology, 113*, 772–776.

Musiek, F., Geurkink, N., Weider, D., & Donnelly, K. (1984). Past, present, and future applications of the auditory middle latency response (MLR). *The Laryngoscope, 94*, 1545–1552.

Musiek, F., & Gollegly, K. (1985). ABR in eighth nerve and low brainstem lesions. In J. Jacobson (Ed.), *The auditory brainstem response* (pp. 181–202). San Diego, CA: College Hill Press.

Musiek, F., Gollegly, K., Kibbe-Michal, K., & Reeves, A. (1989). Electrophysiological and behavioral auditory findings in multiple sclerosis. *American Journal of Otology, 10*, 343–350.

Musiek, F., Johnson, G., Gollegly, K., Josey, A., & Glasscock, M. (1989). The auditory brainstem response interaural latency difference (ILD) in patients with brainstem lesions. *Ear and Hearing, 10*, 131–134.

Musiek, F., Gollegly, K., Verkest, S., & Kibbe-Michal, K. (1987, November). *Auditory P-300 profiles for patients with cerebral lesions.* Paper presented at the meeting of the American Speech, Language, and Hearing Association, New Orleans, LA.

Musiek, F., & Johnson, G. (1987, April). *ABR interaural latency difference in patients with brainstem lesions and symmetrical hearing.* Paper presented at the 22nd Annual Scientific Meeting of the American Neuro-Otology Society, Denver, CO.

Musiek, F., Josey, A., & Glasscock, M. (1986a). Auditory brainstem response in patients with acoustic neuroma: Wave presence and absence. *Archives of Otolaryngology and Head and Neck Surgery, 112*, 186–189.

Musiek, F., Josey, A., & Glasscock, M. (1986b). Auditory brainstem response: Interwave measurements in acoustic neuromas. *Ear and Hearing, 7*, 100–105.

Musiek, F., & Kibbe, K. (1986). Auditory brainstem response Wave IV-V abnormalities from the ear opposite large cerebellopontine lesions. *American Journal of Otology, 7*, 253–257.

Musiek, F., Kibbe-Michal, K., Geurkink, N., Josey, A., & Glasscock, M. (1986). ABR results in patients with posterior fossa tumors and normal pure tone hearing. *Otolaryngology and Head and Neck Surgery*, 94, 568–573.

Musiek, F., Kibbe-Michal, K., & Josey, A. (1987, August). *Selected auditory brainstem response indices in patients with cochlear and eighth nerve lesions matched for hearing loss.* Tenth Biennial International Symposium for the International Evoked Response Audiometry Study Group, Charlottesville, VA.

Musiek, F., Kibbe, K., Rackliffe, L., & Weider, D. (1984). The ABR I-V amplitude ratio in normal, cochlear, and retrocochlear ears. *Ear and Hearing*, 5, 52–55.

Musiek, F., Mueller, R., Kibbe, K., & Rackliffe, L. (1983). Audiologic test selection in the detection of eighth nerve disorders. *American Journal of Otology*, 4, 281–287.

Musiek, F., Weider, D., & Mueller, R. (1982). Audiological findings in Charcot-Marie-Tooth disease. *Archives of Otolaryngology*, 108, 595–599.

Musiek, F., Weider, D., & Mueller, R. (1983). Reversible audiological results in a patient with an extra-axial brainstem tumor. *Ear and Hearing*, 4, 169–172.

Nodar, R., Hahn, J., & Levine, H. (1980). Brainstem auditory evoked potentials in determining site of lesions of brainstem gliomas in children. *The Laryngoscope*, 90, 258–266.

Nodar, R., & Kinney, S. (1980). The contralateral effects of large tumors on brainstem auditory evoked potentials. *The Laryngoscope*, 90, 1762–1768.

Noffsinger, D., Olsen, W., Carhart, R., Hart, C., & Sahgal, V., (1972). Auditory and vestibular aberrations in multiple sclerosis. *Acta Oto-Laryngology*, (Supplement 303), 1–63.

Nuwer, M., Perlman, S., Packwood, J., & Pieter-Kark, R. (1983). Evoked potential abnormalities in the various inherited ataxias. *Annals of Neurology*, 13, 20–27.

Oh, S., Kuba, T., Soyer, A., Choi, I., Bonikowski, F., & Vitek, J. (1981). Lateralization of brainstem lesions by brainstem auditory evoked potentials. *Neurology*, 31, 14–18.

Ozdamar, O., Kraus, M., & Curry, F. (1982). Auditory brainstem and middle latency responses in a patient with cortical deafness. *Electroencephalography and Clinical Neurophysiology*, 53, 224–230.

Paludetti, G., Maurizi, M., & Ottaviani, F. (1983). Effects of stimulus repetition rate on the auditory brainstem response. *American Journal of Otolaryngology*, 4, 226–234.

Parving, A., Solomon, G. Eberling, C., Larsen, B., & Lassen, N. (1980). Middle components of the auditory evoked response in bilateral temporal lesions: Report on a patient with auditory agnosia. *Scandinavian Audiology*, 9, 161–167.

Pederson, K., & Trojaborg, W. (1981). Visual, auditory, and somatosensory pathway involvement in hereditary cerebellar ataxia, Friedreich's ataxia, and familial spastic paraplegia. *Electroencephalography and Clinical Neurophysiology*, 52, 283–297.

Peronnet, F., & Michel, F. (1977). The asymmetry of auditory evoked potentials in normal man and patients with brain lesions. In J. Desmedt (Ed.), *Auditory evoked potentials in man: Psychopharmacology correlates of EPs* (pp. 130–141). Basel, Switzerland: Karger.

Picton, T., Hillyard, S., Krausz, H., & Galambos, R. (1974). Human auditory evoked potentials: Evaluation of components. *Electroencephalography and Clinical Neurophysiology*, 36, 179–190.

Polich, J., Howard, L., & Starr, A. (1985). Effects of age on the P-300 component of the event-related potential from auditory stimuli: Peak definition, variation, and measurement. *Journal of Gerontology, 40,* 721–726.

Pool, K., Finitzo, T., Tzong-Hong, C., Rogers, & Pickett (1989). Infarction of the Superior Temporal Gyrus: A description of auditory evoked potential latency and amplitude topology. *Ear and Hearing, 10,* 144–152.

Prosser, S., & Arslan, E. (1987). Prediction of auditory brainstem Wave V latency as a diagnostic tool of sensorineural hearing loss. *Audiology, 26,* 179–187.

Robinson, K., & Rudge, P. (1975a). Auditory evoked responses in multiple sclerosis. *Lancet, 24,* 1164–1166.

Robinson, K., & Rudge, P. (1977). Abnormalities of the auditory evoked potentials in patients with multiple sclerosis. *Brain, 100,* 19–40.

Rosati, G., Bastiani, P., Paolino, E., Prosser, S., Arslan, E., & Artioli, M. (1982). Clinical and audiological findings in a case of auditory agnosia. *Journal of Neurology, 227,* 21–27.

Rosenhall, U. (1981). Cerebellopontine angle tumors. *Scandinavian Audiology,* (Supplement 13) 115.

Rosenhall, U., Hedner, M., & Bjorkman, G. (1981). ABR and brainstem lesions. *Scandinavian Audiology* (Supplement 13), 117–123.

Rosenhamer, H. (1981). The auditory evoked brainstem electric response (ABR) in cochlear hearing loss. *Scandinavian Audiology,* (Supplement 13), 83–93.

Rowe, M. (1978). Normal variability of the brainstem auditory evoked responses in young and old adult subjects. *Electroencephalography and Clinical Neurophysiology, 44,* 459–470.

Rowe, M. (1981). Brainstem auditory evoked response in neurological disease: A review. *Ear and Hearing, 2,* 41–51.

Rubens, A., Froehling, B., Slater, G., & Anderson, D. (1985). Left ear suppression on verbal dichotic tests in patients with multiple sclerosis. *Annals of Neurology, 18,* 459–463.

Ruth, R., Mills, J., & Jane, J. (1986). Intraoperative monitoring of electrocochleographic and auditory brainstem responses. *Seminars in Hearing, 7,* 307–325.

Satya-Murti, S., & Cacace, A. (1982). Brainstem auditory evoked potentials and disorders of the primary sensoriganglion. In J. Courjon, F. Mauguiere, & M. Revol (Eds.), *Clinical applications of evoked potentials in neurology* (pp. 219–225). New York: Raven Press.

Satya-Murti, S., Cacace, A., & Hanson, P. (1980). Auditory dysfunction in Friedreich ataxia: Result of spiral ganglion degeneration. *Neurology, 30,* 1407–1053.

Scherg, M., & von Cramon, D. (1986). Psychoacoustic and electrophysiologic correlates of central hearing disorders in man. *Psychiatric Neurological Sciences, 236,* 56–60.

Selters, W., & Brackmann, D. (1977). Acoustic tumor detection with brainstem electric response audiometry. *Archives of Otolaryngology, 103,* 181–187.

Selters, W., & Brackmann, D. (1979). Brainstem electric response audiometry aocustic tumor detection. In W. House & C. Luetje (Eds.), *Acoustic tumors* (Vol. 1, pp. 225–235). Baltimore, MD: University Park Press.

Shannon, E., Gold, S., & Himmelfarb, M. (1981). Auditory brainstem responses in cerebellopontine angle tumors. *The Laryngoscope, 80,* 1477–1484.

Shimizu, H. (1968). Evoked response with VIIIth nerve lesions. *The Laryngoscope, 78,* 2140–2152.

Squires, K., & Hecox, K. (1983). Electrophysiological evaluation of higher level auditory processing. *Seminars in Hearing, 4,* 415–432.

Staller, S. (1986). Electrocochleography in the diagnosis and management of Ménière's disease. *Seminars in Hearing, 7,* 267–276.

Starr, A., & Achor, J. (1975). Auditory brainstem responses in neurological disease. *Archives of Neurology, 32,* 761–768.

Starr, A., & Hamilton, A. (1976). Correlation between confirmed sites of neurological lesions and abnormalities of far-field auditory brainstem responses. *Electroencephalography and Clinical Neurophysiology, 41,* 595–608.

Stockard, J., & Rossiter, V. (1977). Clinical and pathological correlates of brainstem auditory response abnormalities. *Neurology, 27,* 316–325.

Stockard, J., Stockard, J., & Sharbrough, F. (1977). Detection and localization of occult lesions with brainstem auditory responses. *Mayo Clinic Proceedings, 52,* 761–769.

Stockard, J., Stockard, J., & Sharbrough, F. (1980). Brainstem auditory evoked potentials in neurology: Methodology, interpretation, clinical application. In M. Aminoff (Ed.), *Electrodiagnosis in clinical neurology* (pp. 370–413). New York: Churchill Livingstone.

Stypulkowski, P., & Staller, S. (1987). Clinical evaluation of the new ECochG recording electrode. *Ear and Hearing, 8,* 304–310.

Tasaki, I. (1954). Nerve impulses in individual auditory nerve fibers of guinea pig. *Journal of Neurophysiology, 17,* 97–122.

Terkildsen, K., Osterhammel, P., & Thomsen, J. (1981). ABR and MLR in patients with acoustic neuromas. Scandinavian Symposium on Brainstem Response (ABR). *Scandinavian Audiology,* (Supplement 13), 103–108.

Thomsen, J., Terkildsen, K., & Osterhammel, P. (1978). Auditory brainstem responses in patients with acoustic neuromas. *Scandinavian Audiology, 7,* 179–184.

Turner, R., & Nielsen, D. (1984). Application of clinical decision analysis to audiological tests. *Ear and Hearing, 5,* 125–133.

Vaughn, H., & Ritter, W. (1970). The sources of the auditory evoked responses recorded from the human scalp. *Electroencephalography and Clinical Neurophysiology, 28,* 360–367.

Verma, N., & Lynn, G. (1985). Auditory evoked potentials in multiple sclerosis. *Archives of Otolaryngology, 111,* 22–24.

Wada, S., & Starr, A. (1983). Generation of auditory brainstem responses: III. Effects of lesions of the superior olive, lateral lemniscus, and inferior colliculus on the ABR in guinea pig. *Electroencephalography and Clinical Neurophysiology, 56,* 352–366.

Weber, B., & Fujikawa, S. (1977). Brainstem evoked response (BER) audiometry at various stimulus presentation rates. *Journal of the American Audiology Society, 3,* 59–62.

Weber, B., Seitz, M., & McCutcheon, M. (1981). Quantifying click stimuli in auditory brainstem response audiometry. *Ear and Hearing, 2,* 15–19.

Whitaker, S. (1986). Sequential electrocochleography and auditory dehydration testing in patients with Ménière's disease. *Seminars in Hearing, 7,* 329–335.

Woods, D., Clayworth, C., Knight, R., Simpson, G., & Naeser, M. (1987). Generators of middle and long latency auditory evoked potentials: Implications from studies of patients with bitemporal lesions. *Electroencephalography and Clinical Neurophysiology, 68,* 132–141.

Yagi, T., & Kaga, K. (1979). The effect of the click repetition rate on the latency of the auditory evoked brainstem response and its clinical use for a neurological diagnosis. *Archives of Otorhinolaryngology, 222,* 91–97.

Zapulla, R., Greenblatt, E., & Karmel, B. (1982). The effects of acoustic neuromas on ipsilateral and contralateral brainstem auditory evoked responses during stimulation of the unaffected ear. *American Journal of Otology, 4,* 118–122.

chapter eight

Auditory evoked potentials in clinical pediatrics

DANIEL M. SCHWARTZ

JAMIE A. SCHWARTZ

Contents

Introduction

With the exception of acoustic immittance, no other clinical assessment technique has had a greater impact on the subspecialty of pediatric audiology than the broad spectrum of auditory evoked potentials. Beginning with the application of late cortical auditory evoked responses to verify suspected congenital hearing loss in difficult-to-test children in the 1950s, auditory clinical electrophysiology has become a pediatric gold standard, both for hearing loss identification and for facilitating the diagnosis of neuropathology in children. Of the four primary classes of auditory evoked potentials (cochlear, brainstem, middle, and late), the short latency

429

brainstem auditory evoked response (BAER) clearly has achieved the greatest success toward providing a reliable, valid, and noninvasive means of assessing the functional status of the peripheral and central auditory network. As such, it has become well accepted in the pediatric community at-large, both for audiological and neurodiagnostic applications. One need only consult any general textbook in pediatrics or its subspecialties in neonatology, neurology, otorhinolaryngology, neurosurgery, anesthesia, and so forth to appreciate the diversity of medical and allied medical professionals that rely on this electrophysiological technique. Moreover, during the past several years there has emerged a small cadre of audiologists who work solely within the area of clinical electrophysiology, with some of them expending their greatest clinical effort in pediatric evoked potentials.

This chapter, like others of its type, focuses on the application of auditory evoked potentials in clinical pediatrics. Unlike other chapters that often serve as excellent general overviews of the topic with particular emphasis on literature citation, we have attempted to write an applied clinical chapter based on our dedicated experience in this field. As such, we hope that the practitioner will be able to apply many of the principles and practices that we have found ultimately successful. We openly admit that much of what is written reflects our professional biases; however, these clinical strategies were derived only after considerable investigation, and importantly, all are based on sound clinical and scientific rationale and/or empirical data. Finally, we have elected to concentrate primarily on the brainstem auditory evoked (BAER) response owing to the many variables that can affect the reliability and validity of the middle and late components with young children. For these later components we review briefly the characteristic features of the response and point out the methodological and conceptual flaws that hamper their use with infants and young children. We hope that this departure from the standard textbook chapter will prove appropriate and meaningful.

Principles of test selection

Although the application of diagnostic tests to differentiate ''normal'' from ''abnormal'' is commonplace in audiology, the mathematical relationship between the properties of these tests to the diagnostic information that they yield is not often considered. Understanding the relationships between results on a diagnostic test and the actual presence or absence of disease serves to (a) increase the likelihood of a correct diagnosis based on the results of a given test and (b) improve the clinician's ability to select the best test for each specific clinical situation. This section discusses concepts in clinical epidemiology that are central to the application of auditory evoked potentials in pediatrics. Appreciation of these principles is important to developing a rational approach to BAER testing, whether it be to screen for hearing loss in newborns or to identify the presence of neuropathology in a child or adult.

Operating characteristics of a test

Although several discussions on the application of clinical epidemiologic concepts to audiology have appeared over the past several years (Jerger, 1985; Schwartz, 1987; Turner & Nielsen, 1984), there continues to be confusion among many audiologists as how best to apply this information clinically. In order for us to outline an effective BAER test protocol, we must therefore first develop a functional appreciation for the rules of test-selection strategy.

A rational approach to testing strategy is based on the interrelationship between test sensitivity and specificity that defines the operating characteristics of any test and that governs the cutoff criterion used to differentiate normal from abnormal. Sensitivity denotes the likelihood that the test (BAER) result will be positive in the presence of disease, whereas specificity refers to the probability of a negative or normal test finding in the absence of the disease or disorder. A perfect test would be one having 100% sensitivity and 100% specificity. Unfortunately, such tests do not exist, particularly those, like the BAER, that require some degree of subjective interpretation. Because sensitivity represents the ratio of the number of diseased patients who failed the test to the total number of diseased patients who were tested, it reflects the true-positive or its reciprocal false-negative (1-sensitivity) rates.

Sensitive tests usually are most helpful as precursors to a comprehensive diagnostic evaluation when clinicians are attempting to reduce the likelihood of a number of disease entities (i.e., rule out disease). They are best applied when the probability of a specific disease is low and the purpose of testing is to identify its presence. Given that sensitive tests are typically positive in the presence of disease, they are the tests of choice when the stakes are high for a false-negative result such as when screening for a particular disease.

Specificity, on the other hand, denotes the ratio of nondiseased patients who pass the test to the total number of nondiseased patients tested. If defines the true-negative rate of any test. Specific tests are more useful, therefore, to confirm an existing impression that the disease already exists because they are rarely positive in the absence of disease; that is, they carry a low false-positive rate.

Clearly, the clinical goal is to select a test that has both high sensitivity (low false-negative rate) and specificity (low false-positive rate); however, it is difficult to achieve one without sacrificing the other, at least to some extent. It is critical, therefore, that test-selection strategies be guided by these concepts so as to optimize the information necessary to make a reliable and valid clinical decision.

> Rule 1. When the penalty is great for a false-negative result and you need to rule out presence of disease or disorder, *the test should be highly sensitive.*

> Rule 2. When a test is used to confirm an existing suspicion that the disease is present and a false-positive finding is harmful, *the test should be highly specific.*

Defining the optimum cutoff criterion

Owing to the interrelationship between test sensitivity and specificity, it is critical to understand the implications of selecting a certain cutoff criterion for differentiating "pass" from "fail" or "normal" from "abnormal." This value will dictate how a given test will operate relative to sensitivity/specificity. This is true whether you have selected a particular click intensity level at which to screen for hearing loss relative to the presence of Wave V, or the maximum I–V interpeak latency interval that you consider within the normal range. Any change in criterion will have a predictable influence on these two test parameters. Thus a criterion that is set to yield the highest sensitivity will do so only at the expense of lowering specificity.

Consider, for example, that your choice of screening click intensity level was 70 dB nHL such that the presence of Wave V denoted a pass, whereas its absence denotes a fail. Using this high a click level will fail all babies with severe-to-profound hearing loss, but alternatively will tend to pass babies who have up to a moderately-severe loss. In other words, this high cutoff screening level will result in few false-positive results (high specificity) but in an unacceptably high number of false-negative findings. The latter, of course, is contrary to the rules for a good screening test. At the opposite end of the spectrum is a situation where you might choose to use 10 dB as the pass–fail intensity criterion. Here, test sensitivity will be 100%, because you will fail every baby with hearing loss, but only at the expense of a high false-positive rate. Of course the same scenario holds true for neurodiagnostic cutoff criteria such as the I–V interpeak interval, interaural Wave V latency difference (IT$_5$), V/I amplitude ratio, and so forth.

The importance of selecting a screening cutoff criterion that will yield a high sensitivity without too great a sacrifice in specificity can be seen from this discussion. Failure to appreciate the influence of cutoff criterion on a test's operating characteristics most certainly will reduce the likelihood of being correct.

Effects of disease prevalence on test performance

Recall from the definitions of sensitivity/specificity that sensitivity represents the proportion of patients with the disease who have a positive test result for the disease; specificity, on the other hand, refers to those without disease who present a negative test finding. In both cases the values give probability figures relative to a test being positive or negative in persons known to have the disease. Of course, in daily practice the clinician is faced with making an opposing deduction, that is, determining whether the disease is present given the results of the test. The probability of disease, given the results of any test, is commonly referred to as the predictive value of the test. Thus positive predictive value is the probability of disease in a patient with an abnormal test result, whereas its reciprocal, negative predictive value, is the probability of not having the disease when the test result is negative or normal. In the case of using BAER to screen for hearing loss in the intensive care nursery, predictive value allows the clinician to answer the question: *If this baby has (does not have) a clearly visible Wave V at 40 dB nHL, what are the chances that he/she has (does not have) normal hearing?* Because predictive value is tied directly to sensitivity/specificity, we can conclude that the more sensitive a test the better its negative predictive value. The opposite is true for specificity and positive predictive value.

Sensitivity and specificity not withstanding, the predictive value of a test also is determined by the prevalence of disease in the population under study. *Prevalence refers to the proportion of persons in a defined population known to have the disease at a given point in time.* Consider, for example, doing screening BAERs on an entirely normal population of babies. Here, any screening failure will represent a false positive. In contrast, if all of the babies had a known hearing loss, any negative test finding would be a false-negative. It can quickly be seen that as the prevalence of disease approaches zero, the positive predictive value of the test is also near zero. Alternatively, as prevalence nears 100%, negative predictive value approaches zero.

Herein lies a major factor to consider in program development. The very notion of searching for a disease in patients who are essentially asymptomatic for the problem dictates a low prevalence rate even among high-risk groups. Thus the positive predictive value of the test is likely to be low even with the most specific of tests.

> Rule 3. When prevalence of disease in the population tested is low, positive predictive value is near zero and the test becomes almost useless for identifying the disease.

Central to this problem is that estimates of disease prevalence are not independent of clinical setting. Because much of what often appears in the research literature comes from data gathered at rather large, often university-affiliated hospitals where the prevalence for serious disease usually is high, statements about the predictive value of any test may, in fact, be misleading when applied to a less highly selective setting. To this end, it appears that interpretation of a positive or negative test result should vary according to clinical setting based on the estimated disease prevalence in that setting.

> Rule 4. Positive test results, even for a very specific test, when applied to a population of patients with a low likelihood of having the disease, will most often be false positive. Negative test results for a highly sensitive test are more likely to be false-negative when applied to patients with a high probability of having the disease.

[For further discussion of test selection principles, refer to Chapter 14 by Turner.]

Pediatric applications of the brainstem auditory evoked response

Since the seminal work of Hecox and Galambos (1974) and Schulman-Galambos and Galambos (1975) the application of brainstem auditory evoked responses in pediatrics has achieved remarkably wide-spread clinical acceptance. Not only has there been a plethora of articles written on the topic, but more important, the technique has been implemented in some form in almost all major metropolitan hospital pediatric programs from the neonatal intensive care unit to the pediatric auditory diagnostic clinic.

In general, BAER testing with children can be divided into three categories, each of which has a specific, but not necessarily mutually exclusive, purpose. These include its roles in neonatal screening, audiological assessment, and neurodiagnostics. (For general overviews of the brainstem auditory evoked response see Hecox & Jacobson, 1984; Picton, Stapells, & Campbell, 1981; Schwartz & Berry, 1985; Schwartz & Costello, 1988; and Chapter 6 in this volume by Durrant & Wolf.)

Audiologic applications of the BAER

Unlike the adult population where the focus of BAER testing has been on neurodiagnostics, its application in pediatrics has emphasized hearing loss identification or estimation. Use of the BAER to identify the presence of hearing loss most certainly represents a screening test, which, by definition, refers to the presumptive identification of a disease or disorder via the application of tests, scales, inventories, examinations, or the like that can be administered rapidly to patients who are either asymptomatic for or predisposed to the disease in question. Conversely, use of a comprehensive latency-intensity series to estimate degree of hearing loss is considered a diagnostic test because it is used to confirm an existing suspicion of hearing loss. In the former case, screening, the rules that govern test selection would dictate the need for a highly sensitive test without too great an increase in the false-positive rate, whereas in the latter there is need for a highly specific test, assuming that the cost is not too great an increase in the false-negative rate. In both circumstances we want to apply a testing strategy that will offer the greatest yield relative to the probability of being correct.

Neonatal hearing screening.   Perhaps no other area of auditory evoked potentials with children has received as much clinical and research interest as its application in neonatal screening. Despite the myriad of papers and oral presentations, however, precious little attention has been given to the formulation of a screening protocol based on concepts related to clinical epidemiology. Rather, the protocol most often described in the literature and presented at BAER workshops or seminars appears to be historic; that is, it seems to be based on the pioneering investigative work of Schulman-Galambos and Galambos (1975). Although this classical study served to promote the use of BAER to screen for hearing loss in the high-risk newborn, the parameters used in data collection did not necessarily represent an optimal screening protocol. It is our opinion, therefore, that prior to implementing a BAER screening program, there must be defensible justification for the protocol.

   Which babies should be screened?   Historically, there has been debate over whether hearing screening should be performed en masse or only with certain high-risk groups. Although most hospital BAER screening programs tend to concentrate on those babies "at-risk" for hearing loss, based on the recommendation of the Joint Committee on Newborn Hearing (1982) and most recently by the Committee on Infant Hearing of the American Speech-Language-Hearing Association (1989), there has been recent impetus on the part of some professionals to recommend mass BAER screening of all newborns. What has not been considered, or certainly has received no mention by these proponents, is that mass screening does not meet most of the basic tenets that underlie screening for disease. To justify screening, the following criteria must be met:

1. It should be common enough to justify the effort to detect it.

2. It should be accompanied by significant morbidity if left untreated.

3. Effective therapy must exist to alter its natural history.

4. Detection and treatment of the presymptomatic state should yield benefits beyond those obtained through treatment in the early symptomatic patient.

When considered in light of the 1:1500–2000 (Northern & Downs, 1978) point prevalence for congenital sensorineural hearing loss among the well baby population, the concept of mass BAER screening does not fulfill the first tenet; namely, the disease in question, hearing loss, is not common enough to justify the effort and cost to detect it. Although supporters of mass neonatal screening argue that this prevalence figure is far greater than that of phenylketonuria (1:14,000), which is routinely screened for at birth, it remains that this inborn error of amino acid metabolism meets essentially all of the other criteria to justify the screening effort. That is, it is accompanied by significant morbidity (brain damage), effective therapy exists to alter its natural history, and detection in the presymptomatic state yields significant benefit in preventing or reducing morbidity. Unfortunately, the same cannot be said for congenital deafness.

Because prevalence of disease has such a significant influence on the predictive value of a screening or diagnostic test, it would seem unjustifiable to apply BAER screening to all well baby newborns given the overall low prevalence among this neonatal population (Rule 3). Consider, for example, that 2,700 well babies were born at the University of Pennsylvania Medical Center in 1987. Based on a prevalence rate for hearing loss of 1:1,500 live births, we would anticipate identifying only one or possibly two newborns with hearing loss. According to a recent advertisement by the Algotek Corp., the estimated cost per test with the Algo 1-plus automated BAER screener is a nominal $30.00. Based on this figure the total expenditure, not including chart notation time, report writing, and so on, would then equal $81,000 to screen all babies or $40,500 for each of the two babies detected to have hearing loss. If we add to this an additional $200.00–$300.00 charge per infant for a diagnostic latency-intensity series to confirm the screening results and to estimate type and degree of loss, along with an additional fee for a behavioral cross-check, the cost of identifying these few newborns is clearly prohibitive. We would anticipate further that the cost per individual screening test is much higher than $30.00 when professional time is involved.

In contrast, consistent with other published reports, the point prevalence of serious sensorineural hearing loss among intensive care infants is estimated at 3%–5% (Alberti, Hyde, Riko, Corbin, & Abramovich, 1983; Dennis, Sheldon, Toubas, & McCaffee, 1984; Simmons, 1980). Obviously this represents a significant increase over the well baby population and thus provides a much greater yield for disease detection at considerably less cost. Applying the nominal $30.00 figure to this select group, the cost for each detection of hearing loss is estimated to be $750.00, which represents a $39,800 savings per detection compared to mass screening.

Although the ideal certainly would be to screen for hearing loss across the neonatal population at-large, the more prudent and certainly cost-efficient clinical strategy would be to apply BAER screening only to specific demographic groups such as high-risk newborns. In this way the positive predictive value becomes acceptably high and screening for the disease is entirely defensible on the basis of cost/benefit ratio.

Where should babies be screened? If one surveys published studies on the application of BAER screening to detect hearing loss in neonates, or talks with professionals who are active practitioners in this area, it becomes clear that the most popular test setting is the intensive care nursery (ICN). Although the logistic of screening in the ICN is perhaps convenient, it does pose some concerns. If the goal of the program is only to screen for hearing loss, it seems inappropriate to evaluate a baby who is critically ill and in an unstable clinical condition. These babies often present with septicemia, receive aminoglycoside therapy, and are at-risk for neuropathology and a host of other variables that may confound BAER interpretation for hearing loss. For sure their predisposition for otitis media with effusion while intubated with an endotrachial tube is sufficient reason not to screen for hearing loss until medical stability is achieved.

In addition, ambient noise levels in the ICN commonly exceed 60 dB, with peak levels in excess of 100 dB SPL (Bess, Peek, & Chapman, 1979; Richmond, Konkle, & Potsic, 1986). It seems rather paradoxical, therefore, that audiologists who are most sensitive to the effects of ambient noise on hearing would elect to screen for hearing loss in such a noisy environment. If we consider still further the electrical hostility of the ICN due to physiological monitors, incubators, warming blankets/mattresses, and the like, one can begin to appreciate how these variables can increase the false-positive rate for BAER hearing screening. Hence, it would seem more reasonable to wait until the baby is clinically stable and to screen for hearing loss either in a controlled test environment such as a sound-isolated and radio frequency (RF) shielded room, or at least to evaluate them in the quieter transitional nursery at about the time of hospital discharge.

If, on the other hand, your reason for screening is to assess neurologic integrity of the critically ill infant to help guide medical management and/or diagnosis, then there is good reason to screen in the ICN. Here, intensity levels in the range of 110–115 dB pSPL are used to maximize neural transmission and as such should not be subject to the confounding influence of the ambient noise levels.

Recommended stimulus transducer. Unquestionably the most popular method of sound delivery in BAER screening or diagnostic testing is the electrodynamic earphone. Until recently (Gorga, Kaminski, & Beauchaine, 1988; Schwartz, Pratt, & Schwartz, 1989), studies on BAER measurements in children were performed with a standard audiometric earphone and cushion assembly (i.e., TDH-39, TDH-49). Although these transducers have indeed been time-honored in almost all aspects of audiology, they too are subject to criticism for pediatric BAER work.

In neonatal screening it is common practice to disassemble the earphone from the headband and either lay the cushion over the baby's exposed or downside ear, or handhold the transducer in place. This approach to signal transduction can result in a variety of measurement and interpretation errors. One of the most common problems is ear canal collapse secondary to the weight and pressure of the earphone diaphragm and cushion. There is no doubt that this alone will increase significantly the rate of false-positive findings. In fact, Gorga, Kaminski, and Beauchaine (1988) recently estimated that as many as 50% of their screening failures were attributed to earphone-induced ear canal collapse. This most likely is also the reason why so many BAER screening studies reported excessively high failure rates ranging from 16%–41% (Cevette, 1984; Cox, Hack, & Metz, 1984; Galambos, Hicks, & Wilson, 1982; Jacobson & Morehouse, 1984; Marshall, Reichert, Kerley, & Davis, 1980; Stein, Ozdamar, Kraus, & Paton, 1983).

An additional problem with the use of an electrodynamic earphone is the increased variability in sound pressure level due to displacement of the transducer from over the baby's external auditory meatus during testing. Because a constant pressure headband is not used, and the infant is prone to changing position or some other body movement while sleeping, there also is opportunity for the earphone to shift position. Not only will this result in a within-subject change in sound pressure level, but a between-subject effect as well. As discussed most recently by Schwartz et al. (1989), this is probably a major reason why so many studies of this type concluded that response variability among infants was so much greater than for adults using identical BAER test protocols.

Along these same lines, Schwartz and co-workers suggested that the poor quality acoustic seal from a hand-held earphone serves as a high-pass filter much the same as a vented hearing aid earmold. They went on to explain that because recent ontological studies (Lippe & Rubel, 1983; Rubel et al., 1984) suggest that low-frequency auditory sensitivity develops before that of the high frequencies, low-frequency leakage around the earphone cushion reduces the available SPL delivered to the infant's cochlea in exactly the frequency region in which they are most sensitive. This too could lead to an erroneous conclusion for hearing loss (false-positive).

To circumvent the many negative characteristics of the electrodynamic earphone in BAER testing with children, or for that matter all patients, we recommend the use of an insert receiver such as the Etymotic Tube-phone[1] or the Nicolet Enhancer.[2] Each of these insert receivers is coupled to the baby's ear via a tiny soft, silicone eartip similar to that used in tym-panometry. In this way there is little or no chance of ear canal collapse, low-frequency leakage is held to a minimum, and both inter- and intra-subject variability is reduced as a result of a better controlled and more constant click SPL.

Finally, owing to the use of a calculated length of tubing between the actual transducer and the eartip, there is a sufficient transmission delay (e.g., 0.9 ms for the ER-3 tubephone™) imposed on the BAER waveform that will negate the smearing effects of stimulus artifact on Wave I at high click intensity levels often seen with earphone measurements.

We disagree with the recommendations of Hall, Kripal, and Hepp (1988) about overcoming the disadvantages of the standard audiometric earphone transducer by using "bone-conduction stimulation for newborn BAERs when air-conduction stimulation [with an earphone] produces a response with delayed absolute latencies" (p. 23). First, this requires an unnecessary second BAER measurement, thus violating the definition of a screening test; that is, if the conductive or mixed loss is of sufficient magnitude to cause absence of Wave V at the screening intensity, then the baby fails and is scheduled for a diagnostic latency-intensity series that should demonstrate a conductive pattern. If, however, Wave V remains present, but simply delayed in latency, the baby passes the hear-

---

[1]™Etymotic Research, Inc., Elk Grove, Illinois.
[2]™Nicolet Biomedical, Inc., Madison, Wisconsin.

ing screen. Second, the problems associated with a hand-held earphone are accentuated even further by attempting to maintain sufficient and constant pressure with a hand-held bone-conduction oscillator. Third, the maximum output of a click transduced through a Radioear B-70A bone-conduction oscillator is equivalent only to 35 dB nHL (Schwartz, Larson, & DeChicchis, 1981). As such, the arguments about the effects of ambient nursery noise become even more critical, particularly in the presence of an unoccluded ear.

Caveat.   Given the reduced undistorted output, bone-conduction BAER is effective only when hearing by bone conduction is assumed to be near normal.

Recommended electrode montage.   Like so many other aspects of BAER testing, choice of electrode montage also seems to have been governed by convention based on early pioneering literature. Clearly the most common recording montage in neonatal screening has been a single channel with the noninverting electrode at the vertex and the inverting electrode either at the ipsilateral earlobe or mastoid (Cz-A1-A2; M1-M2) with ground at the contralateral earlobe/mastoid. Alternatively, some clinicians choose to place the noninverting electrode on the forehead (Fpz) in fear of the fontanelles (Jacobson, Morehouse, & Johnson, 1982). Although placement of the noninverting electrode on the high forehead certainly is adequate, it is perfectly safe to place a recording electrode midway between the anterolateral and posterolateral fontanelles, thereby approximating Cz and optimizing the scalp distribution of the BAER.

In our opinion, a more ideal montage than a single channel for hearing screening represents at least a two channel recording with the inverting electrode of the second channel secured at about the level of the second cervical vertebra (a so-called noncephalic reference site). The result is a much larger amplitude and better resolved Wave V, as illustrated in Figure 8.1. Shown here is an ABR to a 40 dB nHL click recorded from a 33-week gestational age (GA) infant. The top trace represents the Cz-A1 (vertical) response, whereas the bottom BAER reflects the improved Wave V amplitude derived from the noncephalic lead (i.e., Cz-C-2).

To us this second noncephalic reference channel is invaluable to resolve Wave V, particularly when the BAER is used to detect hearing loss. The information provided, particularly when faced with a questionable Wave V at low intensity levels, is more than worth the extra few seconds it takes to prepare another electrode site. Furthermore, it serves as an excellent backup should the ipsilateral ear electrode become displaced.

We also recommend not using the contralateral ear as common. Rather, we prefer to ground somewhere on the forehead, usually Fpz, or at the mid-sternum. This permits continuous recording without having to change the ground electrode when switching the stimulus ear.

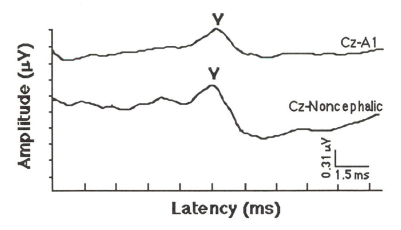

Figure 8.1. Example of the Wave V amplitude increase seen with a noncephalic (Cz-C-2) reference recording compared to the conventional ipsilateral ear montage (Cz-A1, A2). The BAER was recorded from a 33-week-old (gestational age) infant to a 40-dB nHL rarefaction click.

Recently, Weber (1988) indicated that the tenderness of a baby's skin does not permit use of abrasive cleaners and that frequently, babies demonstrate electrode impedance greater than 20 kohms. Such a skin reaction to Omniprep abrasive is extremely rare in our experience. Unless interelectrode impedances are perfectly matched, thereby permitting adequate common mode rejection, high electrode impedances at 20 Kohms surely will lead to unacceptably noisy recordings.

Caveat. If faced with a situation where skin impedance cannot be held to a minimum, regardless of how much or hard the skin is cleansed or abraded, then it is critical to maintain very close intraelectrode impedance balance.

Recommended analog filter setting. In the neurodiagnostic application of the BAER it is common practice to use a high-pass setting of 100 or 150 Hz and a low-pass of 1500 or 3000 Hz. The principle reason for this narrowed bandpass is to reject interfering low-frequency components of the "raw" EEG and myogenic activity that serve to increase the signal-to-noise ratio and thus reduce waveform clarity and reliability.

As a result of the successful use of narrow bandpass filtering in BAER neurodiagnostics, a similar analog filtering strategy also is popular for audiologic application of the BAER. In their suggested strategies for infant BAER assessment, for example, Jacobson et al. (1982), Ruth, Dey-Sigman, and Mills (1985), and Weber (1988) all recommend bandpass filtering between 150 and 3000 Hz based most likely on the convention adopted from the early work of Schulman-Galambos and Galambos (1975), and their desire to negate the possible influences of low-frequency electrical and myogenic noise, and/or instrument limitations. Here again, although adequate, the cost of setting the high-pass filter somewhere around 150 Hz is a major loss of the slow component of the response that contributes greatly to the spectral energy in Wave V (Kavanagh, Domico, Franks, & Jin-Cheng, 1988; Kevanishvili & Aphonchenko, 1979; Laukli & Mair, 1981). Like the use of placing an inverting noncephalic reference electrode, therefore, lowering the high-pass filter from the conventional 100/150 Hz down to 30 Hz for low-intensity work, will lead to a more highly resolved Wave V, as demonstrated in Figure 8.2. Kavanagh and colleagues (1988) recently demonstrated that reducing the high-pass filter from the standard 100 Hz to around 30 to 50 Hz leads to about a 20% improvement in the amplitude of Wave V.

In addition to reducing the high-pass filter, we also see little reason to use 3000 Hz as the low-pass cutoff, given that spectral analysis of the BAER shows little or no contributing energy above 1000 Hz. What one does purchase with a 3000-Hz cutoff frequency is unwanted high-frequency noise. Consistent with the results of Laukli and Mair (1981), we suggest a low-pass filter setting of 1500 Hz for all BAER measurements.

Recommended click rate. Unlike other recording parameters, there appears to be little consensus regarding choice of stimulus repetition rate to be used in neonatal screening. For example, Jacobson et al. (1982) recommended a traditional slow click rate (10.4/s), Dennis et al. (1984) used a rate of 20.1/s, and both Ruth et al. (1985) and Weber (1988) stimulated at a rate of 30/s.

We stimulate at a rate of 37.1/s, which is consistent with Galambos et al. (1982) for several reasons. First, there is little justification for using a slow rate such as the conventional 11.1/s either for hearing screening or estimation of type and degree of sensitivity loss from the latency-intensity function. Although it is true that rates <20/s are best for neuro-diagnostic work because they yield the best definition of Waves I-III, there is no advantage to these slow rates if the only wave of interest is Wave V. In fact, there is considerable disadvantage to using such a slow rate for hearing screening because it increases overall test time significantly.

Consider, for example, using the Jacobson et al. (1982) strategy of 10.4/s. Assuming a very quiet sleeping baby, it would take 12.8 min to average 2,000 repetitions at a single intensity for both ears across a test-retest paradigm. Conversely, the same can be accomplished in 3.59 min using a rate of 37.1/s. Certainly this more than 60% savings in test time has considerable advantage. The ability to screen more babies in less time

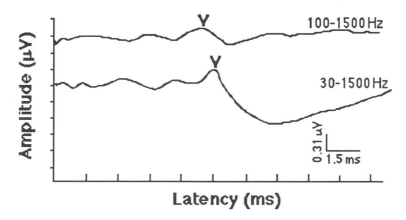

Figure 8.2. Comparison of Wave V morphology and amplitude for a neonatal BAER recorded to a 40-dB nHL rarefaction click under conditions of closed (100–1500 Hz) and open (30–1500 Hz) bandpass filtering.

notwithstanding, foremost among these advantages is that should the baby be active, thus resulting in a noisy response, you can double the number of averages to improve the signal-to-noise ratio in still less time than it would take to average only 2,000 repetitions at a rate of 10.4/s.

Although it is true that increases in click rate will prolong Wave V latency on the order of about 0.2 ms for every 10/s increase in rate, this is easily controlled when establishing the normative data base. Moreover, it remains that by definition, only the presence of Wave V at the criterion screening intensity level is used to denote pass-fail, not its latency. What is more critical is that Wave V amplitude is not affected until click rate is increased above approximately 50/s.

During our early search for an optimal screening protocol we found that, on occasion, a baby would fail the screening at 40 dB nHL at a rate of 57.1/s but pass at a 37.1/s rate. From this observation we concluded that the central auditory system of these babies was characterized by a greater number of unmyelinated neural fibers and more incomplete synaptogenesis than other babies of the same age and physical status. Thus increasing the click rate beyond some value (perhaps 50/s) over-taxes the neural encoding ability of their auditory system. To this end we elected *a priori* to use a nominal rate of 37.1/s and were willing to forego a savings of 50 to 60 s in overall test time as a safeguard against a possible false-positive result. This rate selection is entirely in keeping with the recommendation of Weber (1988) who stated that a rate between 30 and 40/s maintains response clarity without sacrifice of test time.

Recommended stimulus polarity. Without question, alternating polarity is most commonly used in newborn BAER screening (Hall et al., 1988; Jacobson et al., 1982; Ruth et al., 1985). Perhaps the most obvious reason for their choice of polarity is to circumvent the problem of large stimulus artifact that commonly is seen at high stimulus intensity levels when using a standard electrodynamic earphone. Although stimulus artifact has a negative effect primarily on Wave I, and typically is absent at low screening intensities, we presume that continued use of an alternating polarity is one of continuity.

There are several reasons why alternating polarity should not be used. Among these is that phase cancellations during alternating of the two polarities can obscure the "true" BAER, which can cloud interpretation. Along these lines, Schwartz et al. (1989) demonstrated recently that condensation clicks yield smaller BAER amplitudes among infants than rarefaction stimuli. Thus when using alternating polarity clicks, the condensation stimuli will compromise overall response amplitude. This is particularly important in screening work, given that the pass-fail criterion is based on the presence or absence of Wave V at lower intensities.

Because the use of an insert receiver circumvents the problem of stimulus artifact as described previously, and because, on the average, rarefaction stimuli yield better wave amplitude, we recommend at least initial use of rarefaction clicks for all neonatal BAER screening applications.

Caveat. If during screening you are unsure of the exact location of Wave V either in the ipsilateral or noncephalic reference channels and you have followed the protocol described for rate (37.1/s) and bandpass filters (30–1500 Hz), reversing polarity to a condensation click often will help resolve the waveform and prevent a false-positive result.

Recommended analysis epoch. Although it is true that the normal adult BAER occurs within 10 ms poststimulus onset, there is good reason not to use such a short analysis epoch, regardless of the patient's age. This is particularly important for infant screening and/or diagnostics. There are two advantages to lengthening the epoch to 15 ms across all patient populations. First, as illustrated in Figure 8.3, the time interval beyond 10 ms provides for a visual representation of the background noise averaged into the response. Note that in the top trace there remains hills and valleys following Wave V, indicating that the patient was myogenically noisy. Because this noise is undifferentiated from the bioelectric potential of interest (i.e., BAER), it too will be averaged into the resulting waveform, thereby producing spurious amplitudes, poor wave morphology, and poor reproducibility. In contrast, the bottom recording is characterized by a quiet response baseline after Wave V with excellent repeatability, thus supporting excellent signal-to-noise ratio. Of course, the same information can be achieved by introducing a 5-ms delay prior

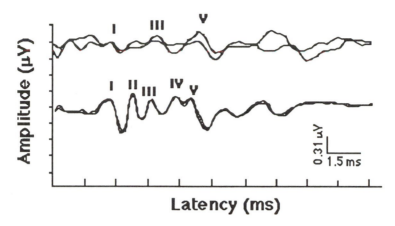

Figure 8.3.   Illustration of the benefits of a 15-ms recording epoch for determining signal-to-noise ratio. The top tracing shows nonrepeatable "hills" and "valleys" following Wave V, representing noise contamination in the BAER. The bottom trace reveals a return to baseline following Wave V, thus supporting a highly quiet recording, which also is evidenced by the excellent reproducibility.

to averaging, which will appear as a prestimulus baseline. To us the 15-ms epoch represents a significantly better approach to estimating background noise level than a no-stimulus control run. In the latter case, the patient might be excessively noisy during testing but highly quiet by the time a no-stimulus input control is obtained. This will lead to the erroneous conclusion that the patient was quiet during testing.

A second justification for lengthening the analysis time to 15 ms that is most salient to neonatal testing is based on the prolonged latency of Waves III and V particularly at low levels of stimulus intensity. If Wave V is present beyond 10 ms due perhaps to neurologic compromise or conductive transmission blockage, a false-positive conclusion for hearing loss will be reached. For these reasons it is recommended that a 10-ms epoch *never* be used. Rather, we concur with Hall et al. (1988) that the analysis time should be at least 15 ms, or should combine a 5-ms prestimulus delay followed by a 15-ms analysis time (i.e., 20-ms epoch).

Recommended pass-fail criterion.   Undoubtedly, the selection of pass-fail criteria represents the single most important aspect of any screening program. Recall that this value will influence test sensitivity/specificity and hence, the false-positive, false-negative rates. Remember also that in screening for any disease, it is most important to select a pass-fail criterion that will yield the highest test sensitivity without too great a sacrifice in specificity. That is, in screening, the cost of a false-negative finding is considerably greater than that of a false-positive one. Here, the baby may become lost to follow-up and the ultimate diagnosis of hearing loss may be delayed well beyond the optimal period for early detection and intervention.

In reviewing the neonatal BAER screening literature it is clear that most investigators and probably the majority of practicing clinicians use a 30 dB nHL pass-fail criterion (Cevette, 1984; Cox et al., 1984; Dennis et al., 1984; Edwards, Picton, & McMurray, 1985; Galambos et al., 1982; Jacobson & Morehouse, 1984; Morgan, Zimmerman, & Dubno, 1987; Ruth et al., 1985; Schulman-Galambos & Galambos, 1975; Weber, 1988). Here again, we presume that use of 30 dB nHL was adopted from the original investigation of Schulman-Galambos and Galambos (1975) on the use of BAER to screen for hearing loss in intensive care newborns. What seems to have been overlooked, however, is that their original data were collected in a double-walled sound treated and temperature controlled test booth with the instrumentation located outside of the chamber. This laboratory condition is in no way similar to the electrically and acoustically hostile intensive care unit. Of additional significance is that our review of the data presented in their Table 2 (p. 460) revealed that of the six infants tested at 34 to 35 weeks GA, an interpretable BAER could be recorded in only one baby at 30 dB nHL, whereas an identifiable Wave V was seen in four of these babies at 40 dB nHL. It is interesting in this regard that in their discussions of false-positive/negative rates in BAER screening, Dennis et al. (1984) and Alberti et al. (1983) argued that increasing screening cutoff criterion from 30 dB nHL to 40 dB nHL would have reduced their false-positive rate significantly without affecting the false-negative rate. This too has been our experience.

Although the recent report from Durieux-Smith et al. (1985) favored a 30 dB nHL pass-fail criterion based on their data from 600 infants, it remains that 472 of these infants were screened in a controlled audiologic test suite and not in the ICN or transitional nursery (TN). In fact, 128 of their babies were seen as outpatients at 3 months of age or older. Of particular note was that despite their ardent support for a 30 dB nHL criterion, the data of Durieux-Smith et al. (1987) indicated that 64% of inpatient babies who failed at 30 dB nHL passed follow-up testing at 40 dB nHL.

We too would agree that 30 dB nHL represents an acceptable screening level under controlled ambient test conditions; however, most hospitals simply do not enjoy the space, time, or staff support to permit testing large numbers of babies in the evoked potential laboratory. It also is true that in many hospitals, like ours, failure to screen a baby prior to discharge almost always will result in that infant being lost to outpatient follow-up.

Based on the principles of clinical epidemiology, therefore, because positive test results, even for a very specific test, will most often be false-positive when applied to a population of patients with a low likelihood of having the disease, use of 30 dB nHL as the cutoff criterion serves only to increase further the likelihood of a false-positive finding. To this end, we argue strongly for a 40 dB nHL cutoff because it purchases a much lower false-positive rate without the expense of a higher false-negative one. Not only will this result in less parental anxiety, but it will be welcomed by the referring neonatologist who rightfully is concerned about any test that carries an unacceptable false-positive rate. Moreover, this 10 dB nHL increase also may help overcome at least some of the aforementioned confounding variables such as: (a) high ambient noise levels in the intensive care nursery, (b) increased possibility of electrical or myogenic interference that could confound response interpretation, (c) reduced SPL secondary to earphone leakage, (d) difference in auditory sensitivity of a newborn versus that of the adults from whom the nHL reference was established, and (e) mild transient conductive hearing loss.

Summary of neonatal ABR hearing screening.   Table 8.1 summarizes the protocol used in the Division of BioelectroDiagnosis and Neural Monitoring, University of Pennsylvania Medical Center for neonatal BAER hearing screening. The philosophical underpinnings of this protocol relate to optimizing Wave V amplitude and morphology for quick reliable detection at a low intensity. The pass-fail criterion of 40 dB nHL was based on the principles of clinical epidemiology and as such permit a highly sensitive screening test while maintaining an acceptably low false-positive rate. We purposely avoided recommending a specific number of samples to be averaged since this is not cast in stone. Rather, we suggest that this number be variable based on response clarity and repeatability. For example, it may be that under quiet recording conditions, a well-formed Wave V will be observed in as few as 800–1,000 sweeps and that an overlapping response also can be seen with the same or even fewer trials. In contrast, as many as 4,000–6,000 averages may be required to resolve Wave V in a noisy baby. Thus in dissonance with common belief, there is no magic number of repetitions that must be obtained. The rule is that you average as many samples as necessary to improve the signal-to-noise ratio sufficiently so as to clarify the response for reliable and valid interpretation.

Brainstem evoked response audiometry

The latency-intensity (L-I) series as exemplified in Figure 8.4 represents the hallmark to brainstem evoked response audiometry (BERA). Unlike

TABLE 8.1
**Neonatal BAER Hearing Screening Protocol Used at the Division
of BioelectroDiagnosis and Neural Monitoring,
University of Pennsylvania Medical Center**

Recording Set Up		Recording Parameters	
Test Site:	Transitional Nursery	Epoch:	15 ms
No. of Channels:	2 (minimum)	Bandpass:	30–1500 Hz
Montage: Channel 1:	noninverting = Cz inverting = A_1, A_2	Stimulus: Duration: Rate:	Click 100 μS 37.1/S
Channel 2:	noninverting = Cz inverting = noncephalic	Polarity: Intensity:	Rarefaction 40 dB nHL
Transducer:	Insert Tubephone™	No. of Sweeps:	Variable RE: S/N Ratio
Ear Tested:	Both		

neonatal BAER hearing screening, which is based on a single intensity cutoff criterion for pass-fail, the L-I series is used to estimate degree and type of hearing loss and as such serves as an electrophysiologic analog to the behavioral pure tone audiogram. (For a detailed description of the L-I series see Hyde, 1985; Schwartz & Costello, 1988.)

The basic approach to brainstem evoked response audiometry is to record Wave V latency across a graded series of intensities down to its visual detection threshold. These latency values are plotted relative to an age-appropriate normal template consisting of the mean Wave V latency ($\pm$2.5–3.0 SD). From this L-I function, type and degree of hearing loss is inferred by the amount of absolute displacement from the normal template and any deviation in the slope configuration. Thus an L-I function that is characterized by a prolonged Wave V latency, regardless of intensity and parallels that of the normal suggests transmission loss secondary to conductive disorder. Conversely, a steep curve most typically is pathognomonic of cochlear disorder and sensorineural hearing loss.

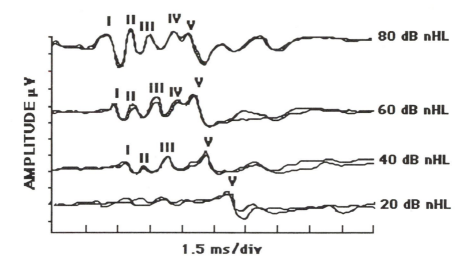

Figure 8.4.   Example of a latency-intensity series for estimating hearing threshold from the BAER.

Optimal recording parameters.   Given that the objective in BAER audiometry with young or difficult-to-test children is to establish Wave V threshold quickly and reliably, many of the recording techniques employed with neonatal screening also are applicable to auditory diagnostic testing. These include a multichannel recording montage, rapid rate of stimulation (37.1/s), and broadband analog filtering (30–1500 Hz). Each of these changes from what might be considered conventional recording parameters is based on optimization of Wave V amplitude and morphology and, as such, will assist greatly in achieving the clinical goal. Consider, for example, the L-I functions displayed in Figure 8.5. Presented on the left are the BAERs obtained with commonly used closed filters. Here, Wave V threshold is 30 dB nHL. The right-hand panel displays recordings from the same child using a broader analog filter bandpass (30–1500 Hz). Observe now that Wave V clearly is identifiable down to 15 dB; that is, threshold was 15 dB better than that seen for the closed filter condition.

Similarly, Figure 8.6 compares Wave V amplitude and threshold for a recording obtained from a noncephalic inverting electrode to that of the ipsilateral earlobe lead-site as suggested by most investigators. The noncephalic referential recording has a broader slope for Wave V, increased amplitude, and a 5-dB nHL better threshold level than the standard vertex to ipsilateral earlobe montage.

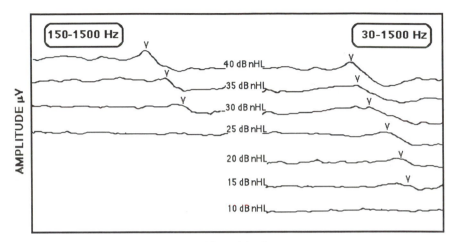

Figure 8.5. Comparison of Wave V amplitude and threshold for a BAER recorded with conventional closed (150–1500 Hz) analog filter settings versus that obtained with open (30–1500 Hz) filters. Note that Wave V threshold is 15 dB lower using a broader filter setting.

Testing strategies in BAER audiometry. Because it is of paramount importance to obtain the most "noise-free" recording possible to ensure a reliable estimate of Wave V threshold, overall test time becomes a critical issue in pediatric BAER evaluation. It often is taught that an L-I series should begin at a high intensity level (e.g., 80 dB nHL) followed by graded 10–20 dB nHL intensity decrements. Yet, by initiating the test sequence at such a high intensity level you increase the risk of arousing the baby immediately, which may result in an inability to obtain the necessary clinical information in a single test session. Furthermore, use of such small intensity decrements serves only to waste precious testing time without adding significant clinical information.

There are two rational, logical, and expedient alternatives to this conventional method that do provide maximum clinical decision-making information within a reasonable time period. One is a modified monaural approach, whereas the other is a binaural strategy.

The modified monaural strategy. Figure 8.7 represents a flowchart of a time-efficient monaural approach to establishing the BAER threshold. Briefly, as is common in pure tone audiometry, the initial presentation level is based on the practitioner's intuition as to the presence of hearing loss. Thus if mild-to-moderate hearing loss is suspected, the BAER is

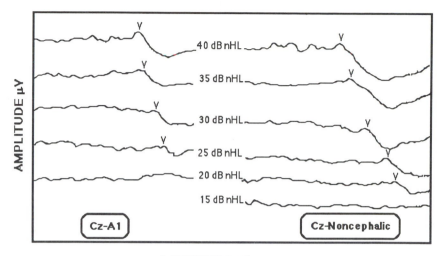

LATENCY (ms)

Figure 8.6. Comparison of Wave V amplitude and threshold for a BAER recorded from a standard ipsilateral ear (Cz-A1) montage versus that from a noncephalic inverting (Cz-C-2) electrode. Note the 5-dB lower Wave V threshold for the noncephalic referential recording.

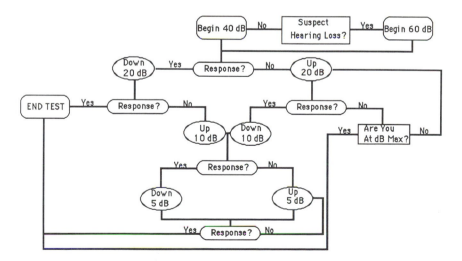

Figure 8.7. Flow chart of a monaural testing strategy for establishing Wave V threshold during brainstem evoked response audiometry.

recorded first to 60 dB nHL clicks, whereas if the child is thought to have normal hearing the initial level is 40 dB nHL. Of course, if there is reason to suspect significant sensitivity loss, then it is more reasonable to begin at the maximum output limits of the evoked potential system, assuming that the transducer is capable of delivering an undistorted transient signal at such a high peak sound pressure level.

Following the flowchart, if a clear and repeatable response is seen at the initial level, intensity is reduced 20 dB nHL and the BAER is repeated. *(Clinical Suggestion: If the response of interest is unquestionably present and the postresponse or prestimulus 5-ms baseline supports a quiet recording, there is no need for a retest. Rather, the extra retest time should be saved for lower intensity recordings near threshold. To be sure, one quiet recording is far better than redundant, poorly repeatable noisy tracings.)* From here, the decisions that follow depend on the starting level. If, for example, it was 40 dB nHL and a response was clear and repeatable at 20 dB nHL, then there is little need to continue. Clearly, establishing the relative BAER threshold below 20 dB nHL will have little impact on the audiologic management of the child. If, however, there was no response at 20 dB nHL, then it becomes necessary to incorporate a bracketing procedure as outlined in the flowchart to determine the BAER threshold. A similar protocol would be used when the beginning test level is 60 dB nHL or greater.

The binaural approach.   Although the binaural strategy advocated by Jerger et al. (1985) has not received widespread clinical application, the underlying basis is well-conceived and justified. The rationale for the binaural strategy is that when test time is limited and the possibility exists that complete monaural assessment may not be possible for any reason, it is more advantageous to establish the BAER threshold in the better ear (which is unknown at the time of testing) than to obtain completely accurate and reliable monaural information that stands the chance of reflecting an estimate of auditory sensitivity only in the poorer ear.

As Jerger et al. (1985) have argued, if time is available only for one threshold run before the child awakens, then having established the binaural threshold at least provides information about hearing in the better ear, thereby permitting the clinician to initiate a suitable intervention strategy. For example, if the binaural threshold was normal, then the clinician need not be overly concerned about significant compromises in language development, because the worse-case scenario would be complete unilateral sensitivity loss. If, on the other hand, the binaural threshold was elevated, then the clinician can begin habilitation with binaural amplification and use a follow-up test session to factor out whether the hearing loss is symmetrical.

For the test protocol the binaural threshold search is initiated using the same decision-making scheme as described for the modified monaural method and illustrated in Figure 8.7 except that both ears are stimulated simultaneously. Once the binaural threshold is defined, monaural symmetry is assessed by recording the BAER independently for each ear at an intensity level 20 dB nHL above that of the binaural threshold. From here, interpretation is based on whether symmetry can be assumed. Thus monaural responses that are essentially equal in latency, amplitude, and morphology would lead to the conclusion that hearing sensitivity is most likely the same in both ears and, hence, no further testing is needed. Conversely, differences between the two monaural responses dictate the necessity for threshold estimation only in the presumed poorer ear. Obviously, any additional testing of the better ear is redundant because the binaural threshold was weighted in favor of that ear. Quite frankly, given the relative ease and time efficiency of the binaural strategy, as well as its philosophical and psychoacoustic underpinnings, one wonders why it has not been adopted by more clinicians for routine pediatric use.

Alternatives to click stimuli. Despite the proven value of the click-evoked BAER as a quasi objective estimate of high-frequency audiometric threshold, such broadband stimuli preclude an accurate frequency-specific correlate to the pure tone audiogram. Particularly troublesome are those children with low-frequency rising audiometric contour where the auditory threshold is elevated below 1000 Hz and rises to normal in the higher frequencies. As a consequence of this lack of place specificity for click stimuli, there has been an ongoing search for alternative methods of stimulus generation and/or presentation that would best serve as the electrophysiologic analog to the pure tone audiogram. Although reproducible BAERs have been measured with linear, cosine-squared and Blackman cosine function gated tone bursts (Davis & Hirsh, 1976; Gorga, Kaminski, Beauchaine, & Jesteadt, 1988; Kodera, Yamane, Yamada, & Suzuki, 1977; Suzuki, Hirai, & Horiuchi, 1977; Suzuki & Horiuchi, 1977), clicks and tonebursts in notched noise (see Stapells, Picton, Perez-Abalo, Read, & Smith, 1985, for review) and by the so-called "derived" high-pass masking technique (Don & Eggermont, 1978; Eggermont & Don, 1980; Laukli & Mair, 1986; Teas, Eldredge, & Davis, 1962), these place-specific strategies remain investigational and open to controversy as to whether they provide low-frequency limited BAER data. (See Schwartz & Costello, 1988, for more detail.)

Caveat. Because we presume that the point prevalence of rising sensorineural hearing loss in children is very low, and because early electrophysiologic identification of these self-limiting low-frequency hearing losses most likely will have little impact on the overall habilitative management of these children, we chose not to include a detailed review of frequency specific (i.e., tonal) BAERs.

The SN$_{10}$ potential.   The description of a scalp-negative slow wave brainstem potential and its application to evoked response audiometry (ERA) by Davis and Hirsh (1979) evolved from the work of Suzuki, Hirai, and Horiuchi (1977) and Suzuki and Horiuchi (1977) on the influence of high-pass filtering and filter rejection rate on the amplitude of Wave V elicited by a low-frequency tone burst. Briefly, these two Japanese studies found that reliable brainstem potentials could be recorded to low-frequency tone bursts if the high-pass filter cutoff was set at or below 50 Hz and the filter slope was 24 dB/octave or greater. Davis and Hirsh (1979) followed suit and identified not only an increase in Wave V amplitude, but a slow wave negative tail following Wave V that could be traced effectively to within 10 dB of audiometric threshold at 500 Hz. The SN$_{10}$ depicted in Figure 8.8 is recorded to a 500-Hz tone burst (linear gating, 2-ms rise/decay, 1-ms plateau) presented at a rate of 31–39/s using a vertical electrode montage. Consistent with the influence of high-pass filtering on the response, the analog bandpass is set at 30–1500 Hz with a rejection rate of 24 dB/octave.

Despite the continued support and praise of this response by Davis and Owen (1985) as a reliable electrophysiologic correlate to low-frequency hearing, it has not been subjected to longitudinal validation nor has it received widespread clinical acceptance. Moreover, the requirement of an external steep reject filter limits the clinical ease of recording the SN$_{10}$ with standard commercially available instrumentation. We also add the same caveat to this response as we did for tonal BAERs.

Neurologic applications of the BAER

In addition to the application of the BAER to hearing assessment and screening, it also serves an important role in the investigation of neurologic integrity across pediatric populations. As such, the BAER has proven to be sensitive to the neurologic sequelae of hypoxic encephalopathy, toxic-metabolic disorders, hydrocephalus, bacterial meningitis, congenital neurodegenerative disorders, brainstem neoplasm, infantile autism, and hypoxic-ischemic insult secondary to traumatic injury.

Neonatal neurologic screening.   Because the BAER interpretation of neuropathology can be complicated by the presence of peripheral hearing loss in many of these high-risk infants, it is fruitful to complement the BAER hearing screening with a neurologic component to screen for possible brainstem disorder. It seems rather paradoxical to us that some audiologists would argue that statements made about an infant's brainstem status based on BAER results goes beyond the expertise of the audiologist while simultaneously advocating its use in the differential diag-

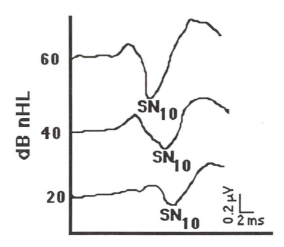

Figure 8.8.   Example of the SN_{10} response for estimating hearing threshold.

nosis of auditory brainstem lesions in adults (Weber, 1988; Jerger, personal communication). To be sure, the neurologist is not holding to the opinion that he or she should not be involved in BAER hearing screening since this is beyond the scope of his or her expertise or broad fund of knowledge.

Where should babies be screened?   The protocol for neurologic BAER screening is modified from that used in hearing screening. Because concern about the neurologic integrity of an intensive care newborn requires immediate attention to help guide medical management or aide in diagnosis, testing cannot be delayed until the baby enters the transitional nursery or can be transported to the evoked potential laboratory. Rather, the BAER often must be recorded in the ICN.

Consistent with the possible confounding effects of ambient noise on the BAER hearing screen results, the electrophysiologist must also pay careful attention to the electrical hostility of the intensive care nursery. This includes eliminating or at least minimizing all possible sources of electrical interference that can enter the amplifiers of the evoked potential system. Indeed there are a variety of routes or paths through which electrical interference can enter the physiologic amplifiers of the evoked potential instrument. Stray electrical signals can (a) be picked up by the patient or by unshielded electrode cables, (b) be conducted to the patient from other monitoring electrodes (e.g., EKG) or by conductance through infusion lines, warming blankets, interarterial catheters, and so forth, (c) leak into the amplifier from nearby power lines (e.g., 60 Hz) or by a common electrical path (i.e., ground loop), and/or (d) be conducted via a magnetic field emanating from the cathode ray tubes of any number of monitors that are in close proximity to the evoked potential system.

In order to minimize the problems of electrical interference, certain precautionary steps should be taken prior to implementing an ICN screening program. Ensuring that all electrical monitoring equipment in the ICN is properly grounded represents the first step toward eliminating the dominant source of interference.

Along the lines of grounding, proper placement of the ground electrode for BAER recording also can alleviate considerable noise interference that can emanate from EKG lead sites. A successful strategy here is to place the ground electrode between the site on the patient where the interference enters (e.g., the upper sternum or shoulder) and the BAER recording electrodes on the head. We are not advocates of using the contralateral ear as a ground site for several reasons, not the least of which is that it precludes multiple channel recording.

Noise can also enter the recording system from a power-cable crossing near the patient or one laid directly over the preamplifier cable of the evoked potential system, or by BAER recording electrodes crossing over EKG leads, infusion lines, and so on. (*Note*: Fluid solutions such as blood, dextrose, saline, electrolytes, and IV medication, serve as excellent electrical conductors that can pass interfering signals through the infant to the recording instrument.) It would behoove the clinician to ensure that neither the electrode head box, cable, nor any electrode leads are crossing over or lying next to power lines, other monitoring electrodes, or infusion tubes. We, at times, also have found it advantageous to shield our braided electrodes in copper mesh and to wrap the array in shrinkable insulated tubing. (*Clinical Suggestion*: Short braided recording electrodes will help reduce electrical interference.)

Finally, it may be necessary to incorporate an isolation transformer into your instrumentation as a means of reducing potential electrical interference. It is wise also to see if certain interfering sources such as warming blankets, heat lamps, apnea monitors, and so forth can be turned off during BAER testing.

Recommended electrode montage.   Consistent with our overall philosophy in BAER testing, the clinical goal for assessing brainstem function in the intensive care newborn is to maximize the type of information that you are seeking. In the case of hearing screening, for example, recall that we advocated at least a two-channel recording montage with the inverting electrode of the second channel secured at about the level of the second cervical vertebra (a so-called noncephalic reference site), a low high-pass filter setting of 30 Hz, a moderately rapid click rate (37.1/s), 40 dB nHL click intensity and tubephone transducers. Each of these parametric manipulations is aimed at improving Wave V resolution and amplitude.

In neurodiagnostics, the testing strategy must be modified because it is critical to assess brainstem transmission, which requires optimization of Wave I, as well as Waves III and V. As such, the electrode montage is again one of multiple recording channels (i.e., Cz-A1, Cz-A2, Cz-C-2); however, a fourth horizontal (A1-A2) channel may be added to help resolve Wave I, if necessary. Hecox and Burkhard (1982) reported that a horizontal configuration will yield up to a 70% increase in the infant Wave I amplitude when compared to a standard vertical electrode arrangement. Although we have not found the horizontal array to be advantageous in all cases, it does provide either supportive or additional information in a sufficient number to warrant inclusion. Moreover, it does not add any testing time.

Represented in Figure 8.9 is a four-channel BAER recorded from a preterm infant in our transitional nursery. Although the ipsilateral recording reveals all of the major peak components, that is, Waves I, III, and V, examination of the horizontal and noncephalic channels demonstrates how different montages can be used to highlight a particular component when peak resolution is poor. Observe, for example, the improvement in Wave I amplitude obtained from the horizontal channel (bandpass filters = 100–1500 Hz). Similarly, although Wave V is seen on the ipsilateral recording, it has better definition on the noncephalic channel (bandpass filters = 30–1500 Hz). We cannot overemphasize the value of multiple recording sites as routine to help clarify specific waveforms when faced with a difficult interpretation.

Recommended analog filter setting.   As discussed previously for BAER hearing screening, choice of filter settings should be predicated on the frequency composition of the desired bioelectric potential as well as on the need for reducing unwanted electrical or myogenic interference. Thus recording channels that are used for special purposes, such as the horizontal (A1-A2) channel to improve Wave I detection, will accommodate bandpass filtering from 100–1500 Hz, given that the primary energy for Wave I lies between 300–1000 Hz (Kavanagh et al., 1988; Kevanishvili & Aphonchenko, 1979; Laukli & Mair, 1981). Likewise, when there is a need to reduce myogenic or low-frequency electrical interference without sacrificing wave amplitude and clarity, narrow bandpass filtering (100–1500 Hz) is recommended. Recall that Wave V has a slow wave component below 100 Hz that is analog filtered if the high-pass setting is the typical 100 or 150 Hz; therefore, it is best to employ a broader passband (e.g., 30–1500 Hz) when Wave V identification is difficult.

Recommended click rate.   Similar to the choice of electrode montage, selection of appropriate stimulus rate also is modified for neurodiagnostic

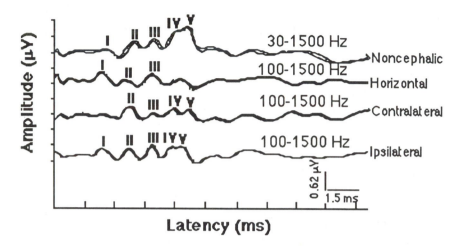

Figure 8.9. Four-channel auditory brainstem response used in neurodiagnostic application. Note how the response from each channel is used to clarify specific ABR wave components.

evaluation. For hearing screening we recommended an intermediate click rate of 37.1/s because the clinical goal was centered on Wave V identification at a low intensity level (40 dB nHL) and an important variable was overall test time. In neurodiagnostic evaluation we are forced to reduce the click rate in order to maximize neural synchrony and, thus, optimize Wave I. It is well recognized that rates in excess of about 20.1/s will have a compromising effect on Wave I amplitude, which is antithetic to the neurodiagnostic evaluation. Although click rates less than 12/s will improve neural synchrony and hence Wave I clarity and amplitude, they often are too slow given the time constraints associated with neonatal screening. We have found that a repetition rate of 17.1/s does not penalize Wave I amplitude when compared to a rate of 11.1/s. Hence, it represents an excellent compromise between too slow and too rapid and allows for significant savings of overall test time. At a conventional rate of 11.1/s it would take 12.0 min to record a BAER for both ears in a test-retest paradigm. At a rate of 17.1/s, however, there would be about a 5-min savings in test time. Although this might appear trivial, it actually translates into a total time advantage of more than 13 min when combined with the 8-min time savings from the hearing screening component. If necessary, one can average more samples to improve signal-to-noise ratio in the same or less time than would be required to record 2,000 averages at 11.1/s. Moreover, it permits evaluation of more infants within the same alloted time period, which increases hospital or clinical practice revenue.

Recommended stimulus polarity. Consistent with the discussion on choice of click polarity for BAER hearing screening, the same arguments against the use of an alternating click holds for neurologic BAER screening (see p. 444). Because the use of insert receivers circumvent the problem of stimulus artifact that most likely was the principal rationale for using alternating polarity stimuli, and because rarefaction stimuli yield better Wave I amplitude in preterm newborns when compared both to condensation and alternating clicks, we again recommend use of rarefaction events for neurologic BAER screening. The data presented in Figure 8.10 are taken from Schwartz et al. (1989) and demonstrate the increased Wave I amplitude achieved with rarefaction versus condensation click stimuli across 40 preterm infants.

Recommended click intensity. Because the primary goal of neurologic BAER screening is to assess the functional integrity of the auditory brainstem pathway, it would seem prudent to stimulate the system at a sufficiently high intensity to optimize neural synchrony and transmission such that the abnormal system will be clearly differentiated from the normal. Yet, when one reviews the salient BAER screening literature, the typical choice of the high-intensity click is 60 dB nHL (Cevette, 1984; Cox et al., 1984; Galambos et al., 1982; Hecox & Galambos, 1974; Jacobson et al., 1982; Mjoen, Langslet, Tangsrud, & Sundby, 1982; Ruth et al., 1985; Stein, Ozdamar, Kraus, & Paton, 1983).

Given that in any neural system there is a direct trade-off between stimulus intensity and response amplitude, and because it is recognized that Wave I amplitude is compromised as signal intensity falls below 70 dB nHL (Schwartz & Berry, 1985), use of 60 dB nHL is contrary to the clinical goal to optimize neural synchrony and transmission. Consequently, we recommend that neurologic BAER screening be done at a high signal intensity such as 110 dB peak SPL (80 dB nHL re: adult norms) and that the signal be transduced through tubephone receivers as described for hearing screening.

Following this strategy, the BAER of the neurologically normal preterm infant consists of a Wave I having a latency and amplitude entirely like that of the adult, with Waves III and V being delayed in latency relative to the adult as illustrated in Figure 8.11. Wave III also is characterized by a broader shape and Wave V by a reduced amplitude and broader slope in the infant ABR. Recall that according to Schwartz and co-workers (1989), the delays in Wave I latency among newborns often reported in the research literature most likely reflect the effects of reduced signal SPL delivered to the infant cochlea through standard electro-dynamic earphones due to displacement of the transducer from over the

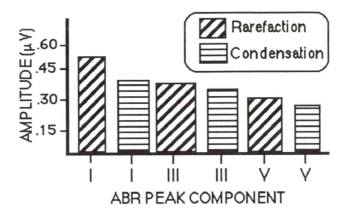

Figure 8.10. Comparison of peak amplitude for Waves I, III, and V for BAERs recorded to rarefaction and condensation clicks in 40 preterm infant ears. Note the larger Wave I amplitude for rarefaction versus condensation stimuli. Adapted from Schwartz et al. (1989).

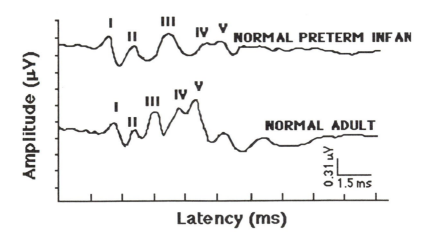

Figure 8.11. Comparison of BAERs recorded from a normal preterm infant (gestational age = 37 weeks) and a normal adult.

baby's external auditory meatus during testing. Because a constant pressure headband is not used, and the infant is prone to changing position or some other body movement while sleeping, there also is opportunity for the earphone to shift position. Furthermore, the poor-quality acoustic seal from a hand-held earphone creates low-frequency leakage around the earphone cushion, which reduces the available SPL delivered to the infants' cochlea in exactly the frequency region in which they are most sensitive. Of course a collapsed ear canal due to pressure from the earphone cushion also could reduce effective transmission of sound to the cochlea, thereby resulting in an abnormal BAER.

Recommended pass–fail criterion.   As with adults, the principal pathophysiologic BAER findings in pediatric neurologic disease are prolongation in conduction times from the peripheral nerve to higher order brainstem nuclei, loss of specific peak components that are not explainable on the basis of hearing sensitivity loss, amplitude abnormalities, and disruptions in wave morphology. Of course, successful interpretation of neurologic disorder in infants requires age-specific normative data; *you cannot use adult norms with infants*.

Among the most salient BAER abnormalities in the neurologically compromised infant is a prolonged central conduction time (I-V interpeak latency). This is exactly the reason why optimization of Wave I is critical, since it represents the electrophysiologic benchmark of the distal aspect of the peripheral VIIIth nerve. In the absence of Wave I, statements about brainstem function are tenuous at best, because any latency delays of rostral peaks III and V may be due to peripheral hearing loss. Among various groups of infants that might display abnormal interpeak intervals (I-III, I-V, III-V) are those with intraventricular hemorrhage involving posterior fossa structures, perinatal asphyxia, hyperbilirubinemia, hydrocephalus, and substance addiction. This later category is particularly interesting in light of the influx of illegal drugs into American society. Figure 8.12 presents an illustrative example of brainstem dysfunction in an otherwise normal preterm infant born to a mother who was a cocaine abuser. The top panel displays a comparative tracing from a typical normal infant of the same gestational age. Observe that the dominant aberrant features are a prolonged I-V interpeak interval and an abnormal V/I amplitude ratio. We have now seen this pattern in several such babies in an ongoing study of cocaine abuse; however, we have not observed the same consistent trend toward BAER abnormality as reported most recently by Shih, Cone-Wesson, and Reddix (1988).

Summary of neonatal BAER neurologic screening.   Table 8.2 summarizes the protocol used at the University of Pennsylvania for neonatal intensive care BAER neurologic screening. The philosophical underpinnings

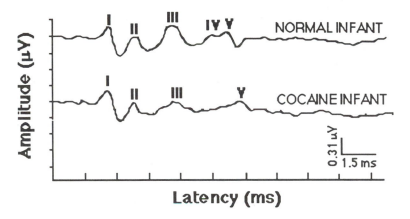

Figure 8.12. Example of an abnormal auditory brainstem response (bottom trace) in a cocaine baby. The BAER from an age-matched normal 35-week gestational age preterm infant (top trace) is shown for comparison.

of this protocol relate to optimizing Wave I amplitude and morphology for calculating brainstem transmission time. The pass–fail criterion relates to prolongations in interpeak latency relative to age-appropriate normative data, abnormal V/I amplitude ratio, and aberrant waveform morphology. We strongly recommend multiple-recording montages accompanied by individual channel bandpass filtering to help define specific peak components. We continue to underscore the importance of a good signal-to-noise ratio and the need to eliminate as much myogenic and electrical interference as possible prior to accepting a given recording.

The BAER in pediatric neurodiagnostics

In general application of the BAER to pediatric neurodiagnostics is not very different from that of adults with the exception perhaps of the pathogenesis of the diseases encountered. Unquestionably the most common neurologic BAER entities in adults are cerebellopontine angle tumors and demyelinating disease, although there are certainly a host of other brainstem lesions (e.g., cerebellar tumors) and vascular disorders (e.g., arteriovenous malformations, basilar artery aneurysm, and stroke) that can alter the BAER. When an acoustic tumor is seen in children it often

TABLE 8.2
Neonatal Neurologic BAER Screening Protocol Used at the Division
of BioelectroDiagnosis and Neural Monitoring,
University of Pennsylvania Medical Center

Recording Set Up		Recording Parameters	
Test Site:	Intensive Care Nursery	Epoch:	15 ms
No. of Channels:	4	Bandpass:	100–1500 Hz[a]
Montage:		Stimulus:	Click
Channel 1:	noninverting = Cz inverting = A_1	Duration:	100 μS
Channel 2:	noninverting = Cz inverting = A_2	Rate:	17.1/S
Channel 3:	noninverting = A_1 inverting = A_2	Polarity:	Rarefaction
Channel 4:	noninverting = Cz inverting = noncephalic	Intensity:	80 dB HL
Transducer:	Insert Tubephone™	No. of Sweeps:	Variable RE: S/N Ratio
Ear Tested:	Both		

[a]Filter bandpass for Channel 4 = 30–1500 Hz.

is part of the complex of neurofibromatosis 2 (bilateral acoustic tumors) which can also have other associated manifestations such as café au lait spots and/or the classic multiple subcutaneous lesions. In such cases the BAER abnormality would be the same as that seen with adults, as discussed by Musiek in Chapter 7.

In children, pontine glioma represents a more common primary pediatric brain tumor. The BAER almost always depicts bilateral central abnormality in the form of absent rostral peak components with maintenance of the peripheral nerve responses (I-II).

A second pediatric neoplastic disorder that can present with significant BAER abnormality is that of cerebellar juvenile astrocytoma because there can be marked midbrain involvement. Here, too, the BAER can be bilaterally abnormal with aberration or complete loss of the rostral components. It is important to remember that these later components represent combined activity from the contralateral brainstem. As such, alterations in peaks III and V may represent an effect of the tumor on the side opposite to the one being stimulated.

Similar to acoustic tumor, multiple sclerosis (MS) is infrequently seen within the first decade; however, there are a myriad of neurodegenerative disorders [e.g., leukodystrophy, Friedreich's ataxia, inborn errors in metabolism (such as phenylketonuria, maple syrup urine disease) that cause dysmyelination of the central nervous system, which will disrupt auditory brainstem transmission along the same lines as MS. Jabbari, Schwartz, MacNeil, and Coker (1981), for example, reported BAER abnormalities in five children with Friedrich ataxia. They noted that although each sibling presented with different BAER manifestations of the disease, the general clinical picture was one of complete absence or poor morphology of rostral components III-V bilaterally. BAER examples associated with other paedoneurologic diseases were described by Hecox, Cone, and Blaw (1981) and Davis, Aminoff, and Berg (1985).

In addition to central nervous system neoplasm, infection, intoxication, and vascular disorder, abnormal BAER patterns can emerge in children with congenital structural defects of the brain such as Arnold-Chiari malformation. This congenital anomaly of the hindbrain is characterized by displacement of the cerebellar vermis into the spinal canal and a distorted, elongated pons and medulla. The BAER pattern seen with Arnold-Chiari malformation can be characterized by prolongations, distortions, or total loss of Waves III-V similar to that seen in patients with cerebellar abnormalities.

Undoubtedly the nosology of congenital neurologic diseases, syndromes, and structural deformities that will affect the BAER is so extensive that a detailed description in a single book chapter is prohibited. It is important to realize also that since the prevalence of these neuropathologies is quite low, the majority of these children will be seen primarily by evoked potential laboratories, such as ours, that are based in large, often medical school-affiliated tertiary care hospitals tied in some way to a children's hospital. Audiologists working in community or university hearing and speech centers or those affiliated with a private otolaryngology practice most likely will not encounter such children; however, they should develop at least an academic appreciation for the pathophysiology of these disease entities.

Application of the BAER in acute pediatric care

During the past decade the monitoring of sensory evoked potentials in comatose adult patients suffering from closed head injury has become routine in many trauma centers. Much of this work has been directed toward correlating the initial BAER classification upon admission to the head trauma facility to the final neurologic outcome (Cant, Hume, Judson, & Shaw, 1986; Greenberg & Becker, 1976; Greenberg, Becker, Miller, & Mayer, 1977; Greenberg, Newlon, & Becker, 1982; Greenberg, Newlon, Hyatt, Narayan, & Becker, 1981; Greenberg, Stablein, & Becker, 1981; Hall, Haungfu, & Gennarelli, 1982). (For detailed reviews see Hall, 1985; Hall & Tucker, 1986, 1988; Hall & Mackey-Hargadine, 1986.)

In addition to adults, the BAER also has been applied to a lesser extent in the pediatric acute care setting. Depending on specific areas of the country, the most common reason for acute pediatric trauma is either closed head injury secondary to motor vehicle or bicycle accident or hypoxic-ischemic insult due to near drowning. In each of these cases the BAER is particularly useful for assessing brainstem function when routine neurological exam is precluded due to coma.

We are not of the opinion that sensory evoked potentials are accurate predictors of neurologic outcome in head injured patients. Of course there are exceptions. These are patients whose BAERs are classified as Grades III or IV (Figure 8.13) wherein the initial recording is significantly abnormal relative to interpeak latency prolongation greater than 5.0 ms, distorted morphology, loss of one or more peak components, or electrical silence with the exception of a peripheral nerve response. If, on the other hand, the admitting BAER is normal or only mildly abnormal, the correlation to neurologic outcome is poor. Similar experiences were reported most recently by Cant et al. (1986). The one BAER pattern that we are most sure of is that which is characterized only by a peripheral nerve response; that is, Wave(s) I or I and II only as depicted in Figure 8.13. This is the BAER signature of brain death from traumatic head injury.

In contrast to the head injured child, prediction of neurologic outcome is much better for near-drowning children who have suffered a cardiac arrest, thus causing inadequate cerebral perfusion/oxygenation. We recently determined the efficacy of the BAER in predicting neurologic outcome in 47 near-drowning children ranging in age from 7 months to 5 years (mean = 2.1 years) admitted to the Pediatric Intensive Care Unit for cardiac arrest (estimated duration ranged from 3 to 90 min). Following hemodynamic stability, all were placed immediately into barbiturate coma with moderate hyperventilation, hyperoxygenation, and mild hypothermia.

If the initial BAER recorded within 5 to 24 hrs postarrest was normal (re 95% confidence limit) on the basis of I-V interpeak latency and amplitude, we predicted no neurologic compromise. If there was only slight interpeak prolongation (<5.0 ms) after correcting the mild hypothermia, and both absolute and relative amplitude measures were normal, then

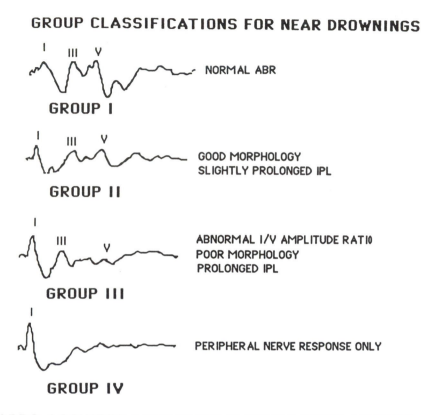

GROUP CLASSIFICATIONS FOR NEAR DROWNINGS

GROUP I — NORMAL ABR

GROUP II — GOOD MORPHOLOGY SLIGHTLY PROLONGED IPL

GROUP III — ABNORMAL I/V AMPLITUDE RATIO POOR MORPHOLOGY PROLONGED IPL

GROUP IV — PERIPHERAL NERVE RESPONSE ONLY

ABRS ACQUIRED LESS THAN 5 HOURS POST ARREST

Figure 8.13. Classification system used to predict neurologic outcome of near drowning children based on BAER results obtained within 5 hrs. following cardiac arrest.

only mild neurologic deficit was predicted. Such deficits were related to feeding ability, ambulation, communicative ability, and personality disturbance. Finally, if there was substantial BAER abnormality either in the form of corrected interpeak latency delay equal to or exceeding 5.0 ms with decreased Wave V amplitude, and/or a V/I amplitude ratio greater than 2:1, or there was a loss of some or all rostral peaks (III-V), then the prognosis for survival was poor or prediction was for severe neurologic compromise requiring chronic care.

Using these guidelines we calculated the operating characteristics of this prognostic-model by defining operationally all of the children who presented with a normal initial BAER as nondiseased. When these data were analyzed without regard to degree of neurologic deficit, sensitivity of the BAER for correct prediction was 94% (false-negative = 6%) and test specificity was a remarkable 100% (false-positive = 0%). Thus these results support the ability of the BAER to predict clinical neurologic outcome in children who have suffered global brain ischemia as a result of cardiac arrest from near drowning.

Summary of the BAER in pediatric neurodiagnostics

As with adults, application of the BAER in pediatric neuroaudiology has proven to play a major role in defining the status of the auditory brainstem. When clinical neurologic signs and symptoms are either normal or equivocal, the BAER can be used to establish the presence and general locus of pathology and/or can help unmask insidious lesion. Even when clinical signs and symptoms point to a diagnosis, the BAER can provide noninvasive objective documentation of neuroelectric abnormality to help confirm the diagnosis.

In addition to its usefulness in differential diagnosis, the BAER has been shown to help monitor changes in the central nervous system in the unresponsive child and to predict long-term neurologic outcome in children who have suffered hypoxic-ischemic insult. As such, the BAER aides in our understanding of the pathophysiology of brain injury and serves as a useful adjunct to other physiologic monitoring devices in the early identification of reversible central nervous system dysfunction.

Beyond the brainstem

Despite the enormous clinical success in recording the far-field brainstem auditory evoked response with young children, investigators have continued to search for other auditory bioelectric potentials that might be used either to complement the BAER in terms of defining more clearly type, degree, and configuration of hearing loss, or as an electrophysiologic window to higher brain function. Unfortunately, much of the applied work in these areas has been plagued by the inescapable effects of central nervous system maturation or to the sensitivity of these potentials to the patient's state of arousal and attention. Consequently, neither the audiologic nor the neurodiagnostic application of middle latency and late cortical responses has enjoyed much success in the pediatric population.

The middle latency response

The middle latency response (MLR) first described by Geisler, Frishkopf, and Rosenblith (1958) actually preceded the BAER as a short latency auditory evoked potential that seemed to correlate with the subject's psychophysical threshold of hearing. Its characteristic waveform in the adult is shown in Figure 8.14, with the most prominent positive peak, P_a appearing around 25 ms poststimulus onset.

During the early to mid 1970s, the application of the tonal MLR as an objective estimate of hearing threshold was zealously exploited by a cadre of young investigators at the University of Wisconsin. Despite repeated early evidence (Goldstein & McRandle, 1976; McRandle, Smith, & Goldstein, 1974; Mendel, Adkinson, & Harker, 1977; Wolf & Goldstein, 1980) that a frequency-specific MLR could be recorded quite reliably and consistently in infants, momentum for its clinical adoption never seemed to materialize. Most likely the advent of the BAER and its rapid acceptance into the neonatal nursery impacted heavily on the fate of the MLR.

Renewed interest in the MLR surfaced upon realization that the transient BAER did not serve as a frequency-specific correlate to the pure tone audiogram and that efforts to use frequency-specific stimuli did not prove initially successful. Then, in 1981, Galambos, Makeig, and Talmachoff described an auditory steady state response (SSR) having an amplitude that was greatest when evoked by low-frequency versus high-frequency tonal stimuli. As such, it appeared to offer the perfect compliment to the BAER. This so-called 40-Hz response was a rapid rate (40/s) variant of the conventional slow rate (< 10/s) MLR. It consisted of successive overlapping P_a components within a 50-ms epoch. From the onset the implication was clear that the 40-Hz event-related potential could be used for predicting low-frequency hearing threshold in children.

Unfortunately, enthusiasm for the audiologic application of the transient or steady state MLR was short lived. Sprague and Thornton (1982) were among the first to provide evidence that the MLRs seen with infants as reported by the University of Wisconsin group (Goldstein & McRandle, 1976; McRandle et al., 1974; Mendel, Atkinson, & Harker, 1977; Wolf & Goldstein, 1980) most likely were response oscillations and distortions introduced by steep analog filtering (48 dB/octave) the EEG within a narrow passband (20–175 Hz). With wide-band (20–2000 Hz) filtering, the MLR was visualized in only 1 of 35 infants and young children. This phenomenon was verified 1 year later by Kileny (1983) and has since been expounded on by Stein and Kraus (1987).

In addition to filter effects, stimulus rate also has been shown to play a major role in the MLR (Fifer, 1985; Jerger, Chmiel, Glaze, & Frost, 1987; Kraus, Smith & McGee, 1987; Stapells, Galambos, Costello, & Makeig,

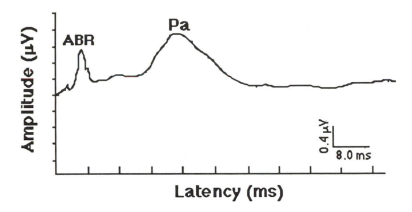

Figure 8.14. Example of a middle latency potential showing the prominent Pa component.

1988); that is, the newborn and young child shows no consistent P_a component, regardless of rate. In some babies, for example, P_a is present only at very slow rates (1–2/s) but its latency can range from 30 to 80 ms (Fifer, 1985; Jerger et al., 1987). In others, P_a or the steady state response simply cannot be appreciated, regardless of rate. To be sure, the 40-Hz response is entirely absent in babies.

The MLR in pediatric neurodiagnostics. It would appear that dependency on neuromaturation precludes recording either the conventional transient or steady state aspects of the MLR with children below at least 12 years of age. Research on the spatio-temporal organization of the MLR in adults has shown that the power of P_a is distributed widely across the scalp to monaural stimulation and achieves its largest amplitude over the midfrontal (Fz) and mid central (Cz) regions (Wood & Wolpaw, 1982; Picton, Hillyard, Krausz, & Galambos, 1974; Ozdamar & Kraus, 1983; Deiber, Irbanez, Fischer et al., 1988; Kraus & McGee, 1988). Two recent studies (Scherg & Von Cramon, 1986; Deiber et al., 1988) have suggested that at P_a maximum amplitude, two dipolar source activities within each temporal lobe overlap partially in time, with the primary one being tangential and the secondary radial. As such, the widely distributed electric field with maximum power at the vertex could result from the summed activity of the two tangential dipoles located within each temporal lobe, respectively. This conclusion is substantiated from the works of Kraus, Ozdamar, Heir, and Stein (1982) and Kileny, Paccioretti, and Wilson (1987) who reported a reduction or absence of P_a amplitude when recorded by an electrode placed over the temporal and/or supratemporal area of the involved hemisphere of patients with surgically confirmed temporal lobe lesion.

On the basis of the accumulated evidence on the scalp topography of the MLR, the recent application of P_a abnormalities in the diagnosis of central auditory processing disorder (CAPD) in children must be interpreted with caution (Jerger & Jerger, 1985; Jerger, Oliver, & Chmiel, 1988). Understanding the neurodevelopmental sensitivity of the MLR in children and knowing that recording from the vertex represents summed electrical activity from both hemispheres, we recommend guarded interpretation from such data. Although the Jerger et al. examples are provocative, the MLR simply is too inconsistent with young children to consider its routine clinical use in the differential assessment of learning disability.

The late vertex potential

First described by P. A. Davis from the awake brain and H. Davis and co-workers from the sleeping brain in 1939, the slow vertex auditory evoked potential is a polyphasic series of waves with latencies ranging from 50 to 300 milliseconds. The prominent N_1-P_2 complex, so known for both their polarity and latency, also has a fronto-central scalp topography. Although the exact generator source(s) is still debated, it is thought to originate in the primary auditory cortices in the supratemporal plane and possibly from adjacent inferior parietal structures. Like the MLR, the slow vertex response (SVR) derives its maximal power over the mid-central region because the dipole in the primary auditory cortex has a vertical orientation.

During the 1950s and 1960s these second- and third-order cortical evoked responses were the topic of considerable audiologic research. Because it was possible to record the SVR to relatively long duration frequency-specific tonal stimuli, it represented the ideal electrophysiological analog to the pure tone audiogram. Unfortunately response amplitude is governed almost entirely by the state of the patient; that is, it is tied directly to depth of sleep. It goes without saying, therefore, that despite the ability to use long duration frequency-specific stimuli for audiometric mapping, it has little pediatric application both for audiologic and neurodiagnostic purposes since it requires an attentive, awake subject—a state that a young child usually is incapable of maintaining for long durations. We refer the interested reader to the classic monograph by Davis (1976), "Principals of Electric Response Audiometry" for a detailed review on audiometric application of the SVR.

In perspective

In this chapter we have attempted to present what we consider to be a rational, defensible clinical approach to the application of auditory evoked potentials in pediatrics. Although our philosophy may be contrary to conventional practice or what routinely is taught in graduate seminars or 3-day workshops, it stems from a considerable amount of critical appraisal, empirical investigation, and years of clinical trial and error.

We have learned that a person cannot become an effective electrophysiologist without a broad fund of knowledge in areas tangential to audiology. Having functional understanding of neuroanatomy, neurophysiology, and the pathogenesis of neurological disease are necessary prerequisites to becoming a successful electrophysiologist. Clearly, appreciation for the principles of clinical epidemiology and the influence of disease prevalence on a test's operating characteristics is critically important to any field that uses laboratory tests.

Throughout this chapter we have made every attempt to explain the reasons that underlie our clinical strategies, an approach that is all too often neglected in book chapter preparation. It is our hope that the techniques and concepts presented herein can be implemented immediately upon completion of this chapter, regardless of the readers' particular professional milieu.

References

Alberti, P. W., Hyde, M. L., Riko, K., Corbin, H., & Abramovich, S. (1983). An Evaluation of BERA for hearing screening in high-risk neonates. *Laryngoscope, 93,* 1115–1121.

ASHA Committee on Infant Hearing. (1989). Audiologic screening of newborn infants who are at risk for hearing impairment. *Asha, 31,* 89–92.

Bess, F. H., Peek, B. F., & Chapman, J. J. (1979). Further observations on noise levels in infant incubators. *Pediatrics, 63,* 100–106.

Cant, B. R., Hume, A. L., Judson, J. A., & Shaw, N. A. (1986). The assessment of severe head injury by short latency somatosensory and brain-stem auditory evoked potentials. *Electroencephalography and Clinical Neurophysiology, 65,* 188–195.

Cevette, M. J. (1984). Auditory brainstem response testing in the intensive care unit. *Seminars in Hearing, 5,* 57–69.

Cox, L. C., Hack, M., & Metz, D. A. (1984). Auditory brainstem response abnormalities in the very low birthweight infant: Incidence and risk factors. *Ear and Hearing, 5,* 47–51.

Davis, H. (1976). Principals of electric response audiometry. *Annals of Otology, Rhinology, and Laryngology, 28* (Supplement), 1–96.

Davis, H., Davis, P. A., Loomis, A., et al. (1939). Electrical reactions of the human brain to auditory stimulation during sleep. *Journal of Neurophysiology, 2,* 500–514.

Davis, H., & Hirsh, S. K. (1976). The audiometric utility of the brain stem response to low-frequency sounds. *Audiology, 15,* 181–195.

Davis, H., & Hirsh, S. K. (1979). A slow brain stem response for low frequency audiometry. *Audiology, 18,* 445–461.

Davis, H., & Owen, J. H. (1985). Brainstem auditory evoked responses. In Owen, J. H., & Davis, H. (Eds.), *Evoked potential testing: Clinical applications* (pp. 55–108). Orlando: Grune & Stratton.

Davis, P. A. (1939). Effects of acoustic stimuli on the waking brain. *Journal of Neurophysiology, 2,* 494–499.

Davis, S. L., Aminoff, M. J., & Berg, B. O. (1985). Brain-stem auditory evoked potentials in children with brain-stem or cerebellar dysfunction. *Archives of Neurology, 42,* 156–160.

Deiber, M. P., Irbanez, V., & Fischer, F., et al. (1988). Sequential mapping favours the hypothesis of distinct generators for Na and Pa middle latency auditory evoked potentials. *Electroencephalography and Clinical Neurophysiology: Evoked Potentials, 71,* 187–197.

Dennis, J. M., Sheldon, R., Toubas, P., & McCaffee, M. A. (1984). Identification of hearing loss in the neonatal intensive care unit population. *American Journal of Otology, 5,* 201–205.

Don, M., & Eggermont, J. J. (1978). Analysis of the click-evoked brainstem potentials in man using high-pass noise masking. *Journal of the Acoustical Society of America, 63,* 1084–1092.

Durieux-Smith, A., Edwards, C. G., Picton, T. W., & McMurray, B. (1985). Auditory brainstem responses to clicks in neonates. *Journal of Otolaryngology,* (Supplement 14), 12–18.

Eggermont, J. J., & Don, M. (1980). Analysis of click-evoked brainstem potentials in humans using high-pass noise masking. *Journal of the Acoustic Society of America, 68,* 1671–1675.

Fifer, R. (1985). *The MLR and SSEP in neonates.* Unpublished doctoral dissertation, Baylor College of Medicine.

Galambos, R., Hicks, G. E., & Wilson, M. J. (1982). The auditory brainstem response reliably predicts hearing loss in graduates of a tertiary intensive care nursery. *Ear and Hearing, 5,* 254–260.

Galambos, R., Makeig, S., & Talmachoff, P. J. (1981). A 40-Hz auditory potential recorded from the human scalp. *Proceedings of the National Academy of Sciences, 78,* 263–264.

Geisler, C., Frishkopf, L., & Rosenblith, W. (1958). Extracranial responses to acoustic clicks in man. *Science, 128,* 1210–1211.

Goldstein, R., & McRandle, C. C. (1976). Middle components of the averaged electroencephalic response to clicks in neonates. In S. K. Hirsh, D. H. Eldredge, I. J. Hirsh, & S. R. Silverman (Eds.), *Hearing and Davis: Essays honoring Hallowell Davis* (pp. 445–456). St. Louis: Washington University Press.

Gorga, M. P., Kaminski, J. R., & Beauchaine, K. A. (1988) Auditory brainstem responses from graduates of an intensive care nursery using an insert earphone. *Ear and Hearing, 9,* 144–147.

Gorga, M. P., Kaminski, J. R., Beauchaine, K. A., & Jesteadt, W. (1988). Auditory brainstem responses to tone bursts in normal hearing subjects. *Journal of Speech and Hearing Research, 31*, 87–97.

Greenberg, R. P., & Becker, D. P. (1976). Clinical applications and results of evoked potential data in patients with severe head injury. *Surgical Forum, 26*, 484–486.

Greenberg, R. P., Becker, D. P., Miller, J. D., & Mayer, D. J. (1977). Evaluation of brain function in severe head trauma with multimodality evoked potentials. Part II. Localization of brain dysfunction in correlation with posttraumatic neurologic condition. *Journal of Neurosurgery, 47*, 163–177.

Greenberg, R. P., Newlon, P. G., & Becker, D. P. (1982). The somatosensory evoked potentials in patients with severe head injury: Outcome prediction in monitoring brain function. *Annals of the New Academy of Sciences, XX*, 683–688.

Greenberg, R. P., Newlon, P. G., Hyatt, M. S., Narayan, R. K., & Becker, D. P. (1981a). Prognostic implications of early multimodality evoked potentials in severely head injured patients: A prospective study. *Journal of Neurosurgery, 54*, 740–750.

Greenberg, R. P., Stablein, D. M., & Becker, D. P. (1981). Noninvasive localization of brainstem lesions in the cat with multimodality evoked potentials: Correlation with human head-injured data. *Journal of Neurosurgery, 54*, 740–750.

Hall, J. W., III, Haungfu, M., & Gennarelli, T. A. (1982). Auditory function in acute severe head injury. *Laryngoscope, 92*, 883–890.

Hall, J. W., III, Kripal, J. P., & Hepp, T. (1988). Newborn hearing screening with auditory brainstem response: Measurement problems and solutions. *Seminars in Hearing, 9*, 15–33.

Hall, J. W., III, Mackey-Hargadine, J., & Allen, S. J. (1985). Monitoring neurologic status of comatose patients in the intensive care unit. In J. T. Jacobson (Ed.), *The auditory brainstem response* (pp. 253–283). San Diego: College Hill Press.

Hall, J. W., & Tucker, D. A. (1986). Sensory evoked responses in the intensive care unit. *Ear and Hearing, 7*, 220–232.

Hall, J. W., & Tucker, D. A. (1988). Auditory brainstem response in the evaluation of peripheral versus central nervous system dysfunction in the pediatric intensive care unit. *Seminars in Hearing, 9*, 47–60.

Hall, J. W., III, & Mackey-Hargadine, J. R. (1986). Sensory evoked responses in the diagnosis of brain death. In M. E. Miner & K. A. Wagner (Eds.), *Neurotrauma: Treatment, rehabilitation and related issues* (pp. 133–154). Boston: Butterworths.

Hecox, K., & Burkhard, R. (1982). Developmental dependencies of the human brainstem auditory evoked response. *Annals of the New York Academy of Sciences, 388*, 538–556.

Hecox, K., & Galambos, R. (1974). Brain stem auditory evoked response in human infants and adults. *Archives of Otolaryngology, 99*, 30–33.

Hecox, K., & Jacobson, J. (1984). Auditory evoked potentials. In J. Northern (Ed.), *Hearing disorders* (pp. 57–73). Boston: Little, Brown.

Hecox, K. E., Cone, B., & Blaw, M. E. (1981). Brainstem auditory evoked response in the diagnosis of pediatric neurologic diseases. *Neurology, 31*, 832–840.

Hyde, M. L. (1985). The effect of cochlear lesions on the auditory brainstem responses. In J. T. Jacobson (Ed.), *The auditory brainstem response* (pp. 13–146). San Diego, CA: College Hill Press.

Jabbari, B., Schwartz, D. M., MacNeil, D. M., & Coker, S. B. (1981). Early abnormalities of brainstem auditory evoked potentials in Friedrich's ataxia: Evidence of primary brainstem dysfunction. *Neurology, 33,* 1071–1074.

Jacobson, J. T., & Morehouse, C. R. (1984). A comparison of auditory brain stem response and behavioral screening in high risk and normal newborn infants. *Ear and Hearing, 5,* 247–253.

Jacobson, J. T., Morehouse, C. R., & Johnson, M. J. (1982). Strategies for infant auditory brainstem response assessment. *Ear and Hearing, 3,* 263–270.

Jerger, J., Chmiel, R., Glaze, D., & Frost, J. (1987). Rate and filter dependence of the middle-latency response in infants. *Audiology, 26,* 269–283.

Jerger, J., & Jerger, S. (1985). Audiologic applications of early, middle, and late auditory evoked potentials. *Hearing Journal, 38,* 31–36.

Jerger, J., Oliver, T., & Chmiel, R. (1988). The auditory middle latency response. *Seminars in Hearing, 9,* 75–85.

Jerger, J., Oliver, T., & Stach, B. (1985). Auditory brainstem response testing strategy. In J. T. Jacobson (Ed.), *The auditory brainstem response* (pp. 371–388). San Diego, CA: College Hill Press.

Jerger, S. (1983). Decision matrix and information theory analysis in the evaluation of neuroaudiologic tests. *Seminars in Hearing, 4,* 121–132.

Joint Committee on Infant Hearing Position Statement 1982. *Ear and Hearing, 4,* 3–4.

Kavanagh, K. T., Domico, W. D., Franks, R., & Jin-Cheng, H. (1988). Digital filtering and spectral analysis of the low intensity auditory brainstem response. *Ear and Hearing, 9,* 43–47.

Kevanishvili, Z., & Aphonchenko, V. (1979). Frequency composition of brain stem auditory evoked potentials. *Scandinavian Audiology, 8,* 51–55.

Kileny, P. (1983). Auditory evoked middle-latency responses: Current issues. *Seminars in Hearing, 4,* 403–413.

Kileny, P., Paccioretti, D. R., & Wilson, A. F. (1987). Effects of cortical lesions on middle-latency auditory evoked responses (MLR). *Electroencephalography and Clinical Neurophysiology, 66,* 108–120.

Kodera, K., Yamane, H., Yamada, O., & Suzuki, J. (1977). Brain stem response audiometry at speech frequencies. *Audiology, 16,* 469–479.

Kraus, N., & McGee, T. (1988). Color imaging of the human middle latency response. *Ear and Hearing, 9,* 159–167.

Kraus, N., Ozdamar, O., Heir, D., & Stein, L. (1982). Auditory middle latency responses (MLRs) in patients with cortical lesions. *Electroencephalography and Clinical Neurophysiology, 54,* 275–287.

Kraus, N., Smith, D. I., & McGee, T. (1987). Rate and filter effects on the developing middle latency response. *Audiology, 26,* 257–268.

Laukli, E., & Mair, I. W. S. (1981). Early auditory-evoked responses: Filter effects. *Audiology, 20,* 300–312.

Laukli, E., & Mair, I. W. S. (1986). Frequency specificity of the auditory brainstem response: A derived study. *Scandinavian Audiology, 3,* 141–146.

Lippe, W., & Rubel, E. W. (1983). Development of place principle: Tonotopic organization. *Science, 219,* 514–516.

Marshall, R. E., Reichert, T. M., Kerley, S. M., & Davis, H. (1980). Auditory functions in newborn intensive care unit patients revealed by auditory brainstem potentials. *Journal of Pediatrics, 96,* 731–735.

McRandle, C., Smith, M., & Goldstein, R. (1974). Early averaged electroencephalic responses to clicks in neonates. *Annals of Otology, Rhinology, and Laryngology, 86,* 293–299.

Mendel, M. I, Adkinson, C. D., & Harker, L. A. (1977). Middle components of the auditory evoked potentials in infants. *Annals of Otology, Rhinology, and Laryngology, 86,* 293–299.

Mjoen, S., Langslet, A., Tangsrud, E., & Sundby, A. (1982). Auditory brainstem responses (ABR) in pre-term infants. *Acta Paediatrica Scandinavia, 71,* 711–715.

Morgan, D. E., Zimmerman, M. C., & Dubno, J. R. (1987). Auditory brain stem evoked responses characteristics in the full-term newborn infant. *Annals of Otology, Rhinology, and Laryngology, 96,* 142–151.

Northern, J. L., & Downs, M. P. (1978). *Hearing in children* (2nd ed.). Baltimore, MD: Williams & Wilkins.

Ozdamar, O., & Kraus, N. (1983). Auditory brainstem and middle latency responses in a patient with cortical deafness. *Electroencephalography and Clinical Neurophysiology, 53,* 224–230.

Picton, T., Hillyard, S., Krausz, H., & Galambos, R. (1974). Human auditory evoked potentials. I: Evaluation of components. *Electroencephalography and Clinical Neurophysiology, 30,* 179–190.

Picton, T. W., Stapells, D. R., & Campbell, K. R. (1981). Auditory evoked potentials from the human cochlea and brainstem. *Journal of Otolaryngology,* (Supplement 9), 1–41.

Richmond, K. H., Konkle, D. F., & Potsic, W. P. (1986). ABR screening of high-risk infants: Effects of ambient noise in the neonatal nursery. *Otolaryngology—Head and Neck Surgery, 94,* 552–560.

Rubel, E. W., Born, D. E., Dietch, J. S., & Durham, D. (1984). Recent advances toward understanding auditory system development. In C. Berlin (Ed.), *Hearing science* (pp. 109–158). San Diego: College Hill Press.

Ruth, R. A., Dey-Sigman, S., & Mills, J. A. (1985). Neonatal ABR hearing screening. *Hearing Journal, 38,* 39–45.

Scherg, M., & Von Cramon, D. (1986). Evoked dipole source potentials of the human auditory cortex. *Electroencephalography and Clinical Neurophysiology, 65,* 344–360.

Schulman-Galambos, C., & Galambos, R. (1975). Brainstem auditory-evoked responses in premature infants. *Journal of Speech and Hearing Research, 18,* 456–465.

Schwartz, D. M. (1987). NeuroDiagnostic Audiology: Contemporary perspectives. *Ear and Hearing,* (Supplement 8), 43S–48S.

Schwartz, D. M., & Berry, G. A. (1985). Normative Aspects of the ABR. In J. T. Jacobson (Ed.), *The auditory brainstem response* (pp. 65–97). San Diego: College Hill Press.

Schwartz, D. M., & Costello, J. A. (1988). Audiologic application of auditory evoked potentials in children. In F. H. Bess (Ed.), *Hearing impairment in children* (pp. 152–175). Parkton, MD: York Press.

Schwartz, D. M., Larson, V., & DeChicchis, A. R. (1981). Spectral characteristics of air and bone transducers used to record the auditory brainstem response. *Ear and Hearing, 6,* 274–277.

Schwartz, D. M., Pratt, R. E., & Schwartz, J. A. (1989). Auditory brainstem responses in preterm infants: Evidence of peripheral maturity. *Ear and Hearing, 10,* 14–22.

Shih, L., Cone-Wesson, B., & Reddix, B. (1988). Effects of maternal cocaine abuse on the neonatal auditory system. *International Journal of Pediatric Otorhinolaryngology, 15,* 245–251.

Simmons, F. B. (1980). Patterns of deafness in newborns. *Laryngoscope, 90,* 448–453.

Sprague, B., & Thornton, A. (1982, November). *Clinical utility and limitations of middle-latency auditory evoked potentials*. Paper presented at the annual convention of the American Speech-Language, Hearing Association, Toronto.

Stapells, D. R., Galambos, R., Costello, J. A., & Makeig, S. (1988). Inconsistency of auditory middle latency and steady-slate responses in infants. *Electroencephalography and Clinical Neurophysiology: Evoked Potentials, 71*, 289–295.

Stapells, D. R., Picton, T. W., Perez-Abalo, M., Read, D., & Smith, A. (1985). Frequency specificity in evoked potential audiometry. In J. T. Jacobson (Ed.), *The Auditory Brainstem Response* (pp. 147–177). San Diego: College Hill Press.

Stein, L., & Kraus, N. (1987). Maturation of the middle latency response. *Seminars in Hearing, 8*, 93–101.

Stein, L., Ozdamar, O., Kraus, N., & Paton, J. (1983). Follow-up of infants screened by auditory brainstem response in the neonatal intensive care unit. *Journal of Pediatrics, 103*, 447–453.

Suzuki, T., Hirai, Y., & Horiuchi, K. (1977). Auditory brainstem responses to pure tone stimuli. *Scandinavian Audiology, 6*, 51–56.

Suzuki, T., & Horiuchi, K. (1977). Effect of high-pass filter on auditory brainstem responses to tone pips. *Scandinavian Audiology, 6*, 123–126.

Teas, D. C., Eldredge, D. H., & Davis, H. (1962). Cochlear responses to acoustic transients: An interpretation of whole-nerve action potentials. *Journal of the Acoustic Society of America, 34*, 1438–1459.

Turner, R. G., & Nielson, D. W. (1984). Application of clinical decision analysis to audiological tests. *Ear and Hearing, 5*, 125–133.

Weber, B. (1988). Screening of high risk infants using auditory brainstem response audiometry. In F. H. Bess (Ed.), *Hearing impairment in children* (pp. 112–132). Parkton, MD: York Press.

Wolf, K. E., & Goldstein, R. (1980). Middle component AERs from neonates to low-level tonal stimuli. *Journal of Speech and Hearing Research, 23*, 185–201.

Wood, C. C., & Wolpaw, J. R. (1982). Scalp distribution of human auditory evoked potentials. II. Evidence for multiple sources and involvement of auditory cortex. *Electroencephalography and Clinical Neurophysiology, 54*, 25–38.

chapter nine

Hearing loss in newborns, infants, and young children

DAN F. KONKLE

JOHN T. JACOBSON

Contents

Introduction

The capability of audiologists to detect and assess hearing impairment in the pediatric population has increased dramatically since the late 1970s. Currently, for example, audiologists are able to detect accurately the presence of hearing loss in newborns only a few hours old, regardless of the severity of the impairment. Ear and frequency-specific information that define hearing sensitivity, audiometric configuration, and type of hearing loss often can be obtained by 6 months of age. Consequently, audiologists no longer must wait until a youngster is 2 to 3 years old before obtaining reliable and valid audiometric data to recommend confidently intervention in the form of amplification or other appropriate rehabilitative strategies.

Concurrent with this increased capability, however, has been an expanding level of responsibility that did not exist prior to the late 1970s. In addition to knowing the most appropriate type of stimuli required to elicit observable responses from pediatric listeners or the rationale for using various types of "play" or "conditioned" audiometry, today's pediatric audiologist must be able to develop and implement programs that maximize appropriate referrals from other professionals, identify and justify those populations that require audiological screening and subsequent follow-up assessment, and establish an array of assessment procedures that are both cost-effective and efficient. Stated differently, whereas advancements in technology coupled with the development of assessment strategies have combined to enhance the audiologist's capability to assess pediatric hearing, these new developments also have resulted in an increasing degree of accountability to devise and implement programmatic strategies that permit maximum and efficient delivery of service, especially as related to early detection and assessment of auditory impairment.

The focus of this chapter concerns various detection and assessment techniques that provide the basis of pediatric audiometry. In addition, however, emphasis is placed on the application of existing techniques into efficient clinical protocols designed to provide cost-effective service. Although it is recognized that there often is considerable overlap among age groups and specific detection or assessment techniques, the organization of material within this chapter is chronological, beginning with the newborn and progressing through school-aged children. In general, these age groups are categorized as birth to 6 months, 6 months to approximately 2 years, and 2 years of age and older. Because of the scope and nature of this chapter, much of the material is presented as an overview. However, a detailed bibliography and suggested readings are available in the reference section of this chapter for those who wish to explore various areas in more depth than presented here. Also, other chapters within this book contain valuable information concerning the use of auditory evoked potentials and middle ear immittance, both of which are important techniques for the detection and assessment of auditory impairment in infants. Again, the reader is referred to this information when appropriate within the context of this chapter.

Fundamental considerations

Importance of early identification of auditory impairment

Hearing loss suffered during the first 3 years of life, either congenital or acquired, conductive or sensorineural, represents a severe deterrent to the acquisition of linguistic skills necessary for subsequent psychosocial, educational, and vocational development (Menyuk, 1977; Osberger, 1986). Thus from a developmental standpoint, it is important to minimize the detrimental influence of hearing loss on language acquisition, especially during the first 3 years of life following birth. This goal can be achieved if there is early identification of the impairment, prompt intervention, and follow-up that combines medical/surgical treatment with the use of appropriate amplification and an intensive program of language stimulation.

It also is important to stress that auditory impairment is a symptom of a disease process, and identification of the hearing loss provides the physician information to assist in diagnosis. Consider, for example, that it is generally agreed that between 30% and 50% of all congenital hearing loss is transmitted genetically via inheritance patterns that, in the majority of cases, are well-documented. Prompt detection of genetic hearing loss, therefore, often allows identification of a specific genetic syndrome and provides the basis for accurate parental counseling. Although not always of genetic origin, approximately 30% of congenital hearing loss is associated with some form of syndrome disorder. Again, early detection of the hearing loss that often is the initial or only symptom of the syndrome permits medical/surgical management of other nonauditory problems that are associated with the syndrome. Finally, early detection of hearing loss and subsequent diagnosis of the disease process promotes better understanding and management of hearing disorders by creating a logical data base for research applications, and, equally important, serves as a guide for family counseling.

Because early detection and subsequent assessment of hearing impairment are prerequisites to early intervention and follow-up, it follows that early detection of an impairment without effective and adequate intervention represents an unjust, and perhaps an unethical, practice. Although this chapter focuses on early detection and assessment, the reader is reminded that prompt intervention is equally, if not more, important to the overall rehabilitation of infants and young children with hearing loss.

Nevertheless, it remains that early detection and assessment are the keys to successful rehabilitation.

Incidence of hearing loss in the newborn population

The incidence of hearing loss in the newborn population is difficult to quantify. Unfortunately, reliable data are not available nor have scientifically sound surveys been conducted upon which to base valid estimates for the number of infants born with educationally significant hearing impairment. Moreover, the limited data that are available convey a wide range of estimates suggesting that severe to profound hearing loss occurs in as few as 1:4,000 or in as many as 1:1,000 live births annually (Carrel, 1977; Catlin, 1978; Coplan, 1987; Fraser, 1971; Jaffe, 1977; Simmons, 1980). Hearing loss of lesser severity has been suggested to approximate 6:1,000 (Carrel, 1977). The American Speech-Language-Hearing Association (ASHA) Committee on Infant Hearing recently reviewed available data and, based on a projected national birth rate of 3.76 million live births annually, conservatively estimated that approximately 6,200 infants will be born each year with either congenital auditory impairment or hearing loss acquired shortly after birth (ASHA, 1988).

Strategies

The terms *detection* and *assessment* have been used frequently in this chapter, but thus far a distinction between the two has not been made. Detection of hearing loss refers to a process whereby a hearing impairment is discovered; however, the severity, type, audiometric configuration, or site of lesion are unspecified. An example of a detection process is a screening test that classifies a listener's hearing as simply normal or abnormal. If the result of the screening test is abnormal, additional audiological work-up is necessary in order to determine the type of impairment (e.g., conductive, sensorineural, or mixed), the magnitude of the loss (e.g., mild, moderate, severe, or profound), the configuration of the loss (e.g., hearing threshold as a function of frequency), and the site of lesion (e.g., cochlear or retrocochlear). This additional (i.e., follow-up) testing often requires the use of several audiological procedures and is referred to as hearing assessment.

The distinction between detection and assessment is important because these two concepts guide the clinical structure of audiological evaluation in the pediatric population. Whereas older children and adults usually are referred for audiological assessment because of symptoms they are able to recognize and report to their parents or physicians, infants and young children seldom have this same level of maturation, and symptoms that would otherwise result in audiological assessment usually go unnoticed. Although procedures such as auditory evoked potentials can be used effectively in the pediatric population to assess auditory impairment, there are various practical and financial restrictions that preclude the assessment of all newborns.

Consequently, clinical programs have focused on the use of detection strategies rather than mass audiological assessment of newborn infants. Moreover, detection of hearing loss in the newborn population has centered on screening specific groups of babies considered to be especially prone to auditory impairment. Typically, screening efforts are concentrated either on babies that require postdelivery management in an Intensive Care Unit (ICU), or those that do not require ICU management but have significant histories for any of several risk factors. In either case, the goal is to screen the infant prior to discharge from the hospital in an effort to promote early identification of hearing loss and to minimize the baby being lost to follow-up. Thus detection of hearing loss in the newborn population is limited to those infants who either are at risk for hearing loss or require ICU management. The criteria used to place an infant at risk for hearing loss have evolved over a period of more than 20 years and have been categorized into a "high-risk register."

High-risk register

The high-risk register is simply a list of factors that place a neonate at a potentially greater risk for hearing loss than those infants who do not present with any of the listed risk criteria. Historically, the concept of a high-risk register is a direct outgrowth of early behavioral auditory identification programs from Scandinavia (Froding, 1960; Wedenberg, 1956) and in North America by Downs and Sterritt (1964, 1967). The essence of the Downs and Sterritt studies provided a suggested protocol for screening newborns using the auropalpebral reflex, a modification of the Moro reflex, which was referred to as a startle response, and the combined observation of head and limb movements.

It is important to note that the intent of initial screening programs was to rule out severe to profound bilateral hearing loss. Using a matrix of observational techniques, Downs and Hemenway (1969) reported the results of the first major screening program in which a total of 17,000 newborns were screened in the Denver metropolitan area. Although this study provided the first attempt at mass infant screening, the protocol and reported results were met with justifiable criticism (Borton & Stark, 1972; Goldstein & Tait, 1971; Goodhill, 1967; Ling, Ling, & Doehring, 1970). Primary concerns focused on the variability of the behavioral protocol as a function of the response features used by Downs and Hemenway and their reported yield of false-positive and false-negative findings.

Although these critiques were not unique to the Downs and Hemenway investigation, they served to focus attention on the growing concern over early identification screening programs and reinforced the need for standardization of testing protocol. In 1969, therefore, the Joint Committee on Newborn Hearing was established and charged with the responsibility of making recommendations concerning newborn screening programs. The Joint Committee, which was composed of members of the American Speech and Hearing Association, the American Academy of Pediatrics, and the American Academy of Ophthalmology and Otolaryngology, issued a statement in 1970 that urged increased neonatal research; however, based on the limited available data the Joint Committee did not endorse routine mass infant hearing screening.

Two years later, in 1972, as a result of a series of longitudinal studies (Downs & Hemenway, 1969; Feinmesser & Tell, 1971; Mencher, 1972) and reports from England (Richards & Roberts, 1967) that suggested deaf infants were prone to factorial categorization, the Joint Committee issued a supplementary statement that gave rise to the now well-recognized "high-risk register" (HRR). The criteria that composed the HRR were given mnemonic reference and described as the ABCD's of deafness (Downs & Silver, 1972). The 1972 criteria included:

A. Affected family: history of hereditary childhood hearing impairment
B. Bilirubin levels: levels greater than 20mg/100ml serum
C. Congenital rubella syndrome: rubella or other nonbacterial intrauterine fetal infection
D. Defects of the ears, nose, or throat; malformed, low-set or absent pinnae; cleft lip or palate; and any residual abnormality of the otorhinolaryngeal system
S. Small at birth: birthweight less than 1500 grams (i.e., approximately 3.5 pounds)

The Joint Committee also recommended that infants who met any one of the criteria should be referred for a detailed audiological assessment during the first 2 months of life.

Following the issue of the ABCD's, subsequent early identification programs used the HRR in conjunction with various screening or assessment protocols. Encouraged by evidence from early newborn screening programs that implemented auditory brainstem response measures

(Galambos, 1978; Jacobson, Mencher, Seitz, & Pasrrott, 1979) and reflected in the success of the HRR in detecting hearing-impaired infants, the Joint Committee issued its most recent position paper (1982) in an attempt to clarify and expand the original 5-item criteria. The current HRR consists of seven factors including two additions to the 1972 statement: asphyxia and bacterial meningitis. Table 9.1 lists the criteria of the current HRR issued by the Joint Committee. A detailed account of this HRR is beyond the scope of this chapter, but the interested reader is referred to Gerkin (1984) for an excellent overview of the criteria, clinical manifestations, prevalence, and associated hearing loss.

The 1982 Joint Committee statement also recommended that any infant manifesting any item of the HRR should be screened under the supervision of an audiologist before the child reaches 6 months of age, and optimally before 3 months of age. The Committee did not specify a preferred method of screening but stated that either behavioral observation or auditory brainstem responses should be used in the screening protocol. Finally, the 1982 statement recommended audiological assessment of all at-risk infants who fail the screening and that medical, audiological, and psychoeducational management be provided to infants subsequently found to have hearing loss.

TABLE 9.1
Factors That Identify Infants At Risk for Hearing Impairment as Advocated by the 1982 Joint Committee on Infant Hearing

- A family history of childhood hearing impairment

- Congenital perinatal infection (e.g., cytomegalovirus, rubella, herpes, toxoplasmosis, syphilis)

- Anatomic malformations involving the head or neck (e.g., dysmorphic appearance, including syndromal and nonsyndromal abnormalities, overt or submucus cleft palate, morophologic abnormalities of the pinna)

- Birthweight less than 1500 gm

- Hyperbilirubinemia at a level exceeding indications for exchange transfusion

- Bacterial meningitis, especially from Haemoplilus influenzae

- Severe asphyxia, which may include infants with Apgar scores of 0 to 3 who fail to institute spontaneous respiration by 10 min and those with hypotonia persisting to 2 hr of age

Since the 1982 Joint Committee statement, there have been several reports that suggest that the current HRR will identify only about 50% of infants with congenital hearing loss (Matkin, 1988; Stein, Clark, & Kraus, 1983). As a result of these findings, some clinics have advocated the use of additional risk factors other than those included in the 1982 statement. Figure 9.1 displays the HRR employed at Geisinger Medical Center (GMC). To date, it is impossible to determine whether any one of the factors included in Figure 9.1, or if potential synergistic effects of two or more of these factors, will prove to be of significant value in detecting early hearing loss.

Neonatal detection and assessment (birth to 6 months)

Recall that the fundamental purpose of the HRR is to identify from a group of newborns those infants who have a high potential (i.e., risk) for auditory impairment. The HRR does not, however, detect hearing loss. Follow-up to the HRR requires that identified infants either be screened or assessed via appropriate audiological techniques.

Behavioral observation audiometry.   Several procedures have been advocated to screen and assess hearing loss in the neonatal population based on observed responses to controlled auditory stimuli. Historically, behavioral audiometric tests have been used most widely in the neonatal population and depend on reflexive reactions such as the auropalpebral, startle, and arousal responses. Audiological procedures that require these so-called behavioral responses commonly are called behavioral observation audiometry (BOA), because the reflexive behavior of the infant in response to auditory stimulation must be observed by one or more examiners.

Although the initial use of BOA generally is attributed to Downs and Sterritt (1967), perhaps the most widely used BOA procedure is that of Mencher (1974). This procedure, commonly termed *the arousal test*, requires the presentation of a noise stimulus (i.e., high-frequency narrow band or white noise) at an intensity of 90 to 100 dB sound pressure level (SPL). The infant is placed in a quiet room (i.e., ambient noise less than 60 dB SPL), unclothed, and evaluated along with two other infants considered not to be at risk for hearing loss. After the infant is in a stage of light sleep, the noise stimulus is presented and the infant's responses are observed by an audiologist and one or two other trained observers. The required response to the stimulus is generalized body movements (i.e., arousal response).

Other BOA procedures have been described by Hoverston and Moncur (1969), Feinmesser and Bauberger-Tell (1971), Thompson and

INFANT HIGH-RISK HEARING LOSS CHECKLIST
Audiology Services
Geisinger Medical Center
Danville, PA 17822

Date _____ Gestational age _____

Baby's Name _____ Birth Date _____ Chart No. _____

Parent(s)' Name _____ Home Address _____

Phone _____ Physician _____ Birth Weight _____

PRENATAL CONDITIONS

1. Rubella or other viral disease during pregnancy _____
2. Any bleeding indicating threatened abortion during pregnancy _____
3. Ototoxic drugs taken during pregnancy _____
4. Toxemia of pregnancy-enclampsia, hypertensive disorders _____
5. Rh incompatibility _____
6. Concurrent maternal diabetes mellitus _____
7. Concurrent maternal syphilis _____
8. Cytomegalic inclusion disease _____
9. Family history of deafness or other congenital abnormality (if yes, explain) _____

PERINATAL CONDITIONS   YES   NO

1. Prolonged labor: longer than 18 hours in primigravida. 8 hours in multigravida _____
2. Precipitate or uncontrolled delivery _____
3. Maternal hemorrhage, abruptio placenta, placenta previa _____
4. Sepsis or other infection present _____
5. Traction on neck, high or mid-forceps delivery, prolapsed cord, abnormal presentation, version and extraction
   _____
6. Fetal distress: passage of meconium, hypoxia, Apgar at 5 min. –7 or less, fetal or neonatal acidosis, respiratory
   distress syndrome _____

NEONATAL CONDITIONS

1. Apnea or cyanosis. Resuscitation requiring more than suctioning or simple stim _____
2. Ototoxic drug used in treating infection in infant _____
3. Hyperbilirubinemia: levels for exchange transfusions _____
4. Prolonged abnormality of central nervous system, e.g., convulsions _____
5. Paralysis _____
6. Birth weight less than 1500 gm (3.3 lbs) or over 5000 gm (11 lbs) _____
7. Discordant twin (smaller twin 25% or lighter and weighing less than 2000 gms) _____
8. Positive family history of hearing loss _____
9. Observed conditions:
      1. skeletal and cranial defects _____
      2. dwarfism _____
      3. malformations of extremities and digits _____
      4. cleft lip/palate _____
      5. underdeveloped maxilae or mandible _____
      6. external ear abnormalities _____

REMARKS: _____
_____
_____
_____
_____

Figure 9.1.   An infant high-risk checklist used to supplement criteria advocated
by the 1982 Joint Committee on Infant Hearing.

Weber (1974), Feinmesser and Tell (1976), and Gerber (1985), among others, but all are similar in that they require high-intensity noise stimuli, a state of quiet or light sleep, and observed reflexive responses. Consequently, there are several important limitations associated with BOA that must be considered when using this technique. First, care should be taken to avoid overinterpretation of BOA results given that responses to high-intensity stimuli preclude generalization about mild or moderate hearing loss. That is, the high-intensity noise will identify only infants with severe or profound hearing losses. Also, the overall health of at-risk or ICU infants may prevent or decrease reflexive responses. Second, examiners must be cautioned against observer bias that can result in high false-positive or false-negative response judgments (Moncur, 1968). Examiner bias can be controlled to some extent when two or more observers are used, especially if one of the observers is masked (i.e., the examiner is unaware of stimulus presentation). Third, reflexive responses typically habituate rapidly in infants older than 2 or 3 weeks of age, thereby minimizing the amount of audiometric information that can be obtained during a test session. Moreover, the presentation of intense noise often results in an agitated infant who will not quiet or go back to sleep. Fourth, although the instrumentation necessary to generate and control stimuli is relatively inexpensive, the time and number of examiners required to conduct BOA may prohibit its use in many clinical settings. Finally, use of BOA as a screening tool has been reported to yield unacceptable operating characteristics, that is, high false-positive and false-negative rates (Feinmesser & Tell, 1976; Jacobson & Morehouse, 1984).

Automated behavioral audiometry.   In order to avoid the problems associated with observer bias during BOA, several techniques have been advocated to automatically record infant responses to acoustic stimulation. Changes in respiration, heart rate, and overall generalized body movement have received the majority of research interest, but clinical applications using these response modes have been confined primarily to motor behavior (i.e., body movement). The reader interested in a review of respiratory and cardiovascular measures of auditory function are referred to Gilchrist (1977) and Mulac and Gerber (1977), respectively. Those procedures concerned with recording motor responses typically use specially designed "movement or pressure sensitive transducers" located in the infant's crib.

These procedures conceptually are similar to BOA, except that motor movement by the infant in response to acoustic stimulation is recorded by the special transducer (e.g., the transducer serves as the observer). The Crib-O-Gram (COG; Simmons & Russ, 1974) and Auditory Response Cradle (ARC; Bennett, 1975) are the two most commonly used of the automated infant testing techniques, but neither has gained wide clinical acceptance.

The COG uses a motion sensitive transducer placed under the mattress to record movement before, during, and after stimulation with a high-frequency noise band presented at 92 dB SPL. The ARC uses a custom-designed crib with motion sensitive devices located both in the mattress and headrest as well as a special respiratory transducer to record breathing behavior. The ARC monitors movement and respiration prior, during, and after stimulation with a noise band centered at about 3400 Hz presented at 85 dB SPL. Both the COG and ARC are under microprocessor control for stimulus presentation and response monitoring; thus the need for personnel is reduced as compared to BOA. Also, because these procedures are automated, testing can be conducted continuously during any part of the day. The amount of time necessary to test an infant with the COG is between 1.5 and 3 hr depending on the number of positive and negative responses to presented stimuli, whereas the testing time for the ARC has been reported to range from 5 to 10 min (Shepard, 1983).

Except for the issue of observer bias, automated procedures have the same limitations as those previously described for BOA. Specifically, automated techniques are not sensitive to mild or moderate hearing loss and relatively high over-referral rates have been reported (Durieux-Smith & Jacobson, 1985; Durieux-Smith, Picton, Edwards, Goodman, & MacMurray, 1985; Galambos, Hicks, & Wilson, 1982).

Auditory evoked potentials.   The application of auditory evoked potentials to detect and assess hearing status in neonates has gained popularity rapidly since the late 1970s. Many clinicians, including the authors of this chapter, consider the evolution and application of evoked potential technology to auditory assessment the single most important and exciting development to occur in the area of pediatric audiometry during the past decade. This observation is supported by the inclusion of an entire chapter in this book devoted solely to the use of auditory evoked potentials in hearing assessment of infants and young children (see Chapter 8). Given the depth of treatment of this topic in Chapter 8 (also see Cox, 1985; and Fria, 1985), the following discussion is restricted to an overview of programmatic considerations.

There are a variety of auditory evoked potentials that have been advocated for detection and assessment of auditory function, but the most commonly used is the auditory brainstem response (ABR). The ABR has been used both as a method to screen for hearing loss as well as to assess auditory function (Cox, 1985; Fria, 1985). Whereas the 1982 statement of the Joint Committee on Infant Hearing did not recommend a specific procedure to screen hearing of the at-risk infants, the ASHA Committee on Infant Hearing has endorsed the use of the ABR as a valid and reliable screening tool (ASHA, 1989). It is important to stress, particularly for the pediatric population, that ABR does not provide a direct measure of hearing. That is, the recorded waveform, or the absence of a recordable waveform, does not document that the acoustic signal is perceived by the patient. Rather, the ABR data are used to estimate hearing sensitivity based on clinical norms, instrumentation, age of the patient, general health status, and the established test procedures used within the individual clinical protocol. Nonetheless, ABR has become a powerful and valuable clinical procedure.

When the ABR is used to screen neonates for hearing loss, the following guidelines generally are accepted as important for an effective and efficient program: (a) Screening should be limited to high-risk infants or ICU graduates as compared to mass screening of all newborns, (b) Screening should be conducted when the infant is medically stable and at full-term conceptual age, (c) Responses should be obtained at more than one stimulus intensity, (d) Background ambient noise levels should not exceed 50 dB-A, and (e) Pass/fail criteria should be derived from locally developed age-appropriate norms (Murray, Javel, & Watson, 1985; Richmond, Konkle, & Potsic, 1986). Adherence to these guidelines will result in a failure rate, based on an initial screen, of between 10% to 20% with over-referrals averaging between 10% to 25% (Dennis, Sheldon, Toubas, & McCaffee, 1984; Murray et al., 1985; Sanders et al., 1985). Because both the failure and over-referral rates are influenced by programmatic factors such as pass/fail criteria, it is important that individuals responsible for administering the screening program not only have an understanding of ABR methodology, but they also need to be acquainted with the basic principles that guide the screening process. A subsequent section of this chapter describes screening principles and the means by which screening protocol can be validated. The reader is encouraged to apply this information in addition to the previously noted guidelines in order to maximize screening programs that depend on ABR data.

There are differences in the ABR obtained from neonates as compared to adults. Consequently, special care must be taken when the ABR is used to assess hearing in the pediatric population. Again, readers are referred to Chapter 8 in this book for a detailed discussion of ABR assessment in infants and young children. It is important, however, to emphasize several aspects related to neonatal ABR assessment. In the neonatal and infant populations, morphology of the ABR waveform varies systematically as a function of maturation. Although infant responses are influenced by the same procedural variables that alter adult data (e.g., type of stimuli, presentation rates and intensities, electrode placement, filter settings, and ambient noise), these alterations are confounded further in the neonatal and infant populations both by maturation and health status. Consequently, whereas the normal adult ABR can be conceptualized as a rather static response, the ABR in infants must be considered as a dynamic process. It is recommended, therefore, that individuals unfamiliar with the ABR in neonates and infants obtain intensive experience assessing normal babies and young children before attempting to evaluate those referred for clinical ABR appraisal. The majority of student educational institutions and audiology clinics, however, either do not have access to a normal newborn population or simply do not provide this extensive experience. In such situations, it is incumbent upon examiners to obtain both theoretical knowledge as well as practical experience prior to performing ABR testing on neonates and infants. This is especially important given the importance and value of ABR to assess hearing within the pediatric population.

Middle ear immittance.   Chapters 4 and 5 of this book provide extensive coverage of the principles and applications of acoustic immittance measurements in hearing assessment. Thus the following section does not duplicate the material contained in these chapters; rather, the subsequent discussion focuses briefly on clinical developments that highlight the importance of middle ear immittance measures in pediatric audiological assessment.

Although acoustic immittance measurements have become a standard part of audiological assessment, their use in the neonatal population has been controversial. Initial efforts to examine the use of tympanometry and acoustic reflexes in neonates and young infants revealed that a substantial number of normal hearing babies failed to demonstrate an acoustic reflex (Keith, 1975) and a high percentage of infants younger than 7 months of age with documented middle ear effusion displayed normal tympanometric function (Paradise, Smith, & Bluestone, 1976). These findings were generalized by many physicians and audiologists to contraindicate the use of middle ear immittance measures in the neonatal population. Indeed, this perception still is held by many professionals despite more recent data that support the use of immittance measures.

Currently, for example, it is known that the complex interaction between source and input impedance requires different measurement protocols when assessing the status of infant as compared to adult ears. Whereas the majority of early research used a relatively low-frequency probe tone (e.g., usually 220 Hz), the findings from more recent investigations have shown that when probe tones exceeding 800 Hz are used to monitor the acoustic reflex or tympanometric behavior of infants, the results of both measures are similar to those found with adults (McMillin,

Bennett, Marchant, & Shurin, 1985; Sprague, Wiley, & Goldstein, 1985). Moreover, special attention should be paid to calibration of both the probe tone and the acoustic reflex stimuli because infant ear canals usually contain smaller volumes than do the canals of adults. Consequently, the use of middle ear immittance measures in the neonatal population must reflect both calibration as well as use of higher frequency probe tones in order to obtain useful information. It is especially important that individual clinics develop their own normative data using specific probe tones so that meaningful interpretations of abnormal findings are age appropriate and obtained using consistent methodology. Hopefully, additional research efforts in the future will help provide a data base that will support further the use of this important measurement.

Summary.   The neonatal population was operationally defined as birth to 6 months of age. Detection and assessment of hearing loss in this age group is based on a strategy of screening babies at-risk for hearing loss (e.g., either as the result of being placed on an HHR or by being an ICU graduate) with audiological assessment conducted on those who fail the screening process. Mass screening of all newborns for hearing loss is not recommended at this time primarily because of economical and other practical factors. In addition to babies that fail screening, other infants should receive audiological assessment upon referral for suspected hearing loss. Based on previous experience and available research data, the ABR is recommended as the preferred technique for detection and assessment. BOA and the COG or ARC should be used to obtain supplemental information. Although many clinics do not advocate the use of immittance measures in this population, valuable information can be obtained concerning middle ear status if special attention is given to selection of appropriate probe tones and calibration. Finally, regardless of the specific method or technique used for detection or assessment, it was stressed that examiners need to become familiar not only with the theoretical rationale for various test procedures, but they also need to obtain extensive practical experience testing both normal and hearing-impaired neonates.

Infant detection and assessment
(7 months to 2 years)

Many of the strategies used to detect and assess hearing loss in neonates also have been used when evaluating the infant population. It follows, therefore, that most of the previously discussed advantages and disadvantages associated with various techniques also apply when these strategies are incorporated into the audiological assessment of older babies. In addition, some strategies have been modified to take advantage of the increased maturation level of older infants to improve the relationship between an observed response and the prediction of hearing sensitivity. In general, detection and assessment strategies commonly used in the infant population can be grouped into those that rely on behavioral responses to auditory stimulation, auditory evoked potentials to predict hearing sensitivity, and acoustic immittance measures used to determine middle ear status or to predict hearing levels. Again, because other chapters in this book provide detailed coverage of auditory evoked potentials and immittance measures appropriate for detection and assessment in the infant population, this chapter focuses on behavioral responses. This does not imply that the behavioral approach should be used exclusively or that behavioral techniques are preferred over evoked potentials or immittance procedures. Rather, all procedures are considered essential parts of the infant test battery.

The use of behavioral responses to acoustic stimuli has been the most commonly employed strategy in infant audiometry. A variety of stimuli have been advocated including noise makers, narrow-band noise, warbled pure tones, and speech signals. The most popular response to these stimuli has been observation of a head turn, usually in the horizontal plane, or to a lesser degree, eye movement via searching behavior or cessation of movement. The response has been recorded both under a nonconditioned (i.e., BOA) and under various conditioned paradigms.

Behavioral response audiometry. Although BOA is used for infant assessment in many audiology and pediatric medical clinics, there are at least three major reasons that severely restrict the information obtained with this procedure. First, infant responses at this age level (e.g., usually a head turn localization-type response) have been shown to habituate rapidly, thereby limiting the amount of information that can be obtained during a test session (Moore, Thompson, & Thompson, 1975; Moore, Wilson, & Thompson, 1977; Thompson & Weber, 1974). Second, there is excessive variability both in the lowest intensity levels at which responses can be observed across different stimuli and for the range of intensities associated with normal hearing for a single stimulus. Infants between the ages of 7 and 12 months, for example, will respond better to speech-type stimuli than to noise or tonal signals (Thompson & Thompson, 1972), but the use of speech stimuli restricts the amount of frequency-specific information. Also, the range of responses characteristic of normal hearing infants (i.e., between the 10th and 90th percentiles) often exceeds 30 to 40 dB (Moore et al., 1977). This relatively large range of response variability precludes accurate distinction among normal and mild or moderate hearing loss. Third, regardless of the types of stimuli, responses have been shown consistently to improve with increasing age

(Northern & Downs, 1978). In general, an increase in minimal response levels of about 18 dB can be expected for speech stimuli for infants between the ages of 4 and 7 months and 21 and 24 months (e.g., the intensity level required to observe a response will decrease), whereas responses will improve almost 25 dB over this same age range for warbled pure tone stimuli. Unfortunately, this improvement in response level is variable as a function of age and confounds further the interpretation of observed responses. Consequently, BOA should not be the method of choice for hearing assessment in the infant population.

Operant conditioning of behavioral responses.   An alternative to the use of BOA is the application of systematic reinforcement of behavioral responses via operant discrimination conditioning procedures. This strategy is based on operant conditioning methodology such that the rate of the operant response (i.e., head turn toward the stimuli source) is increased by the use of reinforcement, thus decreasing response habituation. Stated differently, the acoustic stimulus serves to prompt the infant listener that a response will result in positive reinforcement.

Most of the early research using operant conditioning was based on reinforcement of reflexive behavior that was observed during BOA. Suzuki and Ogiba (1960, 1961) advocated a procedure termed Conditioned Orientation Reflex (COR) based on the infant's reflexive head turn toward the source of an acoustic signal. This reflexive behavior was reinforced via a visual stimulus in order to increase the rate of head turn response. In 1969, Liden and Kankkunen suggested a procedure called Visual Reinforcement Audiometry (VRA) that again used visual reinforcement, but differed substantially from COR, because any observed response was reinforced rather than just a selective head turn. Although the practice of reinforcing any observed response never gained wide clinical acceptance, the term VRA has been accepted as a generic descriptor used to refer to the class of procedures that employ visual reinforcement of the head-turn localization response.

Based on the findings of Moore et al. (1975) and Moore et al. (1977), it appears that the most suitable reinforcer for this age group is a complex visual stimulus composed of a motion toy located in a dark Plexiglas cube that can be activated at the same time as a light source so that the cube is illuminated, allowing the infant to see the motion toy. This visual reinforcer is located along with a loudspeaker at a 45° azimuth either side of the infant's midline and at eye level. During the test session, the infant is encouraged to engage passively in play, or to be otherwise distracted from looking at the loudspeaker/reinforcement apparatus. Correct responses to acoustic stimulation (e.g., a head turn toward the loudspeaker) are reinforced on a 100% schedule. The primary advantages associated with this VRA procedure within the infant age range are (a) the rate of response as a function of stimulus presentation is increased substantially compared to a no-reinforcement condition (Moore et al., 1975); (b) intersubject variability is less than 10 dB between the 10th and 90th percentiles (Wilson, Moore, & Thompson, 1976); and (c) the intensities necessary to obtain minimum response levels for infants are essentially equal to those for adult listeners (Wilson et al., 1976). These advantages, compared to the drawbacks associated with BOA, lend strong support to the use of VRA in the detection and assessment of hearing loss in the infant population.

Although VRA typically is used in a sound-field condition, this procedure also can be used to obtain ear specific information when stimuli are transduced via earphones placed on the infant with an appropriate headband (Wilson & Moore, 1978). Also, stimuli can be presented via a bone vibrator, again using an appropriate headband, to obtain an estimate of cochlear reserve. The use of earphones or a bone vibrator, however, requires a cooperative listener, but this cooperation often can be obtained when the examiner is willing to spend a "little more time" to gain the confidence of the infant. Finally, it is strongly recommended that examiners gain experience with VRA by using this procedure with normal infants prior to testing those suspected of having hearing loss or who otherwise are difficult to test. In this manner, the examiner will have a basis on which to recognize normal behavior and hearing and thus be able to judge confidently responses that may reflect hearing loss.

Summary.   Detection and assessment of hearing loss in infants is accomplished via a test battery consisting of immittance measures, auditory evoked potentials, and behavioral assessment using VRA procedures. As compared to BOA, VRA offers two primary advantages: (a) increased response rate that maximizes the amount of information that can be obtained during a test session; and (b) decreased intersubject variability, making it easier to predict normal hearing sensitivity and to quantify mild and moderate hearing loss. When VRA is used in conjunction with immittance and evoked potential measures, it is possible to quantify with acceptable clinical accuracy the majority of cases of auditory impairment.

Assessment and detection in the young child (2 years and older)

By the time an individual has reached the age of a young child, he or she usually has matured sufficiently to become more interactive within the test environment. Nonetheless, efficient and effective detection and assessment of hearing loss in this age population requires the use of special audiological techniques. The most commonly used procedures to test the young child include play audiometry, tangible reinforcement operant conditioning audiometry (TROCA), and visual reinforcement operant conditioning audiometry (VROCA). As with all populations and as stressed previously, immittance measures are considered to be a vital part of the audiological assessment. Auditory evoked potentials also are used for assessment within this age group, but these measures usually are reserved for the most difficult to test child who often is characterized by severe cognitive delay, restricted motor ability, or neurologically limited response levels.

Play audiometry. Perhaps the most widely used procedure to detect and assess hearing in children aged 2 years and older is play audiometry. This technique is similar to testing conducted with adults, except that the response required from the listener is cast into a game (i.e., play format) rather than a simple hand raise or pushing of a button. Typical responses include placing a block in a box, putting a ring on a peg, or stacking blocks on top of each other. The listener is taught, or if necessary conditioned, to perform the play-type task in response to acoustic stimuli. In this manner, the response serves as a positive reinforcer. Conversely, inappropriate responses are discouraged by taking time-out from the game (e.g., a form of mild negative reinforcement). The test session consists first of establishing the relationship between the acoustic stimulus and the chosen response to ensure that the child understands and can perform the task. During this phase, it often is necessary to use abundant social reinforcement. Once the examiner is confident that the child can perform the listening/response task, thresholds are obtained either in the sound field, under earphones, or with signals presented via a bone vibrator.

It is recommended that at least one parent be present in the test room during play audiometry. Although many children of this age will readily separate from their parents, having a parent in the test room often provides a degree of security for the child (e.g., the child can sit on the parent's lap or the parent can be seated close to the child if necessary), and equally important, the parent can observe first hand the test session including the child's responses to various stimuli. Also, it is important to recognize that play audiometry is limited by the listener's ability to "play the game." Thus if it becomes apparent during the initial learning phase of the session that the child is not able to perform the task or grasp the relationship between the acoustic stimulus and the response task, it is best to opt for another procedure such as VRA. Although limited, findings from clinical research suggest a relatively low success rate for play audiometry with very young or multiply handicapped children (Matkin, 1977; Thompson & Weber, 1974). Also, many examiners tend to be overdependent on play audiometry and use the procedure even when a child is able to be tested using adult response formats.

Tangible and visual reinforcement operant conditioning audiometry. Tangible reinforcement operant conditioning audiometry (TROCA) is an automated test procedure that originally was developed as a technique to test mentally retarded children (Lloyd, Spradlin, & Reid, 1968; Spradlin & Lloyd, 1965). This procedure depends on the use of tangible reinforcers such as cereal, candy, trinkets, and so on that are dispensed automatically whenever the child correctly responds to an acoustic stimulus. The response consists of relatively low-level activity, either depressing a button or pushing a bar, that does not require fine motor skills. The specific procedures that guide positive (i.e., reinforcer dispensed) and negative (i.e., no reinforcer dispensed or time out) reinforcement schedules vary among clinics that use TROCA; however, it generally is agreed that such schedules need to be flexible to accommodate the individual needs of specific children. Although TROCA is not used commonly in most clinics, it may provide useful information when assessing distractible and hyperactive children. Another advantage of TROCA is that once the response is brought under stimulus control via conditioning, only minimal reconditioning is required during subsequent test sessions.

Visual reinforcement operant conditioning audiometry (VROCA) is essentially the same as TROCA, except that a visual stimulus is used to reinforce correct responses. VROCA differs from VRA in that the response used for VROCA requires pushing a button or bar rather than the reflexive head turn. Also, a variety of visual reinforcers can be used with VROCA instead of the motion toy/light source. VROCA can be an excellent technique when used with current microcomputer graphics and, as with TROCA, is valuable if more than one session will be required for assessment.

Summary.   Detection and assessment of hearing loss in young children 2 years of age and older can be accomplished using a combination of conditioned procedures such as play audiometry, TROCA or VROCA, auditory evoked potentials, and acoustic middle ear immittance measures. It generally takes more time to condition a child initially using TROCA or VROCA compared to play audiometry, but clinical assessment may require the use of several techniques (including various reinforcers) to obtain sufficient audiometric data on a young child.

Special considerations

Screening principles and validation

The preceding discussions often have stressed the relationship between screening for hearing loss and the detection and assessment of auditory impairments, especially within the neonatal and infant populations. Since the inception of hearing screening programs, the field of audiology has endeavored to improve techniques that increase the accuracy of correctly identifying hearing impairment. Whether screening programs are administered in the newborn nursery or the school setting, past experience has shown that mass testing is neither an efficient nor cost-effective method of evaluation. The result has been the selective elimination of those within the target population who probably have normal hearing (i.e., ear disease is absent) from screening, thereby concentrating on those who are at-risk for hearing loss. Whereas the basic principles of screening are well-known in the area of epidemiology, they remain relatively obscure to the hearing health care community. The following section describes screening principles and the means by which screening protocol can be validated:

> The presumptive identification of unrecognized disease or defect by the application of tests, examinations or other procedures which can be applied rapidly. Screening tests sort out apparently well persons who probably have a disease from those who probably do not. A screening test is not intended to be diagnostic. (Last, 1986, p. 96)

By necessity, a screening program must be simple, inexpensive, and ultimately both valid and reliable. The application of newborn auditory screening programs illustrates both strengths and limitations of this basic tenant. Recall that an important facet of a newborn screening program, for example, is the use of the HRR. The register is a relatively precise method of dividing the newborn population (i.e., target population) into two distinct groups: those who show little predisposition to hearing loss and those who are at a greater risk for auditory impairment. The process, which usually involves a parental questionnaire and a chart review, is simple, inexpensive, and easily managed. Once a newborn has been identified as being at-risk for hearing loss, however, the testing techniques used to detect or assess hearing, whether they be behavioral (i.e., BOA, COG, or ARC) or electrophysiological (i.e., auditory evoked responses) are time-consuming, expensive, and their results often are suspect to the rigors of clinical decision analysis. Consequently, it is important to ask if HRR yields a substantial number of hearing-impaired infants as compared proportionally to the general population, or if an intermediate screening step would improve significantly the yield of either group?

School screening programs have similar difficulties justifying their existence. Pure tone screening is a simple technique carried out by an audiologist, speech/language pathologist, or frequently a school nurse. Yet, test results and the referral process are often the subject of much criticism. The questions of adequately trained testing personnel, noisy testing environments, and self-resolving middle ear effusion have done much to cloud the issue of school screening programs. Unfortunately, the use of acoustic immittance measures in this population has not improved the dynamics of school screening. Given these concerns, the question is whether the administration of a screening program is a valid and reliable tool for identifying and eventually treating a disease process.

Regardless of the type of hearing screening employed or its setting, the primary objective of the program is to identify accurately hearing loss in those individuals who are truly impaired while ruling out disease in normal hearing subjects. With appropriate screening techniques and their application to selected populations, a screening test should identify high-risk individuals who are predisposed to disease development or who are asymptomatic and can be treated effectively (Wallace & Everett, 1986). If a screening test frequently passes hearing-impaired individuals or too often fails normal hearing listeners, the screening test is an invalid measure and its continued use is both theoretically and economically unjustified. The practical application of a screening program requires the understanding of testing procedures, the pass–fail result outcome, and the referral and treatment of those identified. Finally, test validity is a measurable entity that is based on test results that are diagnostically confirmed.

Principles of Test Selection.   Although not limited to screening, a suitable method of describing test results applies to principles of decision matrix analysis. This test analysis involves a series of operating characteristics that summarize test results and relates test outcome to the actual presence or absence of the disease process (i.e., hearing loss).

The most frequently constructed design uses a 2 × 2 matrix shown in Figure 9.2. The four components of the matrix are: true-positive (TP), the number of hearing-impaired individuals who fail the screen; true-negative (TN), the number of normal hearing individuals who pass the screen; false-positive (FP), the number of normal hearing individuals who fail the screen; and false-negative (FN), the number of truly impaired individuals who pass the screen. A screening test of choice could result in a high proportion of true-positive findings and, conversely, low false-positive rates (e.g., those with the disease would be identified, whereas normal hearing subjects would pass the screen). The cumulative findings of the actual screening pass/fail results are submitted to this matrix model, allowing the calculation of test performance validity.

Operating characteristics.   The validity of a screening test is dependent on diagnostic confirmation for every individual screened. This is one of the major flaws in most screening programs because few provide follow-up services for initial test passes. Thus it is extremely difficult to substantiate the true number of false-negative findings. With this limitation, test validity is determined by the relationship of three components: (a) sensitivity—the ability of a test to correctly identify patients with hearing loss; (b) specificity—the ability of a test to correctly identify those with normal hearing; and (c) disease prevalence—the total number of hearing-impaired patients in a given population (Galen & Gambino, 1977).

Test sensitivity usually is expressed as a percentage of the total number of truly impaired individuals who fail the test. Stated differently, when a test functions at a 60% sensitivity rate, 6 of every 10 patients who are hearing impaired are correctly identified. The remaining 4 hearing-impaired patients are improperly classified. This concept is demonstrated in Figure 9.3, which used a hypothetical group of 1,000 screened school-

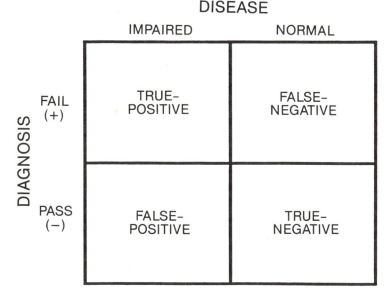

Figure 9.2. Illustration of a 2 × 2 matrix commonly used to categorize test results into true-positive, true-negative, false-positive, and false-negative outcomes.

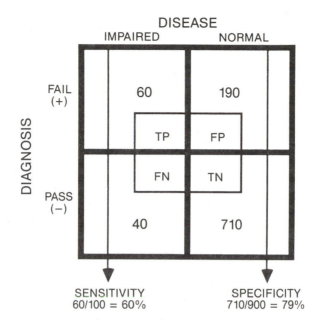

Figure 9.3. Hypothetical outcome of a screening program conducted on a group of 1,000 children illustrating test sensitivity and specificity (see text for details).

aged children. In this example, a total of 100 children are truly impaired; however, only 60 failed the test and were correctly identified. The true-positive rate for this example is 60% (60/100). The remaining 40% who passed the screen represent the false-negative rate. In hearing screening it is most desirable to use a test that offers the highest possible rate of sensitivity. If, for example, a child passes a school screening but presents with significant hearing impairment, the abnormality may hold serious behavioral, developmental, and educational consequences if undetected.

Test specificity also commonly is expressed as a percentage representing the number of normal subjects who pass the test as a function of the total number of normal subjects. If all children with normal hearing passed a school screen, the test would perform at a 100% specificity rate. As the test begins to fail normal hearing children, however, the rate of specificity will decrease. If 7 of 10 normal hearing children passed the screen, the test would operate at a rate of 70% specificity. The remaining 3 normal hearing children would be subjected to subsequent diagnostic follow-up. In the example presented in Figure 9.2, 710 of 900 normal hearing children passed the school screen, resulting in 79% test specificity

(710/900). Those 190 normal hearing children who failed the screen rendered a 21% false-positive rate. This situation may result in parental stress and anxiety; however, misclassification usually is ameliorated by further diagnostic assessment.

By comparing the information presented in Figure 9.3 to the illustration in Figure 9.2, it can be seen that the terms *sensitivity* and *specificity* represent true-positive and true-negative rates, respectively. The remaining cells reflect a reciprocal relationship between sensitivity and the false-negative rate and similarly, between specificity and the false-positive rate. Thus as specificity increases, the false-positive rate will correspondingly decrease. Sensitivity and specificity describe a test's ability to estimate disease (i.e., hearing loss) or nondisease (i.e., normal hearing) in a select population and are of primary consideration in the determination of which screening test to apply for specific populations. If time only permits the use of either pure tone audiometry or acoustic immittance measures in a school screening program, operating characteristics can provide the statistical means to determine the appropriate test for the given condition.

The final operating characteristic that will influence test validity is disease prevalence. The term *prevalence* is similar but not identical to disease *incidence*. Both terms describe the frequency with which the disease occurs. Prevalence is a census measure that expresses the presence of diseased patients per 100,000 population at the time of investigation (MacMahon & Pugh, 1970). In contrast, incidence rate is the frequency of new outbreak of a disease condition in a population for a given period of time (Last, 1983). The relationship between prevalence and incidence is clarified by the following example. The incidence of an acute disease such as middle ear effusion in infants and young children may be high because large numbers routinely contract the disease. The prevalence, however, usually is low because the disease has a relatively short duration. Conversely, the incidence of a chronic disease such as sensorineural hearing loss may be low in infants and young children, but the prevalence in the general population is substantial. Although a small percentage of children are identified as sensorineural hearing impaired each year, the impairment is irreversible, can be acquired in later life, and therefore is cumulative. The effects of prevalence on test performance are described subsequently in this section.

Principles of test interpretation.   As just discussed, sensitivity and specificity are measures of a test's ability to detect the presence or absence of a disease and are important considerations in the selection of a screening test. From the perspective of clinical test interpretation, however, our concern is not with these operating characteristics, because we have no advanced knowledge of whether those screened are normal or hearing-impaired. Rather, test interpretation is focused on predictive values and pass/fail criteria.

The calculation of predictive values provides a means of interpreting test results of patients who are correctly identified with disease or as healthy by the test (Last, 1986). The predictive value of a positive test outcome (PVP) is defined as the percentage of all positive results that are true-positive when the test is applied to a population composed of both healthy and diseased subjects. The predictive value of a negative test (PVN) represents the percentage of all negative results that are true-negative. Predictive values are dependent on test-operating characteristics and disease prevalence in the population under study. Once measures of sensitivity and specificity are determined, it is then possible to establish probability statements regarding the presence or absence of hearing impairment because predictive values are related directly to test outcome. Figure 9.4 illustrates how predictive value measures can be derived from the test outcome data presented in Figure 9.3. Of the 250 children who failed the school screen, 60 were true-positive. The remaining 190 children were false-positive, leaving a PVP of 24.0% (60/250). The PVP result indicates that approximately 75% (190/250) of all children who failed the test were false-positive. Simply stated, 76 out of every 100 positive results were incorrect. The predictive value of a negative test result (PVN) was 95% (710/750), which suggests that this test correctly identified 710 of the normal hearing children. Thus for participants who were determined to have passed the screen, only 5 of every 100 negative results were false-negative.

As stated previously, disease prevalence within the target population will influence predictive values. Table 9.2 presents a hypothetical example of such an event. By decreasing the prevalence of the disease from 5% (50/1000) to 1% (10/1000) to 0.1% (1/1000) while maintaining relatively high operating characteristics (sensitivity and specificity at 90%), predictive values change dramatically. The PVP result decreased from 32.1 to 8.3 to less than 1.0%; whereas, in this case, the PVN remained constant. When disease prevalence is similar to the yield of severe-to-profound hearing-impaired infants reported in the general population (i.e., approximately 1:1,000), the false-positive rate is an alarming 99%. Even the best of tests will result in a low PVP when disease prevalence is low. This concept stresses the importance of applying screening tests to high prevalence populations (i.e., such as infants at risk for hearing loss or ICU graduates). To do otherwise typically will result in false-positive rates that will be so high that test administration may be indefensible.

A second important aspect related to test interpretation concerns pass/fail criteria. Is is unlikely that any test, screening or diagnostic, will separate all patients with disease from those who do not have the disease.

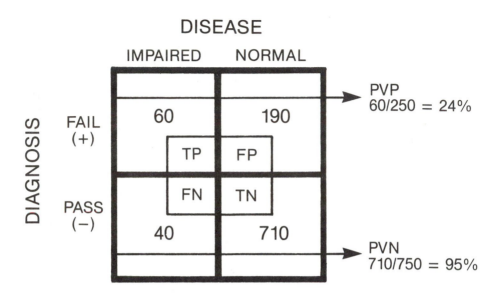

Figure 9.4. Hypothetical outcome of a screening program conducted on a group of 1,000 children illustrating positive and negative predictive values (see text for details).

TABLE 9.2
Effects of Disease Prevalence on Predictive Value When
Sensitivity and Specificity Remain Constant (90%)

Disease Prevalence	Test Results	Impaired	Normal	Total	Predictive Value
5%	Positive	225.0	475.0	700	32.1%
	Negative	25.0	4275.0	4300	99.4%
	Total	250.0	4750.0	5000	
1%	Positive	45.0	495.0	540	8.3%
	Negative	5.0	4455.0	4460	99.9%
	Total	50.0	4950.0	5000	
0.1%	Positive	4.5	499.5	504	<1%
	Negative	0.5	4495.5	4496	100%
	Total	5.0	4995.0	5000	

In reality, there always will be those screened who are incorrectly labeled. This concept of integration of normal and pathological patients has been coined the "theory of overlapping distributions" (Thorner & Remein, 1967). The selection of a pass/fail cutoff point within the overlapping distribution will affect the yield of identified patients with disease and, hence, the operating characteristics of the test. The determination of pass/fail criteria is a critical factor in the establishment of eventual test outcome.

Figure 9.5 illustrates the concept of overlapping distribution in a hypothetical population of children screened for hearing loss. Assume that an initial pass/fail criterion of 35 dB was selected (i.e., a predetermined intensity level) that resulted in a certain proportion of patients who passed the screen and a certain number who failed the screen. Given this outcome, the operating characteristics and predictive values associated with the test can be calculated. It is important to note, however, that such calculations only will be valid for the 35-dB pass/fail criterion. If the cutoff (i.e., pass/fail criterion) was adjusted higher to 50 dB or lower to 20 dB, the test performance values would change despite the same proportion of normal to hearing-impaired children within the population. If the cutoff was adjusted to 50 dB, for example, more hearing-impaired children would pass the screen (e.g., decreased sensitivity), but the false-negative rate would reciprocally increase. Conversely, the specificity rate would increase (i.e., more normal hearing children pass the screen), whereas the false-positive rate would decrease. It follows, therefore, that lowering the pass/fail criterion to 20 dB will result in an overall decrease in specificity and the false-negative rate, but the false-positive rate would increase. An understanding of the concepts just illustrated in conjunction with prior knowledge about the target population will assist in the selection of appropriate pass/fail criteria. Unless careful consideration is given to these factors, however, the entire screening process becomes more of an exercise in guesswork than a defensible and rational program.

Summary. An ideal screening test design would clearly differentiate between diseased and normal subjects; however, the possibility of such an occurrence is unlikely. Because it is economically unfeasible to mass screen, once a population has been targeted for screening, the selection and continued implementation of a screening tool will depend heavily on the various measures of test validity. The use of operating characteristics provide information about the number of individuals correctly identified as hearing-impaired or normal as measured against predetermined pass/fail criteria. Predictive values that are dependent on the disease prevalence describe the test's ability to correctly separate true-positive and true-negative results from those with and without disease. Finally,

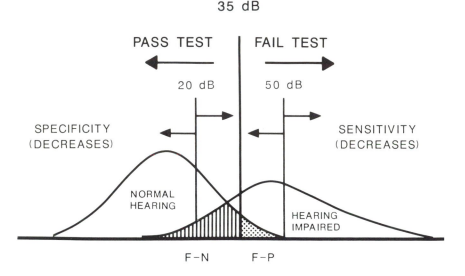

CUT–OFF POINT

35 dB

PASS TEST | FAIL TEST

20 dB   50 dB

SPECIFICITY   SENSITIVITY
(DECREASES)   (DECREASES)

NORMAL
HEARING
                               HEARING
                               IMPAIRED

F–N   F–P

Figure 9.5. Illustration of the relationship between pass/fail criteria and the concept of overlapping distribution (see text for details).

the validation of any test measure must account for the diagnostic confirmation of all individuals screened regardless of initial test outcome. For further discussion of principles of test selection, operating characteristics, and test interpretation, see Chapter 14.

Calibration and stimulus selection

Chapter 16 of this book specifically deals with the importance of instrument calibration. Other chapters, including this one, frequently describe the use of various acoustic stimuli used for hearing assessment. Unfortunately, however, national or international standards are not available for many of the acoustic signals that are advocated, especially those often recommended for pediatric assessment. Sound field thresholds or minimal response levels, for example, are highly dependent on the acoustic parameters of the stimulus, yet normative reference sound pressure levels for such commonly used signals as speech spectrum noise, narrow-band noise, or warbled pure tones are not nationally available. In the absence of standardized criteria, it becomes particularly important that clinics establish their own normative data for various clinical procedures and stimuli.

Detailed consideration of this topic is beyond the scope of this chapter, but given the importance of stimulus selection and calibration, the following general observations appear warranted. First, pure tone stimuli should be avoided for sound field assessment, given that it is difficult to maintain a specific location for active young listeners. Instead, complex signals such as frequency modulated (FM) warble tones or narrow bands of noise should be used with the qualification that such signals have suitable characteristics. Walker, Dillon, and Byrne (1984) recommended that FM warble tones should have a modulation rate of about 20 Hz driven by triangular or sinusoid waveforms; whereas narrow-band noise stimuli should have bandwidths, expressed as a percentage of the centered frequency, ranging from 30% for low frequencies (250 Hz) to approximately 10% for higher frequencies (4000 Hz), and complex rather than simple filtering is appropriate to obtain steep filter slopes. Second, care must be taken to ensure that the test environment remains consistent over time. Listener orientation relative to the sound source should be the same for specific test procedures, furniture within the test room should not be rearranged unless a change in location will not influence acoustic parameters of the test signal being used, and testing should be conducted with the listener located in the far (i.e., reverberant) field from the loudspeaker. Also, the actual test room should be as nonreverberant as possible in order to minimize unwanted intensity variations. Third, careful acoustic measurements of stimuli need to be made within the sound field in order to verify that signals are optimal and have not changed from the findings of initial or previous measurements. Although the manufacturers of most audiological instrumentation provide guidelines suggesting calibration levels for their particular instruments, it is the responsibility of the individual conducting the test procedure to verify that stimuli criteria are maintained. The process of selecting and calibrating stimuli often requires compromise and subsequent care in interpretation of results, but if approached in a logical and informed manner the audiological results obtained from pediatric listeners can be just as reliable and valid as those from adults.

Conclusions

Detection and assessment of hearing loss in the pediatric population represents the first step in a long and expensive process of aural rehabilitation for children with documented hearing impairment. This chapter stressed the importance of developing efficient and effective audiological strategies based on the level of current technology and available research findings. It is clear that the responsibility for providing efficient and cost-effective programs rests primarily with those individuals responsible for assessment and detection. It is our strong contention that individuals responsible for administering various test procedures need to obtain extensive experience with normal hearing and normal functioning neonates, infants, and children prior to expanding testing to the hearing-disordered population. Too often, even experienced pediatric audiologists have only limited experience assessing normal hearing children. Finally, it must be remembered that assessment is an ongoing process that may require the application of knowledge derived from several professions.

References

ASHA Committee on Infant Hearing. (1988). Guidelines for the identification of hearing impairment in at risk infants age birth to 6 months. *Asha, 30,* 61–64.

ASHA Committee on Infant Hearing. (1989). Audiologic screening of newborn infants who are at risk for hearing impairment. *Asha, 31,* 89–92.

Bennett, M. J. (1975). The auditory response cradle: A device for the objective assessment of auditory state in the neonate. *Symposium Zoological Society of London, 37,* 291–305.

Borton, T. E., & Stark, E. W. (1972). Routine neonatal hearing screening: A dissent (Letter to the Editor). *Hospital Practice, 7,* 17–29.

Carrel, R. E., (1977). Epidemiology of hearing loss. In S. Gerber (Ed.), *Audiometry in infancy* (pp. 3–16). New York: Grune & Stratton.

Catlin, F. L. (1978). Etiology and pathology of hearing loss in children. In F. Martin (Ed.), *Pediatric audiology* (pp. 3–34). Englewood Cliffs, NJ: Prentice-Hall.

Coplan, J. (1987). Deafness: Ever hear of it? Delayed recognition of permanent hearing loss. *Pediatrics, 79,* 206–213.

Cox, L. C. (1985). Infant assessment: Developmental and age-related considerations. In J. T. Jacobson (Ed.), *The auditory brainstem response* (pp. 297–316). San Diego, CA: College Hill Press.

Dennis, M. J., Sheldon, R., Toubas, P., & McCaffee, M. (1984). Identification of hearing loss in the neonatal intensive care unit population. *American Journal of Otolaryngology, 5,* 201–205.

Downs, M. P., & Hemenway, W. G. (1969). Report on the hearing screening of 17,000 neonates. *International Audiology, 8,* 72–76.

Downs, M. P., & Silver, H. K. (1972). A.B.C.D.'s to H.E.A.R.: Early identification in nursery, office, and clinic of the infant who is deaf. *Clinical Pediatrics, 11,* 563–566.

Downs, M. P., & Sterritt, G. (1964). Identification audiometry for neonates: A preliminary report. *Journal of Auditory Research, 4,* 69–80.

Downs, M. P., & Sterritt, G. (1967). A guide to newborn and infant hearing screening programs. *Archives of Otolaryngology, 85,* 15–22.

Durieux-Smith, A., & Jacobson, J. T. (1985). Comparison of auditory brainstem response and behavioral screening in neonates. *Journal of Otolaryngology,* (Supplement 14), 47–58.

Durieux-Smith, A., Picton, T., Edwards, C., Goodman, J. T., & MacMurray, B. (1985). The crib-o-gram in the NICU: An evaluation based on brain stem electric response audiometry. *Ear and Hearing, 6,* 20–24.

Feinmesser, M., & Bauberger-Tell, L. (1971, May). *Evaluation of methods of detecting hearing impairment in infancy and early childhood.* Paper presented at the conference on Newborn Hearing Screening, Bureau of Maternal and Child Health, San Francisco.

Feinmesser, M., & Tell. L. (1971). *Progress report: Evaluation of methods for detecting hearing impairment in infancy and early childhood* (U.S.P.H.S.—M.C.H.S. Project 06-48D-2). Jerusalem, Israel: Department of Otolaryngology, Hadassah Hospital.

Feinmesser, M., & Tell. L. (1976). Neonatal screening for detection of deafness. *Archives of Otolaryngology, 102,* 297–299.

Fraser, G. R. (1971). The genetics of congenital deafness. *The Otolaryngologic Clinics of North America, 4,* 227–247.

Fria, T. J. (1985). Identification of congenital hearing loss with the auditory brainstem response. In J. T. Jacobson (Ed.), *The auditory brainstem response* (pp. 317–334). San Diego, CA: College Hill Press.

Froding, C. A. (1960). Acoustic investigation of newborn infants. *Acta Oto-Laryngologica, 52,* 31–41.

Galambos, R. (1978). Use of auditory brainstem response (ABR) in infant hearing testing. In S.E. Gerber & G. T. Mencher (Eds.), *Early diagnosis of hearing loss* (pp. 243–258). New York: Grune & Stratton.

Galambos, R., Hicks, G., & Wilson, M. (1982). Hearing loss in graduates of a tertiary intensive care nursery. *Ear and Hearing, 3,* 87–90.

Galen, R. S., & Gambino, S. R. (1977). *Beyond normality: The predictive value and efficiency of medical diagnosis.* New York: John Wiley.

Gerber, S. E. (1985). Stimulus, response, and state variables in the testing of neonates. *Ear and Hearing, 6,* 15–19.

Gerkin, K. (1984). The high risk register for deafness. *Asha, 26,* 17–23.

Gilchrist, D. B. (1977). Respiratory measures. In S. E. Gerber (Ed.), *Audiometry in infancy* (pp. 117–132). New York: Grune & Stratton.

Goldstein, R., & Tait, C. (1971). Critique of neonatal hearing evaluation. *Journal of Speech and Hearing Disorders, 36,* 3–18.

Goodhill, V. (1967). Detection of hearing loss in neonates (editorial). *Archives of Otolaryngology, 85,* 1.

Hoverston, G., & Moncur, J. (1969). Stimuli and intensity factors in testing infants. *Journal of Speech and Hearing Research, 12,* 687–702.

Jacobson, J. T., Mencher, G. T., Seitz, M. R., & Pasrrott, V. (1979). Infant hearing screening: Theory and practice. *Human Communication, 4,* 203–212.

Jacobson, J. T., & Morehouse, C. (1984). A comparison of auditory brainstem response and behavioral screening in high risk and normal newborn infants. *Ear and Hearing, 5,* 247–253.

Jaffe, B. F. (1977). Middle ear and pinna anomalies. In B. F. Jaffe (Ed.), *Hearing loss in children* (pp. 294–309). Baltimore: University Park Press.

Joint Committee on Infant Hearing, Position Statement. (1982). *Pediatrics, 70*, 496–497.

Keith, R., (1975). Middle ear function in neonates. *Archives of Otolaryngology, 101*, 376–379.

Last, J. M. (1983). *A dictionary of epidemiology*. New York: Oxford University Press.

Last, J. M. (1986). *Public health and preventive medicine*. Norwalk, CN: Appleton-Century-Croft.

Liden, G., & Kankkunen, A. (1969). Visual reinforcement audiometry. *Acta Oto-Laryngologica, 67*, 281–292.

Ling, D., Ling, A. H., & Doehring, D. G. (1970). Stimulus response and observer variables in the auditory screening of newborn infants. *Journal of Speech and Hearing Disorders, 13*, 9–18.

Lloyd, L. L., Spradlin, J. E., & Reid, M. J. (1968). An operant audiometric procedure for difficult-to-test patients. *Journal of Speech and Hearing Disorders, 33*, 236–245.

MacMahon, B., & Pugh, T. F. (1970). *Epidemiology: Principles and methods*. Boston: Little, Brown.

Matkin, N. (1977). Assessment of hearing sensitivity during the preschool years. In F. H. Bess (Ed.), *Childhood deafness, assessment and management* (pp. 127–134). New York: Grune & Stratton.

Matkin, N. (1988). Re-evaluating our evaluations. In F. H. Bess (Ed.), *Hearing impairment in children* (pp. 101–111). Parkton, MD: York Press.

McMillin, P., Bennett, M., Marchant, C., & Shurin, P. (1985). Ipsilateral and contralateral acoustic reflexes in neonates. *Ear and Hearing, 6*, 320–324.

Mencher, G. T. (1972, August). *Screening infants for auditory deficits: The university of nebraska neonatal hearing project*. Paper presented at the Eleventh International Congress of Audiology, Budapest, Hungary.

Mencher, G. T. (1974). A program for neonatal hearing screening. *Audiology, 13*, 495–500.

Mencher, G. T. (1975). Nova Scotia conference of the early identification of hearing loss: A review. *Human Communication, 3*, 5–20.

Menyuk, P. (1977). Cognition and language. *Volta Review, 78*, 250–257.

Moncur, J. (1968). Judge reliability in infant testing. *Journal of Speech and Hearing Research, 11*, 348–357.

Moore, J. M., Thompson, G., & Thompson, M. (1975). Auditory localization of infants as a function of reinforcement conditions. *Journal of Speech and Hearing Disorders, 40*, 29–34.

Moore, J. M., Wilson, W. R., & Thompson, G. (1977). Visual reinforcement of head-turn responses in infants under 12 months of age. *Journal of Speech and Hearing Disorders, 42*, 328–334.

Mulac, A., & Gerber, S. E. (1977). Cardiovascular measures. In S. E. Gerber (Ed.), *Audiometry in infancy* (pp. 133–150). New York: Grune & Stratton.

Murray, A. D., Javel, E., & Watson, C. S. (1985). Prognostic validity of auditory brainstem evoked response screening in newborn infants. *American Journal of Otolaryngology, 6*, 120–131.

Northern, J. L., & Downs, M. P. (1978). *Hearing in children* (2nd ed.). Baltimore: Williams & Wilkins.

Northern, J. L., & Downs, M. P. (1984). *Hearing in children* (3rd ed.). Baltimore: Williams & Wilkins.

Osberger, M. (1986). Language and learning skills of hearing-impaired students. *ASHA Monograph 23*.

Paradise, J., Smith, C., & Bluestone, C. (1976). Tympanometric detection of middle ear effusion in infants and young children. *Pediatrics, 58*, 198–206.

Richards, I.D.G., & Roberts, C. J. (1967). The at risk infant. *Lancet, 2*, 711–714.

Richmond, K. H., Konkle, D. F., & Potsic, W. P. (1986). ABR screening of high-risk infants: Effects of ambient noise in the neonatal nursery. *Otolaryngology Head and Neck Surgery, 94*, 552–560.

Sanders, R. A., Durieux-Smith, A., Hyde, M., Jacobson, J., Kileny, P., & Murnane, O. (1985). Incidence of hearing loss in high risk and intensive care nursery infants. *Journal of Otolaryngology, 14*, 28–33.

Shepard, N. T. (1983). Newborn hearing screening using the Linco-Bennett auditory response cradle: A pilot study. *Ear and Hearing, 4*, 5–10.

Simmons, F. B. (1980). Patterns of deafness in newborns. *Laryngoscope, 90*, 448–453.

Simmons, F. B., & Russ, F. N. (1974). Automated newborn hearing screening, the crib-o-gram. *Archives of Otolaryngology, 100*, 1–7.

Spradlin, J. E., & Lloyd, L. L. (1965). Operant conditioning audiometry with low level retardates: A preliminary report. In L. L. Lloyd & D. R. Frisina (Eds.), *The audiological assessment of the mentally retarded: Proceedings of a national conference.* Parsons, Parsons State Hospital and Training Center, KS.

Sprague, B., Wiley, T., & Goldstein, R. (1985). Tympanometric and acoustic-reflex studies in neonates. *Journal of Speech and Hearing Research, 28*, 265–272.

Stein, L., Clark, S., & Kraus, N. (1983). The hearing-impaired infant: Patterns of identification and habilitation. *Ear and Hearing, 4*, 232–286.

Suzuki, T., & Ogiba, Y. (1960). A technique of pure-tone audiometry for children under three years of age: Conditioned orientation reflex (COR) audiometry. *Revue de Laryngologie, Otologie, Rhinologie, 3*, 221–226.

Suzuki, T., & Ogiba, Y. (1961). Conditioned orientation audiometry. *Archives of Otolaryngology, 74*, 192–198.

Thompson, M., & Thompson, G. (1972). Response of infants and young children as a function of auditory stimuli and test method. *Journal of Speech and Hearing Research, 15*, 699–707.

Thompson, G., & Weber, B. (1974). Responses of infants and young children to behavioral observation audiometry (BOA). *Journal of Speech and Hearing Disorders, 39*, 140–147.

Thorner, R., & Remein, Q. R. (1967). *Principles and procedures in the evaluation of screening for disease* (Public Health Service Publication No. 846.) Washington, DC: U.S. Government Printing Office.

Walker, G., Dillon, H., & Byrne, D. (1984). Sound field audiometry: Recommended stimuli and procedures. *Ear and Hearing, 5*, 13–21.

Wallace, R. B., & Everett, G. D. (1986). The prevention of chronic illness. In J. M. Last (Ed.), *Public health and preventive medicine* (pp. 215–239). Norwalk, CA: Appleton-Century-Croft.

Wedenberg, E. (1956). Auditory tests on newborn infants. *Acta Oto-Laryngologica, 46*, 446–461.

Wegman, M. (1986). Annual summary of vital statistics 1985. *Pediatrics, 78*, 983–994.

Wilson, W. R., Moore, J. M., & Thompson, G. (1976, November). *Sound-field auditory thresholds of infants utilizing visual reinforcement audiometry (VRA).* Paper presented at the annual meeting of the American Speech and Hearing Association, Houston, TX.

Wilson, W. R., & Moore, J. M. (1978, November). *Pure-tone earphone thresholds of infants utilizing visual reinforcement audiometry (VRA).* Paper presented at the annual meeting of the American Speech and Hearing Association, San Francisco, CA.

chapter ten

Audiologic assessment of the elderly

FRED H. BESS

MICHAEL J. LICHTENSTEIN

SUSAN A. LOGAN

Contents

Introduction

The number of elderly people in the United States is growing steadily. Individuals over 65 years of age currently approximate 30,000,000, and by the year 2030 this figure is expected to exceed 50,000,000 (Bess, Logan, Lichtenstein, & Hedley, 1987). This continual increase in age longevity is due in part to the general population's awareness of the benefits of a healthy life style (i.e., exercise and eating habits), as well as to the success in controlling infectious diseases and managing chronic illnesses. Hence, a critical need has developed for the health professions to meet the long-term health care needs of the elderly population. One of these health care needs is rehabilitation of hearing impairment.

Sensorineural hearing loss is a frequent by-product of the aging process. Hearing impairment ranks as one of the three most prevalent,

511

chronic conditions, following only arthritis and hypertension. Prevalence studies indicate that 25%–40% of individuals over 65 years of age exhibit some degree of hearing impairment, and about 90% of those over 80 are hearing-impaired (Feller, 1981; Herbst, 1983; Glass, 1986; Lichtenstein, Bess, & Logan, 1988a). Thus it is estimated that the number of hearing-impaired individuals in middle and later life is considerable, ranging somewhere between 7.5 and 11.5 million. The hearing loss progresses with each succeeding decade and usually begins around 30 years of age (Glorig & Nixon, 1962; Jerger, 1973).

The magnitude of the problem is demonstrated clearly in Table 10.1. This table illustrates the results from three different studies in terms of the percentage of hearing-impaired persons for a given age range and sex. The studies include the Health Examination Survey (HES; 1960–62), the Wilkins Study (which conducted a home interview survey on some 31,000 individuals in 1947), and the Health Interview Survey (conducted

TABLE 10.1

Percentage of People Reported as Hearing-Impaired in Three Different Studies (Health Examination Survey [HES], 1960–62; Wilkins [WIL], 1947; Health Interview Survey [HIS], 1971)

Age Group (in years)	Male			Female			Both Sexes		
	HES	WIL	HIS	HES	WIL	HIS	HES	WIL	HIS
18–24	1.2	1.2	—	0.4	0.9	—	0.8	1.0	—
25–34	1.4	1.8	5.1	1.3	1.5	3.4	1.3	1.6	4.2
35–44	3.7	2.1	—	2.2	2.9	—	2.9	2.5	—
45–54	4.1	4.9	14.0	4.6	4.6	9.0	4.3	4.7	11.4
55–64	10.6	6.2	—	10.1	6.4	—	10.3	6.4	—
65–74	30.5	12.4	28.0	26.2	12.1	19.0	28.2	12.2	23.1
74–79	48.7	28.0	44.0	47.4	25.0	36.0	48.0	26.0	39.8

Note. Table is adapted from Davis (1983).

in the United States on 134,000 people from 44,000 households in 1971). All three studies show a significant increase in the prevalence of hearing impairment with increasing age. It also is noted that the prevalence rates are different for each study. This is mostly due to methodological differences. Interview surveys typically underestimate the prevalence of hearing impairment, especially for those over 55 years of age. Finally, there appears to be a slight trend for males to exhibit a greater prevalence of hearing loss in the different age ranges than females.

Hearing loss among older persons is also reportedly associated with the psychologic features of withdrawal (Weinstein, 1985), negativism (Alpiner, 1978), isolation (Weinstein, 1985), depressive symptoms (Herbst, 1983), frustration (Weinstein, 1985), and anxiety and loneliness (Bess, Lichtenstein, & Logan, in press; Maurer & Rupp, 1979; Hull, 1980). In addition, hearing impairment has been associated with the functional problems of poor general health, reduced mobility, and reduced interpersonal communications (Herbst, 1983).

This chapter is concerned with the audiologic findings associated with aging. Toward this end, the chapter covers the pathological changes in the auditory system associated with aging, the early identification of hearing loss in the elderly, and the audiometric findings commonly found in the aged.

Anatomic and physiologic effects of aging on the auditory system

Hearing loss due to aging, or presbycusis (from the Greek *presbys*, old, and *akouein*, to hear), has no clearcut etiology; however, several different variables in addition to the aging process are thought to be involved. During the life span of an individual, the auditory system can encounter insult from a variety of exogenous and endogenous sources including noise exposure, genotype, vascular disease, systemic disease, faulty diet, neoplastic problems, inflammations, concussive damage, nutrition, ototoxic drugs, heavy metals, solvents, industrial reagents, pollutants, hyperlipidemia, and tobacco (Hawkins & Johnsson, 1985). Of these, noise is perhaps the most common factor that causes cochlear damage and thus complicates the study of presbycusis. Interestingly, elderly populations living in quiet rural regions exhibit less hearing loss than do similar groups from highly industrialized communities.

The seminal work in cochlear pathology and presbycusis was performed by Schuknecht (1955, 1964, 1974). Histological evidence, case history data, and audiological measurements were combined and correlated to delineate four specific types of presbycusis. They include: (a) *sensory*—a degeneration of hair cells and supporting cells at the base of the cochlea with subsequent cochlear fiber degeneration; this type of presbycusis produces an abrupt high-frequency sensorineural hearing loss. (b) *Strial* or *metabolic*—a degeneration of the stria vascularis, resulting in changes in cochlear electrical potentials and possible effects upon energy production in the organ of corti. Strial presbycusis produces a flat audiometric configuration usually accompanied by very good speech recognition. (c) *Neural*—a loss of cochlear neurons, resulting in problems of transmission information coding; neural presbycusis results in poorer speech recognition than expected from the audiometric data. Although Schuknecht (1974) urged that more histopathological evidence for central auditory nervous system (CANS) degeneration would be useful, he presented no direct evidence for CANS involvement. He stated, however, that individuals with neural presbycusis tend to have diffuse CANS degeneration including motor control problems, memory loss, and intellectual deterioration. *Mechanical* or *cochlear conductive*—a hypothetical type of presbycusis resulting from alterations to cochlear mechanics produced by mass/stiffness changes or spiral ligament atrophy. Cochlear conductive presbycusis supposedly would produce a straight line audiometric loss with descending bone-conduction thresholds; speech recognition is inversely related to the steepness of the audiometric configuration.

According to Schuknecht (1974) one or more of these different types of presbycusis can occur in a given individual, thus complicating the relationship between audiometric configuration and histological correlates. In fact, Suga and Lindsay (1976) could not specify correlations between audiometric configuration and site of cochlear involvement; they stated that neural ganglion cell degeneration was the most common finding.

In addition to the Schuknecht data there are other forms of presbycusic pathophysiology reported in the literature. For example, Nadol (1979) mentioned loss of several outer hair cell afferent synapses, although light microscopy showed presence of outer hair cells and normal myelinated fibers. Thus normal light microscopy exams of the cochlea does not guarantee the presence of functional hair cell fibers' synapses. Synaptic damage also has been implicated as a potential factor in noise-induced hearing loss (Saunders, Dean, & Schneider, 1985).

Hawkins and Johnsson (1985) noted two additional types of peripheral presbycusis, *hyperstotic* and *vascular*. It has been suggested that with age, the internal auditory meatus can show hyperstosis (abnormal growth of bony tissue). This new growth could then compress the eighth nerve and internal auditory artery, causing dysfunction/degeneration of the eighth nerve fibers and inner ear tissue. Johnsson and Hawkins (1972) analyzed a series of human temporal bones and reported substantial devascularization involving the capillaries and arterioles of the inner ear, particularly in the regions of the spiral lamina and lateral wall.

Although there is a considerable body of evidence to suggest cochlear degeneration in elderly patients with hearing loss, many believe that there is also central auditory nervous system dysfunction involved in the aged. Some researchers even believe that cognitive, linguistic, and speed of information processing beyond the central auditory nervous system will affect speech perception performance in the elderly. Nevertheless, although CANS involvement in presbycusis is hypothesized there is little direct evidence to support this assumption. In fact, Hawkins and Johnsson (1985) stated that "there is a sad, virtually complete lack of investigations in which audiological, otopathological and neuropathological findings in the same patient are compared and correlated" (p. 118). Figure 10.1 illustrates the various types of presbycusis described in the literature and their associated sites of pathologic changes.

Identification and evaluation of the elderly hearing impaired

Early identification of the elderly hearing impaired

Early identification and intervention is considered an important rehabilitative strategy for the elderly hearing impaired. Indeed, there is some evidence to suggest, albeit indirect, that the earlier the hearing loss is identified and hearing aid rehabilitation ensues, the greater the potential for hearing aid success (Davis, 1983; Salomon, 1986). The following review highlights some of the more important issues concerned with screening the elderly population.

Principles of screening.   Screening for a chronic condition involves the examination of asymptomatic persons to determine if they are likely, or unlikely, to have the target disorder of interest (Morrison, 1985). Once a screening test is positive, the individual must be further evaluated to determine the presence or absence of the condition. Hearing impairment in the aged is a prototypic disorder for screening: It is a common, progressive, easily detected disorder, for which the belief is held that early identification and rehabilitation will ameliorate its consequences.

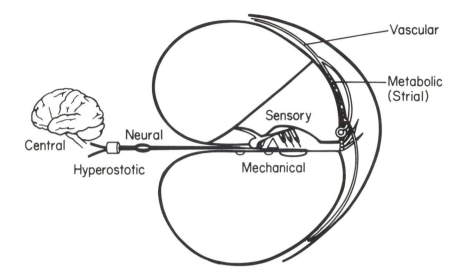

Figure 10.1. Cross-section of the human cochlea to illustrate the types of presbycusis and the accompanying sites of pathological change. (Redrawn with permission from "Otopathological changes associated with presbycusis" by J. E. Hawkins & L. G. Johnsson, 1985, *Seminars in Hearing, 6.* 115–134.)

To judge the effectiveness of a screening program, seven questions must be answered (Cadman, Chambers, Feldman, & Sackett, 1984). The data to answer all seven questions regarding hearing impairment in the aged are not available, but they provide a framework for assessment and future investigation. The questions are:

1. *Has the effectiveness of the program been demonstrated in a randomized trial?* Yes. Mulrow and colleagues (1990) randomly assigned 194 elderly patients to either a hearing aid or to a waiting list. Following a 4-month trial period, hearing aids were found to be associated with significant improvements in social and emotional function and communication. Improvements also were seen in the areas of cognition and depression.

2. *Are efficacious treatments available?* Yes. Hearing aids, though not curative, provide the amplification necessary to overcome the hearing deficit. Overall efficacy, however, must be judged by the aged subjects' use of and satisfaction with the aid.

3. *Does the burden of suffering warrant screening?* Yes. As noted earlier, hearing impairment consistently and strongly is associated with functional deficits and impairments beyond just the ability to communicate. Depending on the definition used, hearing impairment affects 25% to

40% of persons over 65 years of age. Moreover, hearing impairment is associated with depression and dementia (Herbst & Humphrey, 1980; Weinstein & Amsell, 1986), and there is evidence that impaired hearing results in faster cognitive declines in persons with Alzheimer's disease (Uhlmann, Larson, & Koepsell, 1986).

4. *Is there a good screening test?* Yes. Traditional physical diagnostic tests such as the finger rub and whispered voice have been validated recently and are diagnostically useful (Uhlmann, Rees, Psaty, & Duckert, 1989). The use of other instruments, a hand-held audioscope and a self-administered questionnaire, have also been validated (Lichtenstein et al., 1988a).

5. *Does the program reach those who could benefit?* Possibly. Most older persons will see a primary care physician on an annual or biannual basis. Screening tests could be administered in the physician's office. The ability of a screening program to reach other aged subjects (home bound, institutionalized, or those who do not see physicians) remains to be demonstrated.

6. *Can the health care system cope with the program?* Unknown. If hearing aid rehabilitation results in reduced functional disability and improved quality of life, there will be increased pressure to provide and pay for these services. Resource analyses are needed before public policy can be changed to cover the large segment of the aging population that would be eligible for rehabilitation.

7. *Do persons with positive screenings comply with advice and interventions?* Unknown. In one study, 59% of persons had complied with further hearing assessment with pure tone audiometry, regardless of the outcome of a screening test (Lichtenstein et al., 1988a). This figure may be higher if only persons with a positive screen are referred for evaluation. Further information is needed on how well older persons adapt to and use hearing aids once they are prescribed.

These questions are applicable for any screening program, not just one involving hearing impairment. Although progress is being made to investigate these problems, hearing function should be assessed in aged persons as part of a standard physical examination when an aged person visits his or her primary care physician.

Description of screening instruments

Principles of diagnostic test performance. When a patient presents to a caregiver with a complaint, the clinician's first task is to make a diagnosis. This involves a process where information is obtained that is both valid (true) and reliable (the same result is obtained when the information is obtained on more than one occasion). A diagnostic test is any information that may be used to sort out the patient's problem. The primary care provider should be familiar with how useful the testing methods are in ruling in or out a particular diagnosis. This section covers some principles of how to assess the usefulness of two diagnostic tests for detecting hearing impairment in the aged.

Figure 10.2 sets the stage for understanding the diagnostic process. For any problem in a population, we wish to be able to distinguish those persons *with* the characteristic (A + B) from those *without* the characteristic (C + D).

The usefulness of a diagnostic test must be evaluated against an independent standard, the results of which everyone agrees determine the presence or absence of the characteristic. For example, in evaluation for hearing impairment, pure tone audiometry is the gold standard for evaluating screening tests.

When the diagnostic test is compared against the independent standards, the following 2 × 2 table is generated:

		INDEPENDENT GOLD STANDARD		
		CHARACTERISTIC		
		PRESENT	ABSENT	
DIAGNOSTIC TEST	POSITIVE	A	C	A + C
	NEGATIVE	B	D	B + D
		A + B	C + D	A + B + C + D

From this table and Figure 10.2 the following proportions may be calculated.

- PREVALENCE = A + B / A + B + C + D: The proportion of persons in the population with the characteristic.

- PRETEST PROBABILITY: Another use for prevalence, this represents the a priori probability that the characteristic is present. For example, the prevalence of hearing impairment in aged women is about 30%; when an older woman walks into the office, she has a 30% chance of being hearing impaired, and this is true before any diagnostic tests are performed on her.

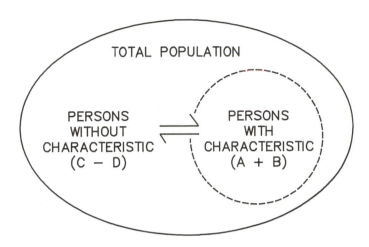

Figure 10.2. Schematic diagram for understanding diagnostic tests. The affected subset with the target disorder (A + B) is part of a larger population (A + B + C + D). A good screening test should distinguish between those with the target disorder (A + B) from those without the target disorder (C + D).

- SENSITIVITY = A /A + B: The proportion of persons *with* the characteristic correctly identified by the test. Sensitivity is affected by severity of the characteristic (the more advanced the condition, the higher the sensitivity).
- SPECIFICITY = D /C + D: The proportion of persons *without* the characteristic correctly identified by the test.
- POSITIVE PREDICTIVE VALUE = A / A + C: The proportion of persons with positive tests who have the characteristic. The posttest probability that, given a positive test, the characteristic is present. Positive predictive values are dependent on sensitivity, specificity, and prevalence.
- NEGATIVE PREDICTIVE VALUE = D / B + D: The proportion of persons with negative tests who do not have the characteristic. The posttest probability that, given a negative test, the characteristic is absent. Negative predictive values also are dependent on sensitivity, specificity, and prevalence.
- TEST ACCURACY = A + D / A + B + C + D: The proportion of persons, with or without the characteristic, correctly identified by the test. In screening, the most valuable tests are those that have the highest accuracy (i.e., they minimize false-positive and false-negative results).

For further discussion of this topic, refer to Chapter 14 by Turner.

Principles of screening instruments

Pure tone measures. The Welch-Allyn Audioscope is a hand-held instrument that delivers a 20-, 30-, or 40-dB hearing level (HL) tone at 500, 1000, 2000, and 4000 Hz (see Figure 10.3). To use the audioscope the largest ear speculum needed to achieve a seal within the external auditory canal is selected. The tympanic membrane is then visualized—if obstructed by cerumen, the impaction must be removed before testing. Then the tonal sequence is initiated, with the subject indicating whether he or she heard the tone by raising a finger.

The audioscope has been validated in the elderly against pure tone audiometry (Lichtenstein et al., 1988a) using the definition for hearing impairment proposed by Ventry and Weinstein (1983): The subjects

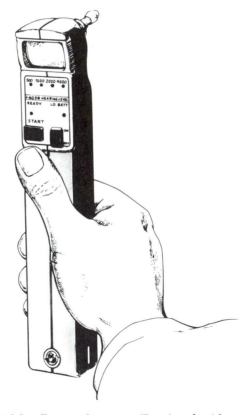

Figure 10.3. The Welch-Allyn Audioscope. (Reprinted with permission from "Validation of screening tools for identifying hearing-impaired elderly in primary care" by M. J. Lichtenstein, F. H. Bess, & S. A. Logan, 1988, *Journal of the American Medical Association, 259,* p. 2876.)

were considered hearing-impaired if (a) they had a 40-dB loss at either 1000 *or* 2000 Hz in both ears, or (b) they had a 40-dB loss at 1000 *and* 2000 Hz in one ear. Subjects were tested in physicians' offices and in a hearing center.

The sensitivities and specificities of the audioscope by signal frequency and site of testing are shown in Table 10.2. The prevalence of having a 40-dB deficit by audiogram increases from 14% to 16% for 500 Hz to 63% to 69% for 4000 Hz. In general, the sensitivity of the audioscope was slightly better and the specificity markedly better at each frequency in the hearing center than in the physicians' offices.

Between-occasion and between-observer agreement for the audioscope results were tested using the kappa statistic, which is a measure of the observed agreement not due to chance (Sackett, Haynes, & Tugwell, 1985). The between-location agreement of audioscope results are listed in Table 10.3 by frequency and ear. The kappa values ranged from .41 for the left ear at 500 Hz to .74 for the left ear at 2000 Hz.

The performance of the audioscope against the audiogram definition of hearing impairment is shown in Table 10.4. Using this definition the prevalence of hearing impairment was 30%. The sensitivity of the audioscope in the physician's office and the hearing center was identical, 94%.

TABLE 10.2

Sensitivity and Specificity of Audioscope by Signal Frequency and Test Site

Signal Frequency (Hz)	Failure To Hear %	Physicians' Offices			Hearing Center		
		N	Sensitivity %	Specificity %	N	Sensitivity %	Specificity %
Right Ear							
500	13.7	175	79	76	172	92	93
1000	18.3	175	91	69	172	97	85
2000	31.4	175	87	88	172	79	96
4000	63.0	173	89	78	172	89	91
Left Ear							
500	16.1	174	79	77	172	89	94
1000	16.7	174	93	70	172	97	87
2000	32.8	174	88	89	171	88	93
4000	69.0	171	83	72	170	87	87

TABLE 10.3
Between Location Agreement of Audioscope Results:
Physicians' Offices Versus Hearing Center

| | Kappa Statistic* | |
Frequency (in Hz)	Right Ear	Left Ear
500	.50	.41
1000	.50	.51
2000	.71	.74
4000	.65	.62

*All values are statistically significant at $p < .0001$.

However, the specificity of the audioscope was significantly lower in the physician's offices compared to the hearing center (72% vs. 90%). The lower specificity in the physicians' offices probably arises from higher ambient background noise levels in these settings. Thus the audioscope is a sensitive, repeatable test for the detection of elderly hearing impaired. Its moderate specificity in the primary care setting would have the effect of an increase in false-positive identification of hearing impairment.

Self-perception scales. The Hearing Handicap Inventory for the Elderly—Screening Version (HHIE-S) is a self-administered 10-item questionnaire designed to detect emotional and social problems associated with impaired hearing (Table 10.5; Ventry & Weinstein, 1983). Subjects respond to questions about circumstances related to hearing by stating whether the situation presents a problem. A "no" response scores 0, "sometimes" scores 2, and "yes" scores 4. Total HHIE-S scores range from 0 to 40.

Test–retest repeatability for the HHIE-S as determined using Pearson product-moment correlation is .84 ($p < .001$) indicating a high degree of repeatability.

The performance of the HHIE-S scores against the audiogram definition of hearing impairment is illustrated in Figure 10.4. Sensitivities and specificities were determined for the performance of the audioscope and HHIE-S by examining the distributions of test results in those with and without hearing impairment as defined by the audiogram. The received operating curves for the HHIE-S at the physicians' offices and the hearing center are virtually superimposable (Figure 10.4). Using a cutoff of 8, the sensitivity of the HHIE-S was 72% and 76%, and specificity was 77% and 71% in the hearing center and physicians' offices, respectively. Above a score of 24, the specificity of the HHIE-S was 98% in the hearing center and 96% in the physicians' offices. The corresponding sensitivities were 24% and 30%.

TABLE 10.4
Sensitivity and Specificity of the Audioscope for Detecting
Hearing Impairment When Compared to the Audiogram

Location	Prevalence of Hearing Impairment %	Number of Persons	Sensitivity %	Specificity %
Physicians' Offices	30	174	94	72
Hearing Center	30	171	94	90

Note. Pure tone test at 40 dB HL at 1000 and 2000 Hz in each ear. Hearing impairment defined as either the (a) inability to hear tone at one frequency in *each* ear or (b) inability to hear both frequencies in one ear.

TABLE 10.5
Hearing Handicap Inventory for the Elderly (Screening Version)

Does a hearing problem cause you to feel embarrassed when you meet new people?

Does a hearing problem cause you to feel frustrated when talking to members of your family?

Do you have difficulty hearing when someone speaks in a whisper?

Do you feel handicapped by a hearing problem?

Does a hearing problem cause you difficulty when visiting friends, relatives, or neighbors?

Does a hearing problem cause you to attend religious services less often than you would like?

Does a hearing problem cause you to have arguments with family members?

Does a hearing problem cause you to have difficulty when listening to television or radio?

Do you feel that any difficulty with your hearing limits/hampers your personal or social life?

Does a hearing problem cause you difficulty when in a restaurant with relatives or friends?

Note. This table is adapted from Ventry and Weinstein (1983).

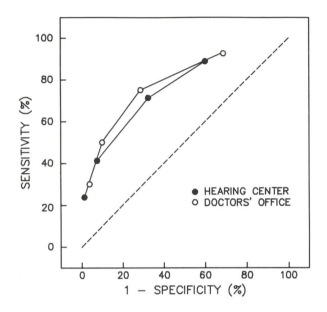

Figure 10.4. Receiver operating curves for HHIE–S scores against audiogram measures of hearing impairment. Hearing impairment defined by the criteria of Ventry and Weinstein (see text). From left to right, the four plotted points on each curve indicate HHIE–S cutoff points of 24, 16, 8, and 2. Solid circles indicate hearing center results, open circles represent results from physicians' office. (Reprinted with permission from "Validation of screening tools for identifying hearing-impaired elderly in primary care" by M. J. Lichtenstein, F. H. Bess, & S. A. Logan, 1988, *Journal of the American Medical Association, 259,* p. 2877.)

The likelihood ratios for different levels of the HHIE–S are given in Table 10.6. In this group the pretest probability of having a hearing impairment was 30%. For those with HHIE–S scores of 0 to 8, the likelihood ratio was 0.36, with a posttest probability of hearing impairment calculated as 13%. For those with scores of 26 to 40, the likelihood ratio was 12.00 with a posttest probability of 84%. The HHIE–S shows a similar level of performance against different definitions of hearing impairment as well. Similar likelihood ratios are found for speech frequency pure tone averages, high-frequency pure tone averages, and speech recognition thresholds (all at 25 dB HL in the better ear; Lichtenstein et al., 1988b). Thus the HHIE–S is a valid repeatable screening test with a robust performance against different definitions of hearing impairment.

Combining the audioscope and HHIE–S results. Both the audioscope and HHIE–S are repeatable valid measures of hearing impairment. The audioscope is very sensitive but moderately specific in the physicians'

TABLE 10.6
Probability of Hearing Impairment Given a Hearing Handicap Inventory
for the Elderly (HHIE-S) Score

HHIE-S	Pretest Probability of Hearing Impairment	Likelihood Ratio (95% Confidence Interval)	Posttest Probability of Hearing Impairment
0–8	30%	0.36 (0.19–0.68)	13%
10–24	30%	2.30 (1.22–4.32)	50%
26–40	30%	12.00 (2.62–55.00)	84%

Note. The HHIE-S was completed at the hearing center. Pure tone test at 40 dB HL at 1000 and 2000 Hz in each ear. Hearing impairment defined as either the (a) inability to hear tone at one frequency in *each* ear or (b) inability to hear both frequencies in one ear.

offices. The HHIE–S is moderately sensitive but highly specific at scores greater than 24. The greatest test accuracy in identifying hearing impairment was found when the two tests were combined (Table 10.7). Persons should be considered in need of referral if they fail the audioscope *and* have an HHIE score greater than 8 *or* they pass the audioscope *and* have an HHIE score greater than 24.

Physical diagnostic maneuvers.   Traditional maneuvers for detecting hearing impairment in the elderly also have diagnostic utility (Uhlmann, Rees, Psaty, & Duckert, 1989). The performance of a 512-Hz tuning fork, 1024-Hz tuning fork, a finger rub, and whispered voice have been tested against pure tone audiometry in demented and nondemented subjects. In this study ears were considered hearing-impaired if the average loss at 500, 1000, 2000, and 3000 Hz was greater than or equal to 40 dB HL. The results are given in Table 10.8. In demented patients, at set sensitivities, the observed specificities are comparable to those found with the audioscope; however, among nondemented subjects, the specificities are lower. The tests also were found to be repeatable (Table 10.8), but this may depend on the setting in which the tests are performed and differences between observers in administering the tests. Compared to the traditional physical diagnostic tests, the audioscope delivers a standard signal at a standard distance (right at the external auditory canal). The HHIE–S offers the advantage of removing observers from the screening process and relying on self-report. All the studied tests are useful screening tools for hearing impairment; to determine which (if one is better than the others) would require a direct comparative study performed under field conditions.

TABLE 10.7
Sensitivity, Specificity, and Predictive Values for Diagnostic Tests
in the Diagnosis of Elderly Hearing Impaired

Test	Sensitivity %	Specificity %	Predictive Values (%)[a]		Test Accuracy %
			Positive	Negative	
Audioscope	94	72	60	97	79
HHIE-S Score					
> 8	72	77	58	86	74
> 24	41	92	67	78	76
Combined Audioscope Failed and HHIE-S Score > 8					
or Audioscope Passed and HHIE-S Score > 24	75	86	70	89	83

Note. HHIE-S = Hearing Handicap Inventory for the Elderly—Screening Version. [a]Predictive values apply at hearing impairment prevalence of 30%.

Audiologic characteristics associated with aging

The aging auditory system typically exhibits a loss in threshold sensitivity and a debasement in the ability to understand comfortably loud speech. The audiologic manifestations can reflect the pathological changes occurring within the auditory system. Because one or more types of presbycusis often are present, however, it is difficult to determine site of lesion from the audiometric data.

Pure tone threshold measures.   The hearing loss among those individuals over the age of 60 years primarily affects the high frequencies, especially those above 1000 Hz. The hearing sensitivity changes that are known to occur as a function of age are shown in Figure 10.5. These data, taken from the Framingham Heart Study (Mościcki, Elkins, Baum, & McNamara, 1985), represent the mean audiometric configurations in the better ear (0.5, 1, 2 kHz) as a function of age for both males and females. The study sample is composed of 935 males and 1,358 females. Both males and females are seen to exhibit hearing loss sensitivity for those persons

TABLE 10.8
Sensitivities (Sens) and Specificities (Spec) of Physical Examination Tests in Detecting Hearing Impairment

Test	Distance*	Spec	Distance*	Spec	
	Demented Patients (68 Ears)				Test/Retest Reliability (38 ears)
	Sens = 90%		Sens = 80%		
512-Hz Tuning Fork	40	53%	27	82%	0.66
1024-Hz Tuning Fork	36	63%	23	95%	0.38
Finger Rub	8	85%	3	95%	0.89
Whispered Voice	19	78%	14	89%	0.67
	Nondemented Patients (68 Ears)				Test/Retest Reliability (44 ears)
	Sens = 90%		Sens = 80%		
512-Hz Tuning Fork	40	56%	34	64%	0.87
1024-Hz Tuning Fork	45	44%	31	69%	0.58
Finger Rub	21	44%	16	49%	0.90
Whispered Voice	29	70%	21	82%	0.78

*Distance of test from ear in centimeters.

60 years of age and older, especially in the high-frequency regions (2000–8000 Hz). Furthermore, threshold values for males are poorer than for females. It generally is thought that these differences are due to the noise exposure males experience throughout their lifetimes.

A problem that consistently has plagued the study of threshold change with age has been the influence of environmental factors that can contaminate the threshold sensitivity data. That is, the influence of high noise levels and other variables are also known to damage the auditory system. Rosen, Bergman, Plester, El-Mofty, and Salti (1962) studied hearing thresholds as a function of age in members of a Mabaan tribe in the Sudan. The members of the tribe were essentially living in a noise-free environment. Rosen et al. reported that the subjects, who ranged in age from 10 to 90 years, exhibited much less hearing loss than do people the same age in the western countries.

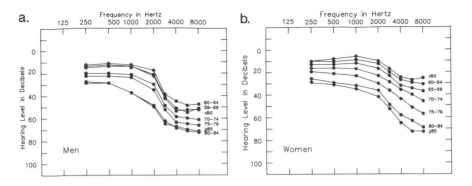

Figure 10.5. Mean audiometric thresholds in the better ear for males and females as a function of age. (Redrawn from "Hearing in the elderly: An epidemiologic study of the framingham heart study cohort" by E. K. Mościcki, E. F. Elkins, H. M. Baum, & P. M. McNamara, 1985, *Ear and Hearing, 6,* p. 186.)

Although the hearing loss typically is sensorineural, there is some data to suggest that a conductive component can be related to the phenomenon known as presbycusis (Glorig & Davis, 1961; Milne, 1977; Nixon, Glorig, & High, 1962). In general, the air-bone gap is reported to increase with increasing hearing loss. The air-bone gap at the high frequencies, particularly 4000 Hz, has been reported to increase from 10 dB at 50 years of age to 40 dB by 80 years of age (Glorig & Davis, 1961; Marshall, Martinez, & Schlamen, 1983). The cause of the observed conductive component is not clearly understood. Glorig and Davis (1961) suggested that the air-bone gap was due to an age-related increase in the stiffness of the cochlear partition. The conductive loss also may be attributed to the changes that can occur in the middle ear (i.e., stiffness of the ossicular chain and tympanic membrane). Another possible cause of the conductive component may be the tissue reduction in the elderly, which produces changes in the properties of the mastoid. Finally, it is possible that the conductive component in the high-frequency region could be due to ear canal collapse or to the use of an earphone with a hard cushion that has a poor fit to the auricle (Bess & Humes, 1990; Gordon-Salant, 1987).

Speech recognition measures. One also sees changes in speech recognition thresholds (SRT) with increasing age. The changes in the SRT correspond with the changes in the pure tone measures. An example of the decrease in SRT with increasing age is shown in Figure 10.6.

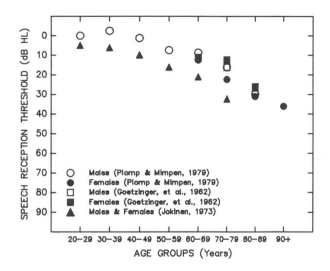

Figure 10.6. Speech recognition thresholds (SRT) as a function of age. Data taken from several studies. (Reprinted with permission from "Basic hearing evaluation" by S. Gordon-Salant, 1987, in H. G. Mueller & V. C. Geoffrey (Eds.), *Communication disorders in aging* (pp. 301–333), Washington, DC: Gallaudet University Press.)

It has long been reported that older persons experience considerable difficulty understanding comfortably loud speech, especially in a background of competing noise. Furthermore, this difficulty with speech understanding is thought to increase with increasing age, especially for persons over the age of 60 years. When speech recognition is assessed in quiet, however, it is difficult to differentiate between young individuals and elderly when the presentation level of the speech material and the degree of hearing loss is controlled. That is, most studies that report poor speech recognition in quiet among the elderly presented the speech material at a fixed intensity level, usually 25–40 dB SL. Because the subjects demonstrated high-frequency sensorineural hearing losses, a presentation level of 25 to 40 dB SL often was insufficient to obtain a maximum speech recognition score. In fact, Jerger and Hayes (1977) illustrated that PB-max scores in quiet remain relatively stable at 50 through 59 years of age and exhibit only a slight decrease above 59 years. Hence, a fixed presentation level is not recommended in the speech recognition assessment of older individuals. According to Gordon-Salant (1987), "an arbitrary presentation level of 95 dB SPL or the use of an adaptive estimate of the PB-max level is preferred" (p. 309).

Several studies have demonstrated that when elderly subjects are matched with a young control group for hearing loss, few differences in speech recognition scores under quiet conditions are found (Kasden, 1970; Surr, 1977; Townsend & Bess, 1980). Bess and Townsend (1977) reported similar findings in a sample of patients with flat audiometric configurations with hearing losses greater than 49 dB HL. For those subjects 70 years of age and older, however, and with hearing losses greater than 50 dB HL, there was a marked breakdown in speech recognition.

The breakdown in speech understanding among the aged appears to be exacerbated even among normal hearers when the listening task is made more difficult through degradation of the speech signal. Jerger and Hayes (1977) examined speech recognition as a function of age with a sentence identification task (synthetic sentence identification—SSI) using an ipsilateral speech competition (message to competition ratio of 0). Sentence recognition performance decreased systematically with age beginning at 30 to 39 years. Jerger and Hayes noted that sentence recognition performance in competition for older persons was much poorer than for monosyllabic materials in quiet. They attributed this finding to a "central aging effect." Shirinian and Arnst (1982) confirmed the findings of Jerger and Hayes with SSI materials but reported that speech recognition problems in the elderly occurred only at the higher speech intensity levels. This "rollover" effect has been reported in subjects with eighth nerve disorders and central auditory dysfunction (Jerger, Neely, & Jerger, 1980). Dubno, Dirks, and Morgan (1984) demonstrated that elderly subjects with normal and mild hearing losses experienced considerable difficulty in speech understanding under varying signal-to-babble (S/B) ratios. The patients with mild hearing loss performed much poorer than did the aged normal hearers. Figure 10.7 illustrates the S/B ratios required for 50% recognition in four groups of subjects: normal hearing and less than 44 years of age, normal hearing and older than 65 years of age, mild sensorineural hearing loss and less than 44 years of age, and mild sensorineural hearing loss and older than 65 years of age. High-predictability (PH) and low-predictability (PL) sentences from the Speech Perception in Noise (SPIN) test were the principal materials. It is seen that more favorable S/B ratios are needed for subjects as the speech material increases in difficulty (PH sentences vs. PL sentences). Furthermore, more favorable S/B ratios are needed for the older subjects, even those with normal pure tone sensitivity. These data support the assumption that performance in noise deteriorates with age, with or without increases in threshold sensitivity.

It appears that the breakdown in speech recognition is even greater when the temporal domain of the speech signal is altered (Bosatra & Russolo, 1982; Jerger, 1973; Konkle, Beasley, & Bess, 1977). Konkle et al. examined the effect of time compression on word recognition in four age groups ranging from 54 to 84 years of age. All of the subjects had similar

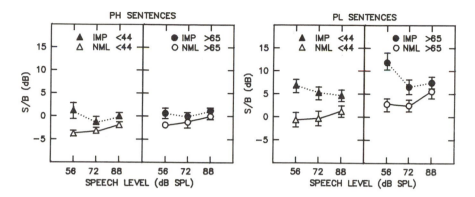

Figure 10.7. Signal-to-babble ratios needed for 50% recognition of sentence material (SPIN—PH and PL) in four groups of subjects: young normal (NML) and hearing-impaired (IMP) listeners (left panels) and older normal (NML) and hearing-impaired (IMP) listeners (right panels). (Redrawn with permission from "Effects of age and mild hearing loss on speech recognition in noise" by J. R. Dubno, D. D. Dirks, & D. E. Morgan, 1984, *Journal of the Acoustical Society of America, 76,* pp. 87–96.)

pure tone data and word recognition scores in quiet of 90% or better. The findings from this study are summarized in Figure 10.8. This figure presents the mean word recognition scores for the different age groups at several conditions of time compression and sensation level. It is seen that word recognition decreases with increasing time compression, age, and decreasing sensation level. Konkle et al. theorized that this degradation in speech understanding under time-compressed conditions was related to senescent changes in the central auditory mechanism.

Jerger, Jerger, Oliver, and Pirozzolo (1989) examined the contributions of peripheral, central, and cognitive factors to the speech recognition problems of the elderly population. Elderly subjects (N = 130) received a comprehensive audiologic and neuropsychologic evaluation. These data were used to determine the central auditory and cognitive status of the elderly patients. The prevalence of central auditory processing problems was 50%, whereas the prevalence for cognitive deficits was evident in 41% of the population. The study revealed that speech understanding problems in the aged cannot be totally explained by peripheral hearing loss or cognitive decline and suggested that central deficits are a contributing factor. More specifically, central auditory problems can be evident when there is no cognitive decline and cognitive abnormality can exist independent of central auditory deficits.

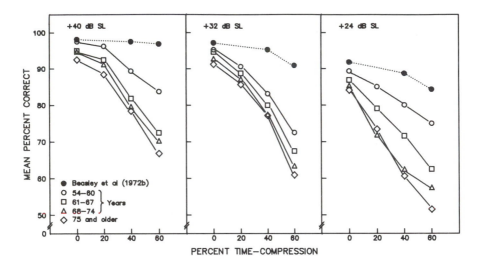

Figure 10.8. Mean word recognition scores for the four different age groups as a function of time compression and sensation level. (Redrawn with permission from "Intelligibility of time-altered speech in relation to chronological aging" by D. F. Konkle, D. S. Beasley, & F. H. Bess, 1977, *Journal of Speech and Hearing Research, 20,* p. 112.)

Acoustic immittance measures. Since about 1970 the measure of acoustic immittance at the tympanic membrane has become an important component in the hearing evaluation. This sensitive and objective diagnostic tool is used to identify the presence of fluid behind the tympanic membrane, to evaluate Eustachian tube and facial nerve function, to predict audiometric findings, to determine the nature of the hearing loss, and to assist in the diagnosis of different auditory disorders (Bess & Humes, 1990). Importantly, acoustic immittance measures are influenced by the aging process. In order to interpret accurately immittance test results, the audiologist must recognize the manner in which age affects the various parameters of acoustic immittance.

Tympanometry and static acoustic immittance. There is limited information available on tympanometric measurements in the elderly population. The presence of excessive negative pressure has been reported among older persons and is thought to be due to poor Eustachian tube function in this population (Nerbonne, Schow, & Gosset, 1976). Such data suggest that elderly individuals should be checked for Eustachian tube dysfunction as part of their basic audiologic evaluation.

It generally is recognized that static acoustic immittance decreases with increasing age (Alberti & Kristensen, 1970; Hall, 1979; Jerger, Jerger, &

Mauldin, 1972) as shown in Figure 10.9. The data in Figure 10.9, taken from Hall (1979), illustrate the systematic decrease in static immittance with increasing age as well as the standard deviations for each group. This decrease in static compliance among the elderly can limit its clinical utility in certain otopathologic conditions such as otosclerosis. Hall (1979) reported that static compliance measures fail to differentiate between otosclerotic patients and individuals over 60 years of age.

Acoustic reflex.   There are a number of studies that have investigated the effect of age on the acoustic reflex. The acoustic reflex is elicited among normal subjects between 80 and 100 dB HL. Of course, the threshold will be elevated for subjects with sensorineural hearing loss. Jerger and co-workers (Jerger et al., 1972; Jerger, Jerger, Mauldin, & Segal, 1974) reported that the acoustic reflex threshold generally decreases from 96 dB HL to about 84 dB HL in subjects between 3 and 80 years. In support of these data, Osterhammel and Osterhammel (1979) noted that the acoustic reflex declines at approximately 3.5 dB per decade when expressed in sensation level; however, no differences were seen when the data were expressed in terms of Hearing Level. Quaranta, Cassano, and Amoroso (1980) reported that 55% of their elderly subjects showed absent or abnormal acoustic reflexes on both ipsilateral and contralateral

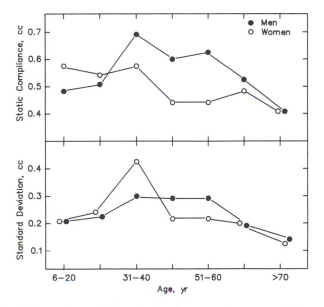

Figure 10.9. Illustration of the effects of age and sex on static compliance. (Redrawn with permission from "Effects of age and sex on static compliance" by J. Hall, 1979, *Archives of Otolaryngology, 105,* pp. 153–156.)

stimulation. Despite the apparent disagreement among research reports, studies suggest that if age effects exist they are at best minimal for pure tone stimuli (Jerger et al. 1972; Silverman, Silman, & Miller, 1983). In Chapter 5 Wilson and Margolis offer a review of the acoustic reflex threshold research in older persons and discuss reasons for disagreement among the various studies.

Age is, however, known to influence the acoustic reflex amplitude. Hall (1982) examined individuals ranging in age from 20 to 80 years and reported that the maximum reflex amplitude decreased by about 56% over this age range. The amplitude changes typically are greater for uncrossed reflexes as opposed to crossed reflexes. The uncrossed and crossed acoustic reflex amplitudes for a 1000-Hz signal in three different age groups as a function of signal level are shown in Figure 10.10. It can be seen that the crossed and uncrossed reflexes decrease with increasing age. At the higher intensity signals the differences in amplitude become more apparent but are somewhat less pronounced for the crossed acoustic reflex. The basis for such age effects is not altogether clear. One possibility is the evidence of age-related dysfunction in the middle ear musculature. Decreased middle ear efficiency would be reflected in reduced capacity

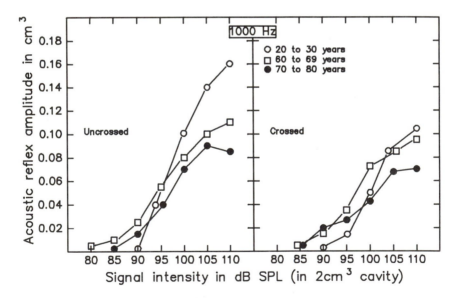

Figure 10.10.   Crossed and uncrossed acoustic reflex amplitude (1000-Hz signal) in three age groups. (Redrawn with permission from "Acoustic reflex amplitude. II: Effect of Age-Related Auditory Dysfunction" by J. Hall, 1982, *Audiology, 21*, pp. 386–399.)

for maximal contraction. Another possibility may be related to age changes in the innervation of the stapedious muscle, which of course would diminish the reflex amplitude (Hall, 1979).

Auditory brainstem response. The measurement of auditory brainstem responses (ABR) is considered now an important component of the audiologic test battery. It typically is used in the identification and estimation of hearing impairment of those patients who cannot be tested in a behavioral format (i.e., newborns and infants) or as a special auditory test in neuro-otologic diagnosis. Although the stability and reliability of brainstem responses are considered quite good for the general population, there are a number of extrinsic (i.e., stimulus rate, stimulus intensity, filter setting) and intrinsic (i.e., age, gender, hearing loss) variables that can affect the ABR response. More specific to this discussion, the influence of age and gender on ABR responses has been studied by many investigators and is the subject of some disagreement. For example, Jerger and Hall (1980) reported that latency increased by approximately 0.2 ms over the age range of 25 to 55 years. Furthermore, the Wave V amplitude decreased by about 10% over the same age range. The ABR Wave I-V interval also is reported to increase over the age range of 60 to 86 years, implying that there may be brainstem involvement (Hall, 1990). Rowe (1978) compared the ABR responses for young adults to an older population and found that the elderly group exhibited latency delays on the order of 0.30 ms to 0.50 ms relative to the younger population. According to Thomsen, Terkildsen, and Osterhammel (1978) the Wave V latency increases at approximately 0.10 ms per decade of life.

In contrast to the above studies, Schwartz and co-workers (submitted 1989) examined the brainstem auditory evoked response data from a large sample of normal hearing adults (120 men and 120 women) across a wide age span (15–88 years) and reported that age had no influence on absolute or interpeak latency. Unlike previous investigators who focused their data analysis on measures of central tendency, Schwartz et al. developed bivariate plots of age versus latency and amplitude and calculated the variance contributing to the regression model. Based on such an analysis, the authors concluded that audiologists need not be concerned with the patient's age in the interpretation of clinical data if latency is the principal diagnostic variable. They did conclude, however, that age does have an effect on the Wave I amplitude but not Waves III and V. This effect was noted to be more pronounced with men than women. Finally, Schwartz et al. emphasized that because elderly individuals tend to be more anxious and noisy, audiologists should maintain an optimal signal-to-noise ratio so that contaminating myogenic activity will not obscure Wave I.

Self-assessment scales. An imperfect relationship exists among hearing impairment, hearing disability, and hearing handicap. *Hearing impairment* or *hearing loss* usually denotes a change for the worse in auditory structure or auditory function, outside the range of normal hearing (ASHA, 1981). *Hearing disability* occurs when there is a change in hearing function that causes problems with the perception of speech and environmental sounds (Salomon, 1986). The term *hearing handicap* is used to denote a change in hearing that interferes with performing activities of daily living (Salomon, 1986; Weinstein, 1984). It is possible for a person with mild to moderate loss to experience no disability or handicap; conversely, individuals with marginal hearing loss may perceive themselves as having a significant disability or handicap. Because of the varying response to a hearing impairment, self-assessment techniques have been advocated as a supplement to our pure tone classification schemes (Bess, Lichtenstein, Logan, Burger, & Nelson, 1989; Schow & Nerbonne, 1982; Ventry & Weinstein, 1983). An understanding of the relationship among hearing impairment, hearing disability, and hearing handicap will offer insight into the impact of hearing impairment in the aged and the rehabilitative needs of this population.

Self-assessment scales and questionnaires allow the audiologist to delve into the patient's and family's perception of their communication difficulties, monitor their progress, and locate their hearing needs outside of the standard audiometric test battery. These tools not only can provide an objective method for evaluating the patient's progress in a rehabilitation paradigm but also provide the professional information for counseling the hearing-impaired and his or her "significant others." The following review summarizes some of the more common self-assessment scales used in audiologic practice. Some of these scales tap only information regarding the perception of difficulty relating to hearing loss; whereas others delve into the vocational, emotional, and social consequences of hearing loss.

Hearing Handicap Scale.   The Hearing Handicap Scale (HHS) Forms A and B (High, Fairbanks, & Glorig, 1964) was developed to evaluate the effectiveness of rehabilitation procedures. The instrument was designed to probe for a person's everyday hearing experiences. Each form contains 20 items and the test takes only about 5 minutes to administer. The questions require only a low level of reading ability. The items are rated on a 5-step continuum from *almost always* to *almost never.*

Hearing Measurement Scale.   Several years after the introduction of the Hearing Handicap Scale, the Hearing Measurement Scale (HMS) was developed (Noble, 1978; Noble, 1979; Noble & Atherly, 1970). This test measures auditory disability for persons with acquired sensorineural hearing loss. It contains 42 scoring items divided into the following seven subcategories: (1) speech-hearing, (2) acuity for nonspeech sounds, (3) localization, (4) reaction to handicap, (5) speech distortion, (6) tinnitus, and (7) personal opinion of hearing loss. The items are weighted to give a measure of disability.

The Denver Scale of Communication Function. The Denver Scale of Communication Function (Alpiner, Chevrette, Glascoe, Metz, & Olsen, 1974) was developed to evaluate the client's communication function before and after therapeutic management. There are 25 questions that cover communication in the following areas: family, self, social–vocation, and communication. Both pre- and post-therapeutic responses are plotted on a grid so that the client can view his or her rehabilitative progress.

Hearing Performance Inventory. The Hearing Performance Inventory (Giolas, Owens, Lamb, & Schubert, 1979) asks the client to rate his or her ability to function in specific listening situations. The original inventory contained 158 items and took almost 1 hour to administer and score. The following areas were probed: understanding speech, signal intensity, response to auditory failure, social aspects of hearing loss, and occupational difficulties. In scoring the inventory the percentage of difficulty was obtained by adding the numerical responses (1 to 5) for all the items answered, dividing by the number of items attempted, and multiplying by 20. The revised HPI (Lamb, Owens, & Schubert, 1983) has 90 items and takes slightly over half an hour to administer and score. Some of the categories could be retaken following intervention from amplification as a measure of validating hearing aid performance.

The McCarthy-Alpiner Scale of Hearing Handicap. The McCarthy-Alpiner Scale of Hearing Handicap (McCarthy & Alpiner, 1980) is a 34-item questionnaire. Form A is for the client to fill out, and Form B is for a family member to use. The only difference in the two forms is a change in the pronoun. The scale was developed to assess the psychological, social, and vocational aspects of hearing loss. The results of the validation study showed a difference in perception between the hearing-impaired person and his or her family. The findings suggest the need to include the family member in the rehabilitation process.

Hearing Handicap Inventory for the Elderly. The Hearing Handicap Inventory for the Elderly (HHIE; Ventry & Weinstein, 1982) was developed to assess the impact of hearing loss on the emotional and social adjustment of the elderly client. The authors wanted a tool that would assess the handicap imposed by a hearing impairment. The questions were developed to be easy to read and pertinent to the life of an elderly individual. There are 25 items—13 items explore the emotional consequences of hearing loss and 12 items pertain to the social and situational effects. Patients respond to questions regarding their hearing by acknowledging whether the situation presents a problem. A *no* response scores 0, a *sometime* scores 2, and a *yes* scores 4. Ventry and Weinstein interpreted a score of 18% or greater as suggesting a self-perceived handicap that should lead to further intervention. A 10-item screening version of the HHIE, known as the Hearing Handicap Inventory for the Elderly—Screening Version (HHIE–S), was described earlier in this chapter.

Self-Assessment of Communication (SAC). The Self-Assessment of Communication questionnaire (Schow & Nerbonne, 1982) is a 10-item self-report questionnaire that assesses (a) difficulties communicating in different situations, (b) emotional responses to the person's hearing impairment, and (c) the perception of the attitudes of others toward the person's hearing abilities. Clients respond to the questions by circling one of five response choices ranging from *never* to *practically always*. Total scores on the SAC range from 10 to 50 and a score over 18 constitutes a fail. The Significant Other Assessment of Communication (SOAC) contains the same 10 items as does the SAC with only pronoun changes. It is used to obtain the impressions of a family member or significant other of the client's hearing difficulty.

Global Functional Scale—The Sickness Impact Profile. The scales discussed to this point are all communication-specific because the questions are weighted toward communication difficulties caused by the hearing loss. More recently, attempts have been made to assess the impact of hearing loss on more global measures of function such as functional health status and psychosocial well-being.

Measures of functional health status provide us with insight into the prognosis of a condition, the impact of intervention on general health, and the ramifications of a disease on an individual's life quality (Bess et al., 1989). One measure of functional health status is the Sickness Impact Profile (SIP). The SIP is a 136-statement standardized questionnaire that assesses function in a behavioral context (Gilson et al., 1975; Bergner, Bobbitt, Pollard, Martin, & Gilson, 1976; Bergner, Bobbitt, Carter, & Gilson, 1981). The statements are weighted and grouped into 12 subscales: ambulation, mobility, body care/movement, social interaction, communication, alertness, emotional, sleep/rest, eating, work, home management, and recreation/pastimes. In addition there are three main scales: Physical (combining ambulation, mobility, body care/movement), Psychosocial (combining social interaction, communication, alertness, emotional), and Overall (combining all 12 subscales). The higher the SIP score, the greater the perceived functional impairment. The SIP is a valid, reliable tool that has been applied in a number of areas to measure sickness-related dysfunction (Carter, Bobbitt, Bergner, & Gilson, 1976; Pollard, Bobbitt, Bergner, Martin, & Gilson, 1976). As examples, the SIP has been used in studies of end-stage renal disease (Hart & Evans, 1987), survivors of myocardial infarction (Bergner, Hallstrom, Bergner, Eisenberg, & Cobb, 1985), chronic obstructive pulmonary disease (McSweeney, Grant, Heaton, Adams, & Timms, 1982), and rheumatoid arthritis (Deyo & Inui,

1984). In addition, SIP scores have been associated with level of hearing impairment: As hearing worsens in the elderly, SIP scores increase (Bess et al., 1989).

Functional impact of hearing loss in the elderly

Investigators who have used communication-specific interview scales to assess the functional impact of hearing loss on older individuals have reported repeatedly that the hearing-impaired elderly experience a wide variety of listening complications (Weinstein, 1985; Ventry & Weinstein, 1982; Schow & Nerbonne, 1982). An important question, however, is this: Does hearing loss in the elderly produce only a local disturbance in a person's ability to hear and understand speech, or does the impairment produce wider ripple effects that have an impact on some of the more basic areas of human performance? A major study was conducted in Great Britain to examine the social and psychological implications of hearing impairment among adult populations (Herbst, 1983). In part, this study contrasted hearing-impaired with normal hearing elderly across several different life dimensions including general health, use of welfare services, experience of loneliness, and interactions with friends and family and the experience of hearing impairment. Some of the pertinent findings from this study include the following: (a) Hearing loss appears to be associated with poor general health and is closely linked with such factors as reduced mobility as well as reduction in activities and number of excursions outside the home. (b) Hearing impairment causes a significant reduction in interpersonal interplay and contacts. (c) Hearing impairment appears to be associated with reduced enjoyment of life. And (d) elderly hearing impaired are more likely to be depressed. In support of Herbst's findings, Bess et al. (1989; in press) analyzed the impact of hearing impairment on individuals over 65 years of age screened in primary care practices. Functional and psychosocial impairment was measured using the Sickness Impact Profile (SIP), a standardized questionnaire for assessing sickness-related dysfunction. The findings of this study are summarized in Figure 10.11. These data reflect the average SIP scores for three different dimensions on the functional measure including physical, psychosocial, and an overall score. For the Physical Scale the mean SIP score increased from 3.3 in individuals with no hearing impairment to 18.9 among those with a loss of 41 dB HL or greater in the better ear. The comparable contrast in the Psychosocial Scale are 4.0 and 16.8. For the Overall Scale the contrasts are 5.3 and 17.1, respectively. In addition, Bess and co-workers conducted a step-wise multiple linear regression to adjust for baseline differences in age, race, sex, educational level, number of illnesses, presence of diabetes and ischemic heart disease, number of medications,

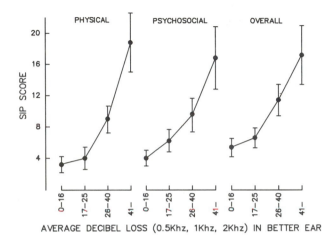

Figure 10.11. Mean physical, psychosocial, and overall Sickness Impact Profile (SIP) scores plotted by level of hearing impairment (average dB loss at 500, 1000, 2000 Hz in the better ear) in 153 elderly subjects. The intervals plotted around the means represent one standard error. (Reprinted with permission from "Hearing impairment as a determinant of function in the elderly" by F. H. Bess, M. J. Lichtenstein, S. A. Logan, M. C. Burger, & E. Nelson, 1989, *Journal of the American Geriatrics Society, 37,* p. 126.)

near visual acuity, and mental status between the hearing-impaired and nonhearing-impaired elderly. In these multivariate analyses the score of each SIP scale served as the dependent variable. The regression coefficient was reported as a change in SIP score per change in hearing level. After adjustment for confounding variables, higher SIP scores were observed on all three main scales with every 10 dB increase in hearing loss, suggesting strong evidence for a relationship between degree of hearing impairment and functional capacity.

In contrast to the studies by Herbst (1983) and Bess et al. (1989), Salomon, Vesterager, and Jagd (1988) reported that life satisfaction, self-perception, and general activity level were not influenced by hearing level.

Several studies have explored the relationship between dementia and deafness. These studies demonstrated that a high percentage of patients with some degree of senile dementia also exhibited significant hearing loss (Herbst, 1983). These studies concluded, however, that hearing loss does not cause dementia, but rather the two conditions coexist among elderly patients. Weinstein and Amsell (1986) reported further that there was a trend among patients with dementia to have more severe hearing losses. Finally, Herbst and Humphrey (1980) showed a significant relationship between depression and hearing impairment. They concluded that "while deafness is not a major cause of depression in old age it is certainly a contributing factor and one that may be more readily ameliorated than many others" (p. 905).

Management issues in the elderly

The primary rehabilitation tool for the elderly hearing impaired population is amplification. Nevertheless, only 13%–18% of the elderly hearing impaired actually receive hearing aids (Gallup, 1980; Humphrey, Herbst, & Faurgi, 1981). A primary reason for the elderly not receiving amplification is that primary care physicians and "caring others" often fail to recognize hearing impairment. Even if a patient complains of hearing loss, there is a 50% chance that he or she will not be referred for rehabilitation (Bess et al., 1987; Herbst, 1983). In spite of these data, it is estimated that 58% of all hearing aid users are 65 years of age or older (Cranmer, 1986; Davies & Mueller, 1987). In addition, over 65% of individuals wearing amplification are first-time hearing aid users (Cranmer, 1986). Many potential hearing aid patients obtain their initial information regarding amplification from newspaper advertisements, magazines, and friends. Hence, they have already formed an opinion as to the style and type of hearing aid they desire prior to the hearing aid evaluation.

A review of the hearing aid selection process for the elderly hearing-impaired patient is beyond the scope of this chapter. Some issues concerning the specific amplification needs of the elderly, however, are worthy of comment.

When selecting a hearing aid for the elderly patient the audiologist should consider the following areas: (a) the patient's choice of style, (b) vision, (c) ability to manipulate the different types of hearing aids, (d) cost, and (e) amplification requirements. It is important to discuss with the elderly hearing impaired the various hearing aid styles available and which instruments will be most appropriate for a given individual. If a person with a severe hearing loss desires a canal style hearing aid, the limitations of these instruments should be brought to his or her attention.

Another important aspect to consider during the prefitting process with the elderly patient is visual status. Given that visual acuity decreases dramatically with older age, it is worthwhile to obtain information regarding the patient's corrected visual status by using near and far vision eye charts or by simply inquiring about visual status.

In addition to amplification restrictions many older persons have a decreased sense of touch as well as some restricted movement and decreased dexterity. Hence, it is important for the audiologist to determine whether the patient can adjust the controls and change the hearing aid battery on a particular hearing aid style before proceeding with the evaluation.

Although the majority of elderly patients are fitted with in-the-ear style hearing aids, the type and style of hearing aid selected should depend on the patient's ability to operate the aid, not just the degree and configuration of the hearing loss. For persons who cannot manipulate the traditional types of hearing aids, manufacturers have provided audiologists with several options. Some hearing aid manufacturers provide raised volume controls on all in-the-ear instruments, whereas with others this is an option. One hearing aid manufacturer has developed a post-auricular hearing aid with a large volume control that is easier to feel and to adjust. The entire design of the hearing aid is modified for the older adult. Recently, a remote control volume control device was developed that allows the hearing aid user to manipulate the gain by a hand-held control.

Finally, the cost of the instrument needs to be weighed against the flexibility for providing the most appropriate electroacoustic response.

Because of the degrading effects of distance, noise, and reverberation, optimum speech understanding cannot be achieved in some listening situations with only a hearing aid. Under such conditions, assistive devices can offer help through direct sound amplification as well as visual and vibrotactile alerts (Bess & Humes, 1990).

The life-style of the older individual will help dictate the need for particular assistive devices. If the individual is still employed and active in the community, the needs will be different from the person who is bedridden. For example, if the person is retired, the interest in recreation may take precedence over meetings and conferences. Ross (1986) reported that telephone listening ranks first in importance with hearing-impaired individuals, followed by television and large space listening.

Individuals who rarely leave their homes rely on television as an important source of information. Assistive listening devices are available to enhance listening to television. These devices have either hardwire connections to the television or a remote system such as infrared. The decision as to the appropriate device for improved television listening depends on cost, clarity, and ease of operation.

Assistive devices also can prove to be valuable with use of the telephone. There are many telephone devices available that are portable and easy to use that provide the patient with sufficient amplification to make the caller easier to understand. Individuals with significant speech understanding problems may benefit from purchasing a telecommunication device for the deaf. It may also be advantageous to enhance the telephone ring and replace it with a louder or visual signal so that the person will know when to answer the phone.

Churches, synagogues, and public facilities are now using assistive listening devices to enhance speech understanding for the hearing impaired. The FM wireless system, infrared systems, and electromagnetic loops are available for group listening. If the patient's church has a loop system, then the need for a telephone switch should be discussed. To be effective with dispensing assistive devices it is important to first let older adults describe their specific needs, show them the options that are available, and guide them in making educated choices.

Finally, many active older adults choose to travel either by automobile or bus. An assistive device can enhance communication in the automobile by improving the signal-to-noise ratio reaching the ear. A direct connection from a microphone to a behind-the-ear hearing aid is efficient; however, because many hearing aid users have in-the-ear models, an inexpensive FM system may be more desirable.

Conclusion

It is estimated that one out of every three individuals over the age of 65 exhibits a significant hearing impairment. When one considers the growing number of elderly people in this country it becomes clear that the audiologist will play an important role in the management of hearing problems with that population. This chapter has focused on the early identification of hearing loss among the elderly population. In addition to the basic audiologic test battery this chapter has emphasized the value of self-assessment scales. The use of such scales can be of significant benefit in learning more about the patient's communication difficulty, monitoring progress, and objectively assessing the value of amplification. Finally, some brief comments relative to the management issues concerned with elderly hearing impaired patients have been reviewed.

Acknowledgment

The authors gratefully acknowledge Dorothy Adams, who typed the manuscript, Don Riggs, who prepared the figures, and Mark Hedrick, who provided assistance with several sections of this chapter.

References

Alberti, P., & Kristensen, R. (1970). The clinical application of impedance audiometry. *Laryngoscope, 80,* 735–746.

Alpiner, J. G. (1978). Rehabilitation of the geriatric client. In J. G. Alpiner (Ed.), *Handbook of adult rehabilitative audiology* (pp. 141–165). Baltimore: Williams & Wilkins.

Alpiner, J. G., Chevrette, W., Glascoe, G., Metz, M., & Olsen, F. (1974). *The Denver Scale of Communication Function.* Unpublished study, University of Denver.

American Speech-Language-Hearing Association. (1981). On the definition of hearing handicap. *Asha, 23,* 293–297.

Bergner, L., Hallstrom, A. P., Bergner, M., Eisenberg, M. S., & Cobb, L. A. (1985). Health status of survivors of cardiac arrest and of myocardial infarction controls. *American Journal of Public Health, 75,* 1321–1323.

Bergner, M., Bobbitt, R. A., Carter, W. B., & Gilson, B. S. (1981). The Sickness Impact Profile: Developments and final revision of a health status measure. *Medical Care, 19,* 787–805.

Bergner, M., Bobbitt, R. A., Pollard W. E., Martin, D. P., & Gilson, B. S. (1976). The Sickness Impact Profile: Validation of a health status measure. *Medical Care, 14,* 57–67.

Bess, F. H., & Humes, L. E. (1990). *Audiology: The fundamentals.* Baltimore: Williams & Wilkins.

Bess, F. H., & Townsend, T. H. (1977). Word discrimination for listeners with flat sensorineural hearing losses. *Journal of Speech and Hearing Disorders, 42,* 232–237.

Bess, F. H., Logan, S. A., Lichtenstein, M. J., & Hedley, A. (1987). Early identification and referral of hearing-impaired elderly. In M. S. Robinette & C. D. Bauch (Eds.), *Proceedings of a symposium in audiology* (pp. 1–27). Rochester, MN: Mayo Clinic/Mayo Foundation.

Bess, F. H., Lichtenstein, M. J., Logan, S. A., Burger, M. C., & Nelson, E. C. (1989). Hearing impairment as a determinant of function in the elderly. *Journal of the American Geriatric Society, 37,* 123–128.

Bess, F. H., Lichtenstein, M. J., & Logan, S. A. (in press). Functional impact of hearing loss on the elderly. *ASHA Reports.*

Bosatra, A., & Russolo, M. (1982). Comparison between central tonal tests and central speech tests in elderly subjects. *Audiology, 21,* 334–341.

Cadman, D., Chambers, L., Feldman, W., & Sackett, D. (1984). Assessing the effectiveness of community screening programs. *Journal of the American Medical Association, 252,* 1580–1585.

Carter, W. B., Bobbitt, R. A., Bergner, M., & Gilson, B. S. (1976). Validation of an internal scaling: The Sickness Impact Profile. *Health Service Research, 74,* 516–528.

Cranmer, K. (1986). Hearing instrument dispensing. *Hearing Instruments, 6,* 4–14.

Davies, J. W., & Mueller, H. G. (1987). Hearing aid selection. In H. G. Mueller & V. C. Geoffrey (Eds.), *Communication disorders in aging: Assessment and Management* (pp. 408–436). Washington, DC: Gallaudet University Press.

Davis, A. (1983). The epidemiology of hearing disorders. In R. Hinchcliffe (Ed.), *Hearing and balance in the elderly* (pp. 1–43). Edinburgh: Churchill Livingstone.

Deyo, R. A., & Inui, T. S. (1984). Toward clinical applications of health status measures: Sensitivity of scales to clinically important changes. *Health Service Research, 19,* 275–289.

Dubno, J. R., Dirks, D. D., & Morgan, D. E. (1984). Effects of age and mild hearing loss on speech recognition in noise. *Journal of the Acoustical Society of America, 76,* 87–96.

Feller, A. B. (February, 1981). *Prevalence of selected impairments: United States—1977* (DHHS publication No. 81-1562, Vital and Health Statistics, Series 10, No. 134). Washington, DC: National Health Center for Statistics.

The Gallup Organization, Inc. (1980). *A survey concerning hearing problems and hearing aids in the United States.* Princeton, NJ: Author.

Gilson, B. S., Gilson, J. S., Bergner, M., Bobbitt, R. A., Kressel, S., Pollard, W. E., & Vesselago, M. (1975). The Sickness Impact Profile: Development of an outcome measure of healthcare. *American Journal of Public Health, 65,* 1304–1310.

Giolas, T. G., Owens, E., Lamb, S. H., & Schubert, E. D. (1979). Hearing Performance Inventory. *Journal of Speech and Hearing Disorders, 44,* 169–195.

Glass, L. E. (1986). Rehabilitation for deaf and hearing-impaired elderly. In S. J. Brody & G. E. Ruff (Eds.), *Aging and rehabilitation* (pp. 218–237). New York: Springer.

Glorig, A., & Davis, H. (1961). Age, noise and hearing loss. *Annals of Otology, Rhinology, and Laryngology, 60,* 407–516.

Glorig, A., & Nixon, J. (1962). Hearing loss as a function of age. *Laryngoscope, 72,* 1596–1610.

Gordon-Salant, S. (1987). Basic hearing evaluation. In H. G. Mueller & V. C. Geoffrey (Eds.), *Communication disorders in aging* (pp. 301–333). Washington, DC: Gallaudet University Press.

Hall, J. (1982). Acoustic reflex amplitude. I. Effects of age and sex. *Audiology, 21,* 294–309.

Hall, J. (1979). Effects of age and sex on static compliance. *Archives of Otolaryngology, 105,* 153–156.

Hall, J. (1990). *Handbook of auditory evoked responses.* Boston, MA: College-Hill Press.

Hart, L. G., & Evans, R. W. (1987). The functional status of ESRD patients as measured by the Sickness Impact Profile. *Journal of Chronic Diseases, 40,* 117S–130S.

Hawkins, J. E., & Johnsson, L. G. (1985). Otopathological changes associated with presbycusis. *Seminars in Hearing, 6,* 115–134.

Herbst, K. G., & Humphrey, C. (1980). Hearing impairment and mental state in the elderly living at home. *British Medical Journal, 281,* 903–905.

Herbst, K. R. G. (1983). Psychosocial consequences of disorders of hearing in the elderly. In R. Hinchcliffe, (Ed.), *Hearing and balance in the elderly* (pp. 174–200). Edinburgh: Churchill Livingstone.

High, W. S., Fairbanks, G., & Glorig, A. (1964). Scale for Self-Assessment of Hearing Handicap. *Journal of Speech and Hearing Disorders, 29,* 215–230.

Hull, R. H. (1980). Aural rehabilitation for the elderly. In R. Schow & M.A. Nerbonne (Eds.), *Introduction to aural rehabilitation* (pp. 311–348). Baltimore: University Park Press.

Humphrey, C., Herbst, K., & Faurgi, S. (1981). Some characteristics of the hearing-impaired elderly who do not present themselves for rehabilitation. *British Journal of Audiology, 15,* 25–30.

Jerger, J. (1973). Audiological findings in the aging. *Advances in Otology, Rhinology, and Laryngology, 20,* 115–124.

Jerger, J., & Hall, J. (1980). Effects of age and sex on auditory brainstem response. *Archives of Otolaryngology, 106*, 387–391.

Jerger, J., & Hayes, D. (1977). Diagnostic speech audiometry. *Archives of Otolaryngology, 103*, 216–222.

Jerger, J., Jerger, S., & Mauldin, L. (1972). Studies in impedance audiometry. I: Normal and sensorineural ears. *Archives of Otolaryngology, 96*, 513–523.

Jerger, J., Jerger, S., Mauldin, L., & Segal, P. (1974). Studies in impedance audiometry. II: Children less than 6 years old. *Archives of Otolaryngology, 99*, 1–9.

Jerger, J., Jerger, S., Oliver, T., & Pirozzolo, F. (1989). Speech understanding in the elderly. *Ear and Hearing, 10*, 79–89.

Jerger, J., Neely, J., & Jerger, S. (1980). Speech, impedance and auditory brainstem audiometry in brainstem tumors. *Archives of Otolaryngology, 106*, 218–223.

Johnsson, L. G., & Hawkins, J. E., Jr. (1972). Vascular changes in the human inner ear associated with aging. *Annals of Otology, Rhinology, and Laryngology, 81*, 361–376.

Kasden, S. (1970). Speech discrimination in two age groups matched for hearing loss. *Journal of Auditory Research, 10*, 210–212.

Konkle, D. F., Beasley, D. S., & Bess, F. H. (1977). Intelligibility of time-altered speech in relation to chronological aging. *Journal of Speech and Hearing Research, 20*, 108–115.

Lamb, S. H., Owens, E., & Schubert, E. D. (1983). The revised form of the Hearing Performance Inventory. *Ear and Hearing, 4*, 152–159.

Lichtenstein, M. J., Bess, F. H., & Logan, S. L. (1988a). Validation of screening tools for identifying hearing-impaired elderly in primary care. *Journal of the American Medical Association, 259*, 2875–2878.

Lichtenstein, M. J., Bess, F. H., & Logan, S. L. (1988b). Diagnostic performance of the Hearing Handicap Inventory for the Elderly (Screening Version) against differing definitions of hearing loss. *Ear and Hearing, 9*, 209–211.

Marshall, L., Martinez, S. A., & Schlamen, M. E. (1983). Reassessment of high-frequency air-bone gaps in older adults. *Acta Oto-Laryngologica, 109*, 601–606.

Maurer, J. F., & Rupp, R. R. (1979). Hearing and aging: Tactics for intervention. New York: Grune & Stratton.

McCarthy, P. A., & Alpiner, J. G. (1980). *The McCarthy-Alpiner Scale of Hearing Handicap*. Unpublished manuscript.

McCarthy, P. A., & Alpiner, J. G. (1983). An assessment scale of hearing handicap for use in family counseling. *Journal of the Academy of Rehabilitative Audiology, 16*, 256–270.

McSweeney, A., Grant, I., Heaton, R. K., Adams, K. M., & Timms, R. M. (1982). Life quality of patients with chronic obstructive pulmonary disease. *Archives of Internal Medicine, 142*, 473–478.

Milne, J. M. (1977). The air-bone gap in older people. *British Journal of Audiology, 11*, 1–6.

Morrison, A. S. (1985). Screening in chronic disease. *Monographs in Epidemiology and Biostatistics, 7*, 1–182.

Mościcki, E. K., Elkins, E. F., Baum, H. M., & McNamara, P. M. (1985). Hearing loss in the elderly: An epidemiologic study of the Framingham Heart Study Cohort. *Ear and Hearing, 6*, 184–190.

Mulrow, C. D., Aqualar, C., Endicott, J. E., Tuley, M. R., Valez, R., Charlip, W. S., Rhodes, M. C., & Hill, J. A. (1990). *Improved function in elderly individuals with hearing impairment: Results of a randomized trial.* Manuscript submitted for publication.

Nadol, J. (1979). Electron microscopic findings in presbycusic degeneration of the basal turn of the human cochlea. *Otolaryngology and Head and Neck Surgery, 87,* 818–836.

Nerbonne, M., Schow, R., & Gosset, F. (1976). *Prevalence of conductive pathology in a nursing home population* (Laboratory Research Reports). Pocatello: Idaho State University, Department of Speech Pathology and Audiology.

Nixon, J., Glorig, A., & High, W. (1962). Changes in air and bone conduction thresholds as a function of age. *Journal of Laryngology and Otology, 74,* 288–299.

Noble, W. G., & Atherly, G. R. C. (1970). The hearing measure scale: A questionnaire for the assessment of auditory disability. *Journal of Auditory Research, 10,* 229–250.

Noble, W. G. (1978). *Test Manual for the Hearing Measurement Scale.* University of New England, Armidele N,S,W. Australia.

Noble, W. G. (1979). The Hearing Instrument Scale as a paper-pencil form: preliminary results. *Journal of the American Auditory Society, 5,* 95–106.

Osterhammel, D., & Osterhammel, P. (1979). Age and sex variations for the normal stapedial reflex thresholds and tympanometric compliance values. *Scandinavian Audiology, 8,* 153–158.

Pollard, W. E., Bobbitt, R. A., Bergner, M., Martin, D. P., & Gilson, B. S. (1986). The Sickness Impact Profile: Reliability of a health status measure. *Medical Care, 14,* 146–155.

Quaranta, A., Cassano, P. & Amoroso, C. (1980). Presbyacousie et reflexmetrie stapedienne. *Audiology, 19,* 310–315.

Rosen, S., Bergman, M., Plester, D., El-Mofty, A., & Salti, M. (1962). Presbycusis: Study of a relatively noise free population in the Sudan. *Annals of Otology, Rhinology, and Laryngology, 71,* 727–743.

Ross, M. (1986). Thoughts on ALDS. *Hearing Instruments, 87,* 16–21.

Rowe, M. (1978). Normal variability of the brain-stem auditory evoked response in young and old adult subjects. *Electroencephalography and clinical neurophysiology, 44,* 459–470.

Sackett, D. L., Haynes, R. B., & Tugwell, P. (1985). *Clinical epidemiology: A basic science for clinical medicine.* Boston/Toronto: Little, Brown.

Salomon, G. (1986, November). Hearing problems in the elderly. *Danish Medical Bulletin.* Special Supplement Series, No. 3, 1–22.

Salomon, G., Vesterager, V., & Jagd, J. (1988). Age-related difficulties: I. Hearing impairment, disability, and handicap—a controlled study. *Audiology, 27,* 164–178.

Saunders, J. C., Dean, S. P., & Schneider, M. E. (1985). The anatomical consequences of acoustic energy: A review and tutorial. *Journal of the Acoustical Society of America, 78,* 833–860.

Schow, R. L., & Nerbonne, M. A. (1982). Communication screening profile: Use with elderly clients. *Ear and Hearing, 3,* 135–147.

Schuknecht, F. (1955). Presbycusis. *Laryngoscope, 65,* 407–419.

Schuknecht, H. F. (1964). Further observations on the pathology of presbycusis. *Archives of Otolaryngology, 80,* 369–382.

Schuknecht, H. F. (1974). *Pathology of the ear.* Cambridge, MA: Harvard University Press.

Schwartz, D. M., Morris, M. D., Spydell, J. D., Grim, M. A., Schwartz, J. A., & Civitello, B. A. (1989). *The brainstem auditory evoked response (BAER) in patients with high frequency cochlear hearing loss: New perspectives on an old clinical problem.* Manuscript submitted for publication.

Shirinian, M., & Arnst, D. (1982). Patterns in performance-intensity functions for phonetically balanced word lists and synthetic sentences in aged listeners. *Archives of Otolaryngology, 108,* 15–20.

Silverman, C. A., Silman, S., & Miller, M. H. (1983). The acoustic reflex threshold in aging ears. *Journal of the Acoustical Society of America, 73,* 248–255.

Suga, F., & Lindsay, J. R. (1976). Histopathological observations of presbycusis. *Annals of Otology, Rhinology and Laryngology, 85,* 169–184.

Surr, R. K. (1977). Effect of age on clinical hearing and evaluation results. *Journal of the American Audiology Society, 3,* 1–5.

Thomsen, J., Terkildsen, K., & Osterhammel, P. (1978). Auditory brainstem responses in patients with acoustic neuromes. *Scandinavian Audiology, 7,* 179–183.

Townsend, T. H., & Bess, F. H. (1980). Effects of age and sensorineural hearing loss on word recognition. *Scandinavian Audiology, 9,* 245–248.

Uhlmann, R. F., Larson, E. B., & Koepsell, T. D. (1986). Hearing impairment and cognitive decline in senile dementia of the Alzheimer's type. *Journal of the American Geriatric Society, 34,* 207–210.

Uhlmann, R. F., Rees, T. S., Psaty, B. M., & Duckert, L. G. (1989). *Validity and reliability of auditory screening tests in demented and non-demented older adults. Journal of General Internal Medicine, 4,* 90–96.

Ventry, I. M., & Weinstein, B. (1982). The Hearing Handicap Inventory for the Elderly: A new tool. *Ear and Hearing, 3,* 128–134.

Ventry, I. M., & Weinstein, B. (1983). Identification of elderly people with hearing problems. *Asha, 25,* 37–42.

Weinstein, B. E. (1984). *A review of hearing handicap scales. Audiology, 9,* 91–109.

Weinstein, B. E. (1985). *Hearing problems in the elderly: Identification and Management.* New York: The Brookdale Institute on Aging and Adult Human Development, Columbia University.

Weinstein, B. E., & Amsell, L. (1986). Hearing loss and senile dementia in the institutionalized elderly. *Clinical Gerontologist, 4,* 3–15.

chapter eleven

Behavioral assessment of the central auditory nervous system

JANE A. BARAN

FRANK E. MUSIEK

Contents

Introduction

In this chapter we present a historical perspective on the development of central auditory testing. This is followed by a brief overview of the anatomy and physiology of the central auditory nervous system (CANS) and a more in-depth discussion of the major behavioral tests currently employed in neuroaudiological assessments. We then present several case illustrations that demonstrate the use of many of these behavioral tests in the assessment of CANS pathology. Finally, we discuss the implications of behavioral CANS testing for the future, as well as outline some of the major research needs as we see them.

Historical perspective

The beginning of central auditory testing can be traced back to the 1950s when Bocca and his colleagues (Bocca, Calearo, & Cassinari, 1954; Bocca, Calearo, Cassinari, & Migliavacca, 1955) first used a monaural distorted speech test to assess the central auditory function of individuals with CANS lesions. These researchers recognized that traditional auditory tests, such as pure tone threshold and speech recognition tests, were not sensitive to the auditory problems that were being experienced by patients with lesions of the CANS. Specifically, they noted that patients with temporal lobe lesions complained of subjective differences in both the quality and clarity of the sounds perceived in the ear contralateral to the affected hemisphere in spite of normal peripheral auditory findings. In an attempt to find a test that would be sensitive to these complaints, these investigators developed a monaural low-redundancy speech test and administered it to 18 patients with confirmed temporal lobe lesions. Their results revealed asymmetrical test performance, with depressed scores being noted in the ear contralateral to the damaged hemisphere. Since the time of the introduction of the low-pass filtered speech test, several other monaural speech tests have been introduced. These have included band-pass filtered speech, compressed speech, speech recognition in noise, performance-intensity functions, and interrupted speech tests.

Binaural interaction tasks, also referred to as binaural integration tasks, were first used to assess CANS function in subjects with brain pathology in the late 1950s. Sanchez-Longo and colleagues (Sanchez-Longo & Forster, 1958; Sanchez-Longo, Forster, & Auth, 1957) demonstrated impaired sound localization ability in the auditory field contralateral to temporal lobe lesions in a group of brain damaged adults. Subsequently, Pinheiro and Tobin (1969, 1971) found that patients with temporal or parietal lobe involvement typically demonstrated abnormal interaural intensity differences (IIDs), whereas patients with frontal or occipital lobe lesions showed normal IIDs. Though it is believed that the critical neural events involved in the processing of the IID occur at the brainstem level, the perception of the location of the sound appears to be a cortical function (Pickles, 1985). Other binaural interaction tasks, which were touted as being particularly sensitive to brainstem pathology, appeared in the late 1950s and early 1960s. These included binaural fusion, rapidly alternating speech perception, and masking level differences.

In the early 1960s, Kimura (1961a, 1961b) introduced a dichotic digits test in which digit triads were presented simultaneously to both ears of a group of patients with unilateral temporal lobe lesions. Kimura noted depressed recognition scores for the contralateral ears of her subjects when the stimuli were presented in a dichotic test paradigm. If, however, the stimuli were presented in a noncompeting condition, no deficits were noted unless the left or dominant hemisphere was affected. In this case, bilaterally depressed scores were typically noted.

Based on these findings and some earlier physiological evidence provided by Rosenzweig (1951), Kimura (1961a, 1961b) developed a model that could be used to explain the function of the CANS in the perception of dichotically presented stimuli. Her model is based on the premise that the contralateral auditory pathways in humans are stronger and more numerous than the ipsilateral pathways. In situations where only monaural input is provided to the auditory system, either pathway is capable of initiating the appropriate neural response. In dichotic situations, however, the weaker ipsilateral pathways are believed to be suppressed and the stronger contralateral pathways take precedence. Thus if one hemisphere is compromised, one would expect reduced performance in the contralateral ear whenever the test stimuli are presented in a competing dichotic manner. In addition, ipsilateral deficits are expected if the left, or dominant hemisphere for speech is affected. Though other theories have been advanced in an attempt to explain dichotic speech perception (Sidtis, 1982; Speaks, Gray, Miller, & Rubens, 1975), Kimura's model remains the most popular. Since the introduction of dichotic digits, several other dichotic speech tests have been introduced. These have included dichotic words, competing sentences, and dichotic CVs (consonant-vowels).

In the early to mid 1960s, several researchers began to use temporal ordering or sequencing tasks in the assessment of CANS disorders (Milner, 1962; Milner, Kimura, & Taylor, 1965; Shankweiler, 1966). Results of these early investigations showed that subjects with temporal lobe pathology demonstrated deficits in the perception of temporal sequences.

In the early 1970s, Swisher and Hirsh (1972) used a test paradigm in which they presented two tones of different pitches and with various onset time differences to either the same ear or to opposite ears of their subjects. Their subjects consisted of two groups of normal control subjects (young and old adults) and three groups of brain-injured adults. The subjects were asked to indicate the order of the two tones. The authors found that subjects with left hemisphere damage and fluent aphasia required the longest intervals to order stimuli, particularly if the stimuli were presented to the same ear. Subjects with right hemisphere damage and no aphasia required smaller time intervals (approximating those for normal subjects) to make temporal order judgments if the two stimuli were presented to the same ear. They did, however, show greater deficits than the normal subjects when the tonal stimuli were presented to opposite ears.

Lackner and Teuber (1973) presented dichotic clicks that varied in terms of their onsets to the two ears of subjects with cortical involvement. They found that subjects with left hemisphere damage required a longer silent interval between stimuli in order to perceive separation than did subjects with right hemisphere damage.

More recently, Efron and associates (Efron, 1985; Efron & Crandall, 1983; Efron, Crandall, Koss, Divenyi, & Yund, 1983; Efron, Dennis, & Yund, 1977; Efron, Yund, Nichols, & Crandall, 1985) have conducted a series of experiments with nonspeech auditory signals that demonstrated contralateral ear deficits in individuals with temporal lobe lesions for a variety of auditory tasks (e.g., gap detection, sound lateralization, and temporal ordering tasks). These researchers found consistent contralateral ear effects not only in subjects with posterior temporal lobe involvement, but also in subjects with anterior temporal lobe resections that reportedly involved portions of the temporal lobe previously believed to have no role in auditory processing. Based on some of their early findings, Efron and Crandall (1983) suggested the existence of a contralaterally organized efferent pathway in each temporal lobe that when activated significantly enhances one's ability to perceive auditory stimuli on the contralateral side of auditory space. It is interesting to note that Seltzer and Pandya (1978) had previously discovered such an efferent multisynaptic pathway in the Rhesus monkey.

One of the more popular temporal ordering tests used today is the frequency pattern sequences test developed by Pinheiro and Ptacek (Pinheiro & Ptacek, 1971; Ptacek & Pinheiro, 1971). This test is composed of 120 test sequences, with each sequence containing three tone bursts. In each sequence, two of the three tone bursts are of the same frequency, whereas the third tone is of a different frequency. Typically, the subject is asked to describe verbally each sequence heard, and a percent correct identification score is derived for each ear. Patients with lesions of either hemisphere or of the interhemispheric pathways have difficulty describing the monaurally presented sequences (Musiek, Kibbe, & Baran, 1984; Musiek & Pinheiro, 1986, 1987; Musiek, Pinheiro, & Wilson, 1980; Pinheiro, 1976; Pinheiro, Weidner, Suren, & Gaydos, 1977). It is interesting to note that some of these same investigators have shown that if split-brain subjects are asked to "hum" the sequences they can do so with close to 100% accuracy (Musiek et al., 1984; Musiek et al., 1980). These results suggest that some processing of the stimuli occurs in both hemispheres and that the auditory interhemispheric connections must be intact if a verbal report of the test sequences is required.

In a recent investigation, Divenyi and Robinson (1989) demonstrated the involvement of the left hemisphere in the processing of spectral, as well as temporal, information. These investigators administered seven nonlinguistic auditory tests to three subject groups, including (a) 11 aphasic subjects with left cerebrovascular accidents (CVAs), (b) 4 nonaphasic subjects with right CVAs, and (c) 11 normal control subjects. Their seven auditory tests included frequency discrimination, gap detection, gap discrimination, frequency sweep discrimination, temporal order discrimination, detection of tones in noise with and without frequency uncertainty, and a tone-by-narrowband-masking test to establish frequency selectivity contours. These researchers noted the expected deficits in certain temporal processing functions (e.g., discrimination of frequency transitions and temporal order) in the left CVA group, but also found that spectral processing functions were affected in this same group of subjects. Based on their specific findings, these authors suggested that left hemisphere lesions are likely to result in some deficits in the spectral analysis of separate auditory events, but that the major impact will be evident in the subject's ability to readjust the spectral focus of listening.

When Divenyi and Robinson compared the test results for their right-CVA and left-CVA subjects, significant differences were noted on four of the seven tests administered. All of them were pitch-related. For the most part the differences could be attributed to the highly abnormal performance of the right-CVA group on these tests, as compared to the moderately abnormal performance of the left-CVA group. Based on these findings the authors propose the existence of a bilateral cortical representation for most, if not all, of the auditory functions studied. They do, however, acknowledge the prominence of the right hemisphere in the processing of spectral information.

Finally, these researchers found that in their aphasic patients there was an orderly deterioration in test performance on four of the seven auditory tasks as the level of linguistic comprehension (as measured by a variety of language tests) decreased, and that as a group, nonfluent aphasics did better than did fluent aphasics on six of the seven tests administered. Acknowledging the limitations of their study in terms of subject numbers, these researchers suggest that there is some evidence in their data to suggest that a generic auditory dysfunction may either parallel, or underlie, the linguistic auditory comprehension dysfunctions often associated with aphasia, as well as the fluency of aphasia.

The foregoing comments provide a very cursory discussion of the development of the field of CANS assessments involving behavioral assessment tools. We hope that this review has placed the development of the field in perspective for the reader. Additional information regarding the development of CANS testing can be found in Musiek and Baran (1987). In the remainder of this chapter, we attempt to provide more in-depth information on the behavioral tests that are currently employed in CANS assessments. We also discuss some of the important variables that can affect one's selection of the tests to be administered and their test results.

Defining the central auditory nervous system

The importance and popularity of clinical evaluation of the CANS have increased steadily over the past several years. This is in large part the result of recent advances in technology for measuring evoked potentials and the advent of cochlear implants. There also has been a renewed interest in the behavioral assessment of the CANS sparked by exciting research findings. At the present time the field of audiology possesses both the technology and knowledge that should enable us to meet the demanding challenge of assessing the auditory status of neurologically involved patients. However, the full clinical value of central auditory testing may not be realized if the audiologist does not possess detailed knowledge of the central auditory system. Before anyone becomes involved in the assessment of central auditory function he or she should have a thorough understanding of the anatomy and physiology of the CANS.

Because of space limitations, we will not be able to discuss in detail the neuroanatomy and neurophysiology of the CANS at this time. We will, however, provide a basic overview of the system. The reader is encouraged to seek out other sources for more detailed information about the CANS (Musiek, 1986a, 1986b; Musiek & Baran, 1986; Pickles, 1982; Thompson, 1983).

The ascending pathways of the CANS originate at the cochlear nucleus complex, which is located at the posterior-lateral aspect of the pontomedullary junction. The other nuclei in the ascending auditory pathways of the brainstem include the superior olivary complex (caudal-most pons), the nuclei of the lateral lemniscus (mid pons), the inferior colliculus (mid brain), and the medial geniculate complex (caudal-posterior thalamus). The projections from the medial geniculate take several subcortical routes to the cortex. Currently, the details of these are not well-known. However, there are at least two main fiber groups that project to Heschl's gyrus, which is located in the superior temporal lobe, and to the insula. In addition to the superior temporal lobe and the insula, the posterior-inferior frontal lobe and the inferior parietal lobe have areas that are responsive to acoustic stimulation. Throughout the CANS there are several points where several of the ascending auditory fibers cross over and course contralaterally, thereby increasing the intrinsic redundancy of the CANS. The first major crossover occurs at the level of the superior olivary complex. It is for this reason that lesions above this level rarely result in significant losses in terms of threshold sensitivity or speech recognition abilities.

The corpus callosum also contains auditory fibers. These inter-hemispheric fibers serve to connect the auditory portions of the two hemi-spheres. Some early primate work by Pandya and colleagues (Pandya, Karol, & Heilbornn, 1971), together with some recent studies of central auditory fui.ction in partial split-brain patients (Baran, Musiek, & Reeves, 1986; Musiek et al, 1984), have shown that the interhemispheric auditory fibers are located in the posterior half of the corpus callosum.

The final portion of the auditory system includes the descending efferent auditory pathways that course caudally from the cortical regions to the cochleas. The descending pathways travel both ipsilaterally and contralaterally, taking an anatomical course that is similar to that of the ascending tracts. Their function, however, is very different from the ascending sensory fibers. Because the central auditory pathways represent the largest portion of the auditory system, it is important that the audiologist possess knowledge not only about the structure and function of the CANS, but also about how lesions and/or pathology in these areas can affect overall auditory functioning.

Value of including electrophysiological and behavioral tests

The focus of this chapter is on the use of behavioral tests in the assessment of central auditory disorders. However, we feel we would be remiss if we did not at least mention the benefits of including some electro-physiological tests in the assessment of certain CANS disorders. In many instances these electrophysiological tests are more sensitive to certain CANS lesions than are any of the behavioral tests that currently are available. For instance, the auditory brainstem response (ABR) is better than most behavioral tests for the evaluation of brainstem lesions involving the pons, but it is of no value in assessing cortical or interhemispheric lesions. On the other hand, many of the behavioral tests that we will cover in this chapter are more sensitive to cortical lesions than are any of the electrophysiological procedures that are currently in vogue. We, therefore, are not advocating that both electrophysiological and behavioral approaches be used in every CANS assessment, but rather that both approaches be considered for a given individual. Final decision regarding which procedures should be used will depend on the presenting complaints of the client, any existing medical documentation that may indicate the probable site of lesion, and the audiologist's own insights into the problem and his or her past experience with CANS assessments. A detailed discussion of the various electrophysiological procedures that can be used in CANS assessments is beyond the scope of this chapter. However, these procedures are covered elsewhere in this text. They include acoustic reflexes (Chapter 5), auditory brainstem response audiometry (Chapters 6 and 7), and middle late and late auditory evoked potentials (Chapters 6 and 7).

Monaural low-redundancy speech tests

Monaural low-redundancy speech tests have been used extensively in the assessment of subjects with CANS pathology. The stimuli for these tests typically are degraded by electroacoustically modifying the frequency, temporal, or intensity characteristics of the undistorted signal. In the following section we discuss some of the more popular monaural low-redundancy speech tests that are used today.

Filtered speech tests

Bocca and his colleagues (Bocca et al., 1954; Bocca et al., 1955) first used a low pass filtered speech (LPFS) test to assess CANS functioning in patients with cerebral tumors affecting the temporal lobe. Their results revealed reduced performance in the contralateral ear for the majority of patients tested. Since the time of these early investigations, several other investigators have used low-pass and bandpass filtered speech tasks to assess CANS function in individuals with intracranial lesions or pathology (Baran et al., 1986; Bocca, 1958; Calearo & Antonelli, 1968; Gilroy & Lynn, 1974; Hodgson, 1967; Jerger, 1960a, 1960b, 1964; Korsan-Bengtsen, 1973; Lynn, Benitez, Eisenbrey, Gilroy, & Wilner, 1972; Lynn & Gilroy, 1971, 1972, 1975, 1976, 1977; Musiek & Geurkink, 1982; Musiek et al., 1984; Musiek, Wilson, & Pinheiro, 1979). These studies varied greatly in terms of the test stimuli employed and the frequency cutoff and filter rolloff characteristics used. In general, the results of these studies revealed contralateral deficits in subjects with temporal lobe lesions (Bocca, 1958; Hodgson, 1967; Jerger, 1960a, 1960b, 1964; Korsan-Bengtsen, 1973; Lynn & Gilroy, 1972, 1977) and essentially normal results with no obvious ear differences with involvement of the interhemispheric pathways (Baran et al., 1986; Gilroy & Lynn, 1974; Lynn et al., 1972; Lynn & Gilroy, 1971, 1972, 1975, 1977; Musiek et al., 1984; Musiek et al., 1979). In subjects with brainstem lesions, no consistent pattern of performance has been noted (Calearo & Antonelli, 1968; Lynn & Gilroy, 1977; Musiek & Geurkink, 1982). Contralateral ear deficits have been reported for some subjects, whereas ipsilateral deficits, bilateral deficits, or normal results were noted for other subjects. It appears that factors, such as the level and size of the lesion, as well as whether it is an extra- or intra-axial lesion, may determine the laterality effects of brainstem lesions (Musiek & Geurkink, 1982).

Lynn and Gilroy (1977), in an attempt to determine the sensitivity and specificity of low-pass filtered speech, studied 34 patients with temporal lobe lesions and 27 patients with parietal lesions. Seventy-four percent of the temporal lobe lesioned patients demonstrated the expected contralateral ear deficit on this test, whereas 74% of the parietal lobe patients demonstrated normal performance.

The most widely used filtered speech test today is the low-pass filtered speech test of Willeford's (1976) central auditory processing test battery. The test consists of two 50-item lists of the Michigan consonant-nucleus-consonant (CNC) words that were selected because they were highly intelligible to adults even when filtered. The stimuli were low-pass filtered with a cutoff frequency of 500 Hz and an 18 dB per octave rejection rate. Stimuli are presented monaurally at 50 dB relative to the pure tone average. Clients are asked to repeat the stimuli perceived, and a percent correct identification score is derived for each ear.

Based on the foregoing test results, it appears that low-pass filtered speech is moderately sensitive to the presence of CANS lesions. The results suggest that filtered speech tests can be useful in documenting the presence of a central lesion; however, they are not useful in locating the specific location of the lesion.

Compressed speech

An accelerated speech test was first used by some Italian researchers (Bocca, 1958; Calearo & Lazzaroni, 1957). These investigators employed a procedure by which they accelerated sentence stimuli, distorting both the time and frequency characteristics of the test stimuli. They found reduced performance in the ear contralateral to lesions in the auditory cortex, whereas diffuse lesions tended to show reduced performance in both ears. Similar results were reported in a number of other investigations (de Quiros, 1964; Korsan-Bengtsen, 1973; Quaranta & Cervellera, 1977).

To date, essentially three methods of accelerating and/or compressing the speech stimuli have been used. These have included (a) having the speaker accelerate his or her speech rate, (b) accelerating the recorded signal via a faster playback rate, and (c) removing segments of the signal electromechanically. A detailed discussion of the various procedures can be found in Beasley and Maki (1976). With the advent of sophisticated computer instrumentation, a fourth method of time compression is possible. This includes computer manipulation and/or generation of time-compressed speech materials.

Beasley and his colleagues (Beasley, Forman, & Rintelmann, 1972; Beasley, Schwimmer, & Rintelmann, 1972) generated tapes of compressed speech stimuli (NU-6 word lists) at several different compression ratios using the method of electromechanical time compression introduced by Fairbanks, Everitt, and Jaeger (1954). These investigators studied the intelligibility of NU-6 word lists as a function of both compression rate (at 0% and from 30% to 70% in 10% increments) and sensation level (8 to 40 dB in 8-dB steps), and provided extensive normative data for their compressed speech test. Their results showed a gradual reduction in the speech recognition scores of normal adults as the compression rate was increased to 70%. At this point, a substantial reduction in performance was noted. As sensation level increased, word recognition scores increased in a curvilinear fashion up to 32 dB SL.

Kurdziel, Noffsinger, and Olsen (1976) used 0%, 40%, and 60% compressed NU-6 word lists in the evaluation of 31 patients with brain lesions (15 had diffuse lesions and 16 had undergone anterior temporal lobe surgery). Reduced performance was noted in the contralateral ear of the patients with diffuse lesions, especially at the 60% compression rate, whereas subjects with discrete lesions (anterior temporal lobe surgery) demonstrated essentially equivalent performance for both ears, with recognition scores at 60% compression being only slightly reduced (10%) compared to recognition scores at 0% compression. Similar results were reported in an earlier study by Rintelmann, Beasley, and Lynn (1974).

In a large study of Vietnam veterans with discrete cerebral lesions, Mueller, Beck, and Sedge (1987) found that performance was poorest for a group of subjects with lesions in Heschl's gyrus, whereas performance in patients with lesions outside the primary auditory area was relatively good. These authors point out, however, that the mean differences in the performances of their pathological subjects (regardless of the location of their lesions) and their controls were small. Also, they failed to note obvious contralateral effects in their subjects. Based on these results, these authors have suggested that the compressed speech test may be relatively sensitive to identifying patients with diffuse lesions, but that the test may be relatively insensitive to discrete lesions.

We have found that compressed speech is a moderately sensitive test for intracranial lesions involving the temporal lobe (Baran et al., 1985). In approximately two-thirds of subjects with confirmed lesions, performance was found to be reduced in one or both ears. The more typical pattern was for reduced performance in the contralateral ear.

We were not able to find any investigations that have employed compressed speech with brainstem lesions. However, two earlier investigations used accelerated speech. In patients with brainstem involvement, reduced performance was noted in one ear for 13 of 14 subjects studied by Calearo and Antonelli (1968). In a subsequent study, Quaranta and Cervellera (1977) reported that none of their nine subjects with brainstem lesions showed reduced performance.

Speech-in-noise

A third method of reducing the redundancy of speech stimuli has involved the addition of an ipsilateral competing noise. Most commonly either white noise or speech spectrum noise is employed, and signal-to-noise ratios (S/Ns) of 0 to +10 dB are most commonly encountered. Stimuli are typically presented at 40 dB relative to the speech reception threshold (SRT).

As early as 1959, Sinha found reduced performance on a speech-in-noise test for contralateral ears in individuals with cortical lesions. Subsequent investigations have revealed abnormal findings for the ipsilateral ear of a patient with an extra-axial brainstem lesion (Dayal, Tarantino, & Swisher, 1966), in one or both ears of patients with intra-axial brainstem lesions (Morales-Garcia & Poole, 1972; Noffsinger, Olsen, Carhart, Hart, & Sahgal, 1972), and for contralateral ears in patients with temporal lobe disorders (Heilman, Hammer, & Wilder, 1973; Morales-Garcia & Poole, 1972).

In their 1972 investigation, Morales-Garcia and Poole used S/Ns of 0 and +5 dB in 32 patients with different types of intracranial lesions. They found that 14 of 15 patients with brainstem lesions had abnormal scores, with mean scores falling 20% below normal for both S/Ns. However, no clear pattern of performance emerged as to laterality effects or to the level of the lesions. In addition, they noted that all 10 of their patients with temporal lobe lesions showed depressed contralateral ear scores for at least one of the S/Ns with normal results in the ipsilateral ear, whereas none of their seven patients with lesions outside the temporal lobe demonstrated a significant contralateral ear deficit.

Olsen, Noffsinger, and Kurdziel (1975) used NU-6 word lists with an ipsilateral white noise (0 dB S/N). These investigators derived not only absolute scores, but also difference scores. Based on their normative data, they determined that difference scores of greater than 40% were significant. Significant mean ear differences were noted for Ménière's patients (41%, N = 24), eighth nerve patients (47%, N = 21), and temporal lobe patients (43%, N = 24). For temporal lobe patients, all abnormal scores were noted in the contralateral ear. However, inspection of the data for this group revealed that in spite of the significant mean ear differences, more than half of the temporal lobe subjects scored within normal limits of variability. Because of the large range of scores and similar findings for different pathology groups, these investigators concluded that speech-in-noise testing may have some usefulness in detecting CANS disorders, but not in specifying site of lesion.

Synthetic sentence identification with ipsilateral competing message

The Synthetic Sentence Identification With Ipsilateral Competing Message Test (SSI-ICM) is composed of 10 third-order approximations of English sentences that are presented along with a competing message consisting of continuous discourse (Jerger & Jerger, 1974). The 10 sentences were originally designed to minimize the subject's reliance on linguistic skills, and they have been carefully controlled for both informational content and length. The sentences are presented to the test ear in the presence of the competing message, and the subject is asked to point to 1 of 10 printed sentences that corresponds to the stimulus presented. The test can be presented in two ways: (a) by varying the message-to-competition ratio, or (b) by keeping the signal-to-competition ratio constant (usually 0 dB) and presenting the sentences at several intensity levels from high to low. If the latter procedure is used in subjects with brainstem involvement, word recognition performance typically decreases as intensity is increased.

The incidence of SSI-ICM abnormality in populations with brainstem involvement is relatively impressive. Jerger and Jerger (1974) reported that 11 of 11 patients with intra-axial brainstem lesions had scores in one or both ears that fell below the normal criteria. In another study of patients with brainstem involvement, an average deficit of 40% was noted for the contralateral ear to the lesioned side of the brainstem (Jerger & Jerger, 1975). Reports using a modification of the SSI-ICM showed that 7 of 13

(Stephens & Thornton, 1976) and 8 of 12 patients (Antonelli, Bellotto, & Grandori, 1987) with brainstem lesions had abnormal results on this test.

The majority of the central auditory tests that appear to be particularly sensitive to brainstem lesions are sensitive to lesions in the low to mid brainstem. For the most part they are likely to miss lesions in the rostral-most portion of the brainstem. The SSI-ICM appears to be sensitive to both rostral and caudal brainstem lesions, though it may also be affected but to a lesser degree by cerebral involvement (Jerger & Jerger, 1974, 1975).

Other low-redundancy monaural speech tests

In addition to the tests discussed above, other investigators have used interrupted speech, expanded speech, and low-sensation level speech tests to study CANS function in pathological cases. These tests have received limited use clinically, and therefore we will not discuss them here. Also, performance-intensity functions have been used to assess CANS function in patients with low brainstem pathology (Jerger, 1973; Jerger & Jerger, 1971). Though this test does not fall under the category of low-redundancy speech tests, abnormal test results have been reported for some individuals with brainstem lesions. The reader who is interested in any of these tests should see Rintelmann (1985).

Dichotic speech tests

As mentioned previously, Kimura (1961a, 1961b) typically is credited with the introduction of dichotic speech tests into the field of central auditory assessment. Since that time, several variations of the dichotic digits test, as well as several other dichotic speech tests, have been introduced. For the most part, these tests have been shown to be particularly sensitive to cortical pathology, though abnormal results also have been reported for subjects with brainstem involvement.

Dichotic digits

In the early 1960s Kimura (1961a, 1961b) administered a dichotic digits test in which dichotic triads were presented simultaneously to each ear to a group of patients with unilateral temporal lobe lesions. She found impaired digit recognition in the contralateral ear when the stimuli were presented in a dichotic paradigm, whereas no deficits were noted in either ear if the stimuli were presented in a noncompeting condition—that is, unless the left or dominant hemisphere was affected. In this case, bilaterally depressed scores typically were noted.

More recently, Musiek (1983a) introduced a revised version of the dichotic digits (DD) test. This version differs from Kimura's original test in that two rather than three digits are presented simultaneously to each ear. The test stimuli consist of the digits from 1 through 10, excluding 7. A total of 20 digits are presented to each ear at 50 dB re: speech reception threshold and a percent correct score is derived for each ear. This new version of the test takes only 4 min to administer and is easily scored. This ease of scoring results in reduced variability among examiners.

There have been several other variations of the dichotic digits test. These have included having the subject report all the test stimuli perceived in one ear first, followed by those perceived in the second ear, or having the subjects add the numbers heard in each ear and report a total figure for each ear. Also, there has been some work with dichotic words. A review of these procedures can be found in Musiek and Pinheiro (1985).

Test results have shown that the dichotic digits test is fairly sensitive to brainstem and cortical lesions. Musiek (1983a) reported that 17 of 21 patients with intracranial lesions (9 brainstem, 12 hemispheric) showed abnormal performance in either one or both ears on the dichotic digits test. In addition, we have demonstrated abnormal test results in several individuals with complete and/or posterior sections of the corpus callosum (Musiek et al., 1984). Other researchers have demonstrated contralateral ear deficits with right temporal lobe lesions and bilaterally depressed scores with left temporal lobe lesions (Mueller, Sedge, & Salazar, 1985; Sedge, Mueller, & Dillon, 1982). In the large study of Vietnam veterans mentioned previously, Mueller et al. (1987) reported that the performance of subjects with cortical damage outside the temporal lobe of either hemisphere on a dichotic digits test did not differ from that of a group of control subjects. However, if right posterior temporal lobe damage was present, a small decrease in mean right ear performance was noted (3.4%) relative to the mean right ear performance of the control subjects, whereas a larger left ear deficit was noted (i.e., a decrease of 9% compared to the mean score for the control subjects). In patients with injury to the left posterior temporal lobe, greater deficits were noted for both ears when compared to the control group; however, no obvious ear differences were noted in that the mean score for the right ear was 15% lower than that for the normal subjects and the left ear score was 16.3% lower. Sparks, Goodglass, and Nichel (1970) reported similar contralateral ear deficits with right hemisphere damage. However, they also reported ipsilateral deficits in a number of subjects with left hemisphere damage. They suggested that the ipsilateral deficits were noted because the lesions were deep and affected the callosal fibers from the right hemisphere.

Therefore, the test results were similar to those expected with right hemisphere lesions.

To date there have been only a few investigations that have studied the dichotic digits performance of individuals with brainstem lesions. Results have revealed that 5 of 13 (Stephens & Thornton, 1976) and 7 of 10 subjects (Musiek & Geurkink, 1982) showed abnormal results on a dichotic digits test.

Results of a comparative study that investigated the relative sensitivity of three dichotic speech tests (dichotic digits, competing sentences, and staggered spondaic words) in the assessment of CANS disorders in 12 subjects with brainstem involvement and 18 with cortical lesions showed that the dichotic digits test yielded slightly more abnormal findings for both groups than did either one of the two remaining tests (Musiek, 1983b). Given the moderately high sensitivity of this test to brainstem, cortical, and interhemispheric lesions, its ease of administration, and its relatively short administration time, this particular test would constitute a good screening tool for CANS disorders. Abnormal findings should alert the audiologist to the need to conduct additional central auditory testing.

Staggered spondaic words

Approximately 1 year after Kimura's introduction of the dichotic speech paradigm into the field of central auditory assessment, Katz (1962) introduced a unique modification of this psychophysical procedure. His Staggered Spondaic Word Test (SSW) is among the best known and most frequently used dichotic speech tests in use today. The test stimuli consist of 40 pairs of spondee words that are presented with a staggered onset. In order to achieve the staggered onsets, the first half of one test item is presented in a noncompeting condition, followed by a competing condition in which the second half of the first spondee and the first half of the second spondee are presented to the two ears in a competing dichotic manner. Finally, the second half of the second spondee is presented in a noncompeting condition. The test stimuli are alternated between the two channels of the audiometer so that the ear receiving the first spondee constantly changes back and forth between the two ears. The procedures for scoring the test are quite complicated and are not used universally. The reader is directed to Brunt (1978) for details regarding test administration and scoring procedures. We frequently use the SSW in our neuro-audiological assessments. However, when we administer this test we typically present the test stimuli at 50 dB re: speech reception threshold and derive percent correct identification scores for the right and left ears under the competing condition only.

Several studies by Katz and associates have demonstrated a close correspondence between SSW test results and site of CANS damage (Katz, 1962, 1968, 1970, 1977; Katz, Basil, & Smith, 1963; Katz & Pack, 1975). The results of these investigations have shown moderately to severely depressed SSW scores (i.e., competing condition) for the contralateral ears in individuals with cortical lesions involving the primary auditory reception areas of either hemisphere, whereas subjects with lesions outside the primary auditory reception areas have shown only mildly depressed contralateral deficits or normal test results. Lynn and Gilroy (1977) also demonstrated depressed scores for 5 patients with anterior temporal lobe lesions and 5 patients with posterior temporal lobe lesions. They noted that patients with posterior lesions tended to demonstrate more severely depressed scores than did those patients with anterior temporal lobe lesions.

Other investigators also demonstrated abnormal test results in patients with both right and left hemisphere lesions (Lynn & Gilroy, 1975; McClellen, Wertz, & Collins, 1973). However, these researchers noted primarily contralateral deficits if the lesion affected the right hemisphere, and smaller ear differences if the lesion affected the left hemisphere. These findings are consistent with those of Mueller et al. (1987) who noted a significant contralateral ear effect in their subjects with right posterior temporal lobe involvement. In this group of subjects mean performance was depressed 10% relative to that of a group of control subjects, whereas mean ipsilateral ear performance was found to be similar to that of the control subjects. When damage was located in the left posterior temporal lobe, scores were found to be bilaterally depressed when compared to the control subjects, that is, 8.8% for the right ear and 8.9% for the left ear.

Results of several investigations with subjects with brainstem lesions have shown mixed results. Jerger and Jerger (1975) studied 10 patients with intra-axial brainstem lesions and 10 control subjects. These investigators found that the pathological group demonstrated mean scores that were 44% and 16% poorer than those of the control subjects for the contralateral and ipsilateral ears, respectively. Stephens and Thornton (1976) reported that 6 of 14 subjects demonstrated abnormal test results, whereas Musiek and Geurkink (1982) reported that approximately 60% of their brainstem subjects revealed abnormal test results. Other investigators (Pinheiro, Jacobson, & Boller, 1982; Rintelmann & Lynn, 1983) reported abnormal results for a small number of additional subjects with brainstem lesions.

Dichotic CVs

In the early 1970s Berlin and his co-workers (Berlin, Lowe-Bell, Jannetta, & Kline, 1972; Berlin et al., 1975) introduced another dichotic speech test, dichotic CVs, into the CANS assessment area. In this test, dichotic CV stimuli are presented to the two ears dichotically while the onsets of the two stimuli are varied. The test stimuli consist of the following CVs: ba, da, ga, pa, ta, and ka. In one part of the test, the alignments of the two stimuli are close to simultaneous, whereas in other instances the onsets of the second or "lagging" stimuli are delayed by a specific length of time relative to the onsets of the leading stimuli. Onset lags of 15, 30, 60, and 90 ms are used. In the earlier investigation, Berlin et al. (1972) found that normal subjects obtained better scores if the onsets of the lagging CVs were delayed by 30 to 90 ms. A similar improvement in performance, however, was not noted for four patients who had undergone temporal lobectomies.

In a subsequent study, Berlin et al. (1975) administered the dichotic CV test to three temporal lobectomy patients and four hemispherectomy patients. They found that in both groups of subjects, weak ear (i.e., ear contralateral to lesion) performance declined to near chance levels following surgery, whereas strong ear (i.e., ear ipsilateral to lesion) performance improved. They reported, however, a significant difference in the amount of improvement noted for the strong ear performance of the two groups. In the lobectomy group a small improvement was noted, but the scores did not begin to approach 100%, whereas in the hemispherectomy group performance rose to nearly 100%. The authors suggested that these differences could be accounted for on the basis of a competition for neural substrate that was still present in the lobectomy group, but that was effectively eliminated in the hemispherectomy group.

Zurif and Ramier (1972) administered dichotic CVs to 20 patients with left hemisphere damage and 20 with right hemisphere damage and noted right brain damaged subjects showed contralateral ear deficits, whereas left brain damaged subjects tended to show similar scores for both ears. Speaks et al. (1975) demonstrated that 10 of 10 subjects with CANS pathology showed depressed contralateral ear scores, whereas Olsen (1977) found that 31 of 40 patients with temporal lobectomies had depressed scores for one or both ears. In Mueller, Beck, and Sedge's 1987 investigation of CANS test results in Vietnam veterans, a substantial reduction in mean performance was noted for the left ear (23.6%) in subjects with right temporal lobe involvement, whereas the mean right ear score did not differ substantially from that of the control group. In subjects with left temporal lobe involvement, a similar, but less pronounced contralateral ear effect (17.7%) was noted. In addition, a small ipsilateral effect (7.2%) was observed.

Limited research has been reported for patients with brainstem involvement. Berlin, Cullen, Berlin, Tobey, and Mouney (1975) demonstrated almost complete suppression of the CVs presented to the left ear of a patient with a lesion in the area of the right medial geniculate body, whereas right ear results were normal.

Synthetic sentence identification with contralateral competing message

The Synthetic Sentence Identification With Contralateral Competing Message test (SSI-CCM) is identical to the SSI-ICM test described previously, except that in this case, the sentences and the competing message are presented to opposite ears rather than the same ear (Jerger & Jerger 1974, 1975). These investigators found that individuals with brainstem lesions generally performed within normal limits on the SSI-CCM version of this test, whereas they tended to show depressed scores in the ear contralateral to the lesion on the SSI-ICM test. On the other hand, patients with temporal lobe lesions typically demonstrated depressed SSI-CCM scores in the contralateral ear (Jerger & Jerger, 1975). Similar findings have been reported for other patients with temporal lobe disorders by Keith (1977) and Jerger and Jerger (1981).

In 1983, Fifer, Jerger, Berlin, Tobey, and Campbell introduced a modification of the SSI-CCM test. This modification of the SSI-CCM, referred to as the Dichotic Sentence Identification test (DSI), uses the original sentences of the SSI-CCM test, but rather than presenting the sentences to one ear and a competing discourse message to the opposite ear, the sentences were paired and presented dichotically. This particular test was designed in the hope of developing a dichotic speech test that would be minimally affected by peripheral hearing loss. To date, there have been only a few investigations that have studied the sensitivity of the DSI to CANS lesions. In their original article, Fifer and his co-workers reported that 5 of 6 subjects with CANS lesions demonstrated abnormal test results in one ear, whereas the sixth subject showed bilateral deficits. Mueller et al. (1987) reported test results for 90 subjects with cerebral lesions. Of these subjects, 22 had damage to the right or left posterior temporal lobe, whereas the remainder of the subjects had damage to structures outside the primary auditory areas. Their results showed that this test yielded sensitivity and specificity ratings that were comparable to those obtained with other dichotic speech tests; namely, DD, SSW, and CVs. This finding, in light of earlier evidence that the test is relatively resistant to the effects of peripheral hearing loss, suggests that the DSI would be a useful dichotic speech test to incorporate in a CANS test battery, particularly if one is assessing an individual with a peripheral hearing impairment. However, more research is needed to support this contention.

Competing sentences

In the late 1960s Willeford, along with some of his graduate students, developed a Competing Sentence test (CS) that is one of the most popular tests of this particular type used in clinics today. The test is composed of 25 sentence pairs that average six to seven words in length. The sentences are presented dichotically with the target sentences presented at 35 dB SL (re: SRT) and the competing sentences presented at 50 dB SL (re: SRT). The subject is instructed to repeat the target sentences and to ignore the competing sentences. A total of 10 sentences are typically presented to each ear, with the remaining 5 sentences used for training or other purposes. One of the major problems with this particular test is that the guidelines for scoring are not well specified in the literature. This leaves open the door for considerable variability in test scores among different testers.

For the most part, this test has been used in the assessment of children with auditory processing disorders; however, there have been some investigations that have looked at the performance of individuals with CANS disorders on this test (Lynn & Gilroy, 1972, 1975, 1977; Musiek, 1983a, 1983b; Musiek & Geurkink, 1982; Rintelmann & Lynn, 1983; Pinheiro, Jacobson, & Boller, 1982). These studies have shown that approximately one-half of the subjects studied with brainstem lesions showed abnormal performance in the ear ipsilateral to the lesion. For subjects with temporal lobe lesions, contralateral deficits were noted for individuals with posterior temporal lobe lesions, whereas for the most part no deficits were noted in subjects with anterior temporal lobe lesions. As mentioned earlier, Musiek (1983b) reported that competing sentences was the least sensitive of three dichotic speech tests (SSW, DD, CS) administered to subjects with intracranial lesions. Similar findings were reported by Lynn and Gilroy (1972, 1975, 1977) when comparing the SSW and CS tests.

A recent procedural variation on the traditional CS test was introduced by Bergman, Hirsch, Solzi, and Mankowitz (1987). In their test, referred to as the Threshold-of-Interference Test, these researchers determined the sensation level at which competing sentences interfered with the subject's ability to repeat target sentences. Their test stimuli included Hebrew sentences that were all three words in length. Target sentences were typically presented at 25 dB relative to the threshold of intelligibility for the sentences, and the level of the competing sentences was increased from threshold level until the subject could no longer repeat the target sentences. The inability of the subject to attend to and repeat the primary message when the level of the competing message was at, or within, 5 dB of the competing message ear's threshold was labeled "complete suppression," whereas partial suppression was defined as a disabling competing message level of 10 to 35 dB SL. These investigators administered the test to 27 subjects with CANS involvement and found that 10 of 17 subjects with right hemisphere damage showed complete left ear suppression, whereas 4 of 10 subjects with left hemisphere damage showed left ear suppression. Two additional subjects with right hemisphere damage showed partial suppression of the left ear targets and one demonstrated mildly depressed scores for both ears with the larger deficit noted in the contralateral left ear. As with the other dichotic tests, contralateral deficits were noted with right hemisphere damage. However, in 4 of 10 cases with left hemisphere damage, ipsilateral left ear deficits were noted. An inspection of the CT scans for these four patients revealed involvement of the callosal fibers traveling from the right side for at least three out of four of these patients. The authors suggest that this test is useful in exposing strong hemispheric suppression, particularly in cases of right hemisphere damage.

Other dichotic speech tests

In addition to the dichotic tests described above, tests such as the Northwestern University Test No. 2 and the Northwestern University Test No. 20 have been used in the assessment of CANS pathology (Jerger, 1964; Noffsinger et al., 1972). In both cases the monosyllabic test stimuli are presented to one ear while a competing message is delivered to the opposite ear. Because these tests have received limited attention in CANS assessment we will not review them here. Additional information regarding these tests can be found in Musiek and Pinheiro (1985).

Binaural interaction tests

Binaural interaction or integration tests encompass those CANS tests that require the interaction of both ears in order to effect closure for dichotic signals that are separated by time, frequency, or intensity factors between the two ears. These tasks were designed to assess the ability of the CANS to take disparate information presented to the two ears, and to unify this information into one perceptual event. This unification is believed to occur in the brainstem. Thus these tests are presumed to be sensitive to brainstem pathology. They can, however, also be affected by cerebral lesions.

Rapidly alternating speech perception

Rapidly alternating speech perception (RASP) tasks require the integration of segments of speech stimuli delivered alternately between the two ears over time. The best-known test in this category is the RASP test developed by Willeford (1976). In this test, segments of sentences are presented to the subject's two ears in an alternating fashion. The alternation rate is 300 ms and a presentation level of 40 dB re: pure tone average is recommended. The ear that receives the first 300 ms of each sentence determines the lead channel. The lead channel is assigned to one ear and 10 sentences are presented. Then the lead channel is switched to the opposite ear and 10 additional sentences are presented. However, testing experience indicates that this procedure may be unnecessary because there is interaction between the ears. Therefore, a binaural score may constitute a more accurate representation.

It seems that the number of alternations per second does not make a difference for normal listeners (Bocca & Calearo, 1963; Lynn & Gilroy, 1977). Bocca and Calearo (1963) employed alternating segments of running speech ranging from about 20 to 500 ms in duration without any disruption in intelligibility. Lynn and Gilroy (1977) selected 300 ms for their work with RASP, but this rate was not based on experienced listeners. However, it is not known what alternation rate would reveal minimum degrees of brainstem involvement.

There is some question as to whether the RASP test is sensitive to other than grossly abnormal brainstem function. Only 6 of 47 subjects tested by Lynn and Gilroy (1977) had clearly positive results. Musiek (1983c), using the Willeford version of the test, reported that 5 of 10 subjects with brainstem involvement demonstrated abnormal performance. Lynn and Gilroy (1977) found that for the most part subjects with cortical and interhemispheric involvement performed normally on their RASP test. They did, however, note that some subjects with diffuse central lesions demonstrated abnormal performance.

Binaural fusion tests

There have been several variations of the binaural fusion test (BF). These tests involve the presentation of bandpass filtered speech to the two ears. Generally the stimuli for these tests are passed through two bandpass filters. Typically, a low bandpass filtered stimulus is delivered to one ear, whereas a high bandpass filtered stimulus is delivered to the opposite ear. In some tests, the ears receiving the bandpass segments are alternated, so that one is able to derive a score for two test conditions; that is, a score is obtained when the low bandpass segment is presented to the right ear and a second score is derived when the left ear receives the low bandpass information. In addition, many researchers and clinicians derive diotic test scores. In this test condition, both bandpass segments are presented to both ears simultaneously. Research findings have shown that the bandpass segments are not highly intelligible when presented monaurally, whereas recognition tends to be quite high when presented together either to the same ear or to opposite ears.

Matzker (1959) used a binaural fusion test with over 1,700 patients with a variety of CANS lesions. His test consisted of 41 two-syllable words that were phonetically balanced. The test stimuli were bandpass filtered into a low pass band (500-800 Hz) and a high pass band (1815-2500 Hz) and vowel recognition rather than word recognition was used as the criterion for correctness. The test was given three times. The first and third presentations were filtered bands, whereas the second presentation was diotic in nature and did not require fusion. Matzker reported that several patients with brainstem lesions had difficulty with the resynthesis of the two frequency bands, whereas patients with cortical lesions tended to perform normally on this test.

Linden (1964) used an adaptation of the Matzker test for resynthesis. In this case, test stimuli consisted of nine Swedish spondaic word lists of 15 items each. The test stimuli were bandpass filtered similarly to those of Matzker, except that the filtering was somewhat more restrictive, especially in the high-frequency band. In addition, rather than scoring for vowel recognition, Linden used word recognition scores. He also tested at several sensation levels, because he found that performance improved in normal subjects with increases in sensation levels; for example, from 35% at 25 dB SL to 89% at 40 dB SL. His findings were reported to be negative, suggesting that the BF test was not sensitive to brainstem lesions. However, Tobin (1985) suggested that if the test results were reinterpreted, 4 of Linden's 18 subjects may have shown some evidence of brainstem involvement.

Smith and Resnick (1972) chose to use phonetically balanced monosyllabic words for their study of BF. They believed that the lower redundancy of the signal would tax the system further, but this fact would limit application of the test to those individuals with at least fair discrimination ability. These researchers used two resynthesis tasks and a diotic task for their test. The two resynthesis scores were compared to the diotic score. If the scores were similar, the results were considered to be normal. If, however, the diotic score was significantly higher than either resynthesis score, the results were considered to be positive for brainstem pathology. The authors presented four cases with brainstem pathology. In all four cases the test results were positive.

One of the more popular BF tests today is the one that is part of Willeford's (1976) test battery. Test stimuli consist of filtered words that were bandpass filtered at 500 to 700 Hz and from 1900 to 2100 Hz with slopes of 36 dB per octave. Presentation levels are 30 dB relative to 500 Hz for the low band and 30 dB relative to 2000 Hz for the high band.

Abnormal test results have been found in 3 of 10 subjects with brainstem lesions by Musiek (1983c) and for a single patient with a gunshot wound to the right pons by Pinheiro et al. (1982). Lynn and Gilroy (1975) reported abnormal findings for patients with brainstem lesions, whereas subjects with cerebral lesions tended to perform normally. These results, however, suggest that the BF test is only moderately sensitive, at best, to brainstem lesions.

Masking level differences

The test protocol for obtaining Masking Level Differences (MLD) involves the presentation of either a pulsed tone, typically a 500-Hz tone, or spondee words to both ears at the same time that a masking noise is being delivered binaurally. The client normally is tested under two conditions. In the homophasic condition, both the speech or pulsed tone and the masking noise are presented to both ears in-phase. In the second, or antiphasic condition, one of the signals is presented 180° out-of-phase between the two ears, whereas the other is held in-phase (Hirsh, 1948; Licklider, 1948).

When administering the MLD test, consideration should be given to several variables. Townsend and Goldstein (1972) found that in the antiphasic conditions the amount of release from masking decreased as the sensation level for the presentation of the signals increased. Pengelly, Mueller, and Hill (1982) noted that there was no difference in the size of the MLD when either a broad-band or narrow-band masker was used in normal subjects. However, in a group of subjects with high-frequency hearing losses, the narrow-band masker produced significantly larger MLDs for a 500-Hz signal. Finally, the size of the MLD also appears to be affected by the duration of the masker. Green (1966) and McFadden (1966) showed that a continuous masker tended to produce larger MLDs than did maskers that were gated to follow the duty cycle of the signal. For further information about these considerations, the reader is referred to Durlach and Colburn (1978) and Tobin (1985).

In the first comprehensive clinical investigation of MLDs, Olsen, Noffsinger, and Carhart (1976) found a greater release from masking could be demonstrated in both normal and impaired subjects if the $S_\pi N_0$, as opposed to $S_0 N_\pi$, antiphasic condition was used. This is the condition in which the masking noise is delivered to the two in-phase, whereas the pure tone or speech signals are delivered out-of-phase. Similar results were reported in a subsequent investigation by Pengelly et al. (1982).

In 1981 Lynn, Gilroy, Taylor, and Leiser reported test results for 26 patients with either brainstem or cortical lesions. Their results showed that patients with low brainstem involvement demonstrated little or no release from masking (i.e., abnormal test results), whereas patients with lesions higher in the CANS tended to perform similarly to a group of normal control subjects. More recently, Noffsinger, Martinez, and Schaefer (1982) demonstrated a close correspondence between MLD and ABR test results. These investigators found that patients with abnormalities in Waves I, II, or III of the ABR yielded small or absent MLDs, whereas patients with abnormalities of Waves IV or V demonstrated normal MLDs.

Other binaural interaction tests

In the late 1950s, Sanchez-Longo and colleagues (Sanchez-Longo et al., 1957; Sanchez-Longo & Forster, 1958) demonstrated impairment of the sound localization ability in the auditory field contralateral to the temporal lobe lesions in a group of brain damaged subjects. These results suggest that the auditory cortex might have a role in forming the concept of auditory space. A subsequent investigation (Pinheiro & Tobin, 1969) using an Interaural Intensity Difference (IID) test paradigm revealed that subjects with central lesions required a larger IID in the ear ipsilateral to the site of lesion than did normal ears or ears with sensorineural hearing losses, whereas the contralateral ear required only an IID of about 4 dB for lateralization. Pinheiro and Tobin (1971) also noted that patients with abnormal IIDs showed neurologic signs of temporal and/or parietal lobe involvement, whereas patients with occipital or frontal lobe lesions tended to demonstrate normal IIDs. These results suggest that the perception of the location of a sound is a cortical function, even though the critical processing for the IID presumably occurs at the brainstem level (Pickles, 1985). For additional information regarding sound localization and lateralization tasks the reader is directed to Tobin (1985).

Temporal ordering tasks

In the 1960s and 1970s, several researchers began to use temporal ordering or sequencing tasks in an attempt to study the relationship between temporal ordering skills and CANS pathology. Unfortunately, few of these research test protocols have gained widespread clinical use.

Early temporal sequencing tasks

In 1962, Milner reported that patients with temporal lobe lesions performed poorly when presented with two sequences of three to five tones and asked to identify which tone in the second series was different than the series of tones in the first sequence. He also noted that patients with right temporal lobectomies made more errors than did subjects with left temporal lobectomies. Similar findings have been reported for other patients with temporal lobectomies for binaurally presented bird songs (Milner et al., 1965) and dichotic melodies (Shankweiler, 1966).

Swisher and Hirsh (1972) studied the ability of subjects with cerebral damage to temporally order two tones. For this investigation they used a test paradigm in which they presented two tones of different pitches and with various onset time differences. The two tones were presented either to the same ear or to opposite ears, and the subjects were asked to indicate the order of the two tones. Participants consisted of young adults, older control subjects, and three groups of brain-damaged subjects, including left brain damaged with fluent aphasia, left brain damage with nonfluent aphasia, and right brain damage with no aphasia. Fluent aphasics required the longest intervals to order stimuli, particularly if the two stimuli were presented to the same ear. In subjects with right hemisphere damage the differences required to make temporal order judgments between the two stimuli presented were smaller and approximated those demonstrated by the control subjects. They did, however, show greater deficits when the tonal stimuli were presented to opposite ears.

Lackner and Teuber (1973) presented dichotic clicks to the two ears that varied in terms of their onsets. Their subjects included 24 veterans with left hemisphere damage and 19 with right hemisphere damage. They found that subjects with left hemisphere damage required a longer silent interval between the stimuli in order to perceive separation.

A number of additional studies in the 1970s revealed temporal ordering deficits for patients with cerebral lesions (Belmont & Handler, 1971; Carmon & Nachshon, 1971; DeRenzi, Faglioni, & Villa, 1977; Karaseva, 1972; Lhermitte et al, 1971). Lhermitte and colleagues (1971) found that patients with bilateral temporal lobe involvement could recognize frequency and intensity differences, but they could not discriminate between two different temporal sequences. Karaseva (1972) found that patients with unilateral damage to the auditory projection areas of the temporal lobe were impaired in the discrimination of rhythmic patterns of clicks in the ear contralateral to the lesion. Contralateral deficits also were reported by Belmont and Handler (1971) for hemiplegics who were asked to indicate the order of stimulation between the two ears when they were stimulated with 500-Hz tones of 200 ms duration separated by delays of 20, 50, or 80 ms in duration. DeRenzi et al. (1977) reported deficits in the ability of a group of brain-damaged subjects to use a verbal memory code to recall serial order information. Finally, Carmon and Nachshon (1971) noted that patients with left hemisphere damage were severely impaired in their ability to point to the locations in correct order for a sequence of three to five bimodal stimuli (consisting of lights and tones) presented in a temporal order, while patients with right hemisphere lesions performed as well as normal subjects.

As mentioned previously, Efron and associates (Efron, 1985; Efron & Crandall, 1983; Efron et al., 1983; Efron et al., 1977; Efron et al., 1985) have conducted a series of experiments with nonspeech auditory signals and have demonstrated contralateral ear deficits in individuals with temporal lobe lesions for a variety of auditory tasks (e.g., gap detection, sound lateralization, and temporal ordering tasks). These authors noted consistent contralateral ear effects in subjects with either posterior temporal lobe involvement or anterior temporal lobe resections. The latter findings were remarkable in that previous to these findings, it was believed that the anterior temporal lobe did not play a role in auditory processing. It is also interesting to note that Efron and Crandall (1983) have postulated the existence of a contralaterally organized efferent pathway that is located within each temporal lobe and that, when activated, significantly enhances our ability to perceive auditory stimuli on the contralateral side of auditory space.

More recently, Blaettner, Scherg, and Von Cramon (1989) introduced a new pyschoacoustic pattern discrimination test. For this test, sequences of noise bursts or click trains are presented dichotically at suprathreshold levels, and the subject is asked to discriminate monaural changes in either the intensity or click pattern. The subject simply indicates his or her response by depressing a button whenever a monaural change is noted. This test was administered to 62 patients with unilateral cerebrovascular accidents. Results indicated that abnormal test results correlated highly (76%) with presence of a cerebral lesion and that isolated lesions of the acoustic radiations and/or of the auditory association areas were sufficient to cause abnormality on this test. As with most behavioral tests, contralateral ear deficits were most prominent. In addition, these researchers found no evidence of ear dominance in normal subjects on this test, nor was size of the laterality effect on this test larger in either the right or left hemisphere lesion groups. It is therefore likely that this test taps a low level of auditory processing at which hemispheric specialization has not yet taken over. This is an important feature because ear dominance may be confounded with lesion effects. A second advantage of this test is that it can be used to assess auditory function in patients who may be incapable of responding verbally.

Frequency pattern sequences

One of the more popular temporal ordering tasks used today is the Frequency Pattern Sequence Test (PATT) developed by Pinheiro and Ptacek

(Pinheiro & Ptacek, 1971; Ptacek & Pinheiro, 1971). It is composed of 120 test sequences, with each sequence containing three tone bursts. In each sequence two of the tone bursts are of the same frequency, whereas the third tone burst is of a different frequency. Thus a total of six different sequences is possible (i.e., high-high-low, high-low-high, high-low-low, low-high-high, low-low-high, low-high-low). The subject is asked to describe verbally each sequence heard. If patients are unable to verbally describe the sequences, they can either hum or manually indicate the sequence heard. Patients with lesions of either hemisphere or of the inter-hemispheric pathways have difficulty describing the monaurally pre-sented test sequences (Musiek et al., 1984; Musiek & Pinheiro, 1986, 1987; Musiek et al., 1980; Pinheiro, 1976; Pinheiro et al., 1977). Some of these same investigators have shown that if asked to hum the sequences, split-brain patients generally perform with close to 100% accuracy. These results suggest some processing of the stimuli occurs in both hemispheres and that the auditory interhemispheric connections must be intact for normal performance if a verbal response is required. For these reasons, perform-ance is most often found to be bilaterally normal or bilaterally depressed. Musiek and Pinheiro (1987) tested three groups of patients with different pathologies (cerebral, brainstem, and cochlear). Their results, depicted in Figure 11.1, revealed that the frequency pattern sequences test was highly sensitive to cerebral lesions (83%) but not as sensitive to brainstem lesions (45%). The specificity of the test was determined to be 88%.

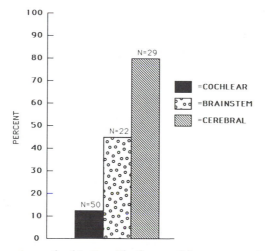

Figure 11.1. Percentage of subjects with abnormal frequency pattern test results (cochlear lesions, N = 50 ears; brainstem lesions, N = 22 patients; cerebral lesions, N = 29 patients). (Adapted with permission from F. E. Musiek & M. L. Pinheiro, Frequency patterns in cochlear, brainstem and cerebral lesions. *Audiology, 26,* 79–88, © by S. Karger AG, Basel, Switzerland, 1987.)

Other temporal ordering tasks

In addition to frequency pattern sequences, Pinheiro and her co-workers also looked at temporally sequenced patterns of tones that varied in terms of intensity and durational features (see Pinheiro & Musiek, 1985). To date, most of the research in this area has involved normal subjects. We have recently begun some preliminary work with the auditory duration pattern sequences tests (Baran, Musiek, Gollegly, Verkest, & Kibbe-Michal, 1987). Our results have shown that the test is highly sensitive to cerebral lesions and generally is not affected by mild-to-moderate hearing loss. In addition, we have noted that many patients who performed normally on the frequency pattern sequences test yielded abnormal results on this task. These results suggest that this test may be tapping different auditory processing skills than does the frequency pattern sequences test.

Neuroaudiological findings in special clinical populations

Split-brain patients

In the late 1960s, two articles appeared in the literature that reported depressed left ear scores on dichotic speech tests for patients who had undergone complete surgical sections of the corpus callosum (Milner, Taylor, & Sperry, 1968; Sparks & Geschwind, 1968). Since that time similar findings have been reported for a number of additional patients with either complete or posterior surgical sections of the corpus callosum (Gazzaniga, Risse, Springer, Clark, & Wilson, 1975; Musiek & Kibbe, 1985; Musiek et al., 1984; Musiek, Reeves, & Baran, 1985; Musiek & Wilson, 1979; Musiek et al., 1979; Springer & Gazzaniga, 1975; Springer, Sidtis, Wilson, & Gazzaniga, 1978). Unfortunately, in many of these investigations no preoperative data were provided. Therefore, it is difficult for the reader to determine if the deficits noted following surgery are related to sectioning of the corpus callosum or to some preexisting hemispheric involvement.

Here at our clinic we have been able to assess the preoperative and postoperative performance of several patients who have had posterior and/or complete commissurotomies (Musiek et al., 1984; Musiek et al., 1980; Musiek et al., 1985; Musiek & Wilson, 1979; Musiek et al., 1979), as well as a number of subjects whose surgical sections were limited to the anterior portion of the corpus callosum (Baran et al., 1986). Our results have shown that patients with posterior and/or complete commissu-rotomies (a) perform normally on a monaural low-redundancy speech test (LPFS), (b) demonstrate left ear deficits on dichotic speech tests (DD and SSW), and (c) show bilateral deficits on a monaural temporal ordering task (PATT). On the other hand, we have found that sectioning of the anterior half of the corpus callosum does not result in similar postsurgical deficits. Figure 11.2 displays the test results for four of our subjects with complete commissurotomies and eight subjects with anterior sections of the corpus callosum.

The differences noted between the test results of these two groups of subjects can be explained on an anatomical basis. Given our test results, as well as the results of some earlier work with primates (Pandya et al., 1971), it appears that the auditory interhemispheric fibers lie in the posterior portion of the corpus callosum. Thus surgical sectioning of this part of the corpus callosum should result in the deficits outlined above given that the necessary interhemispheric transfer of auditory informa-tion would be prevented. The left ear deficits noted on the dichotic speech tests occur because the stronger contralateral pathways from the left ear to right hemisphere (via the corpus callosum) are rendered ineffective by sectioning, whereas at the same time the ipsilateral pathways are being suppressed because of the dichotic nature of the task. The bilateral deficits noted on the frequency pattern sequences test occur because sectioning of the posterior portion of the corpus callosum prohibits the necessary interaction of the two hemispheres. Both hemispheres are involved in the processing of tonal sequences (right hemisphere), which require verbal labeling (left hemisphere). No deficits are noted on the mon-aural low-redundancy speech test because the ipsilateral left ear to left hemisphere pathway is not suppressed during monaural stimulation, and the contralateral right ear to left hemisphere pathway is not affected by the surgical procedure.

The observation of similar test profiles in other pathological subjects could assist in the identification of the site of dysfunction in individuals with CANS lesions that may be affecting the interhemispheric pathways. For example, Damasio and Damasio (1979) reported severe left ear deficits for a group of patients with lesions near the lateral wall of the lateral ventricle at the level of the trigone. These authors concluded that the inter-hemispheric pathways diverge from the geniculocortical pathways by traveling posteriorly and rostrally to arch around the lateral ventricle and join the corpus callosum in its posterior position. These results sug-gest that the interhemispheric fibers may be compromised in at least some hemispheric lesions. Additional evidence of such callosal compromise with hemispheric involvement can be found in an earlier article by Sparks et al. (1970). If you recall, these authors noted ipsilateral ear deficits for

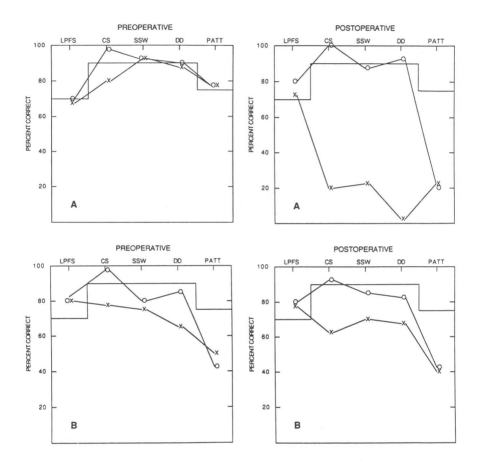

Figure 11.2. Panel A: Mean preoperative and postoperative scores for four patients with complete sections of the corpus callosum on five central auditory tests (LPFS: Low Pass Filtered Speech; CS: Competing Sentences; SSW: Staggered Spondaic Words; DD: Dichotic Digits; and PATT: Frequency Pattern Sequences). Data are presented for the right (O) and left (X) ears. The solid lines cutting across each of the individual figures indicate the lower limits of normal adult performance for each of these tests. (Adapted with permission from F. E. Musiek, K. Kibbe, & J. A. Baran, Neuroaudiological results from split-brain patients. *Seminars in Hearing, 5,* 219–229, © by Thieme Medical Publishers, New York, 1984.) Panel B: Mean preoperative and postoperative scores for eight patients with anterior sections of the corpus callosum. Specifications are the same as described for Panel A. (Adapted with permission from J. A. Baran, F. E. Musiek, & A. G. Reeves, Central auditory function following anterior sectioning of the corpus callosum. *Ear and Hearing, 7,* 359–362, © by Williams & Wilkins, Baltimore, 1986.)

a dichotic digits test in a number of patients with left hemisphere damage. It was suggested that the deficits were the result of deep left hemisphere lesions, which affected the callosal fibers crossing from the right hemisphere.

Ruebens and his associates (Ruebens, Froehling, Slater, & Anderson, 1985) demonstrated severe left ear deficits on dichotic listening tasks in a group of patients with multiple sclerosis. These investigators suggested that the left ear deficits were the result of demyelination of the interhemispheric fibers of the corpus callosum and supported this contention with CT scans demonstrating this callosal abnormality.

Essentially any type of cerebral lesion can compromise the interhemispheric auditory fibers. If only the white matter is involved the neuroaudiological profile should be similar to that of the split-brain patient. However, if a left hemispheric lesion affects both the grey (cortex) and white (corpus callosum) matter, a slightly different profile should emerge. In the latter case, dichotic scores should be abnormal for both ears. This bilateral deficit results from involvement of the left auditory cortex, which causes the classic contralateral right ear deficit and the presence of corpus callosum pathology, which disrupts the transfer of auditory information from the right to left hemisphere causing a left ear deficit. Monaural low-redundancy tasks, such as filtered speech, reveal only a contralateral right ear deficit. This occurs because this task does not require interhemispheric transfer of neural information for verbal report of left ear stimuli as the ipsilateral pathways are not suppressed. Frequency pattern results would reveal bilateral abnormalities because the necessary interhemispheric processing described above cannot be accomplished.

Cases of central auditory deafness

Though cases of central deafness are extremely rare, they can provide a valuable insight into central auditory function and its clinical correlates. Central deafness occurs when the auditory areas in both hemispheres are severely compromised. This type of bihemispheric compromise usually is caused by vascular lesions affecting the middle cerebral artery or one of its main branches. Though these patients do not respond behaviorally to sound, results of tests such as acoustic reflexes and ABRs usually are normal, suggesting normal peripheral auditory function.

In the late 1960s and early 1970s, Jerger and his associates (Jerger, Lovering, & Wertz, 1972; Jerger, Weikers, Sharbrough, & Jerger, 1969) presented audiologic test results for two subjects with tandem bilateral temporal lobe lesions. Both of these subjects demonstrated transient aphasia, but no hearing loss after an initial left-sided episode, and a severe hearing loss after a subsequent right-sided episode. In both cases, the hearing losses reportedly recovered within 3 months of the second episode; however, both subjects continued to demonstrate a marked inability to recognize words or sentences even under ideal listening conditions. Moreover, these investigators noted that if any type of distortion was introduced, recognition declined to near 0%.

Graham, Greenwood, and Lecky (1980) reported similar findings for a third patient who became completely deaf after bilateral temporal lobe embolisms. In addition, these authors provided a comprehensive review of the data presented in 12 earlier case reports. The common symptom noted in all these cases was an auditory agnosia for speech, that is, the patients were unable to comprehend the spoken words even though many of the subjects recognized the stimuli as speech.

Michel, Peronnet, and Schott (1980) reported a case of a 40-year-old male subject with bilateral temporoparietal lobe lesions who had central auditory disorders without aphasic disturbances. Their patient demonstrated deficits for speech recognition tasks, but he could read and write normally. In addition, they found absent late auditory evoked potentials bilaterally.

The foregoing review of the literature demonstrates the critical role that the central (cerebral) auditory mechanism plays in simple, as well as complex, hearing tasks. It also highlights the fact that deficits in audition to any degree can have either a peripheral or central origin. Therefore, the clinician must be alert to the possibility that what may appear to be an apparent peripheral hearing loss may in fact be the audiological manifestation of a central involvement.

Learning disabilities

Central auditory testing of the learning disabled (LD) child began to gain momentum in the early to mid 1970s. Prior to this time, clinical attention primarily was focused on the use of central auditory tests in the assessment of neurologically impaired adults. A great deal of the motivation for testing LD children came about as a result of the development of a test battery by Willeford (1976), which was specifically designed to assess central auditory processing abilities in young children. Here, rather than attempting to document the presence/absence of a lesion, the tests were used to assess the functional integrity of the CANS in an attempt to tease out deficits that could explain any difficulties that the child was having in terms of his or her academic, communicative, and/or social skills. In essence, the goal of central auditory testing with the LD child was to employ tests that would stress the auditory mechanisms at various levels of the CANS in order to identify weaknesses in the system (i.e., by demonstrating age/performance deficits) that could account for the child's problems. It is now commonly accepted that large numbers of children have subtle auditory deficits in spite of normal neurological test results. Therefore, the number of referrals for central auditory assessments has been steadily increasing over the past decade.

Many of the tests detailed in this chapter also have been used with children. Research on monotic low-redundancy tests has included LPFS (Willeford, 1976, 1977a, 1977b, 1980; Willeford & Billger, 1978), compressed speech (Freeman & Beasley, 1976; Orchik & Oelschlaeger, 1977; Willeford, 1975, 1980), speech-in-noise (McCroskey & Kasten, 1980; Willeford & Billger, 1978), and SSI-ICM (Jerger, 1980). Collectively, the results of these investigations have demonstrated (a) that performance on monaural low-redundancy tasks tends to improve with age, suggesting that these skills are maturational, (b) that there is little difference between the right and left ears on these tests, and (c) that there is considerable variability at each age level. Given these considerations, scores are typically considered abnormal only if the scores are severely depressed in one or both ears, or if there is a marked asymmetry between the scores of the two ears.

Dichotic speech tests administered to this population have included dichotic digits, (Musiek, Gollegly & Baran, 1984; Musiek & Geurkink, 1980; Musiek, Geurkink, & Keitel, 1982), staggered spondaic words (Dempsey, 1977, 1983; Musiek & Geurkink, 1980; Musiek et al., 1982; Musiek et al., 1984; Pinheiro, 1977; Protti, 1983; White, 1977; Sweitzer, 1977; Young, 1983), competing sentences (Dempsey, 1977, 1983; McCrosky & Kasten, 1980; Musiek & Geurkink, 1980; Musiek et al., 1982; Pinheiro, 1977; Protti, 1983; Protti & Young, 1980; Welsh, Welsh, & Healey, 1980; Willeford, 1977a, 1977b, 1978, 1980; Willeford & Billger, 1978; Young, 1983), and the SSI-CCM (Jerger, 1980). The results of these investigations have demonstrated an obvious right ear advantage on these dichotic tests in young children and that performance on these tests tends to improve with age. However, generally the more dramatic improvement is noted for the left ear, because even at early ages right ear performance tends to be high. For the most part, test results with LD children have demonstrated depressed left ear scores compared to age-appropriate norms, whereas right ear scores tend to be normal.

Frequency pattern sequences have also been used with children in order to assess the child's pattern perception and temporal sequencing abilities. Pinheiro (1977) demonstrated depressed scores in dyslexic children when she compared their performance to that of normal children on this task. Similar findings also have been reported by Musiek et al. (1982) and Musiek et al. (1984).

Finally, binaural fusion and rapidly alternating speech tests have been used to assess the binaural integration abilities of young children

(Musiek & Geurkink, 1980; Musiek et al., 1982; Willeford & Billger, 1978; Pinheiro, 1977). Results have shown that some children demonstrate difficulties on both tests with the BF test having a higher hit rate than the RASP test. Of all the tests mentioned thus far the RASP appears to be the least sensitive.

The research to date has suggested that the central auditory deficits noted in young children may be related to at least three different causes. Musiek et al. (1984) suggested that in a large number of children referred for testing, the etiology may be related to delays in the neuromaturational development of the CANS. Other investigators have implicated static diffuse neurological involvement (Musiek, Gollegly, & Ross, 1985), whereas others point out that the deficits noted in some children may be related to actual CANS lesions, similar to those noted in adults (Jerger, 1987; Jerger, Johnson, & Loiselle, 1988; Musiek et al., 1985). In addition, researchers have suggested that the central auditory processing disorders observed in many LD children may be differentiated on an auditory-specific perceptual and/or linguistic basis (Jerger et al., 1988).

It is important to note that when testing an LD child it is essential that a variety of tests be used. In many of the studies mentioned above where more than one test was administered, a given child may have performed abnormally on one test and normally on a second test. It is, therefore, important that the audiologist who is attempting to assess these children select tests that assess different processes. It also is important that he or she take into consideration the age appropriateness of the tests to be used and how sensitive the tests may be for a given age group. Recently we have begun testing college-age LD students and have found that some tests, such as compressed speech, which may be sensitive to deficits at younger ages, are not practically useful in the assessment of older students, whereas other tests such as frequency pattern sequences and speech-in-noise testing are more diagnostically useful (Baran & Owen, 1986).

The elderly

The influence of aging on CANS functioning is not well-documented. Much of the reason for this lack of documentation lies in the fact that there are various sites of aging effects in the elderly client, which can complicate the assessment of this individual. For example, Schuknecht (1964, 1974) identified four distinct types of presbycusis. These include (a) sensory presbycusis, related to atrophy of the Organ of Corti and degeneration of the hair cells beginning at the basal end of the cochlea moving toward the apex, (b) neural presbycusis, related to loss of neurons in the auditory pathways and the eighth nerve, (c) stria vascularis atrophy or metabolic presbycusis, related to the degeneration of the stria vascularis in the apical turn of the cochlea, and (d) inner ear conductive-type presbycusis, which probably is related to an increase in the stiffness of the supporting structures of the cochlear duct. These various pathologies manifest themselves in different audiometric configurations, and often more than one may coexist at the same time. Matters are complicated further by the fact that although the binaural hearing thresholds may appear to be similar, both ears may not have the same capacity at suprathreshold levels. Recruitment and problems related to temporal factors may be present. Therefore, one must be aware of the potential confounding effects of a peripheral hearing loss on the central auditory tests being used.

With the elderly client the audiologist may not only be dealing with a cochlear hearing loss but also with a central disability that is not related to a brain lesion. In many presbycusic losses, the central auditory structures, as well as the peripheral hearing mechanisms, are involved. Senile changes in the CANS have been reported for both brainstem and cortical structures (Brody, 1955; Kirikae, Sato, & Shitara, 1964; Smith & Sethi, 1975). In the older patient, central auditory function may be depressed by a general loss of neurons throughout the CANS. Blood flow may be reduced by fatty deposits in the arteries supplying the brain. There may also be age-related changes in the cerebral metabolism that do not affect peripheral hearing. Glucose metabolism and oxygen consumption decrease with aging. The problem that faces the audiologist attempting to conduct central auditory testing with elderly clients is how to account for these differences and their effects on CANS function, which appear to be primarily physiological and not chronological. Therefore, establishing norms by chronological age will not necessarily solve the problem.

There have been a few attempts to study CANS function in the geriatric population. Investigations of elderly patients with no known central lesions demonstrated higher percentages of abnormal findings on LPFS (Bocca, 1958; Bergman, 1980; Kirikae et al., 1964), time compressed or accelerated speech (Calearo & Lazzaroni, 1957; Konkle, Beasley, & Bess, 1977; Sticht & Gray, 1969), SSI (Jerger & Hayes, 1977), MLDs (Findlay & Schuchman, 1976; Tillman, Carhart, & Nicholls, 1973), dichotic nonsense syllables (Dermody, 1975, Kurdziel & Noffsinger, 1977), and interrupted speech (Antonelli, 1970; Bocca, 1958; Bergman, 1971; Kirikae et al., 1964).

The foregoing test results implicate a reduction in the efficiency with which the aging CANS processes difficult auditory stimuli. In addition, the evidence provided in these investigations suggests that this reduced capacity or efficiency is present throughout the CANS from the brainstem to the cortex and the interhemispheric pathways, and that many of these degenerative changes may occur in some individuals as early as the sixth decade of life. Generally, the degenerative changes due to aging are manifest as bilateral deficits on those tests where individual ear scores are obtained. However, ear differences also may occur. If they do, the size of these interaural differences is usually small compared to the general deficit noted for both ears.

The ability to differentiate between age effects and pathological effects is of considerable importance when a clinician is evaluating the elderly client. The differentiation is a relatively easy one to make when age-independent effects manifest themselves in only one ear, because senile changes due to aging alone tend to manifest themselves bilaterally. Unfortunately, widespread CANS disease, some cortical lesions, and some brainstem lesions may also manifest themselves bilaterally. In these cases a clear differentiation of the effects due to aging and those due to a lesion is difficult, if not impossible, to make.

Differentiation of peripheral, brainstem, and cerebral lesions

Effects of peripheral hearing loss

This section is perhaps the most difficult to discuss in this chapter. The best situation for defining a central lesion is to have a patient with normal peripheral hearing. Though this situation does occur in many cases, in many other cases it does not, and one either has to bypass central testing or in some way account for the potential confounding effects of the peripheral hearing loss. It is fair to say that peripheral hearing loss has some effect on practically all central (behavioral) tests. However, some central procedures are affected more by peripheral hearing losses than others. Miltenberger, Dawson, and Raica (1978) showed that filtered speech scores were often abnormal for patients with peripheral hearing loss. Speaks, Niccum, and Van Tassel (1985) reported on the effects of sensorineural hearing loss on dichotic digits, words, and CVs. The digits were found to be influenced the least, whereas CVs were affected the most by deficits in hearing. Fifer et al., (1983) demonstrated that the dichotic sentence identification test was affected less by peripheral loss than several other tests. The frequency pattern sequences test and the auditory duration patterns test also have been shown to be relatively resistant to cochlear hearing loss (Baran et al., 1987; Musiek & Pinheiro, 1987). Generally, the greater the hearing loss, the greater the effect on central tests (Fifer et al., 1983). However, it is difficult to predict for a given individual how much the degree of hearing loss will affect central auditory test results; hence, great caution is suggested. Seldom do we administer central tests to patients with more than a mild bilaterally symmetrical hearing loss and similar speech recognition scores for both ears.

There are some situations in which central interpretation with hearing loss can be made with some degree of confidence. If the hearing loss is bilaterally symmetrical (mild degree) and central test scores are markedly depressed in one ear, then central involvement is a distinct possibility. Also, if one does test an individual with an asymmetrical hearing loss and the central test scores are markedly poorer in the better hearing ear, then central dysfunction is a possibility. If patients with peripheral hearing loss are to be assessed, it is suggested that tests that are most resistant to hearing loss be selected and that the margin for interpretation error be generous!

Need for a test battery

Few behavioral tests can differentiate brainstem from cerebral lesions. As mentioned earlier, MLDs are primarily a test of caudal brainstem function and are not influenced by lesions of the cortex (Lynn et al., 1981). The SSI-ICM is reported to be more affected by brainstem than cerebral lesions (Jerger & Jerger, 1974). Therefore, for patients with good hearing sensitivity and poor scores on either of these two tests, the inference is brainstem involvement. Few other behavioral tests offer much in terms of brainstem/cerebral differentiation. However, the addition of electrophysiological tests into a test battery can be of considerable help. The central auditory nervous system is highly redundant and complex; therefore, the use of a test battery is both prudent and necessary. It is important to select highly sensitive, as well as highly different, tests. Different tests assess different processes, and this is key in identifying dysfunction in a highly redundant system. Background information, both medical and audiological, may provide insight as to whether it is a brainstem or cerebral lesion. If this insight is gained then one can "bias" his or her battery. If a cerebral lesion is expected or needs to be ruled out, a temporal ordering task (e.g., patterns), a dichotic task (digits or CVs or SSW or DSI), and a low-redundancy monaural speech task (e.g., compressed speech) could be used. If a brainstem lesion is suspected, MLDs and SSI-ICM should be included (also ABR and acoustic reflexes). If the clinician is unsure of which way to bias the test selection, it is wise for him or her to use some tests from each category.

Case illustrations

The first case (Figure 11.3) involves a 69-year-old woman with a left-sided brainstem tumor. The lesion was positioned at the lateral aspect of the low to mid pons. Though this patient did have a mild to moderate sensorineural loss, it was bilaterally symmetrical. The results of three dichotic speech tests (staggered spondaic words, competing sentences, and dichotic digits) revealed markedly depressed left ear scores, though all dichotic scores were found to be depressed bilaterally. Given that the audiogram was bilaterally symmetrical, the marked difference between the two ears on these central tests would not be expected unless there was central involvement. Frequency pattern test results were normal bilaterally. These findings are consistent with what was mentioned in the text; that is, frequency patterns are not highly sensitive to brainstem lesions and are often not affected by mild to moderate hearing loss.

The second case (Figure 11.4) is one demonstrating the classical contralateral ear effect. This teenage boy had a large lesion involving the left thalamus and medial segments of the left hemisphere. Involvement of the auditory radiations from the medial geniculate bodies was highly

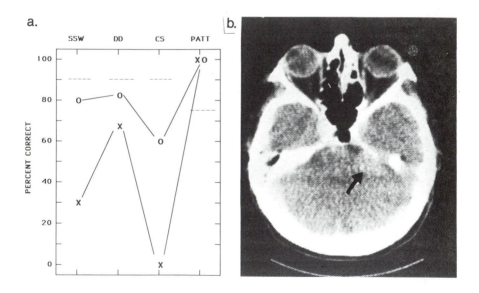

Figure 11.3. Panel A: Central auditory test results for a 69-year-old woman with a mild-to-moderate bilaterally symmetrical sensorineural hearing loss and a left-sided brainstem tumor. Data are presented for four central auditory tests (SSW: Staggered Spondaic Words; DD: Dichotic Digits; CS: Competing Sentences; and PATT: Frequency Pattern Sequences) and for the right (O) and left (X) ears. The dashed lines represent the lower limits of normal adult performance on these tests. Panel B: CT scan for the subject described in Panel A, documenting the presence of a left-sided brainstem tumor located at the lateral aspect of the low to mid pons.

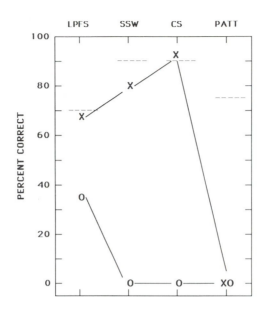

Figure 11.4. Central auditory test results for a teenage boy with normal peripheral auditory test results and a large lesion involving the left thalamus and medial segments of the left hemisphere. Data are presented for four central auditory tests (LPFS: Low Pass Filtered Speech; SSW: Staggered Spondaic Words; CS: Competing Sentences; and PATT: Frequency Pattern Sequences) and for the right (O) and left (X) ears. The dashed lines represent the lower limits of normal adult performance on these tests.

probable. In this case and all subsequent cases, peripheral auditory function was found to be normal. Severe right ear deficits are noted for the two dichotic speech tests (staggered spondaic words and competing sentences). Also, a right ear deficit is noted on the monaural low-redundancy speech test (low pass filtered speech). Frequency pattern test results show bilateral deficits even though only one hemisphere is compromised. This bilaterally depressed score is common with this test in that it is believed both hemispheres must be intact to perform normally on this test (see text for further explanation).

The third case (Figure 11.5) is a woman in her mid forties with a mid, right temporal lobe involvement. Again, a contralateral ear effect is noted for compressed speech and dichotic digits, and though the left ear is worse than the right on frequency patterns, both ears are below normal.

The fourth case (Figure 11.6) is another example of the contralateral ear effect. This case involves a 27-year-old male with a left hemisphere stroke primarily affecting the temporal lobe. Test results are depressed

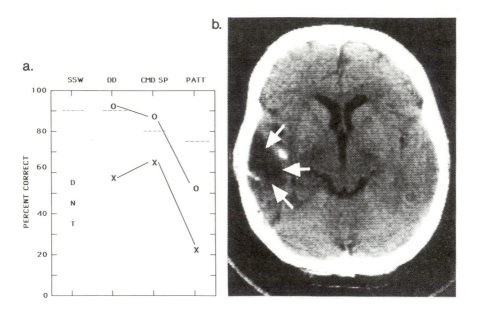

Figure 11.5.   Panel A: Central auditory test results for a woman in her mid forties with normal peripheral auditory test results and a right temporal lobe resection secondary to a tumor. Data are presented for three central auditory tests (DD: Dichotic Digits; CMD SP: Compressed Speech; and PATT: Frequency Pattern Sequences) and for the right (O) and left (X) ears. The dashed lines represent the lower limits of normal adult performance on these tests. Panel B: CT scan documenting the right hemisphere involvement for the subject described in Panel A.

for the contralateral right ear on the staggered spondaic word and competing sentence tests. In addition, a frequency pattern test score obtained in the sound field was found to be moderately depressed. Results for a monaural low-redundancy test (low pass filtered speech) fell within normal limits bilaterally; however, a sizable difference was noted between the performance of the two ears, favoring the left ear.

The fifth case (Figure 11.7) portrays test results for a young woman who had bilateral involvement of both temporal lobes. Note that all central tests (compressed speech, low pass filtered speech, dichotic digits, and frequency pattern sequences) revealed bilaterally reduced scores heralding the consideration of bilateral hemispheric problems.

The sixth case (Figure 11.8) involves a teenage boy with a large lesion involving the cortex and corpus callosum fibers in the left hemisphere. It is evident that all dichotic tests (competing sentences, staggered spondaic words, and dichotic digits) and frequency patterns demonstrate

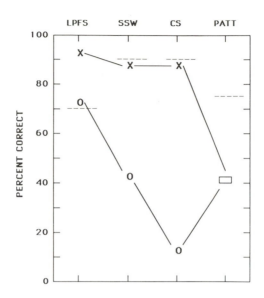

Figure 11.6. Central auditory test results for a 27-year-old man with normal peripheral auditory test results and a left hemisphere stroke primarily affecting the temporal lobe. Data are presented for four central auditory tests (LPFS: Low Pass Filtered Speech; SSW: Staggered Spondaic Words; CS: Competing Sentences; and PATT: Frequency Pattern Sequences) and for the right (O) and left (X) ears. Note that the Frequency Pattern Sequence test results are presented for the sound-field condition (□). The dashed lines represent the lower limits of normal adult performance.

bilateral deficits, whereas only low pass filtered speech results show the contralateral ear effect. The dichotic tests are bilaterally depressed because, as explained in the text, these tests require intact callosal fibers as well as an intact cortex. Filtered speech responses do not require an intact corpus callosum and therefore reflect only the compromise of the left cortex by a contralateral (right) ear deficit.

The foregoing illustrative cases attest to the fact that behavioral central auditory tests can be useful in the identification of CANS pathology, but they may not be particularly useful in the identification of the exact location of a CANS lesion. At the present time there is no evidence establishing a direct relationship between CANS test results and site of CANS pathology. Therefore, the clinician must proceed cautiously when attempting to interpret CANS test results.

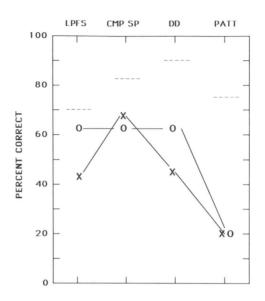

Figure 11.7. Central auditory test results for a young woman with normal peripheral auditory test results and bilateral temporal lobe epilepsy and slight cortical atrophy. Data are presented for four central auditory tests (LPFS: Low Pass Filtered Speech; CMD SP: Compressed Speech; DD: Dichotic Digits; and PATT: Frequency Pattern Sequences) and for the right (O) and left (X) ears. The dashed lines represent the lower limits of normal adult performance.

Concluding remarks

In this chapter we have attempted to highlight the major developments in the field of behavioral assessment of CANS function. This field is relatively new and remains challenging, both to the clinician and to the researcher. Major strides in the assessment of CANS disorders have occurred since the time of Bocca and his colleagues' introduction of LPFS as a CANS assessment tool. Unfortunately, lack of standardization of test procedures, test stimuli, and other related variables, along with often poorly defined subject populations and a paucity of published normative data have limited the usefulness of much of these data. Comparison of test data across research investigations and clinical reports is often difficult, if not impossible to make.

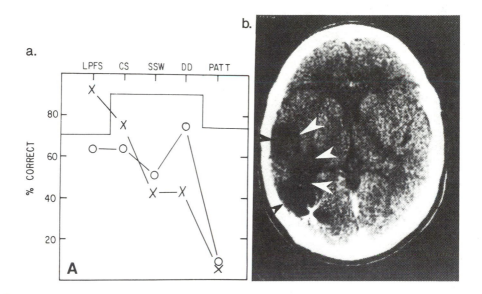

Figure 11.8.   Panel A: Central auditory test results for a teenage boy with normal peripheral hearing and a large left temporal-parietal tumor involving the auditory cortex and corpus callosum. Data are presented for five central auditory tests (LPFS: Low Pass Filtered Speech; CS: Competing Sentences; SSW: Staggered Spondaic Words; DD: Dichotic Digits; and PATT: Frequency Pattern Sequences) and for the right (O) and left (X) ears. The solid line cutting across the upper portion of this figure delineates the lower limits of normal adult performance for each of the central auditory tests. Panel B: CT scan documenting the location of the lesion described in Panel A. (Reprinted with permission from F. E. Musiek & J. A. Baran, Central auditory assessment: Thirty years of challenge and change, *Ear and Hearing, 8,* 22S–35S, © by Williams & Wilkins, Baltimore, 1987.)

Implications for the future and research needs

What is sorely needed at this time is some consensus among researchers and clinicians as to which test protocols and test procedures should be employed when assessing potential CANS disorders. Standardization of procedures and more published normative data should help to advance the field. In addition, more information is needed regarding the sensitivity and specificity of the tests, or test batteries, that we currently use, or will use in the future. In the interest of cost-effectiveness, the clinician needs to develop a test battery that is economical to administer, yet sensitive to the various CANS lesions that he or she is likely to encounter. Careful consideration of some behavioral tests may indicate that they lack the sensitivity needed to be included as a routine part of every test battery. For instance, RASP and BF, both of which appear to have low "hit rates" may be dropped from a test battery and a test such as ABR included, particularly if a low brainstem lesion is suspected.

Also, as mentioned earlier in this chapter, it is important that clinicians and researchers involved in CANS assessments gain a better understanding of the neuroanatomy and neurophysiology of the CANS. Unfortunately, many individuals involved in CANS assessments lack in-depth knowledge of the system. Without this knowledge, inaccurate assessments or misleading research interpretations may result.

Additional studies also should be conducted in order to look at the "hit rates" of some of the tests already studied. Clinicians need to be cognizant of the fact that there is a considerable amount of variability in the subjects being tested. Factors such as size of a lesion, location of lesion, age of onset, time of testing post onset, attention, and motivational factors all can affect test results. Therefore, it is likely that if one were to test the same subject population on two different dates, the results would be different.

To date, most of the studies reported in the literature have been prospective studies, where the clinician/researcher was aware of the location and extent of the lesion prior to testing. More investigations are needed in which the clinician/researcher is blind to the presence/absence of a lesion and its location in order to determine if central auditory tests are useful in the diagnosis of CANS disorders. Also, through the introduction of new diagnostic procedures, such as magnetic resonance imaging (MRI), we may be able to define the location and extent of CANS and ultimately make more accurate correlations to CANS test results.

Finally, with the advent of sophisticated computer technology, many of the CANS tests that have been used to date should be redesigned and restudied. For example, in the case of dichotic speech tests in which the alignment of the signals is vitally important in terms of making the test a truly dichotic test, the use of computer technology should help to make the onsets and offsets of the signals simultaneous. If this can be achieved, then we are likely to see improved sensitivities for these tests.

References

Antonelli, A. (1970). Sensitized speech tests in aged people. In C. Rojskjaer (Ed.), *Speech audiometry* (pp. 66–77). Odennse, Denmark: Danavox Foundation.
Antonelli, A., Bellotto, R., & Grandori, F. (1987). Audiologic diagnosis of central versus VIII nerve and cochlear impairment. *Audiology, 26,* 209–226.

Baran, J. A., Musiek, F. E., Gollegly, K. M., Verkest, S. B., & Kibbe-Michal, K. S. (1987, November). *Auditory duration pattern sequences in the assessment of CANS pathology*. Paper presented at the annual meeting of the American Speech-Language-Hearing Association, New Orleans.

Baran, J. A., Musiek, F. E., & Reeves, A. G. (1986). Central auditory function following anterior sectioning of the corpus callosum. *Ear and Hearing, 7*, 359–362.

Baran, J. A., & Owen, G. A. (1986). *Central auditory test results in college age learning disabled students*. Paper presented at the annual meeting of the American Speech-Language-Hearing Association, Detroit.

Baran, J. A., Verkest, S., Gollegly, K., Kibbe-Michal, K., Rintelmann, W. F., & Musiek, F. E. (1985, November). *Use of time-compressed speech in the assessment of central nervous system disorders*. Paper presented at the 110th meeting of the Acoustical Society of America, Nashville.

Beasley, D. S., Forman, B., & Rintelmann, W. F. (1972). Perception of time-compressed CNC monosyllables by normal listeners. *Journal of Auditory Research, 12*, 71–75.

Beasley, D. S., & Maki, J. (1976). Time- and frequency-altered speech. In N. Lass (Ed.), *Contemporary issues in experimental phonetics* (pp. 419–458). New York: Academic Press.

Beasley, D. S., Schwimmer, S., & Rintelmann, W. F. (1972). Intelligibility of time-compressed CNC monosyllables. *Journal of Speech and Hearing Research, 15*, 340–350.

Belmont, I., & Handler, A. (1971). Delayed information processing and judgment of temporal order following cerebral damage. *Journal of Nervous and Mental Disease, 152*, 353–361.

Bergman, M. (1971). Hearing and aging: Implications of recent research findings. *Audiology, 10*, 164–171.

Bergman, M. (1980). *Aging and the perception of speech*. Baltimore: University Park Press.

Bergman, M., Hirsch, S., Solzi, P., & Mankowitz, Z. (1987). The Threshold-of-Interference Test: A new test of interhemispheric suppression in brain injury. *Ear and Hearing, 8*, 147–150.

Berlin, C., Cullen, J., Berlin, H., Tobey, E., & Mouney, D. (1975, November). *Dichotic listening in a patient with a presumed lesion in the region of the medial geniculate bodies*. Paper presented at the 90th meeting of the Acoustical Society of America, San Francisco.

Berlin, C. L., Cullen, J. K., Hughes, L. F., Berlin, J. L., Lowe-Bell, S. S., & Thompson, C. L. (1975). Dichotic processing of speech: Acoustic and phonetic variables. In M. D. Sullivan (Ed.), *Central auditory processing disorders* (pp. 36–46). Proceedings of a Conference at the University of Nebraska Medical Center, Omaha.

Berlin, C. L., Lowe-Bell, S. S., Jannetta, P. J., & Kline, D. G. (1972). Central auditory deficits after temporal lobectomy. *Archives of Otolaryngology, 96*, 4–10.

Blaettner, U., Scherg, M., & Von Cramon, D. (1989). Diagnosis of unilateral telencephalic hearing disorders: Evaluation of a simple psychoacoustic pattern discrimination test. *Brain, 112*, 177–195.

Bocca, E. (1958). Clinical aspects of cortical deafness. *Laryngoscope, 68*, 301–309.

Bocca, E., & Calearo, C. (1963). Central hearing processes. In J. Jerger (Ed.), *Modern developments in audiology* (pp.337–370). New York: Academic Press.

Bocca, E., Calearo, C., & Cassinari, V. (1954). A new method for testing hearing in temporal lobe tumors. *Acta Oto-Laryngologica, 42,* 289–304.

Bocca, E., Calearo, C., Cassinari, V., & Migliavacca, F. (1955). Testing "cortical" hearing in temporal lobe tumors. *Acta Oto-Laryngologica, 42,* 289–304.

Brody, H. (1955). Organization of cerebral cortex: III. A study of aging in human cerebral cortex. *Journal of Comparative Neurology, 102,* 511–556.

Brunt, M. A. (1978). The staggered spondaic word test. In J. Katz (Ed.), *Handbook of clinical audiology* (pp. 334–356). Baltimore: Williams & Wilkins.

Calearo, C., & Antonelli, A. R. (1968). Audiometric findings in brainstem lesions. *Acta Oto-Laryngologica, 66,* 305–319.

Calearo, C., & Lazzaroni, A. (1957). Speech intelligibility in relation to the speed of the message. *Laryngoscope, 67,* 410–419.

Carmon, A., & Nachshon, I. (1971). Effect of unilateral brain damage on perception of temporal order. *Cortex, 7,* 410–418.

Damasio, H., & Damasio, A. (1979). Paradoxic ear extinction in dichotic listening: Possible anatomic significance. *Neurology, 29,* 644–653.

Dayal, V. S., Tarantino, L., & Swisher, L. P. (1966). Neuro-otologic studies in multiple sclerosis. *Laryngoscope, 76,* 1798–1809.

Dempsey, C. (1977). Some thoughts concerning alternate explanations of central auditory test results. In R. Keith (Ed.), *Central auditory dysfunction* (pp. 293–318). New York: Grune & Stratton.

Dempsey, C. (1983). Selecting tests of auditory function in children. In E. Lasky & J. Katz (Eds.), *Central auditory processing disorders* (pp. 203–222). Baltimore: University Park Press.

de Quiros, J. (1964). Accelerated speech audiometry, an examination of test results. (Trans. by J. Tonndorf). *Transactions of the Beltone Institute of Hearing Research, 17,* 48.

DeRenzi, E., Faglioni, P., & Villa, P. (1977). Sequential memory for figures in brain-damaged patients. *Neuropsychologia, 15,* 43–49.

Dermody, P. (1976, April). *Auditory processing factors in dichotic listening.* Paper presented at the 91st meeting of the Acoustical Society of America, Washington, DC.

Divenyi, P. L., & Robinson, A. J. (1989). Nonlinguistic auditory capabilities in aphasia. *Brain and Language, 37,* 290–326.

Durlach, N. I., & Colburn, H. S. (1978). Binaural phenomena. In E. C. Carterette & M. P. Friedman (Eds.), *Handbook of perception* (Vol. 4, pp. 365–466). New York: Academic Press.

Efron, R. (1985). The central auditory system and issues related to hemispheric specialization. In M. L. Pinheiro & F. E. Musiek (Eds.), *Assessment of central auditory dysfunction: Foundations and clinical correlates* (pp. 143–154). Baltimore: Williams & Wilkins.

Efron, R., & Crandall, P. H. (1983). Central auditory processing: Effects of anterior temporal lobectomy. *Brain and Language, 19,* 237–253.

Efron, R., Crandall, P. H., Koss, D., Divenyi, P. L., & Yund, E. W. (1983). Central auditory processing: III. The "Cocktail Party" effect and anterior temporal lobectomy. *Brain and Language, 19,* 254–263.

Efron, R., Dennis, M., & Yund, E. W. (1977). The perception of dichotic chords by hemispherectomized subjects. *Brain and Language, 4,* 537–549.

Efron, R., Yund, E. W., Nichols, D., & Crandall, P. H. (1985). An ear asymmetry for gap detection following anterior temporal lobectomy. *Neuropsychologia, 23,* 43–50.

Fairbanks, G., Everitt, W., & Jaeger, R. (1954). Methods for time or frequency compression-expansion of speech. *Trans IRE-PGA, AU-2,* 7–12.

Fifer, R., Jerger, J., Berlin C., Tobey, E., & Campbell, J. (1983). Development of a dichotic sentence identification test for hearing impaired adults. *Ear and Hearing, 4,* 300–305.

Findlay, R. C., & Schuchman, G. I. (1976). Masking level differences for speech: Effects of ear dominance and age. *Audiology, 15,* 232–241.

Freeman, B., & Beasley, D. (1976, November). *Performance of reading-impaired and normal reading children on time-compressed monosyllabic and sentential stimuli.* Paper presented at the annual meeting of the American Speech-Language-Hearing Association, Houston.

Gazzaniga, M. S., Risse, G., Springer, S., Clark, E., & Wilson, D. H. (1975). Psychological and neurological consequences of partial and complete commissurotomy. *Neurology, 25,* 10–15.

Gilroy, J., & Lynn, G. E. (1974). Reversibility of abnormal auditory findings in cerebral hemisphere lesions. *Journal of Neurological Sciences, 21,* 117–131.

Graham, J., Greenwood, R., & Lecky, B. (1980). Cortical deafness: A case report and review of the literature. *Journal of Neurological Sciences, 48,* 35–49.

Green, D. M. (1966). Interaural phase effects in the masking of signals of different durations. *Journal of the Acoustical Society of America, 39,* 720–724.

Heilman, K. M., Hammer, L. C., & Wilder, B. J. (1973). An audiometric defect in temporal lobe dysfunction. *Neurology, 23,* 384–386.

Hirsh, I. J. (1948). The influence of interaural phase on interaural summation and inhibition. *Journal of the Acoustical Society of America, 20,* 536–544.

Hodgson, W. (1967). Audiological report of a patient with left hemispherectomy. *Journal of Speech and Hearing Disorders, 32,* 39–45.

Jerger, J. (1960a). Audiological manifestations of lesions in the auditory nervous system. *Laryngoscope, 70,* 417–425.

Jerger, J. (1960b). Observations on auditory behavior in lesions of the central auditory pathways. *Archives of Otolaryngology, 71,* 797–806.

Jerger, J. (1964). Auditory tests for disorders of the central auditory mechanism. In B. R. Alford & W. S. Fields (Eds.), *Neurological aspects of auditory and vestibular disorders* (pp.77–86). Springfield, IL: Charles C. Thomas.

Jerger, J. (1973). Diagnostic audiometry. In J. Jerger (Ed.), *Modern developments in audiology* (pp.75–115). New York: Academic Press.

Jerger, J., & Jerger, S. (1971). Diagnostic significance of PB word functions. *Archives of Otolaryngology, 93,* 573–580.

Jerger, J. F., & Jerger, S. W. (1974). Auditory findings in brainstem disorders. *Archives of Otolaryngology, 99,* 342–349.

Jerger, J. F., & Jerger, S. W. (1975). Clinical validity of central auditory tests. *Scandinavian Audiology, 4,* 147–163.

Jerger, J., & Jerger, S. (1981). *Auditory disorders: A manual for clinical evaluation.* Boston: Little & Brown.

Jerger, J., & Hayes, D. (1977). Diagnostic speech audiometry. *Archives of Otolaryngology, 103,* 216–222.

Jerger, J., Lovering, L., & Wertz, M. (1972). Auditory disorder following bilateral temporal lobe insult: Report of a case. *Journal of Speech and Hearing Disorders, 37,* 532–535.

Jerger, J., Weikers, N. J., Sharbrough, F. W., & Jerger, S. (1969). Bilateral lesions of the temporal lobe: A case study. *Acta-Otolaryngologica, 258* (Supplement), 1–57.

Jerger, S. (1980). Evaluation of central auditory function in children. In R. Keith (Ed.), *Central auditory and language disorders in children* (pp.30–60). Houston, TX: College-Hill Press.

Jerger, S. (1987). Validation of the pediatric speech intelligibility test in children with central nervous system lesions. *Audiology, 26,* 298–311.

Jerger, S., Johnson, K., & Loiselle, L. (1988). Pediatric central auditory dysfunction: Comparison of children with confirmed lesions versus suspected processing disorders. *The American Journal of Otology, 9* (Supplement), 63–71.

Karaseva, T. A. (1972). The role of the temporal lobe in human auditory perception. *Neuropsychologia, 10,* 227–231.

Katz, J. (1962). The use of staggered spondaic words for assessing the integrity of the central auditory system. *Journal of Auditory Research, 2,* 327–337.

Katz, J. (1968). The SSW test: An interim report. *Journal of Speech and Hearing Disorders, 33,* 132–146.

Katz, J. (1970). Audiologic diagnosis: Cochlea to cortex. *Menorah Medical Journal, 1,* 25–38.

Katz, J. (1977). The staggered spondaic word test. In R. Keith (Ed.), *Central auditory dysfunction* (pp. 103–128). New York: Grune & Stratton.

Katz, J., Basil, R. A., & Smith, J. M. (1963). A staggered spondaic word test for detecting central auditory lesions. *Annals of Otology, Rhinology, and Laryngology, 72,* 906–917.

Katz, J., & Pack, G. (1975). New developments in differential diagnosis using the SSW test. In M. D. Sullivan (Ed.), *Central auditory processing disorders* (pp. 84–107). Proceedings of a conference at the University of Nebraska Medical Center, Omaha.

Keith, R. (1977). Synthetic sentence identification test. In R. W. Keith (Ed.), *Central auditory dysfunction* (pp. 73–102). New York: Grune & Stratton.

Kimura, D. (1961a). Cerebral dominance and the perception of verbal stimuli. *Canadian Journal of Psychology, 15,* 166–171.

Kimura, D. (1961b). Some effects of temporal lobe damage on auditory perception. *Canadian Journal of Psychology, 15,* 157–165.

Kirikae, I., Sato, T., & Shitara, T. (1964). A study of hearing in advanced age. *Laryngoscope, 74,* 205–220.

Konkle, D. F., Beasley, D. S., & Bess, F. (1977). Intelligibility of time-altered speech in relation to chronological aging. *Journal of Speech and Hearing Research, 20,* 108–115.

Korsan-Bengtsen, M. (1973). Distorted speech audiometry: A methodological and clinical study. *Acta Oto-Laryngologica (Stockholm), 310* (Supplement), 7–75.

Kurdziel, S., & Noffsinger, D. (1977, November). *Unusual time-staggering effects via dichotic listening with aged subjects.* Paper presented at the annual meeting of the American Speech and Hearing Association, Chicago.

Kurdziel, S., Noffsinger, D., & Olsen, W. (1976). Performance by cortical lesion patients on 40% and 60% time-compressed materials. *Journal of the American Audiological Society, 2,* 3–7.

Lackner, J., & Teuber, H. L. (1973). Alterations in auditory fusion thresholds after cerebral injury in man. *Neuropsychologia, 11,* 409–415.

Lhermitte, F., Chain, F., Escourolle, R., Ducarne, B., Pillou, B., & Chedru, G. (1971). Etude des troubles perceptifs auditifs dans les lesions temporales bilaterales. [Study of the auditory perceptual problems in bilateral temporal lobe lesions]. *Revue Neurologique, 124,* 329–351.

Licklider, J. C. R. (1948). The influence of interaural phase relationships upon the masking of speech by white noise. *Journal of the Acoustical Society of America, 20,* 150–159.

Linden, A. (1964). Distorted speech and binaural speech resynthesis tests. *Acta Oto-Laryngologica (Stockholm), 58,* 32–48.

Lynn, G. E., Benitez, J. T., Eisenbrey, A. B., Gilroy, J., & Wilner, H. I. (1972). Neuroaudiological correlates in cerebral hemisphere lesions: Temporal and parietal lobe tumors. *Audiology: Journal of Auditory Communication, 11,* 115–134.

Lynn, G. E., & Gilroy, J. (1971). Auditory manifestations of lesions of the corpus callosum. *Asha, 13,* 566.

Lynn, G. E., & Gilroy, J. (1972). Neuro-audiological abnormalities in patients with temporal lobe tumors. *Journal of Neurological Sciences, 17,* 167–184.

Lynn, G. E., & Gilroy, J. (1975). Effects of brain lesions on the perception of monotic and dichotic speech stimuli. In M. D. Sullivan (Ed.), *Central auditory processing disorders* (pp. 47–83). Proceedings of a conference at the University of Nebraska, Omaha.

Lynn, G. E., & Gilroy, J. (1976). Central aspects of audition. In J. Northern (Ed.), *Hearing disorders* (pp. 102–116). Boston: Little & Brown.

Lynn, G. E., & Gilroy, J. (1977). Evaluation of central auditory dysfunction in patients with neurological disorders. In R. W. Keith (Ed.), *Central auditory dysfunction* (pp. 177–221). New York: Grune & Stratton.

Lynn, G. E., Gilroy, J., Taylor, P. C., & Leiser, R. P. (1981). Binaural masking-level differences in neurological disorders. *Archives of Otolaryngology, 107,* 357–362.

Matzker, J. (1959). Two methods for the assessment of central auditory functions in cases of brain disease. *Annals of Otology, Rhinology and Laryngology, 68,* 1155–1197.

McClellen, M., Wertz, R., & Collins, M. (1983, November). *The effects of inter-hemispheric lesions on central auditory behavior.* Paper presented at the annual meeting of the American Speech-Language-Hearing Association, Detroit.

McCroskey, R., & Kasten, R. (1980). Assessment of central auditory processing. In R. Rupp & K. Stockdell (Eds.), *Speech protocols in audiology* (pp. 339–390). New York: Grune & Stratton.

McFadden, D. (1966). Masking-level differences with continuous and with burst masking noise. *Journal of the Acoustical Society of America, 40,* 1414–1419.

Michel, F., Peronnet, F., & Schott, B. (1980). A case of cortical deafness: Clinical and electrophysiological data. *Brain and Language, 10,* 367–377.

Milner, B. (1962). Laterality effects in audition. In V. B. Mountcastle (Ed.), *Inter-hemispheric relations and cerebral dominance* (pp. 177–195). Baltimore: John Hopkins Press.

Milner, B., Kimura, D., & Taylor, L. B. (1965, April). *Nonverbal auditory learning after frontal or temporal lobectomy in man.* Paper presented at the annual meeting of the Eastern Psychological Association, Boston.

Milner, B., Taylor, S., & Sperry, R. (1968). Lateralized suppression of dichotically presented digits after commissural section in man. *Science, 161,* 184–185.

Miltenberger, G., Dawson, G., & Raica, A. (1978). Central auditory testing with peripheral hearing loss. *Archives of Otolaryngology, 104,* 11–15.

Morales-Garcia C., & Poole, J. O. (1972). Masked speech audiometry in central deafness. *Acta Oto-Laryngologica, 74,* 307–316.

Mueller, H. G., Beck, W. G., & Sedge, R. K. (1987). Comparison of the efficiency of cortical level speech tests. *Seminars in Hearing, 8,* 279–298.

Mueller, H. G., Sedge, R. K., & Salazar, A. M. (1985). Auditory assessment of neural trauma. In M. Miner & K. Wagner (Eds.), *Neural trauma: Treatment, monitoring and rehabilitation issues* (pp. 155–188). Stoneham, MA: Butterworth.

Musiek, F. E. (1983a). Assessment of central auditory dysfunction: The dichotic digit test revisited. *Ear and Hearing, 4*, 79–83.

Musiek, F. E. (1983b). Assessment of three dichotic speech tests on subjects with intracranial lesions. *Ear and Hearing, 4*, 318–323.

Musiek, F. E. (1983c). The evaluation of brainstem disorders using ABR and central auditory tests. *Monographs in Contemporary Audiology, 4*, 1–24.

Musiek, F. E. (1986a). Neuroanatomy, neurophysiology, and central auditory assessment. Part II: The cerebrum. *Ear and Hearing, 7*, 283–294.

Musiek, F. E., (1986b). Neuroanatomy, neurophysiology, and central auditory assessment. Part III: Corpus callosum and efferent pathways. *Ear and Hearing, 7*, 349–358.

Musiek, F. E., & Baran, J. A. (1986). Neuroanatomy, neurophysiology, and central auditory asessment. Part I: Brainstem. *Ear and Hearing, 7*, 207–219.

Musiek, F. E., & Baran, J. A. (1987). Central auditory assessment: Thirty years of challenge and change. *Ear and Hearing, 8*, 22S–35S.

Musiek, F. E., & Geurkink, N. A. (1980). Auditory perceptual problems in children: Considerations for the otolaryngologist and audiologist. *Laryngoscope, 90*, 962–971.

Musiek, F. E., & Geurkink, N. A. (1982). Auditory brainstem response and central auditory test findings for patients with brainstem lesions: A preliminary report. *Laryngoscope, 92*, 891–900.

Musiek, F. E., Geurkink, N. A., & Keitel, S. (1982). Test battery assessment of auditory perceptual dysfunction in children. *Laryngoscope, 92*, 251–257.

Musiek, F. E., Gollegly, K. M., & Baran, J. A. (1984). Myelination of the corpus callosum in learning disabled children: Theoretical and clinical correlates. *Seminars in Hearing, 5*, 219–229.

Musiek, F. E., Gollegly, K. M., & Ross, M. K. (1985). Profiles of types of central auditory processing disorders in children with learning disabilities. *Journal of Childhood Communication Disorders, 9*, 43–61.

Musiek, F. E., & Kibbe, K. (1985). An overview of audiological test results in patients with commissurotomy. In A. G. Reeves (Ed.), *Epilepsy and the corpus callosum* (pp. 393–399). New York: Plenum Press.

Musiek, F. E., Kibbe, K., & Baran, J. A. (1984). Neuroaudiological results from split-brain patients. *Seminars in Hearing, 5*, 219–229.

Musiek, F. E., & Pinheiro, M. L. (1985). Dichotic speech tests in the detection of central auditory dysfunction. In M. L. Pinheiro & F. E. Musiek (Eds.), *Assessment of central auditory dysfunction: Foundations and clinical correlates* (pp. 201–218). Baltimore: Williams & Wilkins.

Musiek, F. E., & Pinheiro, M. L. (1986, May). *Effect of peripheral and central auditory lesions on auditory pattern perception.* Paper presented at the 109th meeting of the Acoustical Society of America, Cleveland.

Musiek, F. E., & Pinheiro, M. L. (1987). Frequency patterns in cochlear, brainstem, and cerebral lesions. *Audiology, 26*, 79–88.

Musiek, F. E., Pinheiro, M. L., & Wilson, D. H. (1980). Auditory pattern perception in ''split-brain'' patients. *Archives of Otolaryngology, 106*, 610–612.

Musiek, F. E., Reeves, A. G., & Baran, J. A. (1985). Release from central auditory competition in the split-brain patient. *Neurology, 35*, 983–987.

Musiek, F. E., & Wilson, D. H. (1979). SSW and dichotic digit results pre- and post-commissurotomy: A case report. *Journal of Speech and Hearing Disorders*, 44, 528–533.

Musiek, F. E., Wilson, D. H., & Pinheiro, M. L. (1979). Audiological manifestations in split-brain patients. *Journal of the American Audiological Society*, 5, 25–29.

Noffsinger, D., Martinez, C., & Schaefer, A. (1982). Auditory brainstem responses and masking level differences from persons with brainstem lesions. *Scandinavian Audiology*, 15, 81–93.

Noffsinger, D., Olsen, W. O., Carhart, R., Hart, C. W., & Sahgal, V. (1972). Auditory and vestibular aberrations in multiple sclerosis. *Acta Oto-Laryngologica*, 303 (Supplement), 1–63.

Olsen, W. (1977, November). *Performance of temporal lobectomy patients with dichotic CV test materials*. Paper presented at the annual meeting of the American Speech and Hearing Association, Chicago.

Olsen, W. O., Noffsinger, D., & Carhart, R. (1976). Masking level differences encountered in clinical populations. *Audiology*, 15, 287–301.

Olsen, W. O., Noffsinger, D., & Kurdziel, S. (1975). Speech discrimination in noise by patients with peripheral and central lesions. *Acta Oto-Laryngologica*, 80, 375–382.

Orchik, D., & Oelschlaeger, M. (1977). Time-compressed speech discrimination in children and its relationship to articulation. *Journal of the American Audiological Society*, 3, 37–41.

Pandya, D., Karol, E., & Heilbornn, D. (1971). The topographical distribution of interhemispheric projections in the corpus callosum of the Rhesus monkey. *Brain Research*, 32, 31–43.

Pengelly, M., Mueller, H. G., & Hill, B. (1982, November). *Masking level difference: Effects of high-frequency hearing loss and masking stimuli*. Paper presented at the annual meeting of the American Speech-Language-Hearing Association, Toronto.

Pickles, J. O. (1982). *An introduction to the physiology of hearing*. New York: Academic Press.

Pickles, J. O. (1985). Physiology of the cerebral auditory system. In M. L. Pinheiro & F. E. Musiek (Eds.), *Assessment of central auditory dysfunction: Foundations and clinical correlates* (pp. 67–86). Baltimore: Williams & Wilkins.

Pinheiro, M. L. (1976). Auditory pattern reversal in auditory perception in patients with left and right hemisphere lesions. *Ohio Journal of Speech and Hearing*, 12, 9–20.

Pinheiro, M. L. (1977). Tests of central auditory function in children with learning disabilities. In R. W. Keith (Ed.), *Central auditory dysfunction* (pp. 223–256). New York: Grune & Stratton.

Pinheiro, M. L., Jacobson, G. P., & Boller, F. (1982). Auditory dysfunction following a gunshot wound of the pons. *Journal of Speech and Hearing Disorders*, 47, 296–300.

Pinheiro, M. L., & Musiek, F. E. (1985). Sequencing and temporal ordering in the auditory system. In M. L. Pinheiro & F. E. Musiek (Eds.), *Assessment of central auditory dysfunction: Foundations and clinical correlates* (pp. 219–238). Baltimore: Williams & Wilkins.

Pinheiro, M. L., & Ptacek, P. H. (1971). Reversals in the perception of noise and tone patterns. *Journal of the Acoustical Society of America*, 49, 1778–1782.

Pinheiro, M. L., & Tobin, H. (1969). Interaural intensity difference for intracranial lateralization. *Journal of the Acoustical Society of America*, 46, 1482–1487.

Pinheiro, M. L., & Tobin, H. (1971). The interaural intensity difference as a diagnostic indicator. *Acta Oto-Laryngologica* (Stockholm), *71*, 326–328.

Pinheiro, M. L., Weidner, W. E., Suren, S. M., & Gaydos, M. L. (1977, October). *Sequencing of pitch patterns with competing music and competing discourse by patients with right and left hemisphere lesions.* Paper presented at a meeting of the Academy of Aphasia, Montreal.

Ptacek, P. H., & Pinheiro, M. L. (1971). Pattern reversal in auditory perception. *Journal of the Acoustical Society of America, 49,* 493–498.

Protti, E. (1983). Brainstem auditory pathways and auditory processing disorders: Diagnostic implications of subjective and objective tests. In E. Lasky & J. Katz (Eds.), *Central auditory processing disorders* (pp. 117–140). Baltimore: University Park Press.

Protti, E., & Young, M. (1980). The evaluation of a child with auditory perceptual deficiencies: An interdisciplinary approach. *Seminars in Speech, Language and Hearing, 1,* 167–180.

Quaranta, A., & Cervellera, G. (1977). Masking level differences in central nervous system diseases. *Archives of Otolaryngology, 103,* 483–484.

Rintelmann, W. F. (1985). Monaural speech tests in the detection of central auditory disorders. In M. L. Pinheiro & F. E. Musiek (Eds.), *Assessment of central auditory dysfunction: Foundations and clinical correlates* (pp. 173–200). Baltimore: Williams & Wilkins.

Rintelmann, W. F., Beasley, D., & Lynn, G. (1974, April). *Time-compressed CNC monosyllables: Case findings in central auditory disorders.* Paper presented at the meeting of the Michigan Speech and Hearing Association, Detroit.

Rintelmann, W. F., & Lynn, G. E. (1983). Speech stimuli for assessment of central auditory disorders. In D. Konkle & W. F. Rintelmann (Eds.), *Principles of Speech Audiometry* (pp. 231–284). Baltimore: University Park Press.

Rosenzweig, M. (1951). Representation of the two ears at the auditory cortex. *American Journal of Physiology, 165,* 147–158.

Ruebens, A., Froehling, B., Slater, G., & Anderson, D. (1985). Left ear suppression on verbal dichotic tests in patients with multiple sclerosis. *Annals of Neurology, 18,* 459–463.

Sanchez-Longo, L. P., Forster, F. M., & Auth, T. L. (1957). A clinical test for sound localization and its applications. *Neurology, 7,* 653–655.

Sanchez-Longo, L. P., & Forster, F. M. (1958). Clinical significance of impairment of sound localization. *Neurology, 8,* 119–125.

Schuknecht, H. F. (1964). Further observations on the pathology of presbycusis. *Archives of Otolaryngology, 80,* 369–382.

Schuknecht, H. F. (1974). *Pathology of the Ear.* Cambridge, MA: Harvard University Press.

Sedge, R. K., Mueller, H. G., & Dillon, J. D. (1982, November). *Dichotic digit and CV results for individuals with head injuries.* Paper presented at the annual meeting of the American Speech-Language-Hearing Association, Toronto.

Seltzer, B., & Pandya, D. N. (1978). Afferent cortical connections and architectonics of the superior temporal sulcus and surrounding cortex in the Rhesus monkey. *Brain Research, 149,* 1–24.

Shankweiler, D. (1966). Effects of temporal lobe damage on perception of dichotically presented melodies. *Journal of Comparative and Physiological Psychology, 62,* 115–119.

Sidtis, J. (1982). Predicting brain organization from dichotic listening performance: Cortical and subcortical functional asymmetries contribute to perceptual asymmetries. *Brain and Language, 17,* 287–300.

Sinha, S. O. (1959). *The role of the temporal lobe in hearing.* Unpublished master's thesis, McGill University, Montreal, Quebec.

Smith, B. B., & Resnick, D. M. (1972). An auditory test for assessing brain stem integrity: Preliminary report. *Laryngoscope, 82,* 414–424.

Smith, B. H., & Sethi, P. H. (1975). Aging and the nervous system. *Geriatrics, 30,* 109–115.

Sparks, R., & Geschwind, N. (1968). Dichotic listening in man after section of the neocortical commissures. *Cortex, 4,* 3–16.

Sparks, R., Goodglass, H., & Nichel, B. (1970). Ipsilateral versus contralateral extinction in dichotic listening resulting from hemisphere lesions. *Cortex, 6,* 249–260.

Speaks, C., Gray, T., Miller, J., & Rubens, A. (1975). Central auditory deficits and temporal lobe lesions. *Journal of Speech and Hearing Disorders, 40,* 192–205.

Speaks, C., Niccum, N., & Van Tassel, D. (1985). Effects of stimulus material on the dichotic listening performance of patients with sensorineural hearing loss. *Journal of Speech and Hearing Research, 18,* 16–25.

Springer, S. P., & Gazzaniga, M. S. (1975). Dichotic testing of partial and complete split-brain patients. *Neuropsychologia, 13,* 341–346.

Springer, S. P., Sidtis, J., Wilson, D. H., & Gazzaniga, M. S. (1978). Left ear performance in dichotic listening following commissurotomy. *Neuropsychologia, 16,* 305–312.

Stephens, S., & Thornton, A. (1976). Subjective and electrophysiologic tests in brainstem lesions. *Archives of Otolaryngology, 102,* 608–613.

Sticht, T. G., & Gray, B. B. (1969). The intelligibility of time-compressed words as a function of age and hearing loss. *Journal of Speech and Hearing Disorders, 12,* 443–448.

Sweitzer, R. (1977). Team evaluation of auditory perceptually-handicapped children. In R. W. Keith (Ed.), *Central auditory dysfunction* (pp. 341–360). New York: Grune & Stratton.

Swisher, L., & Hirsh, I. J. (1972). Brain damage and the ordering of two temporally successive stimuli. *Neuropsychologia, 10,* 137–152.

Tillman, T. N., Carhart, R., & Nicholls, S. (1973). Release from multiple maskers in elderly persons. *Journal of Speech and Hearing Research, 16,* 152–160.

Thompson, G. (1983). Structure and function of the central auditory system. *Seminars in Hearing, 4,* 81–96.

Tobin, H. (1985). Binaural interaction tasks. In M. L. Pinheiro & F. E. Musiek (Eds.), *Assessment of central auditory dysfunction: Foundations and clinical correlates* (pp. 155–172). Baltimore: Williams & Wilkins.

Townsend, T. H., & Goldstein, D. P. (1972). Supra-threshold binaural unmasking. *Journal of the Acoustical Society of America, 51,* 621–624.

Welsh, L., Welsh, J., & Healey, M. (1980). Auditory testing and dyslexia. *Laryngoscope, 90,* 972–984.

White, E. (1977). Children's performance on the SSW test and Willeford Battery: Interim clinical report. In R. W. Keith (Ed.), *Central auditory dysfunction* (pp. 319–340). New York: Grune & Stratton.

Willeford, J. (1976). Differential diagnosis of central auditory dysfunction. In L. Bradford (Ed.), *Audiology: An audio journal for continuing education* (Vol. 2). New York: Grune & Stratton.

Willeford, J. (1977a). Assessing central auditory behavior in children: A test battery approach. In R. W. Keith (Ed.), *Central auditory dysfunction* (pp. 43–72). New York: Grune & Stratton.

Willeford, J. (1977b). Evaluation of central auditory disorders in learning disabled children. In L. Bradford (Ed.), *Learning disabilities: An audio journal for continuing education* (Vol. 1). New York: Grune & Stratton.

Willeford, J. (1978). Sentence tests of central auditory function. In J. Katz (Ed.), *Handbook of clinical audiology* (pp. 252–261). Baltimore: Williams & Wilkins.

Willeford, J. (1980). Central auditory behaviors in learning disabled children. *Seminars in Speech, Language and Hearing, 1*, 127–140.

Willeford, J., & Billger, J. (1978). Auditory perception in children with learning disabilities. In J. Katz (Ed.), *Handbook of clinical audiology* (pp. 410–425). Baltimore: Williams & Wilkins.

Young, M. (1983). Neuroscience, pragmatic competence, and auditory processing. In E. Laskey & J. Katz (Eds.), *Central auditory processing disorders* (pp. 141–162). Baltimore: University Park Press.

Zurif, E. B., & Ramier, A. M. (1972). Some effects of unilateral brain damage on the perception of dichotically presented phoneme sequences and digits. *Neuropsychologia, 10*, 103–110.

chapter twelve

Pseudohypacusis

WILLIAM F. RINTELMANN
SABINA A. SCHWAN

Contents

Introduction

Most children and adults who are examined by an audiologist or an otologist for a complaint of hearing loss have bona fide disorders of the auditory mechanism that typically require some type of medical treatment, including surgery, and/or audiological management, such as the need for a hearing aid. The preceding chapters have dealt with various aspects of the assessment of hearing based on the assumption that the patient seen by the clinician has an organic disorder that can account for the behavioral symptoms and auditory test results observed. The focus of this chapter, however, is on the child or adult who exhibits a hearing loss in some fashion, but no physical (organic) basis for the hearing disorder is displayed.

In this chapter we consider the problems of terminology, incidence/prevalence, etiological factors, emotional and psychosocial characteristics, and behavioral manifestations related to the disorder in both children and adults. The primary focus of the chapter concerns the detection and assessment of pseudohypacusis via both conventional and special audiologic tests. These include both behavioral and electrophysiological measures for assessing auditory function. Finally, some discussion is concerned with the management of the problem, especially as it relates to children.

Terminology

There is no universally accepted term to describe a hearing loss that cannot be attributed to an organic defect. The terms *nonorganic, functional,* and *pseudohypacusic* are commonly used descriptors of this problem without specifically implying whether the origin of this problem is on a conscious or unconscious basis. If the individual (child or adult) purposefully is exhibiting symptoms of impaired hearing, the problem often is labeled *malingering, feigning,* or is sometimes called *simulated hearing loss.* If, however, the origin of the problem is on an unconscious level, the disorder often is termed *hysterical* or *psychogenic* hearing loss or deafness. Hysterical or psychogenic hearing loss imply that the patient has a severe emotional disorder. Denying the ability to hear on an unconscious level serves as a defense mechanism to avoid resolving the primary emotional conflict.

Some early writers (i.e., Fournier, 1958; Portmann & Portmann, 1961) have stressed the importance of distinguishing between psychogenic deafness and malingering; however, there seems to be general agreement (i.e., Hopkinson, 1973; Kinstler, 1971; Martin, 1985) that it is not the role of audiologists to attempt to determine whether a nonorganic hearing loss is on a conscious or unconscious basis. In fact, there simply are no tests within the audiologist's armamentarium to help make such a distinction.

Goldstein (1966) questioned the validity of psychogenic hearing loss as a clinical entity. He proposed certain criteria that he felt must be met to satisfy the definition of psychogenic hearing loss. Specifically, he felt it is necessary to demonstrate that the patient responds to weaker sounds during electrophysiologic audiometry or under hypnosis than via behavioral audiometry. Also, he stated that the patient's auditory behavior should be consistent between the test situation and his or her daily life activities. Finally, Goldstein argued that a diagnosis of psychogenic deafness can be made only if better auditory sensitivity is displayed behaviorally under all circumstances following successful psychiatric or psychologic therapy or after spontaneous remission of the emotional problem. In short, Goldstein concluded that all patients presenting with nonorganic hearing loss are aware of their simulation, and hence are malingering. He added, however, that feigning probably has a psychogenic basis even when the motive may be related to potential monetary gain.

Hopkinson (1967) and Ventry (1968) disagreed with Goldstein's criteria for validating psychogenic hearing loss. Also, Ventry (1968) objected to Goldstein's thesis that such a clinical entity does not exist and he reported on a case of a veteran with a unilateral psychogenic loss. Thus there clearly is not agreement among experts on whether malingering can be distinguished from psychogenic hearing loss or even if the latter entity exists. More important, however, some clinicians, including the present writers, contend that audiologists need not be concerned with this question, but rather, they should focus on accurately assessing the organic status of the patient's hearing so that appropriate referral and management can be initiated. This topic is considered later in this chapter.

The use of labels like "malingering," "feigning," and "simulation" imply that the patient is willfully lying, and hence, is dishonest. Such terms, therefore, simply should not be used. If an audiologist has occasion to give "medico-legal" testimony, he or she may state that the patient's test results are discrepant or inconsistent without labeling him or her as a malingerer. Furthermore, such reports should include as accurate an estimate as possible about the patient's organic hearing threshold level.

The terms *nonorganic*, *functional*, and *pseudohypacusis* encompass both malingering and psychogenic hearing loss; therefore, use of one of these generic terms is preferable because they avoid the issue of deciding whether the professed hearing loss is on a conscious or unconscious basis. Some writers (i.e., Martin, 1972) prefer the term *nonorganic* because it is immediately clear that the only inference made concerns the organic status of the hearing mechanism. On the other hand, advocates of the term *functional* (Hopkinson, 1973; Ventry & Chaiklin, 1962) point out that *nonorganic* does not provide for the possibility that an actual organic disorder simply has escaped audiologic or otologic identification. Those who prefer the term *functional* stress that in medicine, a functional disease is one in which the organ is not functioning appropriately even though the organ shows no evidence of structural alteration or pathology.

The term *pseudohypacusis* also has several proponents. This word was modified by Carhart (1961) from *pseudo neural hypacusis* used by Brockman and Hoversten (1960) and was subsequently used by Rintelmann and Harford (1963). Goldstein (1966) also preferred the use of this term, but slightly shortened it to *pseudohypacusis*. The above-mentioned writers advocated use of this term because it clearly signifies the condition of a false (pseudo), less than normal auditory sensitivity (hypoacusis or hypacusis). In recent years, the term *pseudohypacusis* has gained in popularity as evidenced by its use by writers who previously preferred the terms *nonorganic* or *functional* (e.g., Martin, 1985). The term *pseudohypacusis* is used primarily for the remainder of this chapter.

It also should be mentioned that some patients may exhibit an exaggerated overlay to an actual organic defect. Such cases also must be considered as pseudohypacusic in that they present the same basic problem of auditory assessment to the audiologist and the otologist.

Incidence/prevalence and etiological factors

Both *incidence* and *prevalence* are terms used to describe the frequency of occurrence of a particular condition or disorder, but they are not synonymous terms. "Incidence is the number of new occurrences of a condition in a population within a specified time period [whereas] prevalence refers to the total number of cases in a population at, or during, a specified period of time" (Moscicki, 1984, p. 39). The only definitive statement that can be made concerning the incidence or prevalence of pseudohypacusis is that it is highly variable depending on the population being examined (Altshuler, 1982; Coles & Mason, 1984). Furthermore, incidence and prevalence are closely linked to potential causative factors. Hence, these two topics are discussed together. A review of the literature on this topic strongly suggests that the highest prevalence figures have been reported in those special populations of adults in which *decibels of hearing loss could be translated into dollars of compensation*. For example, Johnson, Work, and McCoy (1956) reported that the prevalence of nonorganic problems among veterans examined for service-connected hearing loss increased from 10%–15% to nearly 50% in the 10-year-period following World War II. This tremendous increase in pseudohypacusic cases was attributed to essentially three factors: (a) changing the method of compensation from a single lump-sum award to a monthly payment; (b) use of crude hearing tests (i.e., conversation voice) as a basis for verifying the hearing loss;

and (c) inadequate counseling when the hearing loss was initially discovered. In contrast, a prevalence figure for the total 1978 patient population of the Walter Reed Hospital, Audiology and Speech Center was reported as 48 pseudohypacusic cases, or 1.74%, from a total of 2,765 patients (D. Schwartz, personal communication, January, 1979). Ten years later, in 1988, the prevalence of pseudohypacusis among active-duty and retired military personnel who received audiologic evaluations at the Walter Reed Hospital was 1.4% (32 of 2,329 persons tested). In contrast, the prevalence of pseudohypacusis during the late 1980s on Army posts among basic trainees and soldiers in combat arms units was *estimated* to be approximately 4% to 5% (R. Atack, personal communication, January, 1989). However, although records typically are not kept concerning the prevalence of pseudohypacusis in the veterans population, the clinical impression of audiologists queried at two Michigan VA Audiology Centers is that there has been a substantial reduction in the number of pseudohypacusic cases in the past two decades, 1968–1989 (G. Peters & M. O'Shaughnessey, personal communication, January, 1989). One reason given for the reduced prevalence of pseudohypacusis during the 1980s in the military and veterans populations is that since military hearing conservation programs have been established in the past 10–15 years, longitudinal audiologic records are kept for most military personnel; hence, the existence of such detailed "hearing health histories" makes it difficult to suddenly simulate a hearing loss. Furthermore, undoubtedly, the increased sophistication of modern audiology in terms of instrumentation, available tests, and training and experience of personnel has contributed substantially to a significant reduction in the prevalence of this problem during the past two to three decades.

Another concern is the prevalence of pseudohypacusis among some industrial workers who are exposed to high noise levels. Since the enactment of the Occupational Safety and Health Act of 1970 there has been an increasing awareness by the general public concerning the deleterious effects of prolonged exposure to high noise levels. Although this is a legitimate societal concern, the possibility of industrial workers receiving compensation for job-connected hearing loss clearly provides some individuals with the motivation for either feigning a hearing loss or attempting to exaggerate the degree of a bona fide hearing loss (Armbruster, 1982; Coles & Mason, 1984). To illustrate, Barelli and Ruder (1970) obtained data on 162 medico-legal cases and reported that 24% of the 116 workers who had applied for compensation were found to have a nonorganic hearing loss. In another study, Gosztonyi, Vassallo, and Sataloff (1971) reported on the reliability of manual and self-recording audiometric tests of 100 employees in a heavy industry. They found reliable audiometric results from all of the 50 salaried (office) personnel, whereas unreliable and hence invalid audiograms were obtained from 17 (34%) of the hourly (shop) workers. Commenting on the unreliable audiometric results, Gosztonyi et al. (1971) stated "15 were later found to be compensation cases. The unreliable audiograms were deliberate and could be called malingering. In certain instances we also found that workers in relatively quiet departments of the plant were being influenced to complain of hearing loss and file for compensation" (p. 117). Harris (1979) discussed the problem of nonorganic hearing loss in industry and described how to identify the potential malingerer both before and during audiometric testing. He suggested methods of documenting invalid hearing tests among industrial workers and stressed the importance of early detection for immediate resolution of the problem.

Hence, the potential motivation for pseudohypacusis based on the opportunity for a monetary award, which Johnson et al. (1956) considered to be a major causative factor for the increase in the prevalence of this problem for more than a decade after World War II, may prove to be even of larger magnitude in nationwide industrial hearing conservation programs.

Estimates of the prevalence of pseudohypacusis in the "general" adult population are substantially less than in the two special populations (veterans and industrial workers) briefly discussed above. Although most of these prevalence figures are based on somewhat vague estimates, nevertheless, a general notion of the magnitude of the problem can be obtained. For example, Kinstler (1971) reported on a brief survey made in one large western city. He stated that in two otologic groups with large diagnostic caseloads and sizable surgical practices both groups reported a prevalence of under 2%. Kinstler also stated that one otolaryngologist surveyed had many patients who were involved in medico-legal litigation related to traumatic or noise-induced hearing loss. Estimates of pseudohypacusis among these patients was between 5% and 10%. As Kinstler pointed out, the number of functional loss cases will vary in relationship to the proportion of medico-legal cases in an otologist's practice.

Although there is a dearth of prevalence data on adult pseudohypacusics seen in audiology clinics, a survey conducted in 1951 of 30 audiology centers in the United States reported that the percentage of pseudohypacusic civilians "was 0 in 16 of the centers, less than 5 in 11 of the centers, and 5 or more in only 3 of the centers" (Zwislocki, 1963, cited by Hopkinson, 1973, p. 178). Based on the present writers' experience both in university and hospital-based audiology clinics over a period of several years, a prevalence figure of less than 2% in the general adult population (excluding large concentrations of medico-legal cases) appears to be a reasonable estimate for the late 1980s.

The prevalence of pseudohypacusis among children also is difficult to ascertain, again because there are few solid data on which to base an accurate estimate. Most of the reports involving children simply state the number of cases seen without relating these numbers to the total patient population for a given period of time. A few early reports, however, provide some limited clues regarding prevalence figures. The 1951 survey of 30 audiology centers mentioned above (Zwislocki, 1963, cited by Hopkinson, 1973) also attempted to determine the prevalence of pseudohypacusis in children. A negligible percentage was reported by 22 centers, with 6 centers stating less than 5% and only 2 centers reporting more than 5%. Specific prevalence figures collected by Campanelli (1963) for one audiology center revealed that during a 12-month-period 41 school children, or 1.7%, from a total caseload of 2,300 children demonstrated significant "simulated" hearing losses. This sample of children ranged in age from 6 to 17 years, with a mean age of 10.9 years. These children were referred by audiologists and school nurses from school hearing screening programs.

Clearly, the prevalence of pseudohypacusis among both children and adults in the typical patient population seen for audiologic and otologic evaluation is not nearly as great as it is among those special populations in which there is an opportunity to receive direct compensation for a job-related hearing loss. It should be noted, however, that no recent prevalence figures have been reported in the literature for pseudohypacusis in either children or adult populations.

Accidents, not necessarily related to job performance, also can be causative factors resulting in pseudohypacusis. For example, if a patient is sent for a hearing evaluation by his or her attorney because the client (or patient) is involved in a suit over an automobile accident in which he or she allegedly received a traumatic hearing loss, the audiologist should at least consider the possibility of pseudohypacusis. One of us (W. F. R.) recalls a case in which the patient, claiming a severe bilateral hearing loss as a consequence of an auto accident, arrived at our hearing clinic wearing binaural hearing aids. Subsequently, the battery of audiological tests administered to this patient demonstrated normal hearing in both ears.

Motivation or possible etiological factors among children exhibiting pseudohypacusis, too, are based on the possibility of a "reward," in a sense. Contrary to the adult pseudohypacusic where the sought-after gain is often monetary, the reward for children may be for various psychological purposes. Based on several reports in the literature (Barr, 1963; Berger, 1965; Brockman & Hoversten, 1960; Dixon & Newby, 1959; Lehrer, Hirschenfang, Miller, & Radpour, 1964; McCanna & DeLapa, 1981; Rintelmann & Harford, 1963) one of the more common causes among school-age children for exhibiting pseudohypacusis is that a hearing loss serves as an acceptable reason for both parents and teachers to account for poor academic performance. Often such children have failed school hearing screening tests and have a history of middle ear disorders, which initially provides the excuse for poor performance in school. After the middle ear problem has been resolved, and if the academic performance does not improve, some children resort to simulating a hearing loss, probably in an effort to continue to have an excuse for their less than satisfactory school performance. A few children even exhibited nonorganic visual problems in addition to pseudohypacusis (Berger, 1965; Dixon & Newby, 1959; Lumio, Jauhiainen, & Gelhar, 1969; Rintelmann & Harford, 1963).

Another possible factor that can contribute to the display of pseudohypacusis in children, according to several investigators including those mentioned above, is the child's need to gain attention. This can be expressed in various ways such as aggressive behavior at school, strong sibling rivalry at home, or by other forms of manifesting social conflict (Aplin & Rowson, 1986; Lumio et al., 1969; Martin, 1985). Broad in 1980 also reported that another cause of pseudohypacusis in children involves a poor self-image.

A typical pattern for the onset of pseudohypacusis in children found by Rintelmann and Harford (1963) is that the child often initially fails a hearing screening test in school. Such failure may be due to an actual hearing loss, or some children with normal hearing may fail a screening test for various reasons (i.e., poor acoustic environment, audiometers improperly calibrated, etc.). The child may next fail a second screening or pure tone threshold test and subsequently be referred for an otological examination. The child may then be referred to an audiologist, sometimes with the suspicion of pseudohypacusis, but also sometimes for a hearing aid evaluation. Often by the time the child arrives for an examination at an audiology center, he or she has exhibited a hearing loss on two or three tests in a period of a few weeks or months. Thus the pattern has been established for the child to demonstrate a hearing loss in the test situation. Furthermore, if the child has already recognized that a hearing loss may provide certain benefits (i.e., an excuse for poor academic performance), he or she may be quite committed to continuing to show a hearing loss.

Thus it appears that pseudohypacusis in both adults and children can be attributed to some form of gain that may be derived from the hearing loss. The motivating factor for pseudohypacusis in adults often can be directly related to potential monetary gain resulting from the hearing loss. Among children the causative factors usually are less obvious, but they typically can be traced to some form of psychological gain (i.e., providing a reason or excuse for poor school achievement), or serve as a means for getting attention and affection.

It is important that the detection and assessment of pseudohypacusis be accomplished, if possible, before the adult or child becomes strongly committed to exhibiting a hearing loss. For children, especially, it is critical to identify incorrect responses to hearing tests before the child has the chance to recognize that a hearing loss may provide various types of secondary gains such as those discussed above.

Emotional and psychosocial characteristics

Whether pseudohypacusis is displayed on a conscious or an unconscious basis, clearly in either case the child or adult is exhibiting behavior that deviates to some extent from what is considered to be normal. In the preceding discussion, it was pointed out that the causative factors can be almost always related to some form of monetary or psychological gain. Pseudohypacusic children may use their alleged hearing loss to gain attention, to excuse poor school performance, or as a means of expressing hostility at home or in other social environments. By the very nature of the problem of pseudohypacusis, adults too exhibit deviant social behavior. One may ask then: "Are there certain emotional problems or personality characteristics that may be associated with pseudohypacusis?"

Some investigators have reported that pseudohypacusic children often have serious emotional problems (Aplin & Rowson, 1986; Barr, 1963; Berk & Feldman, 1958; Broad, 1980; Dixon & Newby, 1959). Lehrer et al. (1964) conducted extensive psychological evaluations on 10 pseudohypacusic children ranging in age from 11 to 16 years and found that all of the children revealed significant emotional problems that were considered to be associated with pseudohypacusis. The emotional problems typical of these children were as follows: feelings of insecurity and inadequacy resulting in a strong need for attention and approval, hostility toward parents or siblings, and a display of anxious behavior. Each of the children in this study received psychotherapy and the authors reported "a uniformly excellent response to these therapy sessions which were largely supportive in nature" (Lehrer et al., 1964, p. 68). On the other hand, some young children who display inconsistent behavior on audiological tests do not appear to have such emotional problems. These children often are below the age of 8 years or so and based on our experience should probably simply be called difficult-to-test rather than pseudohypacusic.

Many writers have discussed the personality traits and the emotional and social characteristics of adult pseudohypacusics, particularly among the military and veteran populations of World War II. Johnson et al. (1956), Knapp (1948), and Truex (1946), among other researchers, mentioned anxiety, depression, and hypochondriasis as common problems. Gleason (1958) compared the psychological profiles of patients showing inconsistent audiological test results with those displaying consistent audiological behavior in a sample of 278 military patients. He found that 30% of the total sample showed inconsistency during audiological testing and that of this subgroup 86% demonstrated a nonorganic overlay to a true hearing loss. Compared to the group of patients who gave consistent test results, the pseudohypacusic group

> showed poorer intellectual performance, a greater degree of psychiatric and psychosomatic complaints, and deviant social behavior. . . . The group is seen to be heterogenous and composed of three psychological subclasses. The largest element demonstrates emotional immaturity, instability, and an inadequate response to social demands. The next largest group is a neurotic population high in anxiety and feelings of inferiority and lacking in self-confidence. (Gleason, 1958, p. 46)

Cases in the third group, described as "small," were found to be normal psychologically.

Trier and Levy (1965) compared the social and psychological characteristics of pseudohypacusic veterans with a control group having organic hearing disorders. The pseudohypacusics compared to the control subjects revealed a lower socioeconomic status based on lower reported incomes, were somewhat limited in intellectual functioning, and showed poorer emotional stability. The latter was demonstrated on measures of gross emotional disturbance, and in preoccupation with and exploitation of physical symptoms. Furthermore, based on interviews with patients, the authors felt that veterans with functional hearing loss probably lack confidence in their ability to meet the needs of everyday life. Such feelings of general inadequacy can include having doubts about their capabilities of providing financially for themselves and their families. Hence, the possibility of obtaining monthly compensation provides the motivation for exaggerating a hearing loss. Trier and Levy (1965) concluded: "Because social values are generally opposed to the exaggeration of physical symptoms for gain, this behavior is likely to result in a loss of self-esteem" (p. 255).

A comparable psychosocial profile study has not been reported to date to our knowledge for an adult civilian population. Undoubtedly, this is because the cooperation needed from patients (subjects) to gather such data would be difficult to achieve in most civilian settings. Research of this nature is needed in large industrial settings in which workers are filing compensation claims for job-related, noise-induced hearing loss.

Behavioral manifestations

While the audiologist is obtaining a case history, the patient may display certain behavioral characteristics that could alert the clinician to the possibility of pseudohypacusis. These "behavioral clues" have been described frequently in the literature (Altshuler, 1982; Brockman & Hoversten, 1960; Fournier, 1958; Gibbons, 1962; Harris, 1979; Hopkinson, 1973; Johnson et al., 1956; Kinstler, 1971; Martin, 1985; McCanna & DeLapa, 1981; Nilo & Saunders, 1976). Children frequently will respond to the clinician's informal conversation at levels substantially below what one would predict from their voluntary pure tone thresholds (Berger, 1965; Campanelli, 1963; Lehrer et al., 1964). Yet, as soon as formal testing begins, these children have difficulty hearing. This naive behavior seldom is displayed by adults with "confirmed" pseudohypacusis. Features often exhibited, however, by both children and adult pseudohypacusics are normal voice quality, loudness, and pitch with good speech articulation, whereas their voluntary pure tone thresholds usually show severe to profound hearing loss. This too represents naive behavior, because persons with longstanding severe hearing loss typically have defective speech and voice characteristics. The reader should be cautioned, however, that an individual may have a bona fide severe bilateral hearing loss of recent onset, and hence, have reasonably good speech and voice quality when examined.

Several other behavioral signs may raise the suspicion of pseudohypacusis. The patient may explain his or her ability to follow a conversation by claiming excellent lipreading skills, and he or she may continue to follow the conversation while the examiner's head is turned or the lighting in the room is dimmed. Other pseudohypacusics may behave in an opposite fashion, that is, they may display excessive effort to watch the clinician's mouth, cup their hand over their ear while leaning toward the speaker, and talk in an abnormally loud voice. In general, some pseudohypacusics go through excessive contortions in an effort to impress the clinician with how much trouble they have hearing.

Further clues about the possibility of pseudohypacusis may be obtained from the patient's responses to case history information. Elaborate details may be given about the onset and symptoms of the professed hearing loss, which when taken in toto, simply do not fit any known set of symptoms that tend to define a particular type of organic disorder. Also, such patients may go into great detail (more than someone with an organic loss) about how their hearing loss is totally handicapping.

Inappropriate statements and actions regarding hearing aid use can provide additional clues to the clinician. These include (a) exaggerated claims of benefit from amplification, (b) professed daily use of the hearing aid, yet showing lack of familiarity with the aid's operation, and (c) unrealistic statements about battery life and cost.

Other behavioral clues may be gained while administering the battery of audiological tests. Given appropriately calibrated equipment, a cooperative patient, and careful testing procedures, both proper agreement between tests and good test-retest reliability may be expected (Armbruster, 1982). Thus inconsistent responses that exceed expected test-retest reliability (i.e., about 10 dB for pure tone thresholds) should raise the suspicion of the possibility of pseudohypacusis. To account for such discrepancies, the patient may comment frequently during testing about being confused between the test tones and the ringing in his or her ears.

Chaiklin and Ventry (1965) pointed out the value of attending to both false-positive and false-negative responses in the clinical setting. The latter type of response occurs when the subject (patient) fails to respond to signals presented at or slightly above his or her threshold. False-negative responses are considered to be characteristic of pseudohypacusis. By the same token, false-positive responses occur when the subject responds either when the signal is absent or when the stimulus is presented below threshold. False-positive responses are typical of highly motivated patients with bona fide hearing loss. Chaiklin and Ventry (1965) reported that 86% of their adult subjects with true hearing loss exhibited false-positive responses, whereas only 22% of their adult sample with functional hearing loss displayed such responses.

Finally, a word of caution is in order concerning the possibility of over-interpreting the above-mentioned kinds of behavioral manifestations. Most patients seen in an audiology center, including those with job-related noise-induced hearing loss, have true organic hearing disorders. Although the clinician should remain alert to the possibility of pseudohypacusis, drawing such a conclusion without substantial test battery data clearly is not in the best interest of the patient, and hence, is a serious clinical error. Behavioral clues can be useful in helping the audiologist to make a decision about which tests to give; however, such clues should never be used exclusively to arrive at an assessment of hearing. The remainder of this chapter deals mostly with those audiological tests that have proven useful in the detection and assessment of pseudohypacusis.

Conventional audiologic tests

The audiologic tests discussed in this section include both routine and so-called "special" tests, which typically are administered to patients having organic disorders of the auditory system. Hence, these are not special tests for pseudohypacusis per se, and herein lies their primary value. Most audiologists who have infrequent opportunity to test patients suspected of pseudohypacusis do not have the facility necessary to properly administer those tests specifically designed for assessing pseudohypacusis (e.g., the Doerfler-Stewart test) without considerable practice. Thus the fact that pseudohypacusis can be identified and assessed by unique behavior on auditory tests that are commonly employed in a typical audiology center makes these conventional tests especially useful for assessing pseudohypacusis (Rintelmann & Harford, 1963). Such auditory measures include pure tone audiometry, speech audiometry, acoustic immittance, and auditory brainstem response measures.

Pure tone audiometry

One of the most distinguishing characteristics of pseudohypacusis is inconsistency in responses, or poor reliability, on auditory tests including pure tone threshold measures (Chaiklin & Ventry, 1963). As stated earlier, a skilled clinician testing a cooperative patient and using calibrated equipment in a proper acoustic environment should obtain test-retest agreement of pure tone thresholds within ±10 dB. If differences of 15 dB or more are obtained, especially within the same test session, suspicion of pseudohypacusis is in order. A simple technique for measuring consistency of pure tone threshold responses was described by Harris (1958). He suggested using alternately ascending and descending tone presentations in order to increase the difficulty of maintaining a falsely elevated threshold. Although this method is very effective with some pseudohypacusics, others can successfully give consistent responses at suprathreshold levels. In fact, several investigators have reported that some pseudohypacusics demonstrate good test-retest reliability on threshold tests (Berger, 1965; Campanelli, 1963; Lehrer et al., 1964; Shepherd, 1965).

Nilo and Saunders (1976) reported a "modified conventional approach" in which the patient is told a discrepancy in pure tone test results exists. The patient is not placed on the defensive; instead the inconsistencies are blamed on such factors as directions that may have been misunderstood or a patient who may have been nervous. An ascending technique in 2- to 2½-dB steps is then used, with the patient being pressured to respond. The investigators found that with most cases this modified approach gave reliable test results.

Another simple modification of a conventional technique for measuring pure tone thresholds that has been advocated for use with children is the "Yes-No" method (Frank, 1976; Miller, Fox, & Chan, 1968). Pure tone thresholds are obtained with the modified ascending technique (Carhart & Jerger, 1959), but the child is asked to say "yes" when he or she hears a tone and "no" when he or she does not. The critical aspect of this procedure is that the child must give an immediate "no" response as soon as the tone is presented. This technique is not applicable to adults because they understand the fallacy of being asked to say "no" to a tone below an admitted threshold. Some children, however, apparently do not recognize the faulty logic of this technique. As a consequence, the "Yes-No" method has been successfully employed to establish organic thresholds in pseudohypacusic children (Frank, 1976; Miller et al., 1968).

Other modifications of pure tone audiometry also have been used, such as the Variable Intensity Pulse Count Method (VIPCM) described by Ross (1964) as a modification of a procedure used earlier by Dixon and Newby (1959). Using a conventional pure tone audiometer, a variable number of tone pulses are presented above the child's admitted threshold until accurate responses are obtained several times. Next, the variable intensity of the tones includes presentation levels both above and 10–15 dB below the admitted threshold. This process is continued, with the number and intensity of tones randomly varied, until the lowest Hearing Level is found that will elicit three successive responses. Ross found good agreement between the VIPCM pure tone thresholds and the SRTs of pseudohypacusic children. He pointed out that a critical feature of the VIPCM is to instruct the child that he or she will receive a test of counting ability, thereby diverting attention away from the hearing test per se. Obviously, successful use of this test is dependent on the child's ability to count to at least four or five.

For individuals exhibiting a unilateral hearing loss, the absence of a shadow curve due to crossover of the signal to the nontest (normal) ear when masking is not used can be considered as strong evidence for the identification of pseudohypacusis. This is especially true for bone-conduction whereby the interaural attenuation, or crossover of the pure tone stimulus from the test to the nontest ear, is about 0–5 dB. For air-conduction thresholds the crossover or shadow curve response for the test ear should occur somewhere between 35 and 65 dB, depending on frequency, above the threshold of the nontest ear. Hence, when masking is not used, once the signal exceeds the interaural attenuation between ears the tone will be perceived. If a patient actually has a "dead" ear (i.e., no response by air or bone conduction) and a normal ear, the shadow curve audiogram for the poor ear when tested without masking would show a moderate conductive loss with essentially normal bone conduction. Thus if the patient does not respond, this is a clear indication of pseudohypacusis. For further discussion of interaural attenuation and clinical masking, refer to Chapter 3 by Sanders.

The shape of the audiometric configuration has been suggested by some as providing an additional clue for the detection of pseudohypacusis. Doerfler (1951) reported that the "saucer" audiogram usually found between 50 and 90 dB (re audiometric zero) was present in 80% of those patients with functional hearing losses. He attributed this to the notion that a normal listener simulating a hearing loss probably uses a reference level based on comfortable loudness and that the typical saucer audiogram corresponds to the 60-dB equal loudness contour. Johnson et al. (1956) noted that the phenomenon of recruitment will cause the saucer audiogram to be modified for persons with a functional overlay on a high-frequency loss. A functional hearing loss level will vary also with the configuration of a true organic hearing loss. Gelfand and Silman (1985) found that the size of the functional overlay would be the same for all frequencies if hearing were normal or if there were only a mild loss. However, the magnitude of the functional overlay decreased in organic hearing losses as severity of the loss increased.

Other writers (i.e., Aplin & Kane, 1985; Coles & Mason, 1984; Fournier, 1958) have characterized the audiometric pattern as a relatively "flat" loss across frequencies. On the other hand, Ventry and Chaiklin (1965) reported that saucer audiograms were found in only 8% of their pseudohypacusic patients and also were obtained from some cases of true organic loss. Hence, they concluded that the saucer-shaped audiogram is of little use in identifying pseudohypacusis. Finally, it should be noted that saucer or relatively flat audiometric configurations often occur with various types of conductive and sensorineural defects such as otosclerosis and Ménière's syndrome.

Speech audiometry

In routine audiologic assessments, a basic measure of intertest reliability is the comparison between the speech reception threshold (SRT) and the pure tone average of 500, 1000, and 2000 Hz or the two best of these three frequencies. Several investigators have studied the relationship between pure tone and speech thresholds (i.e., Aplin & Kane, 1985; Carhart & Porter, 1971; Siegenthaler & Strand, 1964). Refer to Chapter 2 by Olsen and Matkin for a detailed discussion of this topic. In general, given properly calibrated equipment, careful testing with appropriate threshold procedures, and a cooperative patient, the agreement between the SRT and the appropriate (two or three frequency) pure tone average (PTA) should be within ±6 to 8 dB.

If the SRT-PTA differs by as much as 12 dB or more with lower (better) SRTs, this outcome should raise the suspicion of pseudohypacusis. This SRT-PTA discrepancy in cases of pseudohypacusis was probably first recognized by Carhart (1952) and subsequently has been reported by several investigators (Brockman & Hoversten, 1960; Chaiklin, Ventry, Barrett, & Skalbeck, 1959; Dixon & Newby, 1959; Fournier, 1958). Concerning the efficiency of the SRT-PTA discrepancy for detecting pseudohypacusis, Rintelmann and Harford (1963) found that in a sample of 10 pseudohypacusic children all of the children had SRTs that were substantially better than their PTAs.

Regarding adult pseudohypacusis, Ventry and Chaiklin (1965) evaluated the efficiency of five audiometric measures commonly employed to identify such patients. They reported that the SRT-PTA relationship was the most efficient measure and correctly identified 70% of a sample of 47 subjects. Combined with the pure tone test-retest agreement, these two measures resulted in 85% correct identifications. Later, Conn, Ventry, and Woods (1972) obtained pure tone thresholds via an ascending technique and speech thresholds via both ascending and descending methods from adult normal listeners asked to simulate a hearing loss. They found that the SRT-PTA difference was enhanced (made larger) by using the ascending technique as opposed to the descending technique for measuring the SRT. Hence, they recommended that when pseudohypacusis is suspected, SRTs should be obtained with an ascending technique.

Several writers (i.e., Juers, 1966; Kinstler, 1971) have attempted to explain why SRTs typically demonstrate better hearing than do PTAs in cases of pseudohypacusis. For some children the explanation simply may be that they regard the pure tone test to be the "real" test of their hearing and that when the more common speech signals are presented, they respond as they would in normal conversation. On the other hand, given that a large SRT-PTA difference also is found for the more sophisticated adult pseudohypacusic, another reason must be found to account for this discrepancy. A plausible explanation is that the perceived loudness of spondee words is substantially greater than for pure tones for two reasons. First, the acoustic energy of speech is "broad spectrum" (see Chapter 2), whereas the perceived acoustic energy of a pure tone is that of the fundamental frequency even though some harmonic energy may be present (See Chapter 16). Second, spondaic words that are used for measuring SRT contain strong vowel components, and hence they have an emphasis on low-frequency energy. Because the perceived growth in loudness is greater in the low-frequency region compared to the mid frequencies, this too contributes to the listener's perception of speech stimuli being louder than pure tones. Whatever the reason to account for the SRT-PTA differences found in pseudohypacusis, the fact remains that this audiometric discrepancy is probably the best audiometric clue for alerting the clinician to suspect pseudohypacusis.

Measurement of speech or word recognition (commonly termed *speech discrimination*) is another routinely used audiologic test, which has proven to be useful in identifying pseudohypacusis. If word recognition scores are obtained immediately after measuring SRTs, it is recommended that such tests be given at a low sensation level (SL) re the SRT (Olsen & Matkin, 1978; Rintelmann & Harford, 1963). Often pseudohypacusics will respond to items on a word recognition test at levels fairly close to their admitted SRT, especially if the SRT is substantially above their true organic speech threshold. In fact, Rintelmann and Harford (1963) found that for some pseudohypacusic children, high word recognition scores were obtained at Hearing Levels (re audiometric zero) substantially lower (better) than the admitted PTA. Hence, two important qualitative clues for detecting pseudohypacusis can be obtained via word recognition testing. First, it is obviously not possible to obtain high scores at Hearing Levels below admitted PTAs; and second, high word recognition scores usually are obtained at SLs of +24 dB or higher, depending on the specific test employed and the type of auditory pathology. See Chapter 2 for further discussion of this topic.

Additional clues for identifying pseudohypacusis can be obtained from analyzing the types of responses given both to SRT and word recognition tests. Writers frequently have noted that the types of errors made by pseudohypacusics are different from those made by persons with true organic hearing loss (Fournier, 1958; Johnson et al., 1956). Often pseudohypacusics will repeat only the first half or second half of the spondee word during SRT testing. Also, they may fail to respond to some words after having repeated several spondees at weaker Hearing Levels. Chaiklin and Ventry (1965) did a quantitative analysis of such errors made by pseudohypacusics and based on their findings constructed a spondee error index (SERI). Applying their SERI to a sample of 20 pseudohypacusics, they reported correct identification in 85% of the subjects. Campbell (1965) analyzed the types of errors made on word recognition tests and constructed an index of "pseudo-discrimination loss" for use with a recorded version of the C.I.D.W-22 test. He reported good agreement between the ratings from his index and the independent judgments of three clinical audiologists.

In spite of the encouraging findings of the two studies briefly mentioned above, these methods have received little attention clinically. Lack of interest in such techniques undoubtedly is due to the fact that after the audiologist has taken the time to complete the analysis of the patient's responses, there is still nothing more than qualitative evidence concerning pseudohypacusis. In other words, testing techniques that require substantial time and effort for both administration and interpretation should provide some quantitative information about the patient's true organic level of hearing.

Special audiologic tests

Whether an auditory test is classified as "conventional," implying routine use, or as "special" is somewhat arbitrary. Certain tests may be used frequently in some audiology centers but used only for special purposes in other clinical programs. The tests described in this section are those that generally are regarded as special purpose tests. Some were developed specifically as a test for pseudohypacusis (i.e., the Doerfler-Stewart test), whereas others (i.e., Bekesy and SAL) initially were intended for use in evaluating only patients with true organic hearing disorders. These latter tests (Bekesy and SAL) rarely are used today except for assessment of pseudohypacusis. (see Chapters 1 and 13.)

Automatic audiometry

Automatic audiometry, commonly named Bekesy audiometry after the scientist who first described the instrument (Bekesy, 1947), has been used both in the laboratory and the clinic for various psychoacoustic applications. Its most frequent use was for measuring pure tone thresholds and auditory adaptation.

Jerger (1960) described a procedure for measuring auditory adaptation via Bekesy audiometry that requires the subject (patient) to trace his or her thresholds with both pulsed and continuous pure tones in either a sweep- or fixed-frequency mode of stimulus presentation. He described four types of Bekesy patterns that were associated with normal hearing (Type I) and with various conditions of auditory pathology (Types I, II, III, and IV). For further discussion of this topic refer to Chapter 13 by Hall. In all four types of Bekesy patterns described by Jerger, the threshold tracings with the continuous tonal stimuli are equal to (in sound pressure level or Hearing Level), or poorer than, the threshold tracings with the pulsed stimuli. Later, Jerger and Herer (1961) described a fifth type of Bekesy pattern observed in three cases of pseudohypacusis. This pattern, termed Type V, is the only one in which the continuous tracing shows lower sound pressure levels (better hearing) over some portion of the freuency range tested than the tracing with the pulsed (interrupted) stimulus. Subsequently, the Type V pattern observed in pseudohypacusic children as well as adults was verified by several other investigators (Peterson, 1963; Resnick & Burke, 1962; Rintelmann & Harford, 1963; Stein, 1963).

In the next few years, other studies were reported (Hopkinson, 1965; Price, Shepherd, & Goldstein, 1965; Stark, 1966) that cast some doubt on the interpretation and clinical utility of the Type V Bekesy pattern. These authors used the criterion for a Type V pattern that the continuous tracing be at least 5 dB better than the pulsed tracing. Price et al. (1965) reported that Type V Bekesy tracings were found in 6% of the fixed-frequency Bekesy audiograms of 129 adult normal listeners. Hopkinson (1965) also found that 48% of 52 conductive hearing loss cases had a Type V Bekesy pattern on sweep-frequency tracings. Stark (1966) used fixed-frequency Bekesy audiometry with children ranging in age from 5 through 10 years. He reported Type V patterns for 5% of the 61 normal hearing children and for 8.6% of the 52 children with sensorineural hearing losses. These authors concluded that Type V patterns may be expected in normal, conductive, and sensorineural hearing loss cases.

Rintelmann and Harford (1967) disagreed with the conclusions of the above-cited studies. They argued that the false positive Type V results reported by Price et al. (1965), Hopkinson (1965), and Stark (1966) were caused by arbitrarily and too rigidly defining a Type V pattern based on small decibel separations between continuous and pulsed tracings over a very narrow frequency range (i.e., less than one octave). Also, they argued in favor of using sweep- rather than fixed-frequency tracings. They contended that

> the most appropriate way to define a Bekesy pattern that is distinctive of a certain segment of the clinical population is to examine the Bekesy tracings obtained from a sample of the clinical population in question, arrive at a definition that fits that clinical group, and then finally apply that definition to the other clinical types to determine the amount of overlap that may exist. (Rintelmann & Harford, 1967, p. 735)

These investigators examined the Bekesy sweep-frequency tracings of 33 pseudohypacusics who ranged in age from 8 to 57 years. Based on an analysis of these Bekesy tracings, the following definition of a Type V pattern was proposed—a complete separation of at least 10 dB between continuous and interrupted tracings (with lower sound pressure level by continuous tracings) for at least two octaves. Furthermore, at some point in the frequency range where the break between continuous and pulsed tracings occurs, there must be a peak or maximum separation of at least 15 dB. When this definition was applied to the 33 pseudohypacusic subjects, 25, or 76%, met the criteria for the Type V pattern. To determine the false-positive rate of this definition, Rintelmann and Harford (1967) applied it to the sweep-frequency Bekesy tracings of 32 normal listeners, 50 conductives, and 150 subjects with sensorineural hearing losses. The results showed no Type V patterns in the normal group; one case, 2%, in the conductive group; and four cases, or 3%, in the group of 150 subjects with sensorineural losses. It was concluded that "when defined from an analysis of tracings by documented clinical cases, the Type V Bekesy classification has clinical utility . . . in distinguishing the pseudohypacusic from other clinical entities" (Rintelmann & Harford, 1967, p. 743). The strict criteria described above for classifying Type V patterns have received support from other clinical studies (Ventry, 1971).

In an effort to find a psychoacoustic explanation for the Type V pattern, Rintelmann and Carhart (1964) reasoned that when an individual attempts to simulate a hearing loss via Bekesy audiometry that person must employ some judgment of loudness as his or her gauge for admitting or denying awareness of the signal, because he or she actually will be hearing it all the time. To pursue this notion they administered two types of loudness tracking tasks to normal listeners via sweep-frequency Bekesy audiometry using conventional stimulus parameters (200 ms on and off duration for the pulsed tones; see Chapter 13). The first was the most comfortable loudness task whereby the subjects tracked interrupted and continuous tones according to their "internal standard" for a comfortable level of loudness. The second was a recalled loudness task in which the subjects were required to track the stimuli based on their memory of the loudness of a 1000-Hz tone heard only at the beginning of the task. The authors found that whether a person uses some internal standard for comfortable loudness or attempts to track tones that are changing in frequency according to one's long-term memory of a previously heard tone, in either case continuous tones are traced at substantially lower SPLs than are interrupted tones. Based on these findings Rintelmann and Carhart concluded that a pulsed tone is judged to be less loud than a sustained one at the same sensation level; hence "the Type V Bekesy audiogram is to be expected when a person attempts to establish a false threshold tracing by monitoring the loudness of continuous and interrupted tones" (Rintelmann & Carhart, 1964, p. 92).

Melnick (1967) pursued further the relationship between pulsed and continuous tones when normal listeners tracked loudness via Bekesy audiometry. He conducted a series of studies using both fixed and sweep-frequency. Two listener tasks were used—most comfortable loudness level and tracking loudness of a standard (reference) signal that was presented every 30 s. An important difference between Melnick's technique of loudness matching and the Rintelmann and Carhart recalled loudness task is that Melnick's procedure eliminated the subject's reliance on long-term loudness memory. Melnick's results demonstrated that for the fixed-frequency condition and when the standard signal was presented at frequent intervals during the loudness matching task, only small decibel differences were observed between the pulsed and continuous tracings; however, substantially greater dB differences were found (similar to those of Rintelmann & Carhart, 1964) in the sweep-frequency most comfortable loudness task. Melnick attributed these findings to an ambiguity of the listener's loudness standard rather than a difference in loudness between sustained and pulsed signals. However, there were so many methodological differences concerning signal presentation between the Melnick and Rintelmann and Carhart studies that it is difficult to make overall comparisons between the two studies. At any rate, the important clinical implication of Melnick's results is that when Bekesy audiometry is used with conventional stimulus parameters for pulsed tones (200 ms on and off), one is more apt to find a Type V Bekesy pattern with sweep as opposed to fixed-frequency tracings when a person is attempting to simulate a hearing loss.

Hattler (1968) too studied the effects of loudness memory on the Type V Bekesy pattern. He reasoned that if signal on-duration differences do not affect tracking level (Melnick, 1967), but if loudness memory effects are responsible for the Type V pattern as suggested by the recalled loudness findings of Rintelmann and Carhart (1964), tracking level should be influenced by the duty cycle[1] and not by temporal factors such as on–off-duration or interruption rate. He investigated this notion by having adult normal listeners track a 1000-Hz reference tone with seven different test signals: one continuous and six differentially interrupted 1000-Hz tones. The results of this experiment demonstrated that "tracking levels were inversely related to the signal's duty cycle and were independent of other temporal parameters such as on-duration and interruption rate" (Hattler, 1968, p. 567). Hattler concluded that the Type V Bekesy pattern can be attributed to the differential effects of loudness memory upon pulsed and sustained pure tones. Based on these findings Hattler (1970) developed the lengthened off-time (LOT) test as a screening procedure for pseudohypacusis. He used fixed-frequency Bekesy tracings at 1000 Hz under three signal conditions: (a) a pulsed tone with standard off-time (200 ms on/200 ms off); (b) a pulsed tone with lengthened off-time (200 ms on/800 ms off); and (c) a continuous tone. The LOT test increases the separation between pulsed and continuous tracings for pseudohypacusics, but it has

---

[1]Duty cycle refers to the on–off ratio of the signal, that is, a 50% duty cycle means that (per unit of time) the signal is on half of the time and off half of the time.

no effect on the tracings of normal listeners or patients with organic hearing losses. According to Hattler (1970), results are considered indicative of pseudohypacusis if the pulsed tracing shows at least a 5.5-dB poorer threshold than the continuous tracing. He reported that 95% of a nonorganic group was identified correctly with the LOT test, whereas only 40% of this group was identified correctly with the standard off-time signal. Furthermore, in a group of patients with organic hearing losses, none of the individuals was misclassified by either the standard or LOT pulsed signal when compared to the continuous tracing. Also, Hattler and Schuchman (1970) presented LOT test results of 340 hearing-impaired patients in a clinic population with a high incidence of pseudohypacusis. They reported an overall efficiency (organic and nonorganic patients) of 98.3%. On the other hand, Citron and Reddell (1976) found that the LOT test correctly identified only 7 out of 14, or 50%, from a sample of adult pseudohypacusics.

Behnke and Lankford (1976) demonstrated that the LOT test could be successfully employed with normal hearing children between 7½ and 10½ years of age. They found only a small percentage of false-positive responses at three test frequencies: 4% at 1000 Hz and 3% at 2000 Hz and 4000 Hz. At 500 Hz, however, 14% of the children displayed false-positive results. Hence, the authors recommended that the frequency of 500 Hz should not be used for the LOT test with preadolescent subjects.

Using young adult normal listeners asked to simulate a hearing loss, Martin and Monro (1975) investigated the effects of sophistication and practice on Type V tracings obtained via both LOT and standard off-time fixed-frequency tracings. The findings demonstrated a reduction in the number of Type V patterns observed as listener sophistication increased. Thus the implication of this study is that if a person has some knowledge about the test and a brief practice with the test, it is possible to simulate a hearing loss on the LOT test without producing a Type V tracing. Lankford and Meissner (1977) conducted a study to determine if a manual LOT test would be as effective as the automatic LOT test. They tested 10 nonorganic hearing loss subjects and noted that results of the two procedures were equivalent. The manual technique can be used with most diagnostic audiometers.

Recently, Chaiklin (1990) compared the results of administering both the LOT test and a descending version of the LOT (DELOT) to 24 pseudohypacusic subjects and to 30 subjects who were not pseudohypacusic. He found that the sensitivity (true positive results) of the DELOT was 100% in that all 24 pseudohypacusic subjects were correctly identified, whereas only 17 subjects (70.8%) were correctly identified with the LOT. Concerning specificity (true negative results) only one false positive DELOT result occurred among the 30 nonpseudohypacusic subjects or a

3.3% false positive rate. Specificity could not be compared to the LOT test because the nonpseudohypacusic subjects were selected partly on the basis of negative LOT test results. Chaiklin concluded that the DELOT is a very effective screening test for pseudohypacusis, and he urged that it be used by audiologists who have available Bekesy-type audiometers.

Another modification of Bekesy audiometry advocated for use with pseudohypacusics that has received some attention by audiologists is the Bekesy Ascending Descending Gap Evaluation (BADGE) procedure developed by Hood, Campbell, and Hutton (1964). Three 1-min fixed-frequency tracings are obtained with this test: (a) a continuous ascending (CA) tracing beginning at −20 dB Hearing Level (HL), (b) a pulsed ascending (PA) tracing beginning below threshold, and (c) a pulsed descending (PD) threshold tracing starting at 40–60 dB above the PA threshold or at the maximum output of the audiometer, whichever is lower. Hood et al. (1964) administered the BADGE test at 1000 Hz only and compared the Bekesy tracing gaps for three conditions: PD-PA, CA-PA, and PD-CA. They reported that all three gaps were equally efficient (about 70%) for distinguishing between the organic and nonorganic hearing-impaired veterans tested.

In summary, automatic or Bekesy audiometry can be usefully employed as a qualitative measure for the identification of pseudohypacusis in both children and adults. If conventional stimulus parameters are used for pulsed tones (200 ms on and off), there is ample evidence to support the notion that the method of choice should be sweep and not fixed frequency (Melnick, 1967; Price et al., 1965; Rintelmann & Harford, 1963, 1967; Stark, 1966). Using strict criteria for Type V classification of sweep-frequency tracings, correct identification can be expected in about 75% of pseudohypacusic patients with a low false-positive rate (2–3%) among patients with organic hearing losses (Rintelmann & Harford, 1967). By the same token, fixed-frequency tracings have been found to misclassify normal hearing children (Stark, 1966) and adults (Price et al., 1965) and children with sensorineural hearing losses (Stark, 1966). In addition, fixed-frequency tracings have proven ineffective in detecting pseudohypacusics (Hattler, 1970) and as a measure of normal listeners simulating a hearing loss (Martin & Monro, 1975). When certain modified Bekesy procedures are used, however, fixed-frequency tracings can be quite effective as a screening test for pseudohypacusis. The BADGE test was found to be about 70% efficient in distinguishing between organic and nonorganic hearing loss (Hood et al., 1964), whereas the LOT test has been reported to have an overall efficiency ranging from 50% to nearly 100% (Chaiklin, 1990; Citron & Reddell, 1976; Hattler & Schuchman, 1970). Thus three different Bekesy audiometric procedures have demonstrated fair to good clinical utility for the detection of pseudohypacusis.

Proper use of Bekesy audiometry can produce true positive results (sensitivity) in 70% or more of pseudohypacusic patients, whereas false positive findings (specificity) tends to occur in less than 5% of nonpseudohypacusic individuals. Refer to Chapter 14 for further discussion of evaluating test efficiency.

Sensorineural Acuity Level (SAL) test

The Sensorineural Acuity Level (SAL) test developed by Jerger and Tillman (1960) as a method for measuring the extent of sensorineural hearing loss was received initially with enthusiasm by audiologists as a means for circumventing some of the problems encountered in measuring bone-conduction thresholds. The SAL test is based on the principle that a known level of white noise presented via a bone-conduction vibrator placed at the center of the forehead will produce a smaller threshold shift for a person with a sensorineural hearing loss than for someone with normal hearing or with a conductive loss. The difference between the threshold shifts for a normal ear and for an ear with pathology is the amount of the sensorineural hearing loss. Subsequent research (Tillman, 1963) revealed that the SAL test, like bone-conduction, also was plagued with problems. Its use has had two major limitations: the occlusion effect and the spread of masking. (For further discussion see Chapter 1.) Although the above-mentioned problems tend to restrict the clinical usefulness of the SAL test, Rintelmann and Harford (1963) found it quite effective for the detection and assessment of pseudohypacusis among children. They found that the SAL thresholds demonstrated substantially better hearing than the pure tone thresholds for all 10 children tested. Such findings can be explained by the fact that because a pseudohypacusic individual does not have the "built-in attenuation" provided by a cochlear lesion, the bone-conducted threshold shift produced by the noise is similar to that for a normal ear or one with a conductive loss. Thus if the pseudohypacusic person does not exhibit a conductive loss (which is usually the case), the differences between the air-conduction and SAL thresholds not only helps to confirm the suspicion of pseudohypacusis, but also provides some evidence that the patient's thresholds are at least as good as the SAL results indicate.

The SAL test has the same advantage as the Doerfler-Stewart test for assessing pseudohypacusis; that is, the masking noise disrupts the figurative "yardstick" against which sounds (pure tone or speech) are gauged. Although the SAL test was developed originally by Jerger and Tillman (1960) for use with pure tones, a few investigators have adapted this technique for use with speech stimuli. Bragg (1962) used spondee words to obtain SRT-SAL scores and found close agreement among measures of bone-conduction, pure tone SAL, and the SRT-SAL in subjects with sensorineural hearing loss. Bailey and Martin (1963) reported that speech SAL using spondees showed a closer relationship to postoperative SRTs than either bone-conduction or pure tone SAL thresholds in patients with otosclerosis. Rintelmann and Johnson (1970) using spondees compared speech SAL scores both under earphones and in a sound-field to pure tone SAL scores in three groups of subjects: normal listeners, "plugged" normals, and individuals with sensorineural hearing loss. They found good agreement between the earphone speech SAL score and the 500-, 1000- and 2000-Hz average of the pure tone SAL test. Also, the differences between sound-field and earphone speech SAL scores were consistent with expected minimum audible field-minimum audible pressure differences (i.e., 8.7 dB better via sound-field for the sensorineural group). More recently, Hurley and Mather (1988) reported on the potential clinical use of the SAL test by studying two groups of subjects with feigned hearing loss. Their data demonstrated that this test is useful in predicting audiometric threshold to within 10 dB.

A word of caution is in order for the reader who may wish to consider using either the pure tone or speech SAL test for assessing pseudohypacusis. Like any other auditory test, one must first know the normative value of the particular signal being used. Hence, clinicians must establish their own normative data based on the equipment being used. For further discussion of the SAL test, see Chapter 1 by Wilber.

Doerfler-Stewart test

The Doerfler-Stewart test is based on the notion that if an individual attempts to simulate an elevated speech threshold, complex (sawtooth) noise mixed in the same ear with the test words will cause the pseudohypacusic person to stop responding to the spondees when the noise is actually less intense than required to mask speech. In other words, the noise disrupts the person's figurative loudness yardstick for speech. This test was described initially by Doerfler and Stewart (1946) who recommended using a sawtooth noise with a fundamental frequency of about 128 Hz. They stated that such a noise is psychologically noisier than a white noise at the same sensation level. The norms, reported by Doerfler and Epstein (1956), were established with sawtooth noise. Unfortunately these norms have not been readily available; however, given that the test involves obtaining both a Noise Interference Level (NIL) and a Noise Detection Threshold (NDT), it is appropriate for a clinician to establish his or her own norms with the noise source to be used.

The Doerfler-Stewart test was designed to be administered binaurally; however, it has been used also as a monaural test. The details of the test procedure and interpretation of results have been described elsewhere (i.e., Hopkinson, 1978; Martin, 1985) and will not be reported here. In short, five scores are obtained: (a) SRT-one, (b) SRT-one +5 dB, (c) NIL, (d) SRT-two, and (e) NDT. The interpretation of the Doerfler-Stewart test involves making various comparisons of the above test scores (i.e., NDT-NIL) to the norms for this test.

Surprisingly little published documentation is available concerning the clinical efficiency of the Doerfler-Stewart test, and these sparse data are not in close agreement. Menzel administered the Doerfler-Stewart test to veterans who were examined for compensation purposes and concluded that it is "a sensitive detector of nonorganicity, [and] also serves as an important motivational device in discouraging the would-be malingerer" (Menzel, 1960, p. 54). Ventry and Chaiklin (1965) used the Doerfler and Epstein (1956) norms and found that the Doerfler-Stewart test failed to adequately differentiate functional from nonfunctional subjects. They suggested a revision of the norms to improve the effectiveness of the test, but concluded that the "test's complexity of administration and interpretation weaken its utility as a screening test for functional hearing loss" (Ventry & Chaiklin, 1965, p. 258). Hattler and Schuchman (1971) also used the Doerfler and Epstein procedure for giving the Doerfler-Stewart test. They reported that a major limitation was that it could not be appropriately administered to nearly 65% of 225 nonorganic patients. However, when it could be given it was 77% effective among nonorganic patients but yielded false-positive responses from 20% of the organically-impaired patients.

Modified versions of the Doerfler-Stewart test also have been proposed. Martin and Hawkins (1963) suggested using pure tones instead of spondee words, and white noise in place of sawtooth noise. Also, they eliminated the use of the Noise Detection Threshold from their procedure and hence simplified the scoring of this test. Although the authors did not present any specific findings, they stated that their modified Doerfler-Stewart test has proven to be a rapid and valid method for the detection of pseudohypacusis. Yet another modification using pure tones instead of spondees is the Tone-In-Noise test (Pang-Ching, 1970).

Over the past several years the Doerfler-Stewart test appears to have largely fallen into disuse. This probably is due to the fact that it requires considerable practice for proper administration, and most audiologists see too few pseudohypacusics to gain proficiency with this test. Furthermore, the Doerfler-Stewart test results provide only qualitative information and there are other less complex tests (i.e., SRT-pure tone average difference) that serve the same purpose.

Pure tone and speech Stenger tests

The Stenger test is based on the principle that a tone presented simultaneously to two ears is perceived only in the ear that receives the greater intensity. Hence, this test is most appropriate for persons exhibiting unilateral pseudohypacusis; however, it can be used also for testing pseudohypacusics manifesting an asymmetrical bilateral hearing loss if the admitted threshold difference between ears is at least 40 dB.

The Stenger test, originally administered with a pair of matched tuning forks, was one of the first tests developed specifically for the identification of pseudohypacusis (Stenger, 1907). Since the initial description of this test, various procedures for administering it have been proposed. With regard to appropriate instrumentation, a two-channel audiometer should be used to provide separate attenuation to each earphone, whereby the output from a single audio oscillator can be delivered to both earphones. This latter requirement is especially important because no two oscillators in commercial audiometers will produce the exact frequency set on the frequency dial (see Chapter 16). In other words, if a different pure tone source (oscillator) is used for each earphone, the patient may perceive either a slightly different frequency in each ear or a beating phenomenon. To avoid this problem, the speech Stenger can be used by presenting the same spondee words to each earphone, but at different intensities.

Although several writers have described a test procedure for the Stenger test, there currently is no standardized method for giving this test (Fournier, 1958; Kinstler, 1971; Watson & Tolan, 1949). When using the Stenger as a screening test, Martin (1985) recommended introducing the desired pure tone to the better ear at a level of 10 dB above threshold and at 10 dB below the admitted threshold of the "poorer" ear. If the patient responds to the tone, this suggests that he or she perceived it via the better ear, and hence, the loss in the poorer ear is "real." Such an outcome is called a negative Stenger. On the other hand, if the patient does not respond, this implies that the tone was heard in the professed poorer ear. Hence, such a result is a positive Stenger. In this case, the pure tone is lateralized to the ear receiving the louder signal (poorer ear), and the patient is unaware of the presence of the weaker signal in the better ear. The principle of the Stenger screening test can be applied to a procedure for estimating actual thresholds. Again, begin by presenting the pure tone to the good ear at 10 dB SL while simultaneously giving the tone to the bad ear at 0 dB Hearing Level. The patient should respond. Next, increase the signal level in the bad ear by 5 dB while keeping the level in the good ear constant. Continue raising the level in the bad ear in 5-dB steps until the patient fails to respond. When this "Stenger effect" occurs, the tone has lateralized to the bad ear, which suggests that the signal to the bad ear is approximately at a 15-dB SL or higher. Recall, the tone is still being delivered to the good ear at a 10 dB SL. According to Martin (1985), this procedure for determining the minimum contralateral interference level should provide a reasonable estimate of the organic threshold of the claimed bad ear. The speech Stenger test can be administered by using essentially this same procedure.

Concerning the clinical efficiency of the Stenger test, the findings reported in the literature vary from less than 50% to 100% correct identification. Ventry and Chaiklin (1965) reported that the Stenger test was appropriate for only 55% of their veteran patients and that correct identification of pseudohypacusis was obtained with only 43% of the cases. These findings are in close agreement with those of Hattler and Schuchman (1971) who reported that this test was applicable with 57% of their patients and that it showed only 48% correct identification of pseudohypacusis. They administered the LOT, Doerfler-Stewart, and Stenger tests when applicable to a large sample of pseudohypacusic patients and found the Stenger to be the least efficient of the three tests. In contrast to the above findings, Kinstler, Phelan, and Lavender (1972) reported 83% correct identification for adult pseudohypacusic patients with the pure tone Stenger and 75% successful detection with the speech Stenger test. Peck and Ross (1970) administered the pure tone Stenger by ascending and descending modes to 35 normal hearing young adults who were told to feign a total unilateral loss. Both methods of signal presentation were found to be 100% efficient in detecting unilateral pseudohypacusis. Monro and Martin (1977) also found the pure tone Stenger, using the screening technique, to be 100% effective in detecting feigning unilateral hearing loss in a group of young adult normal listeners. However, Martin and Shipp (1982) found that with sophistication and practice the efficiency was reduced for both the pure tone and speech Stenger tests in providing threshold estimates for young adult normal hearing subjects who were instructed to feign a unilateral hearing loss.

The most likely explanation for the conflicting findings concerning the efficiency of the Stenger test relates to the amount of asymmetry between ears. The importance of this fact was recognized in each of the above-cited studies. For example, Ventry and Chaiklin (1965) noted that both the pure tone and speech Stenger tests were most efficient when the patients exhibited an interaural difference greater than 40 dB. They found very few positive results with smaller differences between ears. Hence, it appears that in order for the Stenger test to be used successfully, either via pure tone or speech, there must be a large interaural discrepancy in the patient's admitted thresholds.

Lombard test

The Lombard is a gross screening test for pseudohypacusis based on the concept of auditory feedback. To explain, a talker regulates his or her vocal intensity to compensate for the background noise level of the environment by listening to his or her own voice. Hence, when the environmental noise level is high, a talker usually will raise his or her voice. This principle serves as the basis for the Lombard test, which is one of the oldest screening tests in existence. Originally, it was administered with mechanical noisemakers, such as the Barany noise box. Now the audiometer serves as the noise source. Masking noise (i.e., white noise) is introduced through earphones (preferably binaurally) and gradually is increased in level while the patient reads a passage aloud. If the loudness level of the patient's voice increases while the masking noise is at a level below his or her admitted threshold, this is a positive Lombard and is indicative of pseudohypacusis.

In cases of unilateral hearing loss, some clinicians have advocated presenting the noise to the better ear, others have suggested applying the noise to the poorer ear, whereas still others have proposed putting the noise first in one ear and then the other (Chaiklin & Ventry, 1963). Based on the findings of Taylor (1949), who probably conducted the first experimental investigation of the Lombard test, binaural application of the noise compared to monaural input appears to enhance the probability of demonstrating the Lombard effect. Hence, it may be advantageous to present noise to both ears when giving the Lombard test, irrespective of whether pseudohypacusis is exhibited as a unilateral or bilateral hearing loss.

The Lombard test has limited value because it does not provide an estimate of the patient's true hearing thresholds, and more important, because many individuals can control their vocal intensity while reading aloud or speaking in the presence of high levels of masking noise. Hence, a negative Lombard finding does not rule out the possibility of pseudohypacusis.

Speech and pure tone delayed auditory feedback

The phenomenon of delayed auditory feedback (DAF), also termed delayed side tone, has been extensively studied in order to gain an understanding of basic sensory monitoring systems (Black, 1951, 1954; Lee, 1950) and to develop additional methods for assessing pseudohypacusis (Tiffany & Hanley, 1952).

Although no standard procedure has evolved for administering the DAF test, it typically involves requiring a subject, wearing earphones,

to read aloud several times measured matched passages into a microphone. The passages, recorded on tape, first are read with no feedback,
next with simultaneous feedback, and then in the delay condition. The
subject is instructed to read at his or her normal rate. A stopwatch is used
to time the reading. Usually, three or more control reading times (without
feedback or with simultaneous feedback) are averaged and compared to
the reading time under the delay condition.

Some investigators have used a single delay time between the
recorded message and the playback message (i.e., 0.18 s) and several sensation levels (i.e., 0, 10, 20, 30, 40, and 50 dB) for presenting the delayed
feedback condition, whereas other experimenters have used several delay
times and one or more sensation levels. Hanley and Tiffany (1954a, 1954b)
found that a delay of 0.175 to 0.2 seconds at sensation levels of 20 to 40
dB above spondee threshold produces substantial changes in reading rate,
voice intensity and quality, and disruption in fluency. These investigators
reported an optimum delay time of 0.18 s and that an 8% difference in
reading rate could be expected when the DAF test is given at 20 to 30
dB above threshold. Based on these findings, it has been suggested that
the DAF test could be regarded as positive when the patient's reading
time in the delay condition varies from the control reading rate by 10%
or more. Furthermore, it has been suggested that the DAF test can be
used not only to detect pseudohypacusis but also to obtain an estimate
of the true organic threshold. On the other hand, Harford and Jerger (1959)
found that hearing-impaired subjects showed the DAF effects at considerably lower SLs than did normal listeners. Hence, for patients with
a pseudohypacusic overlay on a true organic loss, it would be hazardous
to attempt to ascertain speech thresholds from DAF results. This problem,
coupled with the fact that some persons are able to maintain a fairly constant reading pattern regardless of delay time or feedback sensation level,
has had an appreciable negative influence on the clinical utility of the
delayed auditory feedback test.

Recognizing the above-mentioned limitations of the DAF test using
speech stimuli, a comprehensive series of studies were undertaken by
Ruhm and Cooper (1962, 1963, 1964a, 1964b) using a motor task involving key tapping. This technique, proposed earlier by Chase and associates
(Chase, Harvey, Standfast, Rapin, & Sutton, 1959; Chase, Sutton, Fowler,
Fay, & Ruhm, 1961) requires the subject to tap out a simple rhythmic
pattern (i.e., four taps, pause, two taps) with an electromechanical key
that delivers pure tone bursts to the subject's ear with each tap. The key
does not produce any mechanical noise and is hidden from the subject's
visual field. The subject first receives a series of trials with simultaneous
auditory feedback (SAF) in which tapping triggers a synchronous pure
tone pulse (i.e., 50 ms maximum amplitude) to the test ear. After receiv-

ing the SAF series, the tone pulses are presented delayed by some preset duration (i.e., 200 ms) after the subject's tap. If the tone is perceived the DAF effect results in a change in tapping behavior compared to the SAF condition, such as disruption in tapping rhythm, errors in the number of taps, or the use of greater tapping pressure.

Ruhm and Cooper (1962) found that a delay time of 200 ms was most effective in producing disruption in tapping performance at 5 and 10 dB SL. Also, Ruhm and Cooper (1963) found that performance on the DAF task was independent of stimulus frequency from 250 to 8000 Hz. Furthermore, they found that short-term practice had no appreciable effect on DAF performance, but that sophistication (foreknowledge of the task) reduced the effect on tapping performance at threshold but not at 5 dB SL. Later, Cooper and Stokinger (1976) investigated the effect of practice with DAF at moderate sensation levels (+30 and +15 dB) upon key-tapping performance at low SLs (−6, 0, and +6 dB). They found that subjects with prior experience showed greater resistance to the adverse effect of DAF than did subjects without practice. Hence, they recommended that practice should be avoided when giving the pure tone DAF test to clinical patients. However, Monro and Martin (1977) and Martin and Shipp (1982) found for normal listeners feigning a unilateral hearing loss that pure tone DAF at low SLs was very resistant to effects of both previous test knowledge and practice.

In order to use the pure tone DAF technique with clinical patients it is important to know how much deterioration in tapping behavior must occur in order to state with certainty that the change in performance was a result of having heard the delayed pure tone. This question was investigated by Cooper, Stokinger, and Billings (1976). Using subjects with normal hearing (at the test frequency investigated), they established criteria for absolute and relative time error as well as pattern error, which resulted in prediction of the 1000-Hz pure tone threshold within 10 dB in 90% of their subjects.

Concerning the application of the pure tone DAF task to clinical patients, Ruhm and Cooper (1964b) compared estimates of thresholds based on DAF results with those obtained both by conventional and electrodermal audiometry (EDA) in groups of patients with either organic or pseudohypacusic hearing loss. The organic group demonstrated close agreement among all three measures. The pseudohypacusic group also displayed close agreement between the DAF and EDA findings, and both measures showed substantially better hearing than did the conventional voluntary audiometric thresholds. These findings by Ruhm and Cooper (1964b), demonstrating the value of applying the pure tone DAF technique to clinical patients including pseudohypacusics, have been extended and further supported by other investigators. Robinson and Kasden (1973) reported that they were able to establish true thresholds in 34 out of 35 pseudohypacusic patients. Billings and Stokinger (1975) found that the pure tone DAF method was successful in 88% of 100 unselected patients who were examined for medical-legal evaluation. Citron and Reddell (1976) also tested 100 patients referred for the same purpose. They attempted to give the DAF test to 86 patients and were successful in estimating threshold in 75 cases. Of the 11 unsuccessful cases, 5 did not exhibit changes in tapping performance under the delayed feedback condition, and 6 did not tap the pattern as instructed. Finally, Cooper, Stokinger, and Billings (1977) compared DAF time and pattern errors in a group of subjects with normal hearing at 1000 Hz and a sensorineural hearing loss at 4000 Hz. They found no performance difference between frequencies, and hence they concluded that the presence of a hearing loss should not affect the estimate of threshold yielded by DAF test results.

Thus, although the clinical utility of the speech DAF test seems questionable, use of the pure tone DAF technique appears to have considerable merit. Studies with normal listeners have been conducted both to establish the appropriate stimulus parameters for eliciting the DAF effects, and to determine some of the important factors (i.e., practice, SL, etc.) that influence DAF key-tapping performance. These investigations have been briefly reviewed above. Furthermore, sufficient data are available on patient populations to demonstrate that the pure tone DAF test is not only useful for identifying pseudohypacusis, but most important, this technique can provide reasonably close estimates (within 10 dB)[2] of pure tone threshold. In fact, if enthusiasm for clinical research on this test would be renewed, the pure tone DAF test could prove to be one of the most useful, and perhaps even the best, *behavioral* technique for assessing pseudohypacusis.

Other behavioral speech measures

A few other techniques that have been proposed, but which have received only limited application, are mentioned briefly here. The use of rapid interruption and switching of speech from one ear to the other has been suggested by Calearo (1957) as a test for unilateral pseudohypacusis. Although excellent results have been claimed by Calearo for this test, no

---

[2]Threshold estimates yielded by pure tone DAF results can be expected to be 5–10 dB poorer than conventional audiometric thresholds due to the short signal duration (50 ms maximum amplitude tone burst) used in the DAF test. In general, studies on brief tone audiometry have shown that for pure tones, the signal duration must be about 150 ms or longer to achieve the most sensitive threshold value.

specific supporting data have been reported. A somewhat related technique, the swinging (shifting) story or voice test involves switching a story or questions between ears and also (in some versions) binaurally, but without interruption. This test has been described by several writers (Davis & Goldstein, 1960; Newby, 1958; Watson & Tolan, 1949) and more recently by Martin (1985). By switching the story or questions fairly rapidly (i.e., every half second) between ears or from the good ear to both ears to the bad ear, the patient often becomes confused. Because this test provides only qualitative information and puts undue pressure on the patient, coupled with the fact that its clinical effectiveness has not been demonstrated, we believe that there are ample other tests that are more appropriate for evaluating pseudohypacusis. A lipreading test in which monosyllabic homophenous words are presented simultaneously by visual and auditory stimuli was proposed by Falconer (1966). Beginning well above threshold, the words are presented at gradually reduced intensity levels until only visual clues are received. Unaware that homophenous words look alike but sound different, the pseudohypacusic patient will give correct responses that can result only from hearing the words. Hence, according to Falconer, the pseudohypacusic patient may inadvertently exhibit his or her true organic Hearing Level. Although none of the tests mentioned above has received popular acceptance among audiologists, the Falconer lipreading test appears to have potential merit.

Electrophysiological and other direct measures

In this section the following measures are discussed: middle ear muscle acoustic reflex, electrodermal audiometry, auditory brainstem response, and electrocochleography. At the outset it should be emphasized that each of these measures has proven to be useful in assessing the integrity of some portion of the auditory system; however, none of these methods directly measures a person's ability to hear. A major distinction between these procedures and the behavioral methods for assessing auditory function discussed above is that the so-called direct (objective) measures do not necessitate active participation from the patient in the test procedure, but simply require passive cooperation. In a sense, calling these procedures (i.e., auditory brainstem response) objective is somewhat of a misnomer, in that the test results still must be interpreted by the clinician or investigator. Nevertheless, these procedures are called objective (by some) because the patient's role is passive and the particular electrophysiologic response is measured and usually recorded by an instrument.

Acoustic reflex

Acoustic immittance measures (tympanometry, static compliance, and acoustic reflex) have been well established for many years as a routine part of the audiological evaluation (see Chapters 4 and 5). Although the primary application of acoustic immittance (impedance) tests is for the evaluation of organic hearing disorders, it has been recognized for many years that the measurement of middle ear muscle reflex thresholds could be usefully employed in the detection of pseudohypacusis (Jepsen, 1953; Lamb & Peterson, 1967; Sanders, 1975; Thomsen, 1955).

In persons with normal hearing the acoustic reflex usually is elicited with contralateral stimulation at sensation levels ranging from 70 to 95 dB; the reflex is absent in most cases of conductive pathology; and for individuals with cochlear lesions the reflex may be obtained at sensation levels ranging from 15 to 60 dB. Hence, as Wilber (1976) pointed out, there can be dramatic variability in the precise sensation level that will elicit the acoustic reflex from the patient with cochlear pathology. As a consequence, it is difficult to detect pseudohypacusis based on acoustic reflex thresholds unless reflexes are elicited at sensation levels of 10 dB or lower re the patient's alleged pure tone thresholds. The classic example, however, is the patient who exhibits either a unilateral or bilateral profound hearing loss with acoustic reflex thresholds present at Hearing Levels better than the admitted voluntary thresholds. Such a result is not possible physiologically, and hence is strong support for the detection of pseudohypacusis. By the same token, the absence of acoustic reflexes taken as a single measure do not confirm a diagnosis of sensorineural hearing loss.

Acoustic reflex measurements also have been used for estimating thresholds. Jerger, Burney, Mauldin, and Crump (1974) refined and evaluated the procedure of Niemeyer and Sesterhenn (1974) in which acoustic reflex thresholds for pure tones are compared to those elicited by broadband white noise and low- and high-frequency filtered white noise. This procedure, termed SPAR (sensitivity prediction from the acoustic reflex), was intended to provide an estimate of the amount of hearing loss as well as an approximation of the audiometric configuration. If this test had proven to be clinically successful, it could have served an important function in the assessment of pseudohypacusis. Unfortunately, however, subsequent studies (i.e., Jerger, Hayes, Anthony, & Mauldin, 1978) have demonstrated that there are some serious limitations to the employment of the SPAR procedure.

It has been suggested by some (i.e., Wilber, 1976) that the very nature of impedance measures, including tympanometry and acoustic reflex, may serve to deter an individual from exhibiting pseudohypacusis, especially if these tests are administered at the outset of the audiological evaluation. As stated by Wilber (1976), if the unsophisticated patient is made aware by the clinician "that every time the sound occurs there is a needle deflection [of the impedance unit] and, thus, he may infer that we are able to 'see' whether he hears or not" (p. 212). Hence, some clinicians feel that the impedance testing atmosphere per se may discourage the potential pseudohypacusic.

Electrodermal audiometry

Experimental psychologists have employed the technique of psychogalvanic skin response (PGSR) for several decades as a procedure for measuring autonomic nervous system activity associated with affective or emotional states. In the 1940s the first concentrated efforts were made to use PGSR or GSR for the clinical evaluation of hearing (Bordley & Hardy, 1949; Doerfler, 1948; Knapp & Gold, 1950; Michels & Randt, 1947). Much of the impetus for the application of PGSR, later termed electrodermal audiometry (EDA), to the measurement of hearing thresholds (especially in children) came from the extensive work by Bordley, Hardy, and associates at Johns Hopkins University from the late 1940s through the early 1950s.

The EDA procedure is based on a conditioning paradigm in which the conditioned stimulus (pure tone) is presented accompanied by the unconditioned stimulus (mild electric shock). Initially, the shock produces a reduction in skin resistance to a low-voltage electric current. These resistance changes are amplified and graphically recorded. After the subject has been conditioned to the pure tone stimulus, a threshold measurement procedure is begun. A variety of methods have been advocated for measuring pure tone thresholds. Close agreement has been found, approximately ±5 dB, between EDA and voluntary thresholds (Burk, 1958; Doerfler & McClure, 1954). Also, procedures have been reported for measuring EDA speech thresholds with classical conditioning (Ruhm & Carhart, 1958; Ruhm & Menzel, 1959) and with instrumental avoidance conditioning (Hopkinson, Katz, & Schill, 1960). A comparison of the two conditioning methods for obtaining EDA SRTs in normal listeners was conducted by Katz and Connelly (1964). They found that instrumental avoidance was superior to classical conditioning in that acquisition of conditioning was more rapid and extinction was slower.

The primary application of EDA has been for obtaining pure tone thresholds on patients suspected of pseudohypacusis in Veterans Administration (VA) audiology programs. As stated earlier in this chapter, an important motivating factor among veterans for exhibiting pseudohypacusis has been the compensation claims connected with service-related hearing loss. Hence, during the late 1950s through the middle 1960s, EDA was used as a routine test in VA audiology centers with veterans seeking pensions for service-connected hearing loss. With the sharp reduction in the incidence of pseudohypacusis among veterans and military personnel since the late 1960s, the use of EDA with these populations has diminished greatly. However, Stankiewicz, Fankhauser, and Strom (1981) stated that EDA is very useful in a clinical setting and advocate its use in nonorganic hearing loss cases.

It may seem somewhat paradoxical that during the past several years there has been substantial reduction in the clinical application of EDA, whereas at the same time investigators have reported impressive results with this technique for obtaining pure tone thresholds among pseudohypacusic subjects who could be successfully conditioned. However, herein lies a major limitation of EDA. For example, Citron and Reddell (1976) found that among 86 patients seen for medical-legal audiological evaluation 25 could not be conditioned. Also, whereas 88% of those who were tested by EDA demonstrated close agreement (within ±5 dB) with their voluntary thresholds, pure tone DAF results on these same patients were equally accurate. Furthermore, substantially more patients could be tested by DAF than by EDA.

In addition to the problem of not being able to condition some patients for EDA testing, there are other reasons to account for the increased disuse of this technique. The use of an unpleasant electric shock as an integral part of EDA has long been sufficiently disturbing to many audiologists that they simply will not employ this test. Also, within the past several years legal questions have been raised about the use of shock with EDA. Finally, federal regulations and safety standards (i.e., Underwriters Laboratories) concerning maximum allowable current in instruments used with humans may simply prohibit altogether EDA testing in its present form. Thus the future role of EDA, which had its beginning in the 1940s with the "birth of audiology," simply may be to mark a part of the history of hearing assessment.

Auditory brainstem response

Measurement and recording of the evoked electrical activity that originates within the brainstem and higher auditory pathways including the auditory cortex as a consequence of auditory stimulation has received the focus of attention of many auditory physiologists and other investigators since the 1930s. The difficulty in distinguishing evoked electrical potentials resulting from auditory stimulation from the random bioelectric potentials of background noise, however, has delayed the clinical application of auditory brainstem response (ABR) audiometry until the development of small signal averaging computers in the 1960s. Since these small summing computers have become available, many investigators have provided evidence to support the clinical application of ABR as a method for determining pure tone thresholds of patients unable or unwilling to respond appropriately to conventional test procedures (Alberti, 1970; Beagley, 1973; Beagley & Knight, 1968; Hyde, Alberti, & Matsumoto, 1986; McCandless, 1967; McCandless & Best, 1964; McCandless & Lentz, 1968; Sanders & Lazenby, 1983; Shaia & Albright, 1980; Sohmer, Feinmesser, Bauberger-Tell, & Edelstein, 1977). Some of these investigators have reported that ABR thresholds agree within 10 dB of voluntary pure tone thresholds. Others, however, have cautioned that close agreement between ABR and voluntary thresholds is not always found (Rose, Keating, Hedgecock, Miller, & Schreurs, 1972).

Briefly, it should be noted that auditory brainstem responses are distinguished from higher central auditory system responses on the basis of their latencies from the onset of the auditory signal. The "early" or "short" latency responses (1 to 10 ms) are attributed to VIIIth nerve and brainstem activity, the "middle" (10 to 50 ms) to brainstem/primary cortical projection, whereas the "late" (50 to 250 ms) and "very late" (300 ms and longer) responses are considered to represent higher central auditory nervous system activity (see Chapter 6 by Durrant & Wolf).

There clearly is some evidence to support the use of ABR in the assessment of pseudohypacusis (Sanders & Lazenby, 1983). Also, during a recent 3-year period (1987 thru 1989) we used ABR for threshold estimation with 10 pseudohypacusic patients in our own hospital-based audiology clinical setting (Schwan, Rintelmann, Klein, & Schooler, 1989). In every case we were able to demonstrate that auditory evoked responses were elicited at substantially lower (better) Hearing Levels than voluntary pure tone thresholds (see Figure 12.1).

Furthermore, Long Latency Response (50 to 250 ms) evoked potentials to tone bursts also can be used successfully for assessing threshold levels in pseudohypacusic patients. See Figure 6.25 and accompanying text in Chapter 6 for such an example.

Interest in both laboratory and clinical activities concerning ABR and other evoked potentials (reminiscent of impedance studies nearly three decades earlier) has resulted in the use of such measures for the assessment of pseudohypacusis.

Electrocochleography

Electrocochleography (ECochG) is a procedure for measuring and recording the evoked electrical activity that originates within the cochlea and the auditory branch of the VIIIth cranial nerve in response to auditory

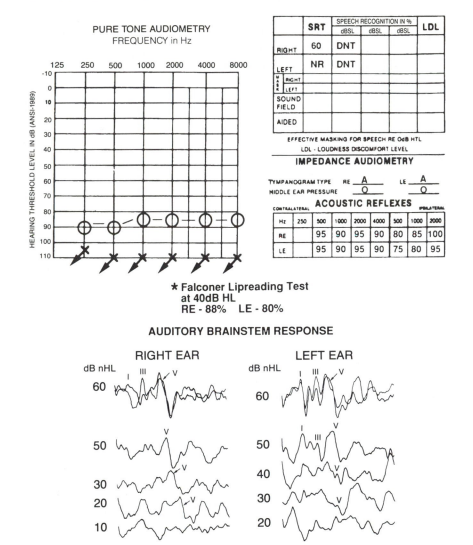

* Falconer Lipreading Test
at 40dB HL
RE - 88%   LE - 80%

Figure 12.1. Audiologic test results of a 26-year-old woman that demonstrate bilateral pseudohypacusis. Voluntary pure tone thresholds were at a severe Hearing Level for the right ear and profound (no response to tonal stimuli) for the left ear. The SRT for the right ear was substantially better than pure tone results. The Falconer Lipreading Test, presented at 40 dB HL to each ear, yielded a score of 88% for the right ear and 80% for the left ear. Acoustic reflexes were present bilaterally at levels at or below admitted pure tone thresholds. ABR results demonstrated an appropriate latency-intensity function for Wave V down to the normal hearing range for the right ear and down to the level of borderline normal or a mild loss for the left ear. Comparison of ABR results with those of behavioral tests clearly demonstrated test findings consistent with pseudohypacusis.

stimuli. Although there are three distinct electrical potentials which could be measured and analyzed, the most commonly recorded potential in ECochG is the compound VIIIth nerve action potential which represents the sum of the synchronous discharges of a number of single unit auditory nerve fibers. Refer to Chapter 6 for a discussion of ECochG.

This procedure, like any electrophysiologic method, can provide important information about the integrity of some portion of the auditory system, but like ABR, it is not a direct measure of hearing per se. Although the use of ECochG for many years was essentially a laboratory procedure, more recently it has been receiving increasing clinical use for a variety of applications (see Chapters 6 and 7).

ECochG also can be applied to patients suspected of pseudohypacusis especially because two noninvasive electrode recording techniques (extra-tympanic and ear canal) recently have proven to be clinically feasible (see Chapter 6). It is difficult to predict the ultimate impact that ECochG may have on the assessment of pseudohypacusis; however, if an audiology clinic has the capability of ECochG testing, this procedure could be an important addition to the test battery for pseudohypacusis.

Test battery protocol and patient management

If the audiologist has some notion in advance that a patient may attempt to exhibit pseudohypacusis, the order and methods of test administration can be structured appropriately. The pseudohypacusic patient usually responds to threshold tasks at suprathreshold levels; therefore, as mentioned previously the patient must use some judgment of loudness as his or her gauge for admitting or denying awareness of the signal because he or she actually will be hearing it all the time. For this reason at the outset of the testing session, the clinician should avoid presenting any auditory signals, pure tone or speech, at high Hearing Levels. Thus an ascending technique should be used to establish first SRTs and then pure tone thresholds in order to obtain the best initial estimate possible of the patient's true organic threshold levels. Recall that in obtaining pure tone thresholds from children, modified techniques (i.e., the Yes-No method) can be utilized. If a large discrepancy is found between the SRTs and the pure tone average thresholds (exceeding 10 dB), typically with better (more sensitive) thresholds for speech, the next test administered should be one that will verify the suspicion of pseudohypacusis and hopefully also provide some quantitative estimate of the patient's hearing ability.

The clinician may choose any one of several tests depending on whether the patient is displaying a unilateral or bilateral loss. For a unilateral loss, the speech Stenger would be a good choice, or for either a unilateral or bilateral loss, the pure tone DAF test, Bekesy audiometry, or the speech SAL test would be appropriate.

Speech recognition scores should be obtained, preferably at low sensation levels re the SRT (i.e., 10 dB). Acoustic reflexes should be measured especially if pure tone thresholds show a profound hearing loss, and typanometry should be obtained if air-bone gaps are found. Other audiological measures comprising the test battery for pseudohypacusis might include the Doerfler-Stewart test, ABR, ECochG, and so forth. Use of such tests, obviously, would depend upon both the availability of the instrumentation and the experience of the clinician. We prefer to use ABR as the final test with all pseudohypacusic patients because it usually gives the best estimate of the patient's true organic Hearing Level within the frequency range of approximately 1000 to 4000 Hz.

Concerning the use of audiological tests for the detection and assessment of pseudohypacusis, the results of a survey by Martin and Sides (1985) indicated that 99% of the audiologists who responded (227 of 230) did have occasion to use various tests for assessing pseudohypacusis. The Stenger, employed by 88% of the respondents, and acoustic immittance measures, used by 87%, were by far the most popular tests. Also, 34% of the respondents used ABR for testing pseudohypacusis. Conventional Bekesy audiometry was employed by 20% of the audiologists, whereas only 6% used the LOT test. The reported frequency of usage of other tests was as follows: the Lombard by 24%, Doerfler-Stewart by 15%, DAF by 9%, EDA by 1%, and "other" tests by 10% of the respondents. Thus it appears that in the middle 1980s the most commonly used special audiologic tests for assessing pseudohypacusis were the Stenger, acoustic immittance measures, and ABR. We expect that these tests plus other electrophysiologic measures will remain popular in the 1990s.

Concerning patient management during the testing session, as soon as inconsistent results are observed, the clinician should attempt to provide the patient (child or adult) with a "graceful way out." It is much easier for the audiologist to provide an adult or child with a way out during initial testing by simply saying something like "I probably didn't explain at first exactly what you should listen to or when you should signal me; but, now you seem to understand and you will do much better." On the other hand, if the adult or child has persisted in displaying inappropriate responses for several test sessions, it is difficult for the patient to change his or her test behavior without considerable embarrassment.

A caution is in order concerning the clinician's attitude toward the patient. Because testing pseudohypacusics can be frustrating even for the clinician experienced in evaluating such patients, one must keep in mind that the purpose of the examination is to evaluate (as well as possible) the patient's hearing—and not to make value judgments about his or her motivation. This principle applies equally whether the clinician is testing a 6-year-old child or a mature adult. Furthermore, the audiologist must recognize that he or she is not involved in a game of matching wits with the patient. The audiologist must maintain an objective clinical attitude with all patients, including pseudohypacusics.

Concerning transmitting the results of an audiological evaluation on an adult pseudohypacusic, in most cases this is accomplished via a written report to the referral source (i.e., an otolaryngologist, attorney, etc.). The only information that usually should be conveyed directly to the patient is that the test results are inconclusive due to certain kinds of inconsistent responses that were found during testing. The amount and type of information, however, and the manner in which it is conveyed obviously varies according to several factors. The counseling ability and experience of the clinician are of paramount importance for this phase of the audiological evaluation.

When testing children, the audiologist may have the responsibility of counseling the parents, providing a written report to the school system, family pediatrician, otolaryngologist, and so forth. Again, this depends on the referral source. If the test results demonstrate that the child has normal hearing, this information should be presented to the parents in such a way that the child does not get blamed for simulating a hearing loss. This can be done by explaining to the parents that children vary greatly in the way in which they respond to formal hearing tests. In other words, statements should be made to play down the significance of the child's behavior on hearing tests. At the same time it should be made clear that the child has normal hearing and that he or she should be treated accordingly. The teacher, too, should be informed of the status of the child's hearing and that the youngster does not need preferential seating in the classroom. The most important notion to convey to both the parents and teacher is that the child should not be confronted with his or her deception of a hearing loss. This approach is supported by other researchers (i.e., Bowdler & Rogers, 1989; Brockman & Hoversten, 1960; Veniar & Salston, 1983).

Also, as indicated earlier in this chapter, some pseudohypacusic children and adults may benefit from a referral to a psychologist or psychiatrist. Such a referral usually should be made by the primary physician who is treating the patient; however, if the audiologist has occasion to make a referral to a psychologist or psychiatrist, the discussion of this referral should be treated in a straightforward fashion in the same manner in which any referral (i.e., to an otolaryngologist) is handled. Finally, it cannot be overemphasized that proper audiological management of pseudohypacusic patients requires experience and skill not only in testing but also in counseling.

Conclusion

Although pseudohypacusis can be identified fairly readily by most audiologists, the problem of determining the patient's true organic hearing ability is a much more difficult task. Several standard tests that are used routinely in audiological evaluations can be employed successfully for the detection of pseudohypacusis. Measures that provide quantitative information, however, about the organic status of the patient's auditory system typically require special equipment and/or some special training or experience on the part of the clinician. In recent years this has become less of a problem with the availability of electrophysiologic measures such as ABR in most clinical audiology settings. Finally, proper audiological evaluation and management of such patients requires appropriate clinical experience based on a thorough knowledge and understanding of the problem of pseudohypacusis.

Afterword

This chapter, like others in this text, has provided comprehensive coverage of the topic with complete reference citations to a large body of literature. However, in revising this chapter from the one that was written about 10 years earlier, it became apparent that no new clinical tests and only a few published studies concerning pseudohypacusis have emerged during the 1980s. On the surface this may seem to be paradoxical given the fact that most audiologists continue to see some pseudohypacusic patients in their clinical practice. However, the increased focus on electrophysiological procedures (e.g., ABR) with demonstrated high clinical efficiency (sensitivity/specificity) has reduced or eliminated the use of some behavioral tests (e.g., Bekesy audiometry) for clinical audiology in general. Furthermore, behavioral tests that require special instrumentation (e.g., LOT, SAL, DAF) or special test procedures (e.g., Doerfler-Stewart) for pseudohypacusic patients, while providing less diagnostic quantitative information than electrophysiologic tests like ABR, have fallen into disuse for obvious reasons. The reader may ask: Why then have the authors of this chapter retained so much discussion on special behavioral tests like Bekesy, SAL, Doerfler-Stewart, Lombard, and Delayed Auditory Feedback? This information has been included because we are committed to the notion that graduate students and young clinicians and researchers should not simply study the latest developments in the field but should also acquire an appreciation of the heritage of their discipline. This can be accomplished only by having some understanding of the evolution of test development and clinical research in one's field. Audiology, compared to most other disciplines, is still fairly young, and students, teachers, clinicians, and researchers should have some understanding and knowledge of how audiology developed and changed during the past 40–plus years since the middle 1940s.

References

Alberti, P. (1970). New tools for old tricks. *Annals of Otology, Rhinology and Laryngology, 79,* 900–907.

Aplin, D. Y., & Kane, J. M. (1985). Variables affecting pure tone and speech audiometry in experimentally simulated hearing loss. *British Journal of Audiology, 19,* 219–228.

Aplin, D. Y., & Rowson, V. J. (1986). Personality and functional hearing loss in children. *British Journal of Clinical Psychology, 25,* 313–314.

Altshuler, M W. (1982). Qualitative indicators of non-organicity: Informal observations and evaluation. In M. B. Kramer & J. M. Armbruster (Eds.), *Forensic audiology* (pp. 59-68). Baltimore: University Park Press.

Armbruster, J. M. (1982). Indices of exaggerated hearing loss from conventional audiological procedures. In M. B. Kramer & J. M. Armbruster (Eds.), *Forensic audiology* (pp. 69-95). Baltimore: University Park Press.

Bailey, H. A. T., Jr., & Martin, F. N. (1963). A method for predicting postoperative SRT. *Archives of Otolaryngology, 77,* 177–180.

Barelli, P. A., & Ruder, L. (1970). Medico-legal evaluation of hearing problems. *Eye, Ear, Nose, and Throat Monthly, 49,* 398–405.

Barr, B. (1963). Psychogenic deafness in school children. *International Audiology, 2,* 125-128.

Beagley, H. A. (1973). The role of electro-physiological tests in the diagnosis of non-organic hearing loss. *Audiology, 12,* 470–480.

Beagley, H. A., & Knight, J. J. (1968). The evaluation of suspected non-organic hearing loss. *Journal of Laryngology and Otology, 82,* 693–705.

Behnke, C. R., & Lankford, J. E. (1976). The LOT test and school-age children. *Journal of Speech and Hearing Disorders, 41,* 498–502.

Bekesy, G. Von (1947). A new audiometer. *Acta Oto-Laryngologica, 35,* 411–422.

Berger, K. (1965). Nonorganic hearing loss in children. *Laryngoscope, 75,* 447–457.

Berk, R. L., & Feldman, A. S. (1958). Functional hearing loss in children. *New England Journal of Medicine, 259,* 214–216.

Billings, B. L., & Stokinger, T. E. (1975). A comparison of pure-tone thresholds as measured by delayed feedback audiometry, electrodermal response audiometry, and voluntary response audiometry. *Journal of Speech and Hearing Research, 18,* 754–764.

Black, J. W. (1951). The effect of delayed side-tone upon vocal rate and intensity. *Journal of Speech and Hearing Disorders, 16,* 56–60.

Black, J. W. (1954). Systematic research in experimental phonetics: 2. Signal reception: Intelligibility and side-tone. *Journal of Speech and Hearing Disorders, 19,* 140–146.

Bordley, J., & Hardy, W. (1949). A study in objective audiometry with the use of a psychogalvanometric response. *Annals of Otology, Rhinology, and Laryngology, 58,* 751–760.

Bowdler, D. A., & Rogers, J. (1989). The management of pseudohypacusis in school-age children. *Clinical Otolaryngology, 14,* 211–215.

Bragg, V. C. (1962, November). *Measurement of sensorineural acuity level using spondee words.* Paper presented at the convention of the American Speech and Hearing Association, New York.

Broad, R. D. (1980). Developmental and psychodynamic issues related to cases of childhood functional hearing loss. *Child Psychiatry and Human Development, 11,* 49–58.

Brockman, S. J., & Hoversten, G. H. (1960). Pseudo neural hypacusis in children. *Laryngoscope, 70,* 825–839.

Burk, K. (1958). Traditional and psychogalvanic skin response audiometry. *Journal of Speech and Hearing Research, 1,* 275–278.

Calearo, C. (1957). Detection of malingering by periodically switched speech. *Laryngoscope, 67,* 130–136.

Campanelli, P. A. (1963). Simulated hearing losses in school children following identification audiometry. *Journal of Auditory Research, 3,* 91–108.

Campbell, R. (1965). An index of pseudo-discrimination loss. *Journal of Speech and Hearing Research, 8,* 77–84.

Carhart, R. (1952). Speech audiometry in clinical evaluation. *Acta Oto-Laryngologica, 41,* 18–42.

Carhart, R. (1961). Tests for malingering. *Transactions of the American Academy of Opthalmology and Otolaryngology, 65,* 437.

Carhart, R., & Jerger, J. F. (1959). Preferred method for clinical determination of pure-tone thresholds. *Journal of Speech and Hearing Disorders, 24,* 330–345.

Carhart, R., & Porter, L. S. (1971). Audiometric configuration and prediction of threshold for spondees. *Journal of Speech and Hearing Research, 14,* 486–495.

Chaiklin, J. B. (1990). A descending LOT—Bekesy screening test for functional hearing loss. *Journal of Speech and Hearing Disorders, 55,* 67–74.

Chaiklin, J. B., & Ventry, I. M. (1963). Functional hearing loss. In J. Jerger (Ed.), *Modern developments in audiology* (pp. 76-125). New York: Academic Press.

Chaiklin, J. B., & Ventry, I. M. (1965). Patient errors during spondee and pure-tone threshold measurement. *Journal of Auditory Research, 5,* 219–230.

Chaiklin, J. B., Ventry, I. M., Barrett, L. S., & Skalbeck, G. S. (1959). Pure-tone threshold patterns observed in functional hearing loss. *Laryngoscope, 69,* 1165–1179.

Chase, R. A., Harvey, S., Standfast, S., Rapin, I., & Sutton, S. (1959). Comparison of the effects of delayed auditory feedback on speech and keytapping. *Science, 129,* 903–904.

Chase, R. A., Sutton, S., Fowler, E. P., Jr., Fay, T. H., Jr., & Ruhm, H. B. (1961). Low sensation level delayed clicks and keytapping. *Journal of Speech and Hearing Research, 4,* 73–78.

Citron, D., III, & Reddell, R. C. (1976). A comparison of EDR, LOT, Pure-tone DAF, and conventional pure-tone threshold audiometry for medical-legal audiological assessment. *Archives of Otolaryngology, 102,* 204–206.

Coles, R. R., & Mason, S. M. (1984). The results of cortical electric response audiometry in medico-legal investigations. *British Journal of Audiology, 18,* 71–78.

Conn, M., Ventry, I. M., & Woods, R. W. (1972). Pure-tone average and spondee threshold relationships in simulated hearing loss. *Journal of Auditory Research, 12,* 234–239.

Cooper, W. A., Jr., & Stokinger, T. E. (1976). Pure tone delayed auditory feedback: Effect of prior experience. *Journal of the American Auditory Society, 1,* 164–168.

Cooper, W. A., Jr., Stokinger, T. E., & Billings, B. L. (1976). Pure tone delayed auditory feedback: Development of criteria of performance deterioration. *Journal of the American Auditory Society, 1,* 192–196.

Cooper, W. A., Jr., Stokinger, T. E., & Billings, B. L. (1977). Pure tone delayed auditory feedback: Effect of hearing loss on disruption of tapping performance. *Journal of the American Auditory Society, 3,* 102–107.

Davis, H., & Goldstein, R. (1960). Special auditory tests. In H. Davis & S. R. Silverman (Eds.), *Hearing and deafness* (pp. 218-241). New York: Holt, Rinehart & Winston.

Dixon, R. F., & Newby, H. A. (1959). Children with non-organic hearing problems. *Archives of Otolaryngology, 70,* 619–623.

Doerfler, L. G. (1948). Neurophysiological clues to auditory acuity. *Journal of Speech and Hearing Disorders, 13,* 227–232.

Doerfler, L. G. (1951). Psychogenic deafness and its detection. *Annals of Otology, Rhinology, and Laryngology, 60,* 1045–1048.

Doerfler, L. G., & Epstein, A. (1956). *The Doerfler-Stewart D-S test for functional hearing loss.* Washington, DC: Veterans Administration. (Unpublished monograph).

Doerfler, L. G., & McClure, C. (1954). The measurement of hearing loss in adults by galvanic skin response. *Journal of Speech and Hearing Disorders, 19,* 184–189.

Doerfler, L. G., & Stewart, K. (1946). Malingering and psychogenic deafness. *Journal of Speech Disorders, 11,* 181–186.

Falconer, G. (1966). A "lipreading test" for nonorganic deafness. *Journal of Speech and Hearing Disorders, 31,* 241–247.

Fournier, J. E. (1958). The detection of auditory malingering. *Translations of the Beltone Institute for Hearing Research, 8,* 3–23.

Frank, T. (1976). Yes-no test for nonorganic hearing loss. *Archives of Otolaryngology, 102,* 162–165.

Gelfand, S. A., & Silman, S. (1985). Functional hearing loss and its relationship to resolved hearing levels. *Ear and Hearing, 6,* 151–158.

Gibbons, E. (1962). Aspects of traumatic and military psychogenic deafness and simulation. *International Audiology, 1,* 151–154.

Gleason, W. J. (1958). Psychological characteristics of the audiologically inconsistent patient. *Archives of Otolaryngology, 68,* 42–46.

Goldstein, R. (1966). Pseudohypacusis. *Journal of Speech and Hearing Disorders, 31,* 341–352.

Gosztonyi, R. E., Vassallo, L. A., Sataloff, J. (1971). Audiometric reliability in industry. *Archives of Environmental Health, 22,* 113–118.

Hanley, C. N., & Tiffany, W. R. (1954a). An investigation into the use of electromechanically delayed side-tone in auditory testing. *Journal of Speech and Hearing Disorders, 19,* 367–374.

Hanley, C. N., & Tiffany, W. R. (1954b). Auditory malingering and psychogenic deafness. *Archives of Otolaryngology, 60,* 197–201.

Harford, E. R., & Jerger, J. F. (1959). Effect of loudness recruitment on delayed speech feedback. *Journal of Speech and Hearing Research, 2,* 361–368.

Harris, D. A. (1958). A rapid and simple technique for the detection of non-organic hearing loss. *Archives of Otolaryngology, 68,* 758–760.

Harris, D. A. (1979). Detecting non-valid hearing tests in industry. *Journal of Occupational Medicine, 21,* 814–820.

Hattler, K. W. (1968). The Type V Bekesy pattern: The effects of loudness memory. *Journal of Speech and Hearing Research, 11,* 567–575.

Hattler, K. W. (1970). Lengthened off-time: A self-recording screening device for nonorganicity. *Journal of Speech and Hearing Disorders, 35,* 113–122.

Hattler, K. W., & Schuchman, G. (1970). Clinical efficiency of the LOT-Bekesy test. *Archives of Otolaryngology, 92,* 348–352.

Hattler, K. W., & Schuchman, G. I. (1971). Efficiency of Stenger, Doerfler-Stewart and lengthened LOT-time Bekesy tests. *Acta Oto-Laryngologica, 72,* 252–267.

Hood, W. H., Campbell, R. A., & Hutton, C. L. (1964). An evaluation of the Bekesy ascending descending gap. *Journal of Speech and Hearing Research, 7,* 123–132.

Hopkinson, N. T. (1965). Type V Bekesy audiograms: Specification and clinical utility. *Journal of Speech and Hearing Disorders, 30,* 243–251.

Hopkinson, N. T. (1967). Comment on pseudohypacusis. *Journal of Speech and Hearing Disorders, 32,* 293–294.

Hopkinson, N. T. (1973). Functional hearing loss. In J. Jerger (Ed.), *Modern developments in audiology* (pp. 175–210). New York: Academic Press.

Hopkinson, N. T. (1978). Speech tests for pseudohypacusis. In J. Katz (Ed.), *Handbook of clinical audiology* (pp. 291–302). Baltimore: Williams & Wilkins.

Hopkinson, N. T., Katz, J., & Schill, H. (1960). Instrumental avoidance galvanic skin response audiometry. *Journal of Speech and Hearing Disorders, 25,* 349–357.

Hurley, R. M., & Mather, J. (1988, November). *Effectiveness of the SAL test in identifying feigned hearing loss.* Poster session presented at the convention of the American Speech and Hearing Association, Boston.

Hyde, M., Alberti, P., Matsumoto, N., & Li, Y. L. (1986). Auditory evoked potentials in audiometric assessment of compensation and medicolegal patients. *Annals of Otology, Rhinology, and Laryngology, 95,* 514–519.

Jepsen, O. (1953). Intratympanic muscle reflexes in psychogenic deafness (impedance measurement). *Acta Oto-Laryngologica* (Supplement), *109,* 61–69.

Jerger, J. (1960). Bekesy audiometry in analysis of auditory disorders. *Journal of Speech and Hearing Research, 3,* 275–287.

Jerger, J., Burney, P., Mauldin, L., & Crump, B. (1974). Predicting hearing loss from the acoustic reflex. *Journal of Speech and Hearing Disorders, 39* 11–22.

Jerger, J., Hayes, D., Anthony, L., & Mauldin, L. (1978). Factors influencing prediction of hearing level from the acoustic reflex. In D. Schwartz & F. Bess (Eds.), *Monographs in contemporary audiology* (Vol. 1, pp. 1–20). Minneapolis MN: Maico Hearing Instruments.

Jerger, J., & Herer, G. (1961). An unexpected dividend in Bekesy audiometry. *Journal of Speech and Hearing Disorders, 26,* 390–391.

Jerger, J., & Tillman, T. A. (1960). A new method for the clinical determination of sensorineural acuity level (SAL). *Archives of Otolaryngology, 71,* 948–955.

Johnson, K. O., Work, W. P., & McCoy, G. (1956). Functional deafness. *Annals of Otology, Rhinology, and Laryngology, 65,* 154–170.

Juers, A. (1966). Nonorganic hearing problems. *Laryngoscope, 76,* 1714–1723.

Katz, J., & Connelly, R. (1964). Instrumental avoidance vs. classical conditioning in GSR speech audiometry. *Journal of Auditory Research, 4,* 171–179.

Kinstler, D. B. (1971). Functional hearing loss. In L. E. Travis (Ed.), *Handbook of speech pathology* (pp. 375–398). New York: Appleton-Century-Crofts.

Kinstler, D. B., Phelan, J. G., & Lavender, R. W. (1972). The Stenger and speech Stenger tests in functional hearing loss. *Audiology, 11,* 187–193.

Knapp, P. H. (1948). Emotional aspects of hearing loss. *Psychosomatic Medicine, 10,* 203–222.

Knapp, P. H., & Gold, B. (1950). The galvanic skin response and diagnosis of hearing disorders. *Psychosomatic Medicine, 12,* 6–22.

Lamb, L. E., & Peterson, J. L. (1967). Middle ear reflex measurements in pseudohypacusis. *Journal of Speech and Hearing Disorders, 32,* 46–51.

Lankford, J. E., & Meissner, W. A. (1977). The manual LOT test. *Journal of the American Audiology Society, 2,* 219–222.

Lee, B. (1950). Some effects of side-tone delay. *Journal of the Acoustical Society of America, 22,* 639–640.

Lehrer, N. D., Hirschenfang, S., Miller, M. H., & Radpour, S. (1964). Non-organic hearing problems in adolescents. *Laryngoscope, 74,* 64–70.

Lumio, J. S., Jauhiainen, J., & Gelhar, K., (1969). Three cases of functional deafness in the same family. *Journal of Laryngology, 83,* 299–304.

Martin, F. N. (1972). Nonorganic hearing loss: An overview and pure tone tests. In J. Katz (Ed.), *Handbook of clinical audiology* (pp. 357–373). Baltimore: Williams & Wilkins.

Martin, F. N. (1985). The pseudohypacusic. In J. Katz (Ed.), *Handbook of clinical audiology* (pp. 742–765). Baltimore: Williams & Wilkins.

Martin, F. N., & Hawkins, R. R. (1963). A modification of the Doerfler-Stewart test for the detection of non-organic hearing loss. *Journal of Auditory Research, 3,* 147–150.

Martin, F. N., & Monro, D. A. (1975). The effects of sophistication on Type V Bekesy patterns in simulated hearing loss. *Journal of Speech and Hearing Disorders, 40,* 508–513.

Martin, F. N., & Shipp, D. B. (1982). The effects of sophistication on three thresholds tests for subjects with simulated hearing loss. *Ear and Hearing, 3,* 34–36.

Martin, F. N., & Sides, D. G. (1985). Survey of current audiometric practices. *Asha, 27,* 29–36.

McCandless, G. (1967). Clinical application of evoked response audiometry. *Journal of Speech and Hearing Research, 10,* 468–478.

McCandless, G. A., & Best, L. (1964). Evoked responses to auditory stimuli in man using a summing computer. *Journal of Speech and Hearing Research, 7,* 193–202.

McCandless, G. A., & Lentz, W. E. (1968). Evoked response (EEG) audiometry in non-organic hearing loss. *Archives of Otolaryngology, 87,* 123–128.

McCanna, D. L., & DeLapa, G. (1981). A clinical study of 27 children exhibiting functional hearing loss. *Language, Speech and Hearing Services in Schools, 12,* 26–35.

Melnick, W. (1967). Comfort level and loudness matching for continuous and interrupted signals. *Journal of Speech and Hearing Research, 10,* 99–109.

Menzel, O. J. (1960). Clinical efficiency in compensation audiometry. *Journal of Speech and Hearing Disorders, 25,* 49–54.

Michels, M. W., & Randt, C. T. (1947). Galvanic skin response in the differential diagnosis of deafness. *Archives of Otolaryngology, 65,* 302–311.

Miller, A. L., Fox, M. S., & Chan, G. (1968). Pure tone assessments as an aid in detecting suspected non-organic hearing disorders in children. *Laryngoscope, 78,* 2170–2176.

Monro, D. A., & Martin, F. N. (1977). Effects of sophistication on four tests for nonorganic hearing loss. *Journal of Speech and Hearing Disorders, 42,* 528–534.

Moscicki, E. K. (1984). The prevalence of 'Incidence' is too high. *Asha, 26,* 39–40.

Newby, H. A. (1958). *Audiology: Principles and practice.* New York: Appleton-Century-Crofts.

Niemeyer, W., & Sesterhenn, C. (1974). Calculating the hearing threshold from the stapedius reflex threshold for different sound stimuli. *Audiology, 13,* 421–427.

Nilo, E. R., & Saunders, W. H. (1976). Functional hearing loss. *Laryngoscope, 86,* 501–505.

Olsen, W. O., & Matkin, N .D. (1978). Differential audiology. In D. E. Rose (Ed.), *Audiological assessment* (pp. 368–419). Englewood Cliffs: Prentice-Hall.

Pang-Ching, G. (1970). The tone-in-noise test: A preliminary report. *Journal of Auditory Research, 10,* 322–327.

Peck, J. E., & Ross, M. (1970). A comparison of the ascending and the descending modes for administration of the pure-tone Stenger test. *Journal of Auditory Research, 10,* 218–220.

Peterson, J. L. (1963). Nonorganic hearing loss in children and Bekesy audiometry. *Journal of Speech and Hearing Disorders, 28,* 153–158.

Portmann, M., & Portmann, C. (1961). *Clinical audiometry.* Springfield, IL: Charles C. Thomas.

Price, L. L., Shepherd, D. C., & Goldstein, R. (1965). Abnormal Bekesy tracings in normal ears. *Journal of Speech and Hearing Disorders, 30,* 139–144.

Resnick, D. M., & Burke, K. S. (1962). Bekesy audiometry in non-organic auditory problems. *Archives of Otolaryngology, 76,* 38–41.

Rintelmann, W. F., & Carhart, R. (1964). Loudness tracking by normal hearers via Bekesy audiometer. *Journal of Speech and Hearing Research, 7,* 79–93.

Rintelmann, W. F., & Harford, E. (1963). The detection and assessment of pseudohypacusis among school-age children. *Journal of Speech and Hearing Disorders, 28,* 141–152.

Rintelmann, W. F., & Harford, E. R. (1967). Type V Bekesy pattern: Interpretation and clinical utility. *Journal of Speech and Hearing Research, 10,* 733–744.

Rintelmann, W. F., & Johnson, K. R. (1970, November). *Comparison of pure-tone versus speech sensorineural acuity level (SAL) test.* Paper presented at the annual convention of the American Speech and Hearing Association, New York.

Robinson, M., & Kasden, S. D. (1973). Clinical application of pure-tone delayed auditory feedback in pseudohypacusis. *Eye, Ear, Nose, and Throat Monthly, 52,* 31–33.

Rose, D. E., Keating, L. W., Hedgecock, L. D., Miller, K. E., & Schreurs, K. K. (1972). A comparison of evoked response audiometry and routine clinical audiometry. *Audiology, 11,* 238–243.

Ross, M. (1964). The variable intensity pulse count method (VIPCM) for the detection and measurement of the pure-tone thresholds of children with functional hearing losses. *Journal of Speech and Hearing Disorders, 29,* 477–482.

Ruhm, H. B., & Carhart, R. (1958). Objective speech audiometry: A new method based on electrodermal response. *Journal of Speech and Hearing Research, 1,* 169–178.

Ruhm, H. B., & Cooper, W. A., Jr. (1962). Low sensation level effects of pure-tone delayed auditory feedback. *Journal of Speech and Hearing Research, 5,* 185–193.

Ruhm, H. B., & Cooper, W. A., Jr. (1963). Some factors that influence pure-tone delayed auditory feedback. *Journal of Speech and Hearing Research, 6,* 223–237.

Ruhm, H. B., & Cooper, W. A., Jr. (1964a). Influence on motor performance of simultaneous delayed and synchronous pure-tone auditory feedback. *Journal of Speech and Hearing Research, 7,* 175–182.

Ruhm, H. B., & Cooper, W. A., Jr. (1964b). Delayed feedback audiometry. *Journal of Speech and Hearing Disorders, 29,* 448–455.

Ruhm, H. B., & Menzel, O. J. (1959). Objective speech audiometry in cases of nonorganic hearing loss. *Archives of Otolaryngology, 69,* 212–219.

Sanders, J. W. (1975). Symposium on sensorineural hearing loss in children: Early detection and intervention. Impedance measurement. *Otolaryngologic Clinics Of North America, 8,* 109–124.

Sanders, J. W., & Lazenby, B. B. (1983). Auditory brain stem response measurement in the assessment of pseudohypacusis. *American Journal of Otology, 4,* 292–299.

Schwan, S. A., Rintelmann, W. F., Klein, L.A., & Schooler, R. J. (1989). Hearing assessment in pseudohypacusis via ABR. *Asha, 31,* 156.

Shaia, F. T., & Albright, P. (1980). Clinical use of brainstem evoked response audiometry. *Virginia Medical, 107,* 44–45.

Shepherd, D. C. (1965). Non-organic hearing loss and the consistency of behavioral auditory responses. *Journal of Speech and Hearing Research, 8,* 149–163.

Siegenthaler, B., & Strand, R. (1964). Audiogram-average methods and SRT scores. *Journal of the Acoustical Society of America, 36,* 589–593.

Sohmer, H., Feinmesser, M., Bauberger-Tell, L., & Edelstein, E. (1977). Cochlear, brain stem, and cortical evoked responses in nonorganic hearing loss. *Annals of Otology, Rhinology, and Laryngology, 86,* 227–234.

Stankiewicz, J., Fankhauser, C. E., & Strom, C. G. (1981). Electrodermal audiometry: Renewed acquaintance with an old friend. *Otolaryngology: Head and Neck Surgery, 89,* 671–677.

Stark, E. W. (1966). Jerger types in fixed-frequency Bekesy audiometry with normal and hypacusic children. *Journal of Auditory Research, 6,* 135–140.

Stein, L. (1963). Some observations on Type V Bekesy tracings. *Journal of Speech and Hearing Research, 6,* 339–348.

Stenger, P. (1907). Simulation and dissimulation of ear diseases and their identification. *Deutsche Medizinsche Wochenschrift, 33,* 970–973.

Taylor, G. J. (1949). An experimental study of tests for the detection of auditory malingering. *Journal of Speech and Hearing Disorders, 14,* 119–130.

Thomsen, K. A. (1955). Case of psychogenic deafness demonstrated by measuring impedance. *Acta Oto-Laryngologica, 45,* 82–85.

Tiffany, W. R., & Hanley, C. N. (1952). Delayed speech feedback as a test for auditory malingering. *Science, 115,* 59–60.

Tillman, T. W. (1963). Clinical applicability of the SAL test. *Archives of Otolaryngology, 78,* 20–32.

Trier, T., & Levy, R. (1965). Social and psychological characteristics of veterans with functional hearing loss. *Journal of Auditory Research, 5,* 241–255.

Truex, E. H. (1946). Psychogenic deafness. *Connecticut State Medical Journal, 10,* 907–915.

Veniar, F. A., & Salston, R. S. (1983). An approach to the treatment of pseudo-hypacusis in children. *American Journal of Diseases of Children, 137,* 34–36.

Ventry, I. M. (1968). A case for psychogenic hearing loss. *Journal of Speech and Hearing Disorders, 33,* 89–92.

Ventry, I. M. (1971). Bekesy audiometry in functional hearing loss: A case study. *Journal of Speech and Hearing Disorders, 36,* 125–141.

Ventry, I. M., & Chaiklin, J. B. (1962). Functional hearing loss: A problem in terminology. *Asha, 4,* 251–254.

Ventry, I. M., & Chaiklin, J. B. (1965). Evaluation of pure-tone audiogram configurations used in identifying adults with functional hearing loss. *Journal of Auditory Research, 5,* 212–218.

Watson, L. A., & Tolan, T. (1949). *Hearing tests and hearing instruments.* Baltimore: Williams & Wilkins.

Wilber, L. A. (1976). Acoustic reflex measurement—procedures, interpretations and variables. In A. S. Feldman & L. A. Wilber (Eds.), *Acoustic impedance and admittance: The measurement of middle ear function* (pp. 197–216). Baltimore: Williams & Wilkins.

Zwislocki, J. (Ed.). (1963). *Critical evaluation of methods of testing and measurement of nonorganic hearing impairment.* Report of Working Group 36, NAS-NRC Committee on Hearing, Bioacoustics and Biomechanics.

chapter thirteen

Classic site-of-lesion tests: Foundation of diagnostic audiology

JAMES W. HALL III

Contents

Introduction

The 30 years from 1948 through 1978 was an exciting period of scientific discovery, clinical application, and professional growth for audiology. During this time, the term *diagnostic audiology* became almost synonymous with site-of-lesion audiometric assessment, in particular the differentiation of cochlear versus eighth nerve pathology. Diagnostic audiology in this era relied on a battery of behavioral test procedures based on pure tone signals. The author, although born at the start of this 30-year period, had the good fortune to experience some of the excitement of diagnostic audiology and classic site-of-lesion test administration and interpretation in the final half dozen years of the era, first during graduate study at Northwestern University and then at Baylor College of Medicine. Each of the classic site-of-lesion tests are related to one of three fundamental auditory phenomena. Alternate binaural loudness balance (ABLB) is

653

related to *abnormal growth of loudness,* a collection of tone decay test versions and Bekesy audiometry procedures are related to *auditory adaptation,* and various versions of short increment sensitivity index (SISI) procedures are associated with *difference limen for intensity.*

The scope of this chapter is specifically restricted to these classic site-of-lesion tests. The chapter begins with a historical review of traditional diagnostic audiometry, with an emphasis on the personalities that contributed to its development, followed by a brief critical description of the major classic site-of-lesion tests. More detailed information on test administration and interpretation can be found among the original sources cited in this article and comprehensive review chapters in the first edition of this textbook (Konkle & Orchik, 1979; Owens, 1979; Sanders, 1979). Each of these original articles introducing the classic site-of-lesion procedures is essential reading for the serious student of audiology. After the test procedures are described, accuracy rates for identification of cochlear versus eighth nerve pathology among them are compared using data compiled by the author (Hall, 1978) from 52 published studies. The chapter concludes with a discussion of factors contributing to the development and demise of the "traditional diagnostic test battery," and an assessment of the impact of site-of-lesion testing on audiology.

Historical overview

Gradenigo and Allen (1893) generally are credited with first applying an auditory test in the differential diagnosis of sensorineural hearing impairment. Using a rudimentary tone decay test, they successfully distinguished cochlear from eighth nerve pathology. Major advances in the development of diagnostic audiology procedures for site-of-lesion assessment are summarized in Table 13.1. In 1936, the concept of cochlear versus retrocochlear differentiation with auditory testing was revived when an Englishman, E. P. Fowler, observed in cases of unilateral sensorineural hearing impairment that an increase in intensity presented to both ears resulted in an unusually rapid growth of loudness in the impaired ear. Fowler coined the term *loudness recruitment* to describe this phenomenon and developed the alternate binaural loudness balance (ABLB) test to assess it. Dix, Hallpike, and Hood (1948) reported in England on the clinical application of ABLB testing in differential diagnosis of cochlear versus eighth nerve disorders. The appearance of this publication, for all practical purposes, marked the beginning of traditional diagnostic audiology. The pent-up demand for a clinical means of distinguishing sensory from neural auditory disorders was clearly evident by the proliferation in the 1950s of studies on what became commonly (and unfortunately) known as loudness recruitment (Eby & Williams, 1951; Fowler, 1950; Goodman, 1957; Hallpike & Hood, 1951; Jerger & Harford, 1960; Kristensen & Jepsen, 1952; Miskolczy-Fodor, 1956).

In this same year (1948), Lüscher and a colleague, Josef Zwislocki (also from Europe) published one of the first of a series of papers reportedly on evaluation of loudness recruitment but, in contrast to ABLB, monaurally with a procedure for estimating difference limen for intensity. The article was followed by numerous subsequent studies, this time of difference limen for intensity in ears with cochlear versus eighth nerve pathology. Perhaps the most important of these for the development of diagnostic audiology was a paper by James Jerger (1952; 1953) describing the results of his master's thesis research at Northwestern University on the difference limen for intensity. Within 7 years, the concept of differences in intensity perception by cochlear versus eighth nerve lesion ears was adapted clinically in the form of the short increment sensitivity index (SISI) procedure (Jerger, Shedd, & Harford, 1959).

The classic site-of-lesion test battery was complete with the introduction of a third type of auditory procedure—the tone decay test—within this same time frame. In 1955, Hood described decreased perception of a continuously presented tone in patients with retrocochlear lesions. Raymond Carhart, at Northwestern University, popularized in 1957 a clinical test for evaluating abnormal auditory adaptation, the threshold tone decay test (TDT). Other investigators then applied the TDT, and later modified versions, for differentiating cochlear versus retrocochlear lesions (Green, 1963; Jerger, 1962a, 1962b; Jerger, Carhart, Lassman, 1958; Olsen & Noffsinger, 1974; Palva, 1964; Rosenberg, 1958, 1971; Sorensen, 1960; Tillman, 1966).

Several years earlier, Nobel prize winner George von Bekesy had described an automatic recording audiometer and a technique for assessing hearing threshold. Bekesy audiometry, as it came to be known, was then applied clinically by Lundborg (1952) and Lierle and Reger (1954, 1955). Bekesy audiometry findings were reported for a patient with a retrocochlear tumor as early as 1955, but it was Jerger's systematic deliniation in 1960 of four distinct Bekesy tracing classifications among 434 patients with normal hearing or conductive, cochlear, or eighth nerve pathology that marked the inclusion of this auditory adaptation technique to the diagnostic audiometry test battery. The diagnostic value of forward (sweeping from low to high frequencies) threshold Bekesy tracings and also reverse tracings (high to low frequencies) was soon confirmed by Jerger and others (Jerger, Jerger, & Mauldin, 1972; Rose, 1962).

TABLE 13.1
Chronologic Summary of Major Advances in Classic Diagnostic Audiology Procedures for Site-of-Lesion Assessment

Year	Procedure	Principle investigator(s)
1930	audiometer (Western Electric)	
1935	monaural loudness balance	Reger
1937	alternate binaural loudness balance (ABLB)	Fowler
1946	impedance audiometry	Metz
1947	Bekesy audiometer	Bekesy
1948	ABLB in site-of-lesion evaluation	Dix, Hallpike, & Hood
1948	difference limen for intensity	Lüscher & Zwislocki
1957	tone decay	Carhart
1959	short increment sensitivity index (SISI)	Jerger, Shedd, & Harford
1960	Bekesy threshold types	Jerger
1969	acoustic reflex decay	Anderson, Barr, & Wedenberg
1970, 1971	auditory brainstem response (ABR)	Jewett & Williston Jewett, Romano, & Williston
1971	performance-intensity functions for PB words	Jerger, J., & Jerger, S.
1972	Bekesy forward-backward	Jerger, J., & Jerger, S., & Mauldin
1974	tone decay	Olsen & Noffsinger
1974b	Bekesy comfortable loudness (BCL)	Jerger & Jerger, S.
1975	suprathreshold adaptation test (STAT)	Jerger, J., & Jerger, S.
1977–1979	ABR in eighth nerve pathology	Selters & Brackmann Clemis & McGee Thomsen, Terkildsen, & Osterhammel, 1978 Terkildsen et al., 1977 Rosenhamer, 1977

Throughout the 1960s and into the mid-1970s a second generation of these classic site-of-lesion procedures emerged, distinguished from their earlier counterparts by administration at suprathreshold intensity levels. Dual objectives of this testing approach were to enhance sensitivity to eighth nerve dysfunction while reducing test time. Among the suprathreshold procedures were the modified SISI (Thompson, 1963), the Olsen and Noffsinger version of the tone decay test (Olsen & Noffsinger, 1974) and two procedures developed by James and Susan Jerger, the suprathreshold adaptation test (STAT) and Bekesy Comfortable Loudness (BCL) test (Jerger & Jerger, 1974b, 1975). One must keep in mind that two major diagnostic procedures that are beyond the scope of this discussion— acoustic reflex measurement (Anderson, Barr, & Wedenberg, 1970; Chiveralls, 1977; Jerger, Harford, Clemis, & Alford, 1974; Lidén & Korsan-Bengtsen, 1973; Olsen, Noffsinger, & Kurdziel, 1975; Sanders, Josey, Glasscock, 1974; Sanders, Josey, Glasscock, & Jackson, 1981; Thomsen, 1955) and performance-intensity functions for phonetically-balanced (PI-PB) word lists (Bess, Josey, Humes, 1979; Jerger & Jerger, 1971)— figured prominently into the diagnostic audiometry test battery by mid-1970, and of course still do (Hall, 1985; Jerger, 1973, 1987).

In retrospect, viability of the traditional diagnostic test battery was challenged first about 1970 with the introduction of two clinically feasible electrophysiologic auditory procedures. As just noted, impedance (immittance) audiometry, in particular measurement of acoustic stapedial reflex threshold and decay (Anderson et al., 1970; Chiveralls, 1977), offered multiple clinical advantages (see Hall, 1985, 1988) including objective, quick, and relatively sensitive differentiation of cochlear versus retrocochlear pathology. Importantly, acoustic reflex measurement in suspected retrocochlear ears is not constrained by hearing status of the opposite ear (as is the ABLB).

Audiology was changed forever by Jewett and Williston's clinical description of a scalp-recorded auditory brainstem response (ABR) in 1970 (Jewett, Romano, & Williston, 1970; Jewett & Williston, 1971). Ironically, primitive instrumentation for measurement of sensory evoked responses was described initially in 1947 by the Englishman Dawson, just as his compatriots Dix, Hallpike, and Hood (1948), along with Lüscher and his colleagues in Germany, were conducting their studies of abnormal growth of loudness and difference limen for intensity in sensorineural hearing impairment (Lüscher, 1951a, 1951b; Lüscher & Zwislocki, 1948). There is little doubt that the infant diagnostic audiology would have failed to thrive had ABR been immediately discovered. Late (vertex) auditory evoked responses were extensively investigated beginning in the late 1950s and throughout the 1960s, in some cases by researchers who also were instrumental in the development of diagnostic audiology (e.g., Jerger & Jerger,

1970). However, the delay of ABR as a clinically available and proven auditory procedure until about 1975 permitted unbridled growth of the classic site-of-lesion test battery. The era of traditional diagnostic audiometry came to an abrupt and unceremonious end around 1978 with the publication of a series of independent studies of ABR in retrocochlear pathology (Clemis & McGee, 1979; Selters & Brackmann, 1977; Terkildsen, Huis in't Veld, & Osterhammel, 1977; Thomsen, Terkildsen, & Osterhammel, 1978). There are various reasons for the clinical preference of ABR over classic site-of-lesion tests, but the remarkably high accuracy in identification of eighth nerve pathology predominated. This point is discussed further in the next section and in Chapter 14 by Turner.

Classic site-of-lesion auditory tests

Alternate Binaural Loudness Balance (ABLB)

Discovery and definition.   Credit for the discovery of abnormal loudness growth, in this century at least, must be given to Fowler (1936, 1937) and Reger (1935), although as pointed out in the historical overview presented above, it was the 1948 description of ABLB findings for 30 patients with unilateral cochlear dysfunction (endolymphatic hydrops) versus 20 patients with eighth nerve pathology (acoustic neuroma) by Dix, Hallpike, and Hood that secured the assessment of this phenomenon in diagnostic audiometry.

The ABLB test compares loudness growth in an impaired ear versus a normal hearing ear. The typical outcome found in patients with unilateral cochlear impairment is an abnormally rapid growth of loudness as a pure tone stimulus intensity is increased above threshold in the impaired ear. The amount of intensity increase above threshold needed to create the sensation of equal loudness (interaural loudness balance) is much less for the impaired ear than for the normal ear. This phenomenon is illustrated in Figure 13.1. Requirements for the ABLB are a unilateral hearing loss (vs. bilateral). Hearing in the noninvolved ear must be normal (e.g., 25 dB HL or better). Another procedure, the monaural loudness balance (MLB) test, was described early on for patients not meeting these two criteria (Reger, 1935). Loudness growth is compared between two frequencies in the same ear, when there is impaired hearing sensitivity at one frequency and normal hearing sensitivity at the other.

For the ABLB, stimulus intensity level is kept constant or fixed in one ear (the reference ear). Intensity level is varied in the other ear, and the patient's perception of loudness is then matched or balanced to the

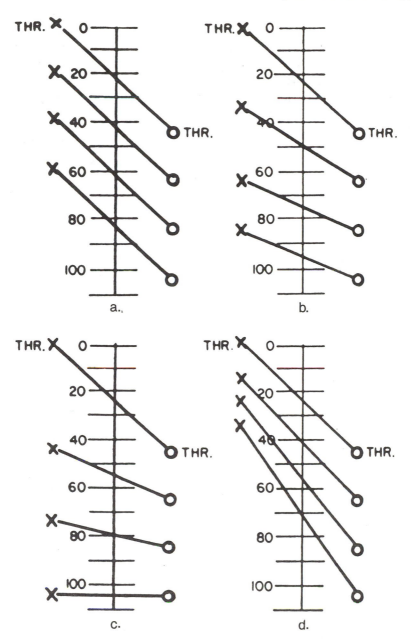

Figure 13.1. Alternate binaural loudness balance (ABLB) results for no recruitment (A), partial recruitment (B), complete recruitment (C), and decruitment (D) plotted as laddergrams. (From J. W. Sanders in *Hearing Assessment* [1st ed., 1979], with permission.)

reference ear. The patient balances loudness as the pure tone signals are rapidly alternated from one ear to the other. A host of test variables may influence the patient's performance on the ABLB, including which ear is used for the reference versus variable stimulus intensity, the psychophysical method used in testing, the duration of tones and rate at which they are alternated, and how many intensity levels are used for loudness balancing (Jerger, 1962a, 1962b). As classically defined (Jerger, 1962), there are three test outcomes. Complete recruitment is present when at equal intensity levels (hearing levels within ± 10 dB) the patient perceives the stimuli to each ear as equally loud (see Figure 13.1). There is no recruitment if loudness is perceived as balanced when the stimulus intensity for each ear is at the same sensation level (SL), that is, the same number of dB above threshold for each ear. Partial recruitment falls between these two rather clearcut outcomes. With another possible but infrequent outcome, termed *derecruitment*, greater intensity is required in the impaired ear (greater SL above threshold) to produce balanced loudness between ears.

Physiologic bases.   There is general consensus that the anatomic locus for abnormal loudness growth, if there is one, resides in the cochlea, more specifically at the hair cell level. However, a rather long list of authors have speculated on an even longer list of possible pathophysiologic mechanisms for the phenomenon. These theories attempt to explain abnormal loudness growth or its absence on the basis of hair cell loss and dysfunction, decoupling of hair cell cilia with the tectorial membrane, eighth nerve function (nerve fiber characteristic frequency tuning curves; adaptation), physiologic differences between outer and inner hair cells as a function of intensity, spread of cochlear activity along the basilar membrane as a function of intensity, and central nervous system mechanisms (Bekesy, 1966; Dix, 1965; Moore, 1982; Pickles, 1982; Salvi, Henderson, Hamernik, & Ahroon, 1983). Perhaps the most plausible current theory of loudness recruitment is explained by Pickles (1982):

> As the stimulus intensity is raised, the number of fibres activated at first rises slowly, while only the tip segments of the curves are activated, and then more abruptly, when the tails of the tuning curves are encountered. In the pathological ear, the tips of the tuning curves are missing, and as the stimulus intensity is raised the number of fibres activated increases rapidly, soon approaching normal levels. (p. 291)

Still, there is no unifying concept or firm experimental evidence to explain abnormal loudness growth as demonstrated by the ABLB.

Critical summary. As the foregoing comments indicate, the pathophysiologic processes, if any, underlying abnormal growth of loudness are not known. It is a clinical axiom that a diagnostic procedure cannot be fully exploited without knowledge of the anatomic and physiologic bases of the procedure. This is a serious clinical limitation. Furthermore, in a germinal paper describing comparison of performances of three procedures (ABLB, Bekesy audiometry, and SISI) in predicting site of lesion, Jerger (1961) observed that,

> Throughout the flurry of claims and denials [about loudness recruitment] some investigators have apparently lost sight of two fundamental considerations: 1. The primary issue is not "recruitment" but site of lesion. . . . One should not be seduced into the erroneous belief that the measurement of recruitment is the primary goal and that any other test is good or bad only to the extent that it agrees with the loudness balance test and 2. In spite of the rather pervasive lack of reticence to cast aspersions on other tests, no one has thought to ask, 'How good is the loudness balance test?' " (p. 146)

It would appear, in retrospect, that much investigative energy and probably hundreds of pages of journal text were frittered away because these two points were generally unappreciated for close to three decades.

Another apparent oversight during the persistent study and clinical application of ABLB was exposed by Sanders (1982). The ABLB (and SISI) are based on a comparison of loudness at a relatively low intensity level in the normal ear versus loudness at a relatively high intensity level in the impaired ear. The typical normal (no recruitment) versus abnormal (complete recruitment) ABLB findings are not necessarily a function of cochlear pathology but, rather, a function of stimulus intensity level. In fact, if masking is presented to one ear to simulate a cochlear impairment, and then the ABLB is carried out with intensity levels in SL above normal unmasked and normal masked threshold levels, the masked normal ear shows evidence of recruitment. Sanders perceptively suggested that we consider a "revised concept of suprathreshold loudness response in the cochlear pathology ear—namely, that loudness recruitment and positive SISI scores are normal loudness responses at high intensity and not the pathologic result of abnormal sensitivity to intensity" (Sanders, 1982, p. 962). A final clinical liability of ABLB (the test's sensitivity and specificity characteristics) are noted in the final section.

Short Increment Sensitivity Index

Discovery and definition. "Differential sensitivity refers to the ear's ability to discriminate changes in intensity. The unit of differential sensitivity is the difference limen. It is defined as that increment in the physical intensity of a sound which a subject perceives as a change in loudness just 50 percent of the time'' (Jerger, 1952, p. 1317). The short increment sensitivity index (SISI) test evolved indirectly from Fowler's description of "loudness recruitment" in 1936 and 1937 and directly from international work on differential sensitivity to intensity changes in the late 1940s and early 1950s (Denes & Naunton, 1950; Doerfler, 1948; Halm, 1949; Lüscher & Zwislocki, 1948). As Jerger (1952) stated in the opening sentence of an article summarizing a master's thesis under the direction of Raymond Carhart, ''The discovery of the recruitment phenomenon has created an entirely new area of study in the clinical evaluation of hearing loss'' (Jerger, 1952, p. 1316).

The study reported in the 1952 Jerger article has dual purposes of simplifying Lüscher's technique and exploring the possible enhancement of the test by presenting the stimuli at 20 dB SL versus 40 dB SL. This latter approach was suggested by the results of doctoral dissertation research by Leo Doerfler at Northwestern University in 1948. Difference limens were abnormally small in patients with histopathologic evidence of cochlear impairment. In addition, difference limen and ABLB test outcomes were consistently equivalent. Further simplification of the technique, in particular, abandoning the search for an exact difference limen in dB in favor of assessing a patient's performance in detecting a fixed intensity increment, led to the conventional SISI test (Jerger, Shedd, & Harford, 1959). There is, perhaps, more published clinical experience with the SISI than with any other single site-of-lesion procedure (see Buus, Florentine, & Redden, 1982; Lamore & Rodenburg, 1980; Owens, 1979, for reviews).

In the conventional SISI, a continuous carrier tone at the test frequency is presented at 20 dB SL and the patient listens for brief (e.g., 200 ms) presentations of an increment of the same pure tone frequency that is 1 dB greater in intensity, superimposed on the carrier tone. The increments are presented periodically (e.g., every 5 s). Before this testing begins, increments of 5 dB and then 2 dB are first presented to acquaint the patient with the task. A 1-dB increment is not perceived by normal hearing subjects but is heard without difficulty by the patient with pure cochlear dysfunction (Jerger, 1955; Jerger et al., 1959; Jerger & Jerger, 1967). Twenty separate presentations of the 1-dB intensity increment are presented at each test frequency for each ear (usually 500, 1000, 2000, and 4000 Hz), and the percentage of increments perceived by the patient is calculated. Patients with cochlear hearing impairment typically can detect over 70% of the increments, whereas normal hearing subjects or patients with retrocochlear pathology yield scores of 30% or less.

Failure of patients with cochlear hearing loss of presumably less than about 50 or 60 dB to produce high SISI scores (above 70%) at the usual 20 dB SL intensity level prompted a second generation of SISI protocols at SLs of 75 to 90 dB (Cooper & Owen, 1976; Owens, 1965; Swisher, 1966; Thompson, 1963; Young & Harbert, 1967). At the higher intensity level, cochlear ears with mild-to-moderate impairment were much more likely to show high SISI scores (referred to as a positive test outcome), and high scores are even typically found in normal ears. Unfortunately, a point not fully appreciated by these investigators was the correspondingly greater proportion of patients with retrocochlear dysfunction who also produced high (positive for cochlear impairment) scores (Sanders, 1982). Finally, a variety of other subject characteristics (e.g., age, degree of hearing sensitivity loss, size of eighth nerve tumor, the presence of auditory adaptation) or stimulus parameters (e.g., increment size, test frequency, contralateral masking) can influence SISI outcome (Bartholomeus & Swisher, 1971; Blegvad & Terkildsen, 1966; Otto & McCandless, 1982; Sanders, 1966).

Physiologic bases. The limited understanding of the physiologic bases of ABLB, noted above, applies as well to SISI. A fundamental difference in the activity of outer versus inner hair cells as a function of stimulus intensity is repeatedly incorporated into theories on the mechanism underlying high SISI scores in cochlear impairment (Swisher, 1966). That is, the outer hair cells have low thresholds (relatively responsive to faint sounds), whereas the inner hair cells are activated exclusively by higher intensity sounds (they have high thresholds for excitation). Cochlear pathology most often affects the low-threshold outer hair cells, thus producing a hearing sensitivity impairment by pure tone audiometry. As stimulus intensity is increased and eventually exceeds the threshold of the inner hair cells, there is a quantum increase in the detectability of the 1-dB intensity increment by the patient with cochlear dysfunction.

The above, briefly described presumed role of inner and outer hair cells was held for many years. Recent studies, however, seriously question this rather simple explanation of the response properties of hair cells, that is, inner hair cells excited by high SPLs and outer hair cells by low SPLs. The interested reader is referred to Dallos, Santos-Sacchi, and Flock (1982) and Pickles (1982), among other sources.

Critical summary. Although the name of this test—short increment sensitivity index—was specifically chosen by Jerger as being descriptive of the nature of the task, rather than an implication of some presumed underlying mechanism, first the difference limen for intensity, and subsequently the SISI, became incorrectly identified as measures of loudness recruitment by various authors. Perhaps because of the influence of SISI test protocol and subject characteristics on outcome and the inextricable neuropathophysiologic link between eighth nerve and cochlear dysfunction in some patients (e.g., cochlear dysfunction secondary to compromised blood supply caused by a tumor of the eighth nerve in the internal auditory canal), high (cochlear) SISI scores do not consistently rule out retrocochlear pathology. Thus the predictive accuracy of SISI in eighth nerve pathology has traditionally been low, often at the level of chance (Sanders, 1982; Schwartz, 1987). Finally, the consideration of the method used in determining stimulus intensity (sound pressure level [SPL] vs. SL) noted for ABLB is equally important for SISI. Normal hearing persons can detect small intensity increments at high intensity levels, and conversely, patients with cochlear impairment do not necessarily detect small increments at low intensity levels (Harbert, Young, & Weiss, 1969; Konig, 1962; Martin & Salas, 1970).

Tone decay tests

Discovery and definition.   As noted at the beginning of this chapter, the clinical observation of tone decay (auditory adaptation) in retrocochlear pathology dates back to 1893, and perhaps even earlier. Availability of the Bekesy audiometer a few years after its description in 1947 led to the description of abnormal tone decay in patients with confirmed eighth nerve tumors by Reger and Kos (1952) and, very soon thereafter, measurement of tone decay with conventional audiometers by others (Carhart, 1957; Hood, 1955; Rosenberg, 1958).

The feature common to all behavioral measures of auditory adaptation is presentation of a continuous tone and determination that threshold for the tone has changed (becomes poorer) over time. There are, however, many different tests for tone decay that are distinguished by variations in measurement technique, such as the intensity level of the tone, criteria for an abnormal change in threshold, and the audiometer used (conventional vs. Bekesy).

Prominent among these different versions of tone decay tests carried out with a standard audiometer are those proposed by Hood (1955), Carhart (1957), Rosenberg (1958), Yantis (1959), Green (1963), Sorensen (1960), Owens (1964), Olsen and Noffsinger (1974) and Jerger and Jerger (1975). The Carhart and Rosenberg tone decay tests were each motivated by the clinical need for simpler and quicker procedures. The Sorensen version was modified slightly from Carhart's test (a 90-s vs. 60-s time period and limited to a test frequency of 2000 Hz). Yantis likewise recommended only a minimal alteration of Carhart's protocol (beginning the test at 5 dB SL vs. threshold). Green included criteria for tonality of the stimulus in addition to audibility in test interpretation. Owens proposed a modification of Hood's test that required classification of the pattern of response (taking into account the degree and speed of adaptation). Olsen and Noffsinger (1974) recommended the Carhart type test, but started at 20 dB SL (rather than at threshold), again to save test time without sacrificing accuracy.

The procedure introduced by the Jergers (suprathreshold adaptation test, or STAT) was developed in the interest of both simplicity and heightened sensitivity to retrocochlear dysfunction. In contrast to previous procedures that are carried out at a designated SL, the STAT stimulus is presented at a fixed SPL (110 dB) with, of course, adequate masking to the nontest ear. A cochlear finding is a patient response for a full 60 s. There are, in addition, three distinct Bekesy adaptation (tone decay) procedures: the Bekesy forward (low to high frequency) threshold test, the Bekesy forward-backward threshold test, and the Bekesy Comfortable Level (BCL) test (Jerger, 1960; Jerger, Jerger, & Mauldin, 1972; Jerger & Jerger, 1974a, 1974b, respectively). The reader is referred to these original articles and to several review papers (Konkle & Orchik, 1979; Sanders, 1982) for detail on methodology and interpretation criteria for these procedures.

Physiologic bases.   Tone decay is not an exclusive feature of eighth nerve pathology. Auditory nerve fibers normally show some degree of auditory adaptation. Tone decay is also found in presumably purely cochlear impairment. Excessive tone decay (loss of audibility) has been reported in patients with a variety of peripheral and CNS diseases, in addition to eighth nerve tumors. Suggested peripheral sites for auditory adaptation are the chemical synapse between hair cell and afferent eighth nerve fibers (Abbas, 1979; Smith, 1977). A definitive physiologic basis for the clinical phenomenon of tone decay is lacking.

Critical summary.   The apparent extensive investigation of tone decay procedures in differentiation of cochlear versus retrocochlear lesions is, in some respects, misleading. To be sure, there are many published studies on the topic but, in the final analysis, the majority are concerned more with rectifying a relatively minor clinical flaw in a previously reported procedure than with probing the pathophysiologic essence of tone decay or rigorously assessing the actual value of any tone decay procedure in accurately and precisely identifying eighth nerve pathology. The literature on ABLB and SISI certainly is subject to the same criticism. It is perhaps the multitude of variations in tone decay procedures that invites such criticism. One possible reason for the persistent interest in tone decay tests was their relatively high predictive accuracy in groups of patients with known eighth nerve pathology in selected studies reported in the 1960s (e.g., 80% by Tillman in 1966). What was not recognized, however, was almost one-half of patients with mild-to-moderate cochlear dysfunction yielded tone decay or Bekesy threshold audiometry findings that were also consistent with eighth nerve pathology (Sanders, 1982).

Accuracy rates among diagnostic audiometry procedures

Audiologic test findings of patients with surgically confirmed eighth nerve tumors are compared to those for patients with other sensorineural dysfunction (presumably sensory, or cochlear) in Table 13.2. These data were abstracted by the author from selected studies reported between 1948 and 1980 (through 1978 for all tests except ABR). A total of 52 published studies reporting findings for 808 patients with confirmed eighth nerve lesions and 3,494 presumably with cochlear dysfunction were surveyed. Most were studies reporting data for a series of patients (e.g., Johnson, 1965, 1977). Papers that simply described case reports or illustrative cases were excluded. Whenever possible, only studies presenting data for both cochlear and eighth nerve pathology were reviewed.

There were at least five inherent limitations in interpreting findings from among these studies. First, none of the studies surveyed applied all of the procedures shown in Table 13.2. In fact, just over one-half of the studies (52%) described data for pure tone audiometry and two classic site-of-lesion tests, and only one-third (33%) of the investigators administered their tests to all patients on whom findings were reported. Second, a mere 11% of the studies evaluated auditory test data as a function of patient age and only 20% made any mention of patient age. Age is, of course, an important factor in the interpretation of virtually all measures of auditory function (Hall, 1984, 1985, 1990). Third, fewer than one-third of the studies presented site-of-lesion test outcome as a function of degree of hearing loss and only 39% even stated the average hearing thresholds for patients. Fourth, although two-thirds (67%) of the studies described data for a group of patients with eighth nerve pathology and also a group with cochlear dysfunction, the groups were rarely matched for age or degree of hearing loss. Furthermore, the proportion of patients in each group invariably did not approximate the actual proportion encountered clinically. Finally, none of the investigators reporting original data calculated positive or negative predictive value for the site-of-lesion tests or test battery (see Chapter 14 by Turner in this text).

Some explanation on test protocol for the procedures displayed in Table 13.2 is needed for evaluation of the data. ABLB data were com-

TABLE 13.2

Accuracy of Diagnostic Audiometry Procedures in Correct Identification of Eighth Nerve and Cochlear Pathology

Procedure	Eighth Nerve		Cochlear	
	N	%	N	%
Short increment sensitivity index (SISI)	720	64	696	92
Tone decay[a]	737	64	2069	91
Alternate binaural loudness balance (ABLB)	620	68	1067	90
Phonetically balanced word recognition	737	69	250	60
Suprathreshold adaptation test (STAT)	20	70	75	83
Bekesy threshold tracing	44	84	327	96
Bekesy comfortable loudness (BCL)	16	80	101	97
Acoustic reflex[b]	126	85	218	84
Auditory brainstem response (ABR)	292	96	793	88

Note. Data for the number of subjects indicated were compiled by the author from studies published through 1980.
[a]Data for Carhart, Rosenberg, and Olsen/Noffsinger procedures were combined.
[b]Acoustic reflex threshold or decay.

piled from five studies for cochlear patients and eight studies for eighth nerve patients. A finding consistent with eighth nerve pathology (accurate prediction or hit rate) was absent recruitment, whereas partial or complete recruitment correctly identified (correct rejection) cochlear dysfunction. SISI data for cochlear dysfunction were compiled from 12 studies and for eighth nerve pathology from 19 studies, all at the conventional low intensity level. Correct identification of eighth nerve pathology was a SISI score of 0% to 30%. Cochlear site-of-lesion was identified by a score of greater than 60%. Data for various versions of threshold tone decay tests (reported by Carhart, 1957; Green, 1963; Hood, 1955; Owens, 1964; Rosenberg, 1958; Sorensen, 1960; Yantis, 1959) were analyzed together. A total of 21 studies reported findings for cochlear dysfunction and 31 studies for eighth nerve pathology. Correct identification of eighth nerve pathology was decay greater than 30 dB, and of cochlear dysfunction less than 30 dB. Data for the 4000-Hz test frequency were included. STAT statistics were derived from one study (Jerger & Jerger, 1975) with 20 confirmed eighth nerve tumors and 75 patients with cochlear dysfunction. Correct identification was a finding of abnormal decay for the former and no decay for the latter. Data for the 4000-Hz test frequency were included.

Threshold forward tracing Bekesy audiometry data for cochlear dysfunction were taken from 10 studies. Twenty-one studies were surveyed for the eighth nerve tumor patients. A cochlear finding was Bekesy Type I or II, and an eighth nerve finding was Type III or IV. There were two studies reporting cochlear findings (little or no discrepancy) for the Bekesy forward-reverse procedure and three studies reporting data (significant forward-backward discrepancy) for patients with eighth nerve pathology. Bekesy Comfortable Loudness (BCL) data were abstracted from a single study (Jerger & Jerger, 1974b). An eighth nerve finding was a positive classification (P1, P2, or P3) and a cochlear finding was a negative classification (N1, N2, or N3).

Acoustic reflex data were based on a combination of threshold measurements (five studies with cochlear data and eight studies with eighth nerve data) and calculation of acoustic reflex decay from three studies with patients having cochlear dysfunction and nine with eighth nerve pathology. Patients showing no acoustic reflex activity were not included in the latter series of data. Findings consistent with eighth nerve pathology were absent reflexes (sensorineural hearing loss less than 70 dB or amplitude decrease of greater than 50% from maximum over 10 s at a sensation level of 10 dB). An abnormal ABR was defined by a difference between ears in Wave V latency of greater than 0.4 ms or a Wave I–V interval exceeding normal expectations (above 2.5 standard deviations of normal value).

As seen in Table 13.2, accuracy was greater for cochlear than eighth nerve dysfunction for all procedures except the acoustic reflex and ABR. Even so, the false-positive rate among patients with cochlear dysfunction (incorrect prediction of eighth nerve pathology) was less than 5% for only the two Bekesy procedures. In clinical practice, many more patients evaluated for possible retrocochlear pathology have cochlear dysfunction than confirmed eighth nerve tumors. Thus a false-positive rate of, for example, 10% can be expected to produce unnecessary alarm and additional medical expense for a large number of patients undergoing diagnostic audiometry. The three original site-of-lesion procedures—ABLB, SISI, and tone decay—each offer a rather poor hit rate for eighth nerve pathology (less than 70% correct identification even in patients with confirmed pathology). It would appear that the Bekesy procedures, including the little-studied BCL, offer the best combination of relatively high hit rate for eighth nerve pathology and relatively low false-positive rate for cochlear dysfunction. The accuracy of the combined acoustic reflex measure (threshold or decay) of 85% in eighth nerve pathology and 84% in cochlear dysfunction exceeds the best of the traditional site-of-lesion procedures. Finally, ABR accuracy rates of 96% to 100% are consistently reported for patients with eighth nerve pathology. With proper appreciation of the limitation imposed by substantial sensorineural hearing impairment on ABR interpretation, the proportion of inaccurate predictions of retrocochlear pathology in patients with cochlear dysfunction can be greatly reduced. The application of ABR in differentiation of cochlear versus retrocochlear auditory dysfunction is discussed in more detail by Musiek in Chapter 7 of this textbook. Also, see Chapter 14 by Turner for a detailed discussion of the concepts of "hit rate," "miss rate," "false alarm," and "correct rejection" applied to audiologic tests.

Discussion and conclusions

It is tempting to valiantly argue, as have others (Brunt, 1985; Green, 1985; Martin, 1985) that the classic site-of-lesion test battery, or at least one or two procedures, still has a role in diagnostic audiometry, albeit a more limited and less glorious role than in years past. Few audiologists would suggest that we regress to a state-of-the-art that is 20 or 30 years outdated, but there is nevertheless a tendency to look back longingly upon the good old days of diagnostic audiology. Nostalgia, however, has no place in modern auditory and otologic neurodiagnosis. Current technology and procedures, including acoustic reflexes and auditory evoked responses, are by no means perfect, but improved neurodiagnosis will be found only in the future and not in the past. In this final section, I will first offer a discussion of factors that contributed to the steady growth and then precipitous decline of traditional diagnostic audiology, at the same time considering what audiology gained and, hopefully, can learn from the experiences during this period.

Acoustic tumors (typically vestibular nerve schwannomas) account for only 10% of intracranial neoplasms (Hall, 1990). The disease is uncommon in the general population and even among patients undergoing evaluation by hearing health care personnel, the prevalence is no greater than 5%. With the exception of neurofibromatosis (particularly neurofibromatosis Type 2), acoustic tumors are unilateral and at worst minimally affect communication abilities. They are extremely rare in children. Why, then, did so many talented audiologists devote so much professional time and effort to developing better techniques for identification of pathology that occurs so infrequently and with such minimal communicative consequence? There are probably several compelling reasons. One was, and still is, the clinical demand for earlier and more accurate diagnosis of potentially life-threatening pathology. Audiologists in the past were obligated to adjust their clinical interests to meet this pressing demand. Audiologists are today likewise adjusting their interests to meet new clinical demands. The professional excitement and diagnostic challenge of this audiologic activity was no doubt also an important factor.

What returns did audiology reap from this substantial professional commitment to site-of-lesion testing? The era of traditional diagnostic audiology began virtually the same time as the profession of audiology. Many of the important American personalities publishing in the area of diagnostic audiology, and cited throughout this chapter, were on the faculty of the major educational programs (e.g., Northwestern University, University of Iowa). The clinical excitement and potential of diagnostic audiology at the formative period of the profession probably was an important attraction for bright, career-oriented prospective audiologists. These people, in turn, were instrumental in establishing and maintaining audiology as an independent clinical profession. Certainly, the rather impressive publication record of these early diagnostic audiologists contributed to the academic credentials of the fledgling profession. For example, James Jerger and his colleagues published no fewer than 21 major papers on the topic from 1952 through 1975.

Two related observations seem to be appropriate at this juncture. First, it might be argued that the close alliance with otolaryngology that resulted from the mutual interest in diagnosis of otoneurologic pathology also thwarted the development of audiology as an autonomous profession primarily focused on the identification and remediation of communicative impairments. Second, a likely reason for the impact of site-of-lesion testing on audiology and, in turn, the influence of audiology in otolaryngology lies in the way research findings were published. The majority of studies in traditional diagnostic audiometry conducted in the United States were first presented at audiology professional scientific meetings (e.g., at American Speech, and Hearing Association national conventions). A survey of the references cited in this chapter shows that the publications by audiologists appeared most often in several otolaryngology journals, especially the *Archives of Otolaryngology*, or at least as often in the *Journal of Speech and Hearing Disorders or Research*. Thus audiologists and otolaryngologists both had easy access to the latest developments in site-of-lesion testing. In contrast, among the references on ABR in neurodiagnosis cited in a recent chapter on the ABR (Hall, 1984), a mere three (less than 0.1%) appeared in the ASHA journals. Technically, the development of computer-based literature searches makes important clinical papers more accessible, although the proportion of clinical audiologists taking advantage of this service is unknown. Within the past 8-10 years, a number of journals have become popular sources of information on neurodiagnosis, notably *Ear and Hearing, Audiology,* and *Electroencephalography and Clinical Neurophysiology.* For the busy clinician, of course, the challenge is to consistently search this literature for relevant publications. Clearly, current information on neurodiagnosis is not as readily accessible to the student or clinical audiologist who relies on the ASHA journals to remain abreast of developments in this area.

The demise of traditional diagnostic audiology was, it appears, due to a combination of at least four factors occurring, by chance, almost simultaneously. Two of these factors have already been mentioned. The almost instantaneous clinical popularity of acoustic reflex measurement and ABR in the early 1970s soon led to irrefutable clinical evidence of superior accuracy in differentiating cochlear versus retrocochlear pathology in comparison to the traditional test battery. With every passing year, up to the present, clinical application of classic site-of-lesion tests has declined directly as a function of the availability of evoked response systems to clinical audiologists. The advent of computerized tomography (CT) in 1975 was also a major factor in the decline of site-of-lesion testing. Computerized tomography offered the physician a far more sensitive and specific means of acquiring structural evidence of eighth nerve neoplasms, and by the middle to late 1980s, magnetic resonance imaging (MRI) provided a means of even greater resolution of anatomical imaging. Hence, the classic test battery became progressively less important as CT and MRI became readily available in most large hospitals. Finally, by 1980 there was a trend toward increased sophistication in evaluating diagnostic tests in all areas of medicine. As epidemiologic concepts such as sensitivity versus specificity, disease prevalence, and positive versus negative predictive value were applied in the evaluation of the classic site-of-lesion test battery, serious and irreparable flaws were immediately evident in the foundations of traditional diagnostic site-of-lesion tests (Schwartz, 1987; Turner, Frazer, & Shepard, 1984; Turner & Nielsen, 1984; Turner, Shepard, & Frazer, 1984; also, see Chapter 14 by Turner).

What have we learned from the accumulative experience with classic site-of-lesion testing and how can we apply it in the future? This question alone could easily be the focus of an entire essay. There probably always will be a clinical demand for early and accurate identification of potentially life-threatening otoneurologic pathology. As long as audiologists are involved in assessing auditory function, they should strive to apply the best procedures at their disposal to meet this demand. Today, the procedure of choice is ABR, but the neurodiagnostic value of even this technique can clearly be improved upon (Hall, 1990). Audiologists must not remain content with existing technology or technique. In the past, there was a constant effort to improve the accuracy or clinical efficiency of the classic site-of-lesion test procedures, and this tradition must continue with current procedures. It is quite possible that the next frontier in neurodiagnosis is brain mapping. Audiologists had best prepare now for this possibility.

The dearth of information on the physiologic bases of the classic site-of-lesion tests, even after 30 years of clinical application, is quite remarkable and no doubt a factor in the ultimate dissatisfaction with these auditory measures. Audiologists would be well-advised to study the pathophysiologic correlates of abnormalities in AERs to assure that they are being fully exploited in neurodiagnosis.

Finally, the test battery concept is still viable in clinical audiology. Even in the era of ABR, acoustic reflex measurement and performance intensity functions for PB word lists and synthetic sentence identification (SSI) materials are the best first-line means of identifying possible retrocochlear dysfunction among *unselected patients*. Furthermore, for patients with severe sensorineural hearing impairment, the finding of no measurable ABR is equivocal and does not contribute to neurodiagnosis. This is one occasion when the audiologist should consider applying a traditional diagnostic audiology procedure. The BCL is particularly recommended by this writer. On balance, the investment in classic site-of-lesion testing yielded valuable dividends to a young profession. If we learn from this professional history, the future of audiology undoubtedly will be brighter.

Acknowledgments

Data reported in this chapter were collected and initially analyzed while the author was affiliated with the Division of Audiology and Speech Pathology, Department of Otorhinolaryngology and Communicative Sciences, Baylor College of Medicine, Houston, Texas from 1973 through 1979. I gladly acknowledge the encouragement and support of Drs. James and Susan Jerger, then and now.

The following audiology students in the Division of Hearing and Speech Sciences at Vanderbilt University contributed to the preparation of portions of this work: Marcia Fort, Emiko McGraw, Kathy Neudahl, Lisa Rider, and Lisa Sells.

References

Abbas, P. J. (1979). Effects of stimulus frequency on adaptation in auditory nerve fibers. *Journal of the Acoustical Society of America, 65,* 162–165.

Anderson, H., Barr, B., & Wedenberg, E. (1970). Early diagnosis of VIIIth-nerve tumours by acoustic reflex tests. *Acta Oto-Laryngologica, 263,* 232–237.

Bartholomeus, B., & Swisher, L. (1971). Tone decay and SISI scores. *Archives of Otolaryngology, 93,* 451–455.

Bekesy, G. Von. (1947). A new audiometer. *Acta Oto-Laryngologica, 35,* 411–422.

Bekesy, G. Von. (1966). Loudness recruitment. *Transactions of the American Otological Society, 53,* 85–93.

Bess, F., Josey, A. F., & Humes, L. (1979). Performance intensity functions in cochlear and eighth nerve disorders. *American Journal of Otology, 1,* 27–31.

Blegvad, B., & Terkildsen, K. (1966). SISI test and contralateral masking. *Acta Oto-Laryngologica, 62,* 453–458.

Brunt, M. A. (1985). Bekesy audiometry and loudness balance testing. In J. Katz (Ed.), *Handbook of clinical audiology* (pp. 273–291). Baltimore: Williams & Wilkins.

Buus, S., Florentine, M., & Redden, R. B. (1982). The SISI test: A review. Part I. *Audiology, 21,* 273–293.

Carhart, R. (1957). Clinical determination of abnormal auditory adaptation. *Archives of Otolaryngology, 65,* 32–39.

Chiveralls, K. (1977). A further examination of the use of the stapedius reflex in the diagnosis of acoustic neuroma. *Audiology, 16,* 331–337.

Clemis, J., & Mastricola, P. (1976). Special audiometric test battery in 121 proved acoustic tumor. *Archives of Otolaryngology, 102,* 654–656.

Clemis, J. D., & McGee, T. (1979). Brainstem electric response audiometry in the differential diagnosis of acoustic tumors. *Laryngoscope, 89,* 31–42.

Cooper, J. C., & Owen, J. H. (1976). In defense of SISIs. *Archives of Otolaryngology, 102,* 396–399.

Dallos, P., Santos-Sacchi, J., & Flock, A. (1982). Intracellular recordings from cochlear outer hair cells. *Science, 218,* 582–584.

Dawson, G. D. (1947). Cerebral responses to electrical stimulation of peripheral nerve in man. *Journal of Neurology, Neuropsychiatry and Psychiatry, 10,* 134–140.

Denes, P., & Naunton, R. (1950). The clinical detection of auditory recruitment. *Journal of Laryngology and Otology, 65,* 375–398.

Dix, M., Hallpike, C., & Hood, J. (1948). Observations upon the loudness recruitment phenomenon with especial reference to the differential diagnosis of disorders of the internal ear and VIIIth nerve. *Journal of Laryngology and Otology, 62,* 671–686.

Dix, M. R. (1965). Observations upon the nerve fibre deafness of multiple sclerosis with particular reference to the phenomenon of loudness recruitment. *Journal of Laryngology and Otology, 79,* 695–706.

Doerfler, L. (1948). Differential sensitivity to intensity in the perceptively deafened ear. *Summary of Dissertations at Northwestern University, 16,* 75–79.

Eby, L. G., & Williams, H. L. (1951). Recruitment of loudness in the differential diagnosis of end-organ and nerve fiber deafness. *Laryngoscope, 61,* 400–414.

Flower, R., & Viehweg, R. (1961). A review of audiologic findings among patients with cerebellopontine angle tumors. *Laryngoscope, 71,* 1105–1126.

Fowler, E. P. (1936). Differences in loudness response of the normal and hard-of-hearing ear at intensity levels slightly above the threshold. *Annals of Otology, Rhinology, and Laryngology, 45,* 1029–1039.

Fowler, E. P. (1937). The diagnosis of diseases of the neural mechanism by the aid of sounds well above threshold. *Transactions of the American Otological Society, 70,* 207–219.

Fowler, E. P. (1950). The recruitment of loudness phenomena. *Laryngoscope, 60,* 680–695.

Goodman, A. C. (1957). Some relations between auditory function and intracranial lesions with particular reference to lesions of the cerebellopontine angle. *Laryngoscope, 67,* 987–1010.

Gradenigo, G., & Allen, S. E. (1893). On the clinical signs of effections of the auditory nerve (German). *Archives of Otorhinolaryngology, 22,* 213–215.

Green, D. S. (1963). The modified tone decay test (MTDT) as a screening procedure for eighth nerve lesions. *Journal of Speech and Hearing Disorders, 28,* 31–36.

Green, D. S. (1985). Tone decay. In J. Katz (Ed.), *Handbook of clinical audiology* (pp. 304–318). Baltimore: Williams & Wilkins.

Hall, J. W. (1978, November). *Diagnostic audiometry in sensorineural hearing loss: A survey and critical review of the literature.* Paper presented at the American Speech and Hearing Association Convention, San Francisco.

Hall, J. W. (1984). Auditory brainstem response audiometry. In J. Jerger (Ed.), *Hearing disorders in adults* (pp. 3–55). San Diego: College-Hill Press.

Hall, J. W. (1985). Acoustic reflex in central auditory dysfunction. In M. L. Pinheiro, & F. E. Musiek (Eds.), Assessment of central auditory dysfunction: Foundations and clinical correlates (pp. 103–130). Baltimore: Williams & Wilkins.

Hall, J. W. III. (Ed.) (1988). Immittance audiometry. *Seminars in Hearing, 8,* 307–406.

Hall, J. W. (1990). *Handbook of auditory evoked responses.* Austin, TX: PRO-ED.

Hallpike, C. S., & Hood, J. D. (1951). Some recent work on auditory adaptation and its relationship to the recruitment phenomenon. *Journal of the Acoustical Society of America, 23,* 270–274.

Halm, T. (1949). Determination of the difference limen and the latest illustration thereof in audiometry. *Journal of Laryngology and Otology, 63,* 464–466.

Harbert, F., Young, I. M., & Weiss, B. G. (1969). Clinical application of intensity difference limen. *Acta Oto-Laryngologica, 67,* 435–443.

Hood, J. D. (1955). Auditory fatigue and adaptation in the differential diagnosis of end-organ disease. *Annals of Otology, Rhinology and Laryngology, 64,* 507–518.

Jerger, J. (1952). A difference limen test and its diagnostic significance. *Laryngoscope, 62,* 1316–1332.

Jerger, J. (1953). DL difference test. *Archives of Otolaryngology, 57,* 490–500.

Jerger, J. (1960). Bekesy audiometry in the analysis of auditory disorders. *Journal of Speech and Hearing Research, 3,* 275–287.

Jerger, J. (1961). Recruitment and allied phenomena in differential diagnosis. *Journal of Auditory Research, 1,* 145–151.

Jerger, J. (1962a). Hearing tests in otologic diagnosis. *Asha, 4,* 139–145.

Jerger, J. (1962b). Comparative evaluation of some auditory measures. *Journal of Speech and Hearing Disorders, 27,* 3–17.

Jerger, J. (1973). Diagnostic audiometry. In J. Jerger (Ed.), *Modern developments in audiology* (2nd ed., pp. 75–115). New York: Academic Press.

Jerger, J. (1987). Diagnostic audiology: Historical perspective. *Ear and Hearing,* (Supplement) *8,* 7–12.

Jerger, J., Carhart, R., & Lassman, J. (1958). Clinical observations on excessive threshold adaptation. *Archives of Otolaryngology, 68,* 617–623.

Jerger, J., & Harford, E. (1960). Alternate and simultaneous binaural balancing of pure tones. *Journal of Speech and Hearing Research, 3,* 15–30.

Jerger, J., Harford, E., Clemis, J., & Alford, B. (1974). The acoustic reflex in eighth nerve disorders. *Archives of Otolaryngology, 99,* 409–413.

Jerger, J., & Jerger, S. (1967). Psychoacoustic comparison of cochlear and VIIIth nerve disorders. *Journal of Speech and Hearing Research, 10,* 659–688.

Jerger, J., & Jerger, S. (1970). Evoked response to intensity and frequency change. *Archives of Otolaryngology, 91,* 433–436.

Jerger, J., & Jerger, S. (1971). Diagnostic significance of PB word functions. *Archives of Otolaryngology, 93,* 573–580.

Jerger, J., & Jerger, S. (1974a). Audiological comparison of cochlear and eighth nerve disorders. *Annals of Otology, Rhinology and Laryngoscope, 88,* 275–285.

Jerger, J., & Jerger, S. (1974b). Diagnostic value of Bekesy comfortable loudness tracings. *Archives of Otolaryngology, 99,* 351–360.

Jerger, J., & Jerger, S. (1975). A simplified tone decay test. *Archives of Otolaryngology, 101,* 403–407.

Jerger, J., Jerger, S., & Mauldin, L. (1972). The forward—backward discrepancy in Bekesy audiometry. *Archives of Otolaryngology, 96,* 400–406.

Jerger, J., Shedd, J., & Harford, E. (1959). On the detection of extremely small changes in sound intensity. *Archives of Otolaryngology, 69,* 200–211.

Jerger, J. F. (1955). Differential intensity sensitivity in the ear with loudness recruitment. *Journal of Speech and Hearing Disorders, 20,* 183–191.

Jerger, S., & Jerger, J. (1983). Evaluation of diagnostic audiometric tests. *Audiology, 22,* 144–161.

Jewett, D. L., Romano, M. N., & Williston, J. S. (1970). Human auditory evoked potentials: Possible brainstem components detected on the scalp. *Science, 167,* 1517–1518.

Jewett, D. L., & Williston, J. S. (1971). Auditory evoked far fields averaged from the scalp of humans. *Brain, 94,* 681–696.

Johnson, E. (1965). Auditory test results in 110 surgically confirmed retrocochlear lesions. *Journal of Speech and Hearing Disorders, 30,* 307–317.

Johnson, E. (1977). Auditory test results in 500 cases of acoustic neuroma. *Archives of Otolaryngology, 103,* 152–158.

Konig, E. R. (1962). Difference limen for intensity. *International Audiology, 1,* 198–202.

Konkle, D. F., & Orchik, D. J. (1979). Auditory adaptation. In W. F. Rintelmann (Ed.), *Hearing assessment* (pp. 207–233). Baltimore: University Park Press.

Kristensen, H. K., & Jepsen, O. (1952). Recruitment in otoneurological diagnostics. *Acta Oto-Laryngologica, 42,* 553–562.

Lamore, P. J. J., & Rodenburg, M. (1980). Significance of the SISI test and its relation to recruitment. *Audiology, 19,* 75–85.

Lidén, G., & Korsan-Bengtsen, M. (1973). Audiometric manifestations of retrocochlear lesions. *Scandinavian Audiology, 2,* 29–40.

Lierle, D. M., & Reger, S. N. (1954). Further studies of threshold shifts as measured with the Bekesy-type audiometer. *Annals of Otology, Rhinology and Laryngology, 63,* 772–784.

Lierle, D. M., & Reger, S. N. (1955). Experimentally induced temporary threshold shifts in ears with impaired hearing. *Annals of Otology, Rhinology and Laryngology, 64,* 263–272.

Lundborg, T. (1952). Diagnostic problems concerning acoustic tumors: A study of 300 verified cases and the Bekesy audiogram in differential diagnosis. *Acta Oto-Laryngologica, 99,* (Supplement), 1–111.

Lüscher, E. (1951a). The difference limen of intensity variations of pure tones and its diagnostic significance. *Journal of Laryngology and Otology, 65,* 486–510.

Lüscher, E. (1951b). The difference limen of intensity variations of pure tones and its diagnostic significance. *Journal of Laryngology and Otology, 65,* 486–510.

Lüscher, E., & Zwislocki, J. (1948). A simple method of monaural determination of the recruitment phenomenon. *Practical Oto-Rhinolaryngology, 10,* 521–522.

Martin, F. N. (1985). The SISI test. In J. Katz (Ed.), *Handbook of clinical audiology* (pp. 292–303). Baltimore: Williams & Wilkins.

Martin, F. N., & Salas, C. R. (1970). The SISI test and subjective loudness. *Journal of Auditory Research, 10,* 368–371.

Metz, O. (1946). The acoustic impedance measured on normal and pathological ears. *Acta Oto-Laryngologica,* Supplement *63,* 1–254.

Miskolczy-Fodor, F. (1956). The relation between hearing loss and recruitment and its practical employment in the determination of receptive hearing loss. *Acta Oto-Laryngologica, 46,* 409–415.

Moore, B. C. J. (1982). *Introduction to the psychology of hearing.* London: Academic Press.

Olsen, W., & Noffsinger, D. (1974). Comparison of one new and three old tests of auditory adaptation. *Archives of Otolaryngology, 99,* 94–99.

Olsen, W., Noffsinger, D., & Kurdziel, S. (1975). Acoustic reflex and reflex decay: Occurrence in patients with cochlear and eighth nerve lesions. *Archives of Otolaryngology, 101,* 622–625.

Otto, W. C., & McCandless, G. A. (1982). Aging and auditory site of lesion. *Ear and Hearing, 3,* 110–117.

Owens, E. (1964). Tone decay in eighth nerve and cochlear lesions. *Journal of Speech and Hearing Disorders, 29,* 14–22.

Owens, E. (1965). The SISI test and VIIIth nerve versus cochlear involvement. *Journal of Speech and Hearing Disorders, 30,* 252–262.

Owens, E. (1979). Differential intensity discrimination. In W. F. Rintelmann (Ed.), *Hearing assessment* (pp. 235–259). Baltimore: University Park Press.

Palva, T. (1964). Auditory adaptation. *Acta Oto-Laryngologica, 57,* 207–216.

Pickles, J. O. (1982). *An introduction to the physiology of hearing.* London: Academic Press.

Reger, S. (1935). Loudness level contours and intensity discrimination of ears with raised auditory threshold. *Journal of Acoustical Society of America, 7,* 73 (Abstract).

Reger, S. N., & Kos, C. M. (1952). Clinical measurements and implications of recruitment. *Annals of Otology, Rhinology and Laryngology, 61,* 810–823.

Rose, D. (1962). Some effects and case histories of reversed frequency sweep in Bekesy audiometry. *Journal of Auditory Research, 2,* 267–278.

Rosenberg, P. (1971). Abnormal auditory adaptation. *Archives of Otolaryngology, 94,* 89.

Rosenberg, P. E. (1958, November). *Rapid clinical measurement of tone decay.* Paper presented at the annual convention of the American Speech and Hearing Association, New York.

Rosenhamer, H. (1977). Observations on electric brain-stem responses in retrocochlear hearing loss. *Scandinavian Audiology, 6,* 179–196.

Salvi, R. J., Henderson, D., Hamernik, R., & Ahroon, W. A. (1983). Neurological correlates of sensorineural hearing loss. *Ear and Hearing, 4,* 115–129.

Sanders, J., Josey, A. F., & Glasscock, M. (1974). Audiologic evaluation in cochlear and eighth nerve disorders. *Archives of Otolaryngology, 100,* 283–289.

Sanders, J. W. (1979). Recruitment. In W. F. Rintelmann (Ed.), *Hearing assessment* (pp. 261–280). Baltimore: University Park Press.

Sanders, J. W. (1982). Diagnostic audiology. In N. J. Lass, L. V. McReynolds, J. L. Northern, & D. E. Yoder (Eds.), *Speech, language, and hearing:* Vol. 3. *Hearing disorders* (pp. 944–967). Philadelphia: WB Saunders.

Sanders, J. W., Josey, A. F., Glasscock, M. E., & Jackson, C. G. (1981). The acoustic reflex test in cochlear and eighth nerve pathology ears. *Laryngoscope, 91,* 787–793.

Schwartz, D. M. (1987). Neurodiagnostic audiology: Contemporary perspectives. *Ear and Hearing, 8,* 43S–48S.

Selters, W. A., & Brackmann, D. E. (1977). Acoustic tumor detection with brainstem electric response audiometry. *Archives of Otolaryngology, 103,* 15–24.

Smith, R. L. (1977). Short-term adaptation in single auditory nerve fibers: Some poststimulatory effects. *Journal of Neurophysiology, 40,* 1098–1112.

Sorensen, H. (1960). A threshold tone decay test. *Acta Oto-Laryngologica,* (Supplement) *158,* 356–360.

Swisher, L. P. (1966). Response to intensity change in cochlear pathology. *Laryngoscope, 76,* 1706–1713.

Terkildsen, K., Huis in't Veld, F., & Osterhammel, P. (1977). Auditory brainstem responses in the diagnosis of cerebellopontine angle tumors. *Scandinavian Audiology, 6,* 43–47.

Thompson, G. (1963). A modified SISI technique for selected cases with suspected acoustic neuroma. *Journal of Speech and Hearing Disorders, 28,* 299–302.

Thomsen, J., Terkildsen, K., & Osterhammel, P. (1978). Auditory brainstem responses in patients with acoustic neuromas. *Scandinavian Audiology, 7,* 179–183.

Thomsen, K. A. (1955). The Metz recruitment test. *Acta Oto-Laryngologica, 45,* 544–552.

Tillman, T. (1966). Audiologic diagnosis of acoustic tumors. *Archives of Otolaryngology, 83,* 574–581.

Turner, R. G., Frazer, G. J., & Shepard, N. T. (1984). Formulating and evaluating audiologic test protocols. *Ear and Hearing, 5,* 321–330.

Turner, R. G., & Nielsen, D. W. (1984). Application of clinician decision analysis to audiological tests. *Ear and Hearing, 5,* 125–133.

Turner, R. G., Shepard, N. T., & Frazer, G. J. (1984). Clinical performance of audiological and related diagnostic tests. *Ear and Hearing, 5,* 187–194.

Yantis, P. A. (1959). Clinical implications of the temporary threshold shift. *Archives of Otolaryngology, 70,* 779–787.

Young, I. M., & Harbert, F. (1967). Significance of the SISI test. *Journal of Auditory Research, 7,* 303–311.

chapter fourteen

Making clinical decisions

ROBERT G. TURNER

Contents

Essential decision making

As in life, decision making is an essential and unavoidable component of clinical work. Even refusal to decide often constitutes a significant decision. Whether interpreting a test or selecting a hearing aid, it is this professional, educated decision that the audiologist "sells" to his patient. The success of the profession of audiology depends on the ability of the audiologist to make appropriate decisions.

How do we make decisions? There are three basic steps: (a) gathering of data, (b) processing of data, and (c) calculating cost-benefit. Let me illustrate with a simple example. It is Friday night and I want to take my family to the movies. First I check the newspaper for times and admission cost. This is the gathering of data. Next I calculate the exorbitant cost for six people. This is the processing of data. Finally, I consider the benefit I would receive relative to the cost of attending. This is the cost-benefit analysis. I decide to rent a video and watch a movie at home. This is an intelligent decision.

The first step, gathering of data is extremely important because the correctness of the decision is a function of the accuracy of the data. The old computer expression applies, "Garbage in, garbage out." Despite its importance, we will not consider this step in detail; the problems of data collection are particular to the problem. The other two steps are of interest to us. How do we analyze data; that is, how do we reduce raw data to useful measures, and how do we determine cost-benefit?

There are two basic strategies for analysis and decision making: analytic/objective and intuitive/subjective. In the analytic/objective technique, the emphasis is on quantifying data, costs, and benefits. Mathematics and logic are applied to the data to produce a quantitative result. A well-defined criterion is applied to the result to determine the decision. The advantage of this approach is that subjectivity and bias are removed from the decision process. In addition, there is little "noise" in the analysis because math and logic are very precise techniques. There are, however, several disadvantages. Some problems are too complex to model and describe. A major problem is the necessity of quantifying all relevant issues. Financial costs are easy to quantify, but how do you assign a number to illness or hearing impairment. Another limitation is the individual's expertise with the tools of quantitative analysis. Not everyone, including audiologists, are facile with calculus, Boolean algebra, or complex number theory. Some problems may be possible to quantify but impossible to analyze. Thus the analytic/objective approach works best with simpler problems that are within the technical capabilities of the individual audiologist.

The intuitive/subjective approach is less well understood but frequently employed. The essence of this technique is that the analysis takes place, not in the conscious mind, but in the sub- or superconscious mind. All of us are familiar with intuition and the ability to make good judgments on the basis of limited data. It just "feels" right. This is clearly the basis for decision making for complex problems in our lives, and the only technique available for problems so difficult that they defy quantitative analysis. If the reader doubts the existence of this subconscious analytic ability, consider speech perception. The process of converting acoustic waveforms into linguistic concepts is an extremely difficult problem of analysis. This process cannot be duplicated by machine, yet, it is performed effortlessly by the human without conscious thought.

The mechanisms of intuitive decision making are not clear. Perhaps we can access, through our subconscious mind, the "answer" or at least data not available to the conscious mind, in some universal store of knowledge. Another possibility is that the subconscious mind has the ability to evaluate and integrate *qualitative* data, permitting the solution of very complex problems. There is an important disadvantage to the intuitive/subjective approach. The decision process cannot be examined by the conscious mind. This makes the process susceptible to undetected error. Decisions may be based on emotion, prejudice, or bias, not a superior form of analysis. There is no way to determine the basis for the decision. In summary, the intuitive/subjective technique works best on complex problems that resist quantitative analysis.

The issue of analytic versus intuitive decision making has important implications for health care. Although both techniques are used, there is a strong tradition of the intuitive approach reflecting medicine's history as the healing arts. Many problems are too complex to permit analytic analysis; however, there are issues that, with effort, can be quantitatively analyzed. How often is the statement, "This decision was based on 20 years' experience!", an excuse to avoid the difficulty of an analytic solution to the problem?

The objective of this chapter is to examine some quantitative techniques of decision making, in particular, those techniques that are relevant to the use of diagnostic tests. Although this is a fairly narrow perspective, diagnostic audiology has, historically, played an important role in the development of the profession.

Diagnostic tests are used in many specialties of health care. For audiology, the classic example of diagnostic tests are those developed to distinguish between cochlear and retrocochlear site-of-lesion. In this context, diagnostic means to distinguish between several possible conditions, not necessarily to identify the etiology of a disease. There are other examples of diagnostic tests in audiology, and some of these will be discussed later. All health care professionals using diagnostic tests face the same problem. How do you appropriately select, administer, and interpret diagnostic tests? This is a basic problem in decision making. Next, we will examine some powerful techniques, called Clinical Decision Analysis, that facilitate our use of diagnostic tests.

Clinical decision analysis

Clinical Decision Analysis (CDA) is a quantitative, systematic approach to clinical decision making. It is concerned with both the processing of data and the cost-benefit analysis. The techniques of CDA are largely derived from the Theory of Signal Detection (TSD). TSD began during World War II as an engineering attempt to extract signals from noise, a prime example being radar. Following the war, psychologists applied TSD to the detection of auditory signals by the human observer.

In the past 20 years, CDA has been applied to a variety of clinical disciplines and problems. The primary emphasis has been on the evaluation of the performance of screening and diagnostic tests. TSD was developed to extract signal from noise, that is, to make a decision as to the presence of a signal in noise. The use of a diagnostic test is an analogous problem because most diagnostic tests are not infallible—there is some "noise" in the test result. Most tests will produce a range of scores for a particular type of patient, and, more important, there will be an overlap in the scores produced by diseased and nondiseased patients. It is this overlap of test scores for the two patient groups that creates a potential for error. A particular score could, with finite probability, be produced by either patient group.

Consider the following situation. A patient, either diseased or nondiseased, receives a diagnostic test. The outcome of the test is either positive or negative for the disease. The test is fallible and makes errors, reflecting the noise in the testing process. There are four possible outcomes of the testing, reflecting the result of the test and the state of the patient. These outcomes are represented by a 2 × 2 decision matrix (Figure 14.1). If the patient is diseased, a positive test is called a hit and a negative result a miss. If the patient is nondiseased, a positive result is a false alarm and a negative result is a correct rejection. The terminology of *hits*, *false alarms*, and so forth, reflect the historical origin of TSD. Different terminology is frequently used in the clinical literature. A hit is a true positive; a miss is a false negative; a false alarm is a false positive; a correct rejection is a true negative. The traditional terminology will be used in this chapter because it is less confusing and more consistent with the historical origin of TSD.

The four elements of the matrix represent the number of hits, misses, false alarms, and correct rejections when the test is given to a number of patients. The hits and correct rejections are correct decisions, whereas misses and false alarms are errors that degrade the performance of the test. For example, 10 diseased and 20 nondiseased patients are tested. The test is positive on 7 out of 10 diseased patients and 2 out of 20 nondiseased patients. Thus there would be 7 hits and 3 misses, 2 false alarms and 18 correct rejections. Note that the number of hits plus misses always equals the number of diseased patients. The number of false alarms plus correct rejections equals the number of nondiseased patients.

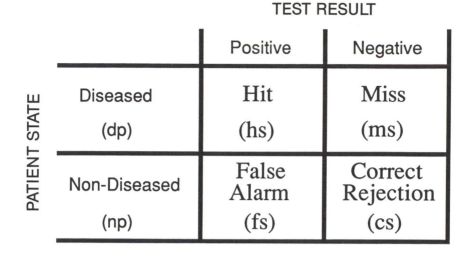

Figure 14.1. Decision matrix for diagnostic tests. dp: number of diseased patients; np: number of nondiseased patients; hs: number of hits; ms: number of misses; fs: number of false alarms; cs: number of correct rejections. Hit rate (HT) = hs/dp; false alarm rate (FA) = fs/np.

Measures of individual test performance

Hit rate and friends

Next we will consider measures of diagnostic test performance. These measures are discussed in detail in Turner and Nielsen (1984). The most basic measures of test performance can be calculated from the decision matrix. These are hit rate (HT), miss rate (MS), false alarm rate (FA), and correct rejection rate (CR). Hit rate (also called true positive rate and sensitivity) is the percentage of diseased patients correctly identified as positive for the disease; miss rate (also called false negative rate) is the percentage of diseased patients incorrectly identified as negative. False alarm rate (also called false positive rate) is the percentage of nondiseased patients incorrectly called positive; correct rejection rate (also called true negative rate and specificity) is the percentage of nondiseased patients correctly identified as negative. These measures are calculated by the following equations:

$$HT = \frac{hs}{dp} \tag{1}$$

$$MS = \frac{ms}{dp} \tag{2}$$

$$FA = \frac{fs}{np} \tag{3}$$

$$CR = \frac{cs}{np} \tag{4}$$

where dp = number of diseased patients, np = number of nondiseased patients, hs = number of hits, ms = number of misses, fs = number of false alarms, and cs = number of correct rejections. (See Table 14.1 for abbreviations used in this chapter.) It should be noted that these measures can be expressed as a percentage or the equivalent decimal, that is, 50% = .50. For most calculations in this chapter, the decimal form should be used. Although all four measures can be calculated, only two, usually HT and FA, need be considered. This is because HT + MS = 100% and FA + CR = 100%; thus MS and CR can always be determined from HT and FA.

HT and FA are easily calculated from clinical data. For example, 100 diseased (dp) and 200 nondiseased patients (np) are tested. The test is positive for 82 (hs) of the diseased patients and 38 (fs) of the nondiseased patients. HT = 82/100 = .82 = 82%; FA = 38/200 = .19 = 19%. If desired, MS = 100% – HT = 18% and CR = 100% – FA = 81%.

The measures of test performance, HT, FA, MS, and CR, can also be expressed as probabilities. HT is the probability of a positive test result given a diseased patient (Pr[+/D]); FA is the probability of a positive result with a nondiseased patient (Pr[+/N]); MS is the probability of a negative result given a diseased patient (Pr[–/D]), and CR is the probability of a negative result given a nondiseased patient (Pr[–/N]).

Probability distribution curve

As shown above, HT and FA can be easily calculated from clinical data, but they are, in fact, determined by the basic properties of the test and the criterion that is selected to determine if the test result is positive or negative. Consider a theoretical test that produces a score from 0 to 100. The test is administered to two groups of patients, one diseased and the other nondiseased. Each group will produce a variety of scores on the

TABLE 14.1
Abbreviations Used in Text

HT/FA: Hit rate/false alarm rate of an individual test (%)

HTn/FAn: Hit rate/false alarm rate of test in n^{th} block of protocol (%)

HBn/FBn: Hit rate/false alarm rate of nth block in a protocol (%)

HTp/FAp: Hit rate/false alarm rate of protocol (%)

HTp(m)/FA(m): Hit rate/false alarm rate of protocol with mid-pos correlation (%)

HTp(z)/FAp(z): Hit rate/false alarm rate of protocol with zero correlation (%)

HTp(+)/FAp(+): Hit rate/false alarm rate of protocol with max-pos correlation (%)

HTs/FAs: Hit rate/false alarm rate of a screening protocol used wth a definitive test (%)

Pr[+/D]: Hit rate; probability of a positive test result with a diseased patient (%)

Pr[+/N]: False alarm rate; probability of a positive test result with a nondiseased patient (%)

Pr[D/+]: Posterior probability of being correct with a positive test result (%)

Pr[N/−]: Posterior probability of being correct with a negative test result (%)

EF: Efficiency; percentage of correct test results (%)

d': Measure of test performance; larger d' means better performance (%)

A': Measure of test performance; large A' means better performance (%)

PD: Disease prevalence; percentage of test population with disease

dp: Number of diseased patients

np: Number of nondiseased patients

hs: Number of hits

ms: Number of misses

fs: Number of false alarms

cs: Number of correct rejections

---

test. We could plot a histogram of scores for each population, that is, the number of patients in a group with a score between 0 and 10, 10 and 20, and so on. Next, we divide the number of patients in each score range by the total number of patients in the group to obtain the probability distribution curve (PDC). Essentially, the PDC gives the probability of obtaining a particular score, or range of scores, for each group of patients. PDCs for a theoretical test are shown in Figure 14.2. Note that there are two PDCs, one for diseased patients and one for nondiseased patients. Also note that the two distributions are different; the probability of a particular score is different for the two populations of patients. For example, the probability of a score from 31 to 40 is 40% for diseased patients and 5% for nondiseased patients. Stated another way, 40% of the diseased patients and 5% of the nondiseased patients had scores from 31 to 40.

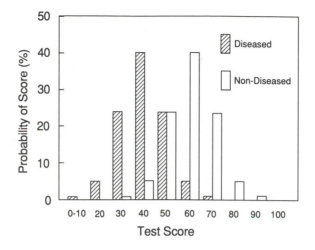

Figure 14.2. Probability distribution curves for a theoretical test. One distribution corresponds to test performance for diseased patients, the other for non-diseased patients. Possible test scores are divided into 10 intervals: 0–10, 11–20, 21–30, . . . 91–100. The number below each cluster of two bars represents the upper limit of test score except for 0–10, which indicates the whole interval. Thus, 40 means the test score interval of 31–40. The two bars above 40 give the probability of diseased and nondiseased patients having a test score in the range of 31–40. That probability is 40% for diseased and 5% for nondiseased patients. (From Turner & Nielsen, 1984, with permission.)

Because the two PDCs in Figure 14.2 do not completely overlap, we may use this test to distinguish diseased from nondiseased. First, however, we must establish a criterion to determine if a test score is positive or negative for disease. Remember, in the clinic, we do not know the type of patient being tested; that is the purpose of the test. In Figure 14.3 we set the criterion at 50. On average, nondiseased patients have higher scores than do diseased patients; therefore, a score greater than 50 is negative and a score less than or equal to 50 is positive for disease. Because there is some overlap in the two PDCs, the criterion divides the PDCs into four regions corresponding to hits, misses, false alarms, and correct rejections. Below the criterion (<50), the diseased patients constitute the hits and the nondiseased patients the false alarms. Above the criterion, the diseased patients are the misses and the nondiseased patients the correct rejections. HT, FA, MS, and CR can be calculated from the PDCs. For example, HT is the total probability that a diseased patient will have a test score less than or equal to 50. From Figure 14.3, we add all of the probabilities below 50 from the diseased distribution: HT = 1% + 5% + 24% + 40% + 24% = 94%.

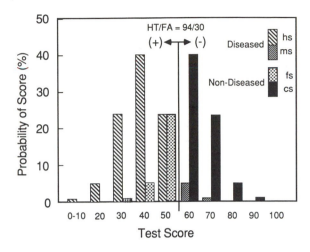

Figure 14.3. Establishing criterion to determine test outcome. Test scores below criterion are positive for disease; scores above are negative. The criterion divides the probability distribution curve for diseased patients into hits and misses, the distribution for nondiseased patients into false alarms and correct rejections. Once the criterion is established, the hit rate (HT) and false alarm rate (FA) can be calculated (HT/FA = 94/30%) for the test. (From Turner & Nielsen, 1984, with permission.)

We can select any criterion for a test; however, different criteria will produce different test performance. HT/FA for various criteria are shown in Figure 14.4 for the PDCs in Figure 14.2. Evident in these calculations are several important results. If criterion is increased (e.g., 50 to 60), there is an increase in HT (94% to 99%), which is good, but there is also an increase in FA (30% to 70%), which is bad. If criterion is reduced (e.g., 50 to 40), the FA will be reduced (30% to 6%), which is good, but so will HT (94% to 70%), which is bad. Thus we see a fundamental property of diagnostic tests; there is a trade-off between HT and FA when we adjust criterion, that is, you never get something for nothing. Although theoretical PDCs can be defined for which HT will increase without increasing FA, this is unlikely with real tests. This trade-off between HT and FA has important clinical consequences.

Another interesting result occurs with extreme criteria. We could set the criterion at 100 and call all results positive for disease. This would produce an HT = 100%, a wonderful result. The problem is that FA would also equal 100%. Likewise, with a criterion of 0, all results would be negative for disease. This would produce an FA = 0%, but also an HT

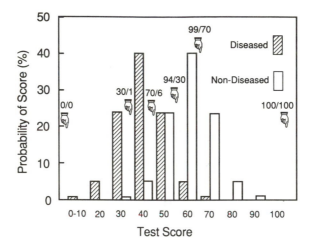

Figure 14.4.   Effect of criterion on hit rate (HT) and false alarm rate (FA). HT/FA can be varied by changing criterion. Each "hand" indicates a criterion; the corresponding HT/FA is shown above each symbol. (From Turner & Nielsen, 1984, with permission.)

= 0%. Thus criterion can be manipulated to increase HT or decrease FA, but there is the trade-off that limits the value of changing criterion.

Because any HT or FA can be obtained by adjusting criterion, both HT and FA are needed to evaluate the performance of a test. Yet, the literature is full of studies where a new test is evaluated only with diseased patients. This produces an HT but no FA, because nondiseased patients must be tested to calculate FA. These studies must be interpreted carefully because of the ability to vary HT with criterion. Obviously, the authors of these studies do not understand the techniques for evaluating diagnostic tests.

ROC curve, d' and A'

Because HT and FA vary significantly with criterion, how can this important relationship be visualized? The receiver operating characteristic (ROC) curve is a plot of HT versus FA for different criteria. The ROC curve can be plotted on linear coordinates or special coordinates called double probability, which are derived from the Gaussian (Normal) distribution. The HT/FA data from Figure 14.4 are plotted on linear coordinates in Figure 14.5. The shape of the ROC curve is determined by the PDCs. One special case occurs when the PDCs are Gaussian with equal variance (GEV), as

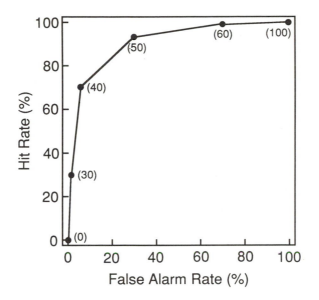

Figure 14.5. Receiver operating characteristic curve plotted on linear coordinates. The six values of HT/FA that are calculated in Figure 14.4 are plotted to form the ROC curve. The number in parentheses next to datum point is the criterion that was used to determine HT/FA.

in Figures 14.2, 14.3, and 14.4. On double probability coordinates (not shown), the ROC curve will be a straight line. The ROC curve is not a straight line on linear coordinates (Figure 14.5).

The ability of a test to distinguish patients is related to the amount of overlap of the PDCs. If in Figure 14.2, the two PDCs completely overlapped, then the test would be useless. For any test score we would have HT = FA, and MS = CR. If there was absolutely no overlap in the PDCs, then the test would be perfect. It would be possible to set the criterion such that HT = 100% and FA = 0%.

A measure of PDC overlap is the parameter, d', which is technically defined for PDCs that are GEV. d' is the difference of the means of the two PDCs divided by their common standard deviation. (The two PDCs have the same variance, therefore, their standard deviation is the same.) When the PDCs completely overlap, there is no difference in the means and d' = 0. The ROC curve corresponds to HT = FA. As the overlap is reduced, d' increased and the ROC curve moves away from the HT = FA diagonal. On linear coordinates (Figure 14.5), the ROC curve approaches the lines FA = 0% and HT = 100%, that is, the upper left corner.

For many tests, including audiological tests, the PDCs are not GEV. This is illustrated by data for speech discrimination scores (SDS) and auditory brainstem responses (ABR) interaural Wave V latency differences (IT5). (The PDCs for these two tests are shown in Turner and Nielsen, 1984, Figures 8 and 9.) The ROC curves for these two tests are plotted on linear coordinates (Figure 14.6) and double probability coordinates (Figure 14.7). These ROC curves differ in shape from those for PDCs that are GEV. This is best shown in Figure 14.7 where the straight lines are ROC curves for PDCs that are GEV. The ROC curves for SDS and IT5 deviate significantly from these lines, indicating that they are not GEV.

The parameter d' is based on the shape of the PDCs, but can also be calculated from HT and FA. Each point on the ROC curve corresponds to a particular value of HT/FA; thus d' can be calculated for each point. The easiest way to determine d' from HT/FA is to use published tables (Swets, 1964). When the PDCs for a test are GEV, there is a single d' reflecting the amount of overlap of the PDCs. This d' does not change with criterion. Each point on the ROC curve corresponds to a different

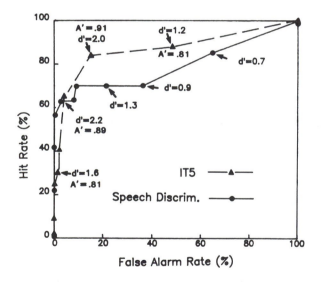

Figure 14.6. Receiver operating characteristic curves for SDS and IT5 plotted on linear coordinates. These curves were derived from probability distribution curves for SDS and IT5 in Figures 8 and 9, Turner and Nielsen (1984). Values of d' are shown for various points on the ROC curves. Values of A' are shown for points on the curve for IT5. Note that d' and A' can vary with criterion for a particular test. (From Turner & Nielsen, 1984, with permission.)

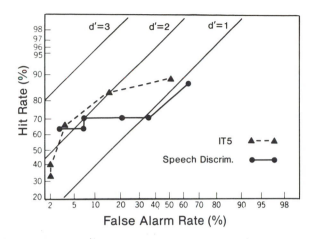

Figure 14.7. Receiver operating characteristic curves for SDS and IT5 plotted on double probability coordinates. Same data as in Figure 14.6. Straight lines correspond to constant values of d'. (From Turner & Nielsen, 1984, with permission.)

HT/FA, but to the same d'. That is why in Figure 14.7 each straight line corresponds to a particular value of d'. If the PDCs are not GEV, then d' will vary with criterion and each point on the ROC curve can have a different d'. This is illustrated in Figure 14.6 where d' is shown for SDS and IT5.

Another measure of test performance, A', is calculated from a single point (HT/FA) on the ROC curve (Robinson & Watson, 1972). This measure is independent of the shape of the PDCs. A' is the average of the maximum and minimum possible areas under ROC curves that can be passed through the known point. A' is an approximation to the area under the actual ROC curve, which is not known. A' varies from 0.5 to 1.0 and is given by

$$A' = 0.5 + \frac{(HT - FA) \times (1 + HT - FA)}{4HT \times (1 - FA)} \tag{5}$$

where the decimal form of HT and FA are used. The larger the A', the better the test. A' can vary with criterion, as in Figure 14.6 where A' is calculated for several points on the ROC curve for IT5. For further discussions of ROC curves, d', and A', see Robinson and Watson, 1972, or Egan, 1975.

Posterior probabilities and efficiency

Consider this situation. We are testing a patient in the clinic and the test result is positive. We know the hit rate of the test, but hit rate is the probability of a positive result given a diseased patient. We do not know if the patient is diseased, but we do know the test result. Hit rate tells us little about the accuracy of the test result. What we want is not hit rate, the probability of a positive result given a diseased patient ($Pr[+/D]$), but the probability that the patient is diseased given a positive test result ($Pr[D/+]$). This probability is called a posterior probability. Another posterior probability is $Pr[N/-]$; this is the probability of a nondiseased patient given a negative test result. These two posterior probabilities are important because they are the probability of being correct given a particular test result. There are two other posterior probabilities, $Pr[D/-]$ and $Pr[N/+]$, which are the probability of being incorrect given a test result.

Because $Pr[D/+] + Pr[N/+] = 100\%$, and $Pr[D/-] + Pr[N/-] = 100\%$, we need calculate only two of the four posterior probabilities. To calculate the posterior probabilities we need HT and FA for the test, plus the prevalence (PD) of the disease in the test population. Prevalence is the percentage of the test population that has the disease at the time of testing. Prevalence is often confused with incidence, which is the percentage of a population that develops a disease in a specified time period (Moscicki, 1984).

The posterior probabilities are calculated by the following equations. The decimal form of HT, FA, and PD must be used.

$$Pr[D/+] = \cfrac{1}{1 + \cfrac{(FA) \times (1 - PD)}{(HT) \times (PD)}} \qquad (6)$$

$$Pr[N/-] = \cfrac{1}{1 + \cfrac{(1 - HT) \times (PD)}{(1 - FA) \times (1 - PD)}} \qquad (7)$$

Posterior probabilities are calculated for several audiological tests that are used to identify retrocochlear site-of-lesion (Table 14.2). Consider first, $Pr[D/+]$, the probability of being correct with a positive test result. This is calculated for three disease prevalences, PD = 2%, 5%, 50%. Two percent and 5% represent the range of prevalences for retrocochlear disease typically found in clinical practice. Fifty percent is used to illustrate the

TABLE 14.2
Posterior Probabilities and Efficiency for Several Audiological Tests[a]

Test	HT/FA	Pr[D/+]			Pr[N/−]		EF	
		2%	5%	50%	5%	50%	5%	50%
ETT	99/5	29	51	95	99+	99	95	97
ABR	95/11	15	31	90	99+	95	89	92
TDT	70/13	10	22	84	98	74	86	79
BEK	49/7	13	27	88	97	65	91	71

[a]All measures in percentages; 2%, 5%, 50% indicate disease prevalence. Abbreviations are spelled out in Tables 14.1 and 14.4. ETT: excellent theoretical test.

effect of prevalence on the posterior probabilities. ABR is considered the best audiological test. With a relatively high prevalence of 5%, the probability of ABR being correct with a positive result is only 31%. With a 2% prevalence, the probability is only 15%. For comparison, consider an excellent theoretical test (ETT) with HT/FA = 99%/5%. Even with this test, which is better than any audiological test, the probability of being correct is only 29% for PD = 2% and 51% for PD = 5%. In contrast, when PD = 50% the probability of being correct is >80% for all tests. We see that when prevalence is low, the probability of a positive result being correct is small, even for tests with excellent performance.

Even with a relative high prevalence of retrocochlear disease of 5%, the probability of being correct with a positive result is only 20% to 30% for audiological tests. Does this low probability mean the tests are of no value? No, these tests provide some information. Without any tests, the probability of identifying an ear as retrocochlear is PD, the prevalence of disease. For PD = 5%, we would be correct 5% of the time if we arbitrarily call an ear retrocochlear. Using ABR, we would be correct 31% of the time. Thus our performance is improved from 5% to 31% by using ABR.

Now consider Pr[N/−], the probability of being correct with a negative test result. When prevalence is low (5%), Pr[N/−] is greater than 97% for all tests. In fact, there is little difference between 2% and 5% and, therefore, only 5% is shown in Table 14.2. Only when prevalence is high is there a significant variation in Pr[N/−] with test performance.

A frequent comment in the literature is that a positive test result is somehow more meaningful than a negative result. For example, in the text, *Hearing Disorders,* it is stated, ''As a general rule, positive findings should be taken at their face value, while negative results should be viewed as failing to support a specific locus of pathology, but not necessarily ruling it out" (Feldman, 1976, p. 37). This is an interesting concept considering the calculations in Table 14.2. The posterior probabilities clearly indicate that the probability of being correct with a positive result is much smaller than the probability of being correct with a negative result. It is difficult to understand the rational for giving more credibility to a positive result.

We can interpret the posterior probabilities in a slightly different way. $Pr[D/+] = 25\%$ means that the probability of being correct with a positive result is 25%. One out of four positive results will actually be diseased. Stated differently, for every diseased patient identified, there will be three nondiseased patients incorrectly called diseased. Thus there will be three false alarms for every hit. Because of the low prevalence of retrocochlear disease (2% to 5%), even ABR will produce two to five false alarms for every patient correctly identified. The audiologist should not be discouraged if patients are incorrectly referred for additional testing because of a positive test result. A large number of false alarms are to be expected when prevalence is low.

Several of the posterior probabilities have been given other names, predictive value and information content, and have been suggested as measures of performance for audiological tests (Jerger, 1983; Jerger & Jerger, 1983). These measures are identical to the posterior probabilities and, thus, provide the same information.

HT/FA and PD can also be used to calculate efficiency (EF). EF is the percentage of total test results that are correct and is calculated by

$$EF = HT \times PD + (1 - FA) \times (1 - PD) \tag{8}$$

The decimal form should be used for HT, FA, and PD. Like the posterior probabilities, efficiency is a function of disease prevalence. When disease prevalence is small, false alarms rate drives efficiency more than hit rate. For example, Bekesy has an efficiency higher than ABR (Table 14.2) for PD = 5%. Even though ABR has a much higher HT (95% vs. 49%), Bekesy has a lower FA (7% vs. 11%). When prevalence is high, for example, 50%, ABR would have a significantly higher efficiency (92% vs. 71%).

It may seem strange that Bekesy could have a higher efficiency than ABR, but consider this. Assume PD = 5%. If we call all ears negative for retrocochlear then we would be correct 95% of the time. Our efficiency would be 95%; the efficiency with no test would be better than with ABR. The problem is that we would identify no diseased ears. With ABR, efficiency would be 89%; we would make fewer correct decisions, but we would identify most of the diseased ears. Essentially, we would be trading false alarms for misses. We would probably make a subjective cost-benefit decision that misses "cost" more than false alarms.

Comparing test performance

Can the measures discussed above be used to determine which test is "best"? The answer to that question depends on the meaning of best. If we mean best in a particular clinic situation, then the answer is usually no. These measures evaluate test performance. The test with the best performance may not be the best test to use because of other issues such as cost of test, morbidity of test, or the availability of necessary equipment. The decision as to the best test is based on a cost-benefit analysis, not simply test performance. The measures described can provide a basis, although somewhat limited, for comparing test performance. It is important, however, to remember the limitations of each performance measure. It is not always possible to rank order tests on the basis of a single measure of test performance.

Sometimes hit rate and false alarm rate can indicate the test with superior performance. For example, if Test 1 has HT/FA = 85%/10% and Test 2 has HT/FA = 75%/15%, then Test 1 is better than Test 2 because Test 1 has *both* a higher HT and a lower FA. If, however, Test 2 has HT/FA = 75%/5%, then Test 1 has a higher HT and FA; it is no longer obvious which test is superior.

In some situations, the ROC curves for two tests can be compared to determine the superior test. If the ROC curve for one test lies in the ROC space above the curve for a second test, then the first test is superior. The test with the upper curve is superior because for any particular value of FA, the upper test will have a greater HT. If the PDCs for the two tests are not GEV, then the two ROC curves can interweave as for SDS and IT5 in Figure 14.6. Thus one test will not always lie above the other test and determining the superior test is more difficult. In the case of SDS and IT5, the curve for IT5 is above the curve for SDS for most values of FA. We can reasonably conclude that IT5 is superior to SDS.

For most audiological tests, the criterion for test interpretation is well defined, and as a result, there is a single value of HT/FA corresponding to the established criterion. This single HT/FA represents one point on the ROC curve. Seldom is there sufficient published clinical data to construct an entire ROC curve. Thus when comparing tests we have only single values of HT/FA for each test. A d' can be calculated from a single HT/FA, but is it appropriate to compare tests using d'? If the tests have PDCs that are GEV, then the meaning of d' is clear and all points on the ROC curve have the same d'. The test with the largest d' is superior. If the PDCs are not GEV, then d' can vary with criterion, and different points on the ROC curve will have different values of d' (Figure 14.6). In addition, the relation of d' to the shape of the PDC is not clear. When two tests are compared, the test with the larger d' may have the smaller d' if a different criterion was used for either test, as with SDS and IT5. Still, d' can be useful when comparing tests on the basis of single values of d'. When restricted to a particular criterion for each test, which is often the case, the test with the larger d' can be considered to have superior performance.

The posterior probabilities provide extremely useful information about test performance, but can they be used to rank order tests? When prevalence is low, the posterior probabilities are biased toward tests with low false alarm rates. Consider two tests with HT/FA = 90%/20% and 10%/2%. With a prevalence of 5%, both tests would have a $Pr[RE/+] = 20\%$, but d' equal to 2.1 and 0.8, respectively. The first test is clearly superior on the basis of d', but both tests have the same posterior probability. The posterior probabilities provide important information, but should not be used to rank order tests.

Application to audiological tests

Cochlear versus retrocochlear

The techniques of clinical decision analysis can be applied to a variety of clinical issues in audiology. We will consider one application in some detail to illustrate the use of the techniques. For many years, a major interest in diagnostic audiology has been the differentiation of cochlear from retrocochlear site-of-lesion. Even though retrocochlear means everything beyond the cochlear, for our purposes we will restrict retrocochlear site-of-lesion to the cerebellopontine angle (CPA) including the VIIIth nerve. We will not consider high brainstem or cortical disease.

The most common tumors of the CPA are acoustic tumors (78%), which are also called acoustic neuromas, neurinomas, neurilemmomas, neurofibromas, or vestibular schwannomas. Other, less frequent, tumors include meningioma, primary cholesteatomas, and glomas body tumors. Acoustic tumors comprise 8% to 10% of all intracranial tumors (Schuknecht, 1974).

In Sweden and Great Britain, statistics indicate about 7 per 1,000,000 (general population) diagnosed cases of acoustic tumor each year (Hirsh & Anderson, 1980). If this statistic were applied to the United States, 20 new cases per year in a city of 3 million people would be expected. The point is that most audiologists will see relatively few patients with acoustic tumors. Considering the small number of cases, we must wonder why this problem has received such educational and research emphasis, often at the expense of more important issues.

The prevalence of retrocochlear disease in a clinic population will be significantly greater than in the general population. Clinic patients are at risk for the disease because of symptoms and case history. In patients suspect for retrocochlear disease, a prevalence as great as 10% (Bauch, Rose, & Harner, 1982) has been reported, although 5% is more typical (Hart & Davenport, 1981). Referral centers for retrocochlear disease will have a higher prevalence; 2% might be more appropriate for a general otolaryngology clinic.

The audiologist's role in the detection of retrocochlear disease results from the nature of the symptoms. The initial symptom of an acoustic tumor is auditory about 77% of the time, either hearing loss (69%) or tinnitus (8%). Vestibular problems occur only 3% of the time. The presenting complaint is auditory in 57% of cases and vestibular in 6% (Hart, Gardner, & Howieson, 1983).

Performance of tests

Many special audiological tests have been developed to identify retrocochlear site-of-lesion. To effectively use these tests, the audiologist must know which tests are available and the performance of these tests. Surprisingly, until the work of Turner, Shepard, and Frazer (1984), only a few studies attempted to evaluate and compare audiological tests (Buxton, 1973; Hall, 1978). Turner et al. reviewed 15 years of the clinical literature to evaluate 26 audiological, vestibular, and radiological tests designed to identify retrocochlear disease. The tests were evaluated using the performance measures discussed in this chapter. The results of this study are summarized in Table 14.3. Test abbreviations are explained in Table 14.4.

The average hit rate (HTa) and the average false alarm rate (FAa) for each test were calculated from the clinical literature. The other measures of performance were calculated using HTa/FAa and an assumed prevalence of 5%. Briefly, Turner et al. used the following procedure to calculate HTa/FAa. A hit rate and false alarm rate were determined for each test evaluated in an individual study. For example, for ABR there were 22 studies that yielded an HT/FA. To determine HTa for ABR, the 22 hit rates were not simply averaged; this would be inappropriate because significantly different numbers of patients were tested in different studies. One HT may be based on 10 patients and another on 100 patients. The HT for each study was weighted by the number of patients in the study. Then an average was calculated using the weighted values of HT from each study. FA was calculated in a similar way.

The data presented in Table 14.3 are the best available performance measures for these tests. These data are, however, estimates of performance subject to certain limitations. The numbers were derived by "averag-

TABLE 14.3
Performance of Audiological, Vestibular, and Radiological Tests[a]

Test	HTa	FAa	d'	A'	Pr[D/+]	EF
ABLB	59	10	1.5	0.84	23	88
SISI	65	16	1.4	0.83	17	83
SISIM	69	10	1.8	0.88	26	89
BEK	49	7	1.4	0.83	28	91
BCL	85	8	2.5	0.94	37	92
FBB	71	5	2.2	0.91	45	94
TDT	70	13	1.6	0.87	22	86
STAT	145	0	b	0.86	100	97
STAT2	54	5	1.7	0.86	35	93
STAT4	70	13	1.6	0.87	22	86
SDS	45	18	0.8	0.73	11	80
PIPB	74	4	2.4	0.92	48	95
ART	73	10	1.9	0.89	28	89
ARD	63	4	2.1	0.89	47	95
ARC	84	15	2.0	0.91	22	85
ABR	95	11	2.9	0.96	31	89
ENGC	85	33	1.5	0.84	12	68
XRP	70	23	1.3	0.82	14	76
XRS	89	4	3.0	0.96	56	96
TOMO	77	16	1.8	0.88	21	84
CAT	40	0	b	0.85	100	97
CTIV	77	3	2.6	0.93	55	96
CTMC	98	2	>4	0.99	75	98
CTGC	97	<1	>4	0.99	90	99
CTHR	98	0	b	>0.99	100	>99
PFC	>99	<1	>5	>0.99	96	>99

[a]Calculations of posterior probability and efficiency based on an assumed prevalence of retrocochlear disease of 5%. All measures are in percentages except A' and d'. Abbreviations are spelled out in Tables 14.1 and 14.4. Data from Turner, Shepard, & Frazer (1984).
[b]Cannot calculate d' when FAa = 0.

ing" the performance of a test as calculated from independent studies. Given that these studies had different authors, the pathology of patients studied, the protocol for administering the test, and the criterion for test interpretation varied somewhat across studies. The performance of a particular test could differ significantly from study to study. For example, the hit rate for the speech discrimination score ranged from 15% to 58% across 12 studies. One could argue that this variability makes it inap-

TABLE 14.4
Abbreviations for Diagnostic Tests

ABLB: Alternate Binaural Loudness Balance
ABR: Auditory Brain Stem Response
ARC: Immittance—Combined Acoustic Reflex and Decay
ARD: Acoustic Reflex Decay
ART: Elevated or Absence Acoustic Reflex Thresholds
BCL: Bekesy Comfortable Loudness
BEK: Bekesy Audiometry
CAT: Computed Axial Tomography
CTIV: CAT with Intravenous Enhancement
CTMC: CAT with Metrizamide Cisternography
CTGC: CAT with Gas Cisternography
CTHR: High Resolution or 4th Generation CAT
COG: Crib-O-Gram
DEF: Definitive Test
ENGC: Electronystagmography—Caloric Response
FBB: Forward Backward Bekesy
HHR: High-Risk Register
MRI: Magnetic Resonance Imaging
PFC: Posterior Fossa Cisternography
PIPB: Performance Intensity—Phonetically Balanced Speech Discrimination
SDS: Traditional Speech Discrimination
SISI: Short Increment Sensitivity Index
SISIM: Modified SISI
STAT 1: Suprathreshold adaptation test; 500, 1000 Hz
STAT 2: Suprathreshold adaptation test; 500, 1000, 2000 Hz
STAT 4: Suprathreshold adaptation test; 500, 1000, 2000, 4000 Hz
TDT: Tone Decay Test
XRP: Plain X-Ray of Petrous Pyramid
XRS: X-Ray With Special Views

propriate to average results across studies. On the other hand, estimates of test performance should not be based on a single study because of the same variation in results. Which individual study should we use to determine performance? If we reject both group averages and individual study results as a basis for determining test performance, then we have no technique left to evaluate diagnostic tests. Even with its limitations, averaging performance data across many studies is an appropriate technique.

Comparison of tests

Can we form any useful conclusions about the performance of the audiological and related diagnostic tests? One way to compare the tests is to plot the HT/FA for each test on the ROC curve (Figure 14.8). Not all tests are shown; some tests were eliminated because the calculation of HT/FA was based on a small number of studies and/or patients. In general, the closer the test is to the upper left corner of the ROC space, the better the test.

The tests can be separated into four groups. Several of the radiological tests, PFC, CTMC, and CTGC, are in the upper left corner and have near definitive performance; that is, HT = 100% and FA = 0%. The second group consists of ABR and, perhaps, CTIV. The remaining tests fall into the third group with the exception of SDS, which forms the fourth group.

Traditionally, the radiological tests in the first group have shown the best performance and have been used as the "gold standard" for ultimate patient diagnosis. Today, magnetic resonance imaging (MRI) is becoming the test of choice for the definitive "gold standard" (Mikhael, Wolff, & Ciric, 1987). The cost and morbidity of these radiological tests have, however, prevented their routine use on every patient. Other tests are still needed to screen for the definitive test. ABR has become the primary screening test. ABR is clearly superior to the remaining tests with a high HT (95%) and a low FA (11%). With additional improvements in the radiological tests, the use of ABR as a screening test may become unnecessary.

Note that ARC has about the best performance in the third group. This is interesting because for many years before ABR, tomograms were the most popular screening test even though ARC was available and was probably the better choice. The SDS is the fourth group and should not be used to identify retrocochlear site-of-lesion.

Test protocols

Clinical necessity?

Often, more than one diagnostic test has been developed to identify a particular disease. If any one test is perfect, that is, HT/FA = 100%/0%, then only that test is needed. Diagnostic tests, however, seldom have perfect performance. The practice has been to use multiple tests. A combination of individual diagnostic tests is a test protocol. The routine use of test protocols results, to a large degree, from the subjective impression that several tests are better than one test. Are several tests better than one? Before addressing this question we should develop a rational for combining tests. We cannot evaluate the value of test protocols until we define what we expect to gain from their use.

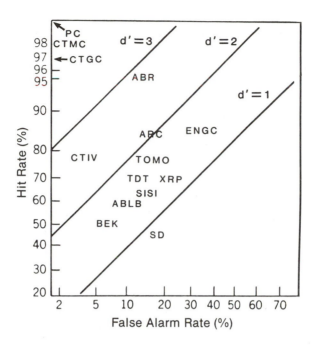

Figure 14.8.   Hit rate (HTa) and false alarm rate (FAa) for selected tests plotted on ROC space using test abbreviations to indicate datum point. Abbreviations are spelled out in Table 14.4. The straight lines indicate constant values of d'. (From Turner, Shepard, & Frazer, 1984, with permission.)

There are four basic justifications for combining tests into a test protocol:

1. *Super protocol*: A super protocol is a protocol with a hit rate higher *and* a false alarm rate lower than any individual test in the protocol. For example, a protocol consists of two tests with HT/FA = 90%/20% and 80%/10%. A super test would have HTp >90% and FAp <10%, for example, 95%/6%. In this case, protocol performance would be superior, by any measure, to that of the individual tests that form the protocol.

2. *Improved performance*: A protocol may not qualify as a super protocol, but the performance, as indicated by some measure such as d' or A', may be better than that of the individual tests. For the example above, we might have HTp/FAp = 90%/10%.

3. *Manipulate hit rate or false alarm rate*: We saw earlier that the hit rate and false alarm rate of an individual test varied with criterion. Hit rate could be increased or false alarm rate decreased but there was always a trade-off. Thus a desired hit rate or false alarm rate could be obtained, but there was little improvement in the performance of the test. It may be possible to use a protocol to obtain a hit rate higher (or false alarm rate lower) than available with any individual test in the protocol. The higher hit rate (or lower false alarm rate) may be advantageous in a particular clinical situation even though the performance of the protocol is no better than that of any individual test. For the example above, we might obtain HTp/FAp = 95/25%.

4. *Screen patients for a definitive test*: Even when tests are available with near perfect performance, such as the definitive radiological tests discussed above, the financial cost, morbidity, and mortality may preclude the use of these tests on every patient. In this case, other tests are needed to screen patients for the definitive test. A protocol consisting of the screening test(s) and a definitive test may be appropriate.

Thus we see that there are reasonable theoretical justifications for using test protocols. The use of a test protocol, however, raises certain important questions: (a) What tests should be used in the protocol?, (b) How should the tests be administered?, (c) How is a criterion determined for the protocol?, (d) How is protocol performance evaluated? We will now consider some basic issues related to the use of protocols.

Formulation and use

The test protocol functions much like an individual test, and in many ways can be treated as one. The purpose of the protocol is to indicate the state of the patient. The simplest result would be positive or negative for a particular disease; however, a protocol may also have more than two outcomes (e.g., positive, negative, uncertain).

There are two basic ways of combining tests into a protocol: parallel and series. Parallel means that several tests are administered and a decision concerning patient management is made on the basis of multiple test results (Figure 14.9, Panel a). When tests are combined in parallel, a criterion is needed to determine if the result of the protocol is positive or negative. The criterion for a protocol differs slightly from the criterion for individual tests. Standard criteria are used to determine if the individual tests are positive or negative. The protocol criterion defines how many individual tests must be positive for the protocol to be positive. For example, five tests are combined in parallel. If all five tests must be positive for the protocol to be positive, then the criterion is "strict." If

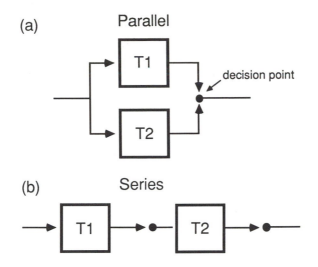

(a) Parallel

(b) Series

Figure 14.9. Two techniques for combining tests (T1 and T2) into a protocol. At a decision point (solid dot), a decision is made about future testing or treatment. That decision is based on a single test result for a series protocol and multiple test results for a parallel protocol. (From Turner, Frazer, & Shepard, 1984, with permission.)

only one test must be positive, then the criterion is "loose." If two, three, or four tests must be positive, then we have established an "intermediate" criterion.

Tests combined in series are performed sequentially with a decision made after each test (Figure 14.9, Panel b). A protocol criterion is not needed for tests combined in series. The protocol is implicit in the design of the series protocol. Tests can be combined in series in two ways: series-positive or series-negative (Figure 14.10).

With a series-positive protocol, a patient is excluded from additional testing with a negative test result, whereas a positive result means that the patient receives the next test (Figure 14.10, Panel a). For a series-positive protocol to be positive, all test results must be positive. Recall that a parallel protocol with a strict criterion required all tests to be positive for the protocol to be positive. Thus a series-positive protocol is analogous to a parallel protocol with a strict criterion. In fact, the performance of a series-positive is identical to the corresponding parallel protocol with a strict criterion. As stated above, the protocol criterion is implicit in the design of a series protocol.

With a series-negative protocol, a positive test result sends the patient for the ultimate treatment (Figure 14.10, Panel b). If a test result is nega-

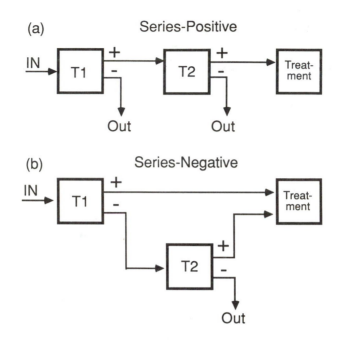

Figure 14.10. Two techniques for combining tests (T1 and T2) into a series protocol. "Out" means that the patient receives no additional testing or treatment. (From Turner, Frazer, & Shepard, 1984, with permission.)

tive, the patient receives the next test. For the series-negative protocol to be positive, only one test must be positive. The series-negative protocol is analogous to the parallel protocol with a loose criterion, and they have the same performance.

Performance measures

How can protocol performance be evaluated? The performance measures developed for individual tests can be used with slight modification. Protocol performance can be described in terms of hit rate and false alarm rate. Once this is known, other measures of performance, for example, d' and efficiency, can be calculated for the protocol.

The most straightforward technique to determine protocol hit rate (HTp) and false alarm rate (FAp) is to calculate them using clinical data. The calculations are similar to those for individual tests. Protocol hit rate is the total number of protocol hits divided by the total number of diseased patients. False alarm rate is the total number of protocol false alarms divided by the total number of nondiseased patients. The posterior probabilities and efficiency for the protocol are calculated using protocol hit rate, protocol false alarm rate, and disease prevalence.

The calculation of protocol performance is illustrated by a simple example. A test protocol is formed by combining two tests in parallel (Figure 14.11). A population of 10 diseased (dp = 10) and 12 nondiseased (np = 12) patients are tested by the protocol. The prevalence in this test population is PD = dp/(dp + np) = 10/22 = 45%. Test 1 has HT/FA = 80%/25%; Test 2 has HT/FA = 60%/17%. Because the two tests are in parallel, all patients receive both tests. First a loose, then a strict criterion will be considered. Test results are shown in Table 14.5.

With a loose criterion, the protocol is positive if one or both tests are positive. For the diseased patients, 9 show a positive result on one or both tests. Thus the number of hits for the protocol is nine, as opposed to eight and six for the individual tests. The hit rate for the protocol (HTp) is 9/10 = 90%. For the nondiseased patients, 4 show a positive test result on one or both tests. The number of false alarms for the protocol is four, compared to three and two for the individual tests. False alarm rate for the protocol (FAp) is 4/12 = 33%.

The same type of calculations are possible for a strict criterion. For the protocol to be positive, both tests must be positive. For the diseased patients, both tests were positive five times for HTp = 5/10 =50%. For the nondiseased patients, both test were positive one time for FAp = 1/12 = 8%. Using HTp and FAp, efficiency and the posterior probabilities can be calculated for both a loose and strict criterion.

Test correlation

When clinical data are available, protocol performance is easily calculated. We shall see later that there has been little clinical evaluation of audiological protocols. Often, the necessary clinical data are not available to calculate protocol performance. Is there any way to theoretically determine protocol performance? Yes, protocol performance can be predicted if we know (a) the design of the protocol, (b) the performance (HT/FA) of the individual tests in the protocol, and (c) the correlation between the individual tests. Before proceeding, let us consider what is meant by test correlation.

Test correlation is the tendency of individual tests in a protocol to identify the same patients as positive or negative. If both tests identify the same patients, then the tests have maximum-positive (max-pos) correlations. If the two tests identify different patients, then the tests have maximum-negative (max-neg) correlations. The two tests can have zero

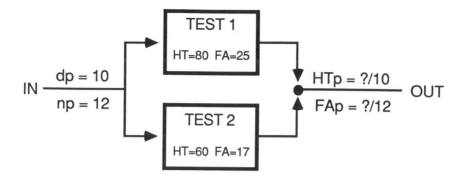

Figure 14.11. Simple test protocol for data shown in Table 14.5. (From Turner, 1988, with permission.)

TABLE 14.5
Test Results for Simple Protocol in Figure 14.11[a]

	DISEASED PATIENTS												
PATIENT	1	2	3	4	5	6	7	8	9	10		TOTAL	HT(%)
Test 1	+	+		+	+		+	+	+	+		8	80
Test 2		+	+		+		+	+		+		6	60
Protocol													HTp(%)
Loose	+	+	+	+	+		+	+	+	+		9	90
Strict		+			+		+	+		+		5	50

	NONDISEASED PATIENTS													
PATIENT	1	2	3	4	5	6	7	8	9	10	11	12	TOTAL	FA(%)
Test 1				+	+					+			3	25
Test 2		+		+									2	17
Protocol														FAp(%)
Loose		+		+	+					+			4	33
Strict				+									1	8

[a]Abbreviations are spelled out in Tables 14.1 and 14.4. Adapted from Turner (1988).

correlation, in which case the patients identified by Test 1 would not provide any information about the patients identified by Test 2. Test correlation can be anywhere from max-neg to max-pos.

Test correlation has a significant effect on protocol performance. This is best illustrated by an example. Twelve diseased patients are to be tested by two tests. Both Test 1 and Test 2 identify 6 out of 12 patients as positive, that is, HT = 50%. The two tests are combined in parallel with a loose criterion; the protocol is positive if either test is positive. For max-pos correlation, the two tests identify the same 6 patients as positive. Even with a loose criterion, the protocol hit rate is 6/12 = 50%, no better than the individual tests. Next we assume max-neg correlation. In this case, the two tests identify different patients. Thus all 12 patients are identified by one test or the other. A loose criterion requires only one test to be positive for the protocol to be positive; thus, HTp = 12/12 = 100%. For this simple example, protocol hit rate can vary from 50% to 100% depending on test correlation. In general, protocol hit rate and false alarm rate will vary significantly with test correlation for any protocol criterion.

Limits on protocol performance

Do we know test correlation for audiological tests? Data suggest that correlation is mid-positive, that is, between zero and max-pos correlation. Let me emphasize, however, that these data are extremely limited. Later in this chapter, we will develop techniques for predicting protocol performance based on the assumption of mid-pos correlation. First, we will calculate limits on protocol performance that do not require a knowledge of actual test correlation.

We have seen that protocol performance is a function of criterion and test correlation. The extremes of criterion are loose and strict; the extremes of test correlation are max-pos and max-neg. The important point is that protocol performance at the extremes of criterion or correlation define limits on protocol performance. For example, if we calculate protocol hit rate for both a loose and a strict criterion, then hit rate for any intermediate criterion would be between that calculated for loose and strict. Likewise, protocol hit rate for any actual test correlation would lie between that calculated for max-pos and max-neg correlation.

The two extremes of criterion and the two of correlation form four combinations of criterion/correlation: loose/max-pos; loose/max-neg; strict/max-pos; strict/max-neg. If protocol performance is calculated for these four conditions, then these calculated values place limits on actual protocol performance for any criterion or test correlation. We can think of criterion and correlation as axes of a two-dimensional space (Figure 14.12).

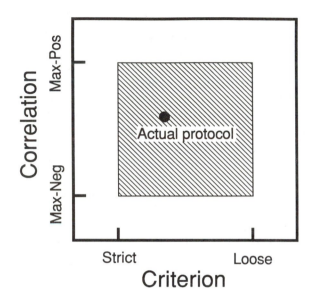

Figure 14.12.   Space defined by extremes of protocol criterion and test correlation. Any real protocol would lie somewhere in this rectangular space depending on actual test correlation and selected criterion.

The four combinations of criterion and correlation define the four corners of a rectangle in that space. Any protocol would define a point in the rectangle based on the selected criterion of the protocol and actual test correlation. We can calculate limits by calculating protocol hit rate and false alarm rate at the four corners, that is, at the extremes of correlation and criterion.

Consider a simple protocol of "N" tests combined in parallel (or the equivalent series protocol). The hit rate and false alarm rate of the nth test in the protocol is indicated by HTn/FAn. If we specify a loose criterion and assume max-pos correlation the protocol performance is given by the following equations:

$$HTp(l/+) = HTx \tag{9}$$

$$FAp(l/+) = FAx \tag{10}$$

where HTx and FAx are the maximum individual hit rate and false alarm rate of the tests in the protocol. For a strict criterion and max-pos correlation, we have

$$HTp(s/+) = HTm \tag{11}$$

$$FAp(s/+) = FAm \tag{12}$$

where HTm and FAm are the minimum individual hit rate and false alarm rate of the tests in the protocol.

If we assume max-neg correlation and specify a loose criterion for the protocol, we have

$$HTp(l/-) = MIN [\Sigma HTn \text{ or } 100\%] \tag{13}$$

$$FAp(l/-) = MIN [\Sigma FAn \text{ or } 100\%] \tag{14}$$

where ΣHTn and ΣFAn mean the sum of the individual hit rates and false alarm rates, respectively. MIN [A or B] is the smaller of A or B. Finally, for a strict criterion and max-neg correlation the equations are

$$HTp(s/-) = MAX [\{\Sigma HTn - 100(N - 1)\} \text{ or } 0\%] \tag{15}$$

$$FAp(s/-) = MAX [\{\Sigma FAn - 100(N - 1)\} \text{ or } 0\%] \tag{16}$$

where MAX [A or B] means the larger of A or B, and $100(N-1)$ means 100% times one less than the number of individual tests. For convenience, hit rate and false alarm rate are expressed as percent, not decimal, for these calculations.

The derivation of these equations may not be obvious to the reader, nor will it be discussed in detail. The equations are easily determined by using simple set theory. One example will illustrate the strategy. Consider a parallel protocol consisting of Test 1 and Test 2. We assume max-pos correlation. The hit rate of Test 1 (HT1) is 80% and the hit rate of Test 2 (HT2) is 60%. Ten diseased patients are tested by the protocol. These 10 patients can be considered a set, labeled Set D (Figure 14.13). Test 1 will identify 8 of the 10 patients because HT1 = 80%. These 8 patients (Set 1) are a subset of the original 10 (Set D), as shown in Figure 14.13. Test 2 will identify 6 patients (Set 2) that are also a subset of Set D. Because the tests have max-pos correlation, these 6 patients identified by Test 2 are a subset of the 8 identified by Test 1. Thus Set 2 is a subset of Set 1.

If we choose a strict criterion, then the protocol will be positive only when both tests are positive. The subset of patients identified by the protocol (Set P) will be the intersection of Set 1 and Set 2 (Set P = Set 1 $\cap$ Set 2). This is true only for the 6 patients identified by *both* tests (Set 2). Thus the protocol hit rate will equal the smallest hit rate of the individual tests.

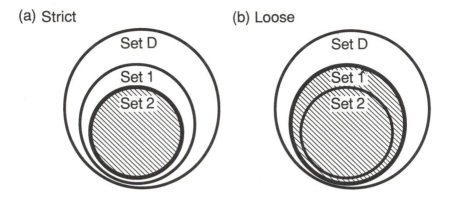

(a) Strict (b) Loose

Figure 14.13. Set D consists of all diseased patients. Set 1 are all patients identified as positive by Test 1; Set 2 are patients identified as positive by Test 2. For this example, test correlation is maximum-positive. Because of correlation, Set 2 is a subset of Set 1. Test 1 and Test 2 are combined in parallel to form a protocol. The cross-hatched area indicates those patients identified as positive by the protocol (Set P) with a strict (a) and a loose (b) criterion.

If we select a loose criterion, then the protocol will be positive if either test (or both tests) is positive. This corresponds to the union of the two sets (Set P = Set 1 $\cup$ Set 2). Because Set 2 is a subset of Set 1, the maximum number of positive patients will be those in Set 1. Thus the protocol hit rate will equal the greatest individual hit rate.

To illustrate the equations developed in this section, we will calculate limits on an example protocol. This protocol is designed to distinguish cochlear from retrocochlear site-of-lesion and consists of the tone decay test (TDT), acoustic reflex-combined (ARC), and auditory brainstem response (ABR) combined in parallel with either a loose or strict criterion. These tests have HT/FA of TDT = 70%/13%, ARC = 84%/15%, and ABR = 95%/11%. Limits on performance are shown in Table 14.6. For a particular criterion, note the large variation in protocol hit rate and false alarm rate with test correlation. This variation is, in general, so large that the limits are not usual for evaluating protocol performance. We cannot say from the data in Table 14.6 if this is a "good" or "bad" protocol. These data do, however, reveal some basic properties of test protocols.

Basic properties

Earlier, we described four theoretical justifications for using a test protocol. The first justification is to create a super protocol. We would like the

TABLE 14.6
Limits on Protocol Performance[a]

| CORRELATION | HTp/FAp | |
	Loose	Strict
Max-Positive	95/15	70/11
Max-Negative	100/39	49/0

[a]Protocol consists of ABR, TDT, and ARC combined in parallel. Calculations of protocol hit rate and false alarm rate at the extremes of criterion and correlation define limits on possible protocol performance. Results for loose and strict criteria are indicated. Abbreviations are spelled out in Tables 14.1 and 14.4.

protocol to have a hit rate higher and a false alarm rate lower than that of any test in the protocol. Again consider the sample protocol of ABR, TDT, and ARC. ABR has the highest individual hit rate, 95%, and the lowest false alarm rate, 11%. Thus for some criterion, we want the protocol to have HTp > 95% and FAp < 11%. From Table 14.6, it is evident that there is no single combination of criterion and test correlation that produce an HTp > 95% and FAp < 11%. With a loose criterion, the protocol hit rate and false alarm rate can be no lower than the largest individual hit rate (95%) and false alarm rate (15%). Likewise, with a strict criterion, the protocol hit rate and false alarm rate can be no greater than the smallest individual hit rate (70%) and false alarm rate (11%). It is never possible to obtain, for any particular combination of criterion and correlation, a protocol hit rate higher than the highest individual hit rate (95%) *and* a false alarm rate lower than the lowest individual false alarm rate (11%). A basic property of test protocols is that a super protocol is not possible and, therefore, cannot be a justification for using a test protocol.

A second justification for a test protocol is improved performance. Is protocol performance always superior to the performance of the individual tests in the protocol? No, performance is not always improved by combining tests. This can be demonstrated by a simple argument. Consider a protocol that consists of a definitive test (HT/FA = 100%/0%) and a test that is not perfect. If used alone, the definitive test will never make an error. If the second test is combined in any way with the definitive test to form a protocol, the protocol will make some errors because the second test will make errors. Clearly, the performance of the protocol is inferior to the performance of the definitive test alone.

The same point can be made from the data in Table 14.6 for the sample protocol. For max-pos correlation and a loose criterion, HTp/FAp = 95%/15%. This is clearly inferior to ABR, which has HT/FA = 95%/11%. ABR has the same hit rate, but a lower false alarm rate. Again we see that protocol performance can be inferior to that of the tests in the protocol.

Protocol performance is not always better; however, is it ever better than the individual tests? For the example protocol of ABR, ARC, and TDT, we can calculate performance measures, d' and A', and compare to that of the individual tests (Table 14.7). Two special test correlations, zero and mid-positive, are also considered. (The techniques for calculating protocol performance with zero and mid-positive correlation will be discussed later in this chapter.) Of the three tests in the example protocol, ABR has the best performance with the highest HT, the lowest FA, and the largest d' and A'. Does the performance of the protocol ever exceed that of ABR? First note that as hit rate of the protocol increases with a loose criterion, so does the false alarm rate. Likewise, as false alarm rate decreases with a strict criterion, so does hit rate. There is the same general trade-off between hit rate and false alarm rate that is evident for individual tests when criterion is changed. No combination of criterion and correlation produce an A' for the protocol that is better than that for ABR;

TABLE 14.7
Comparison of Individual Test Performance to Protocol Performance[a]

TEST	HT/FA	A'	d'
ABR	95/11	.96	2.9
TDT	70/13	.87	1.6
ARC	84/15	.91	2.0

CORRELATION	Loose			Strict		
	HTp/FAp	A'	d'	HTp/FAp	A'	d'
Max-Pos	95/15	.95	2.7	70/11	.88	1.8
Mid-Pos	97.4/24.5	.93	2.6	63/5.6	.88	1.9
Zero	99.8/34	.91	3.3	56/0.2	.89	3.0
Max-Neg	100/39	.90	b	49/0	.87	b

[a]Protocol consists of ABR, TDT, and ARC combined in parallel. Results for loose and strict criteria are indicated. Abbreviations are spelled out in Tables 14.1 and 14.4.
[b]The measure, d', cannot be calculated because HTp = 100% or FAp = 0%.

protocol performance is never as good as that of ABR. Only for zero correlation is d' slightly better for the protocol than for ABR. For all other correlations, ABR has a larger d'.

Later in this chapter, we predict the performance of four protocols assuming mid-positive correlation. These protocols consist of a screening audiological protocol combined with a definitive test. For the present discussion, we will calculate A' and d' for the screening protocols using the predicted values of hit rate and false alarm rate (Table 14.8). We can then determine if screening protocol performance is ever better than individual test performance. Note in Table 14.8 that the first screening protocol, A1, is just ABR; the performance of this protocol is, of course, the same as ABR. Two other protocols, A2 and A4, contain ABR. Is their performance superior to ABR, the best test in the protocol? No, A' and d' for protocols A2 and A4 are less than for ABR. Protocol A3 is of interest because it does not contain ABR. Of the tests in the protocol, PIPB has the largest A' (.92) and d' (2.4). Both A' (.89) and d' (1.9) for the protocol are less than for PIPB. We see that none of the protocols achieved a performance better than that of the best test in the protocol.

TABLE 14.8

Comparison of Individual Test Performance to Screening Protocol Performance[a]

TEST	HT/FA	A'	d'
ABR	95/11	.96	2.9
ABLB	59/10	.84	1.5
ARC	84/15	.91	2.0
PIPB	74/4	.92	2.4
SISI	65/16	.83	1.4
TDT	70/13	.87	1.6

SCREENING PROTOCOL	HTs/FAs	A'	d'
A1. ABR	95/11	.96	2.9
A2. ARC + ABR	82/6	.93	2.5
A3. ABLB*ARC*PIPB*SISI*TDT	92/31	.89	1.9
A4. ABLB*ARC*PIPB*SISI*TDT + ABR	89/8	.95	2.6

[a]Screening protocols the same as in Table 14.13. A + between tests indicates series-positive. An asterick (*) between tests indicates tests in parallel with a loose criterion. The values for HT/FA were taken from Table 14.3; values for HTs/FAs were taken from Table 14.13. Abbreviations are spelled out in Tables 14.1 and 14.4.

What can we conclude about protocol performance? First, it is clear that protocol performance can be inferior to individual test performance. The assumption that performance is always improved by using more tests is incorrect. We evaluated four different audiological protocols and found that, in general, performance was poorer with the protocol. There was, however, one result that suggested improved performance on the basis of d'. It is possible that under some conditions performance might be better than the individual tests. The exact relationship between protocol performance and individual test performance is determined by the design of the protocol and the tests that form the protocol. Some type of theoretical or clinical evaluation is required to demonstrate improved performance with a protocol. This assumption cannot be made a priori.

The third justification for a protocol is to manipulate hit rate and false alarm rate. From Table 14.7, it is evident that a protocol can produce hit rates and false alarm rates not available with the individual tests. For any correlation other than max-pos, hit rate can be increased with a loose criterion, and false alarm rate can be reduced with a strict criterion. Even though protocol performance may be no better than the best test, a higher hit rate, or a lower false alarm rate, may be of clinical value.

The fourth justification for a protocol is to screen for a definitive test. This is a legitimate use of multiple tests and is not affected by protocol properties.

Based on the properties of test protocols, we can state the following conclusions:

1. The super protocol is not possible.
2. Improved diagnostic performance with a protocol is questionable; however, degraded performance is clearly possible.
3. Protocols can be used to manipulate hit rate and false alarm rate. A loose criterion will increase hit rate; a strict criterion will decrease false alarm rate.
4. The legitimate reasons for using a protocol are to manipulate hit rate and false alarm rate, or to screen for a definitive test.

Audiological test battery

Test battery principle

With the development of numerous audiological tests to identify retrocochlear site-of-lesion, there also developed the test battery principle. This principle, which became a fundamental commandment of academic and clinical audiology, is that the audiological tests are never administered or interpreted in isolation, but are combined into a test battery. This philosophy was espoused in many introductory and general texts on audiology. For example, in the *Handbook of Clinical Audiology* (Rosenberg, 1978), we are told, "The audiologist neither expects nor gets complete agreement on all the different tests he performs. . . . The utilization of a large number of tests, therefore, renders clarity to an otherwise muddy series of events. . . . There is also a statistical advantage to the test battery approach when compared with the utilization of but a single examination finding. The multiplicity of judgements in the test battery renders the entire examination more reliable and valid" (p. 159).

This argument has a certain appeal and face validity. The use of multiple diagnostic tests is common in clinical work. The concept that multiple tests "render clarity to an otherwise muddy series of events," sounds analogous to the use of signal averaging to extract a small signal from noise. If multiple averages can reduce noise in an electrical signal, why cannot multiple test results reduce noise in diagnosis? In fact, the use of multiple tests is not analogous to averaging. Averaging a signal in noise always improves the signal-to-noise ratio. We have seen that the use of additional tests does not always improve performance.

The important point is that the test battery concept gained popularity because it seemed right. It was never subjected to rigorous quantitative analysis until the work of Turner, Frazer, and Shepard (1984). This is a classic example of the danger of the intuitive/subjective technique for analysis. The test battery principle was proposed, accepted, and practiced for many years because, subjectively, the rational for the test battery was appealing. The test battery principle is not fundamentally unreasonable; the use of multiple tests is sometimes appropriate, as outlined above. The problem is that assumptions were made and conclusions drawn without clinical data and theoretical support. In addition, being reasonable is not equivalent to being correct.

The test battery principle was most popular in the 1960s and 1970s. By the development of ABR in the late 1970s, audiologists were questioning the concept. Audiologists were told to use a test battery, but there was little information as to which tests to use, how the battery should be constructed, or how to interpret multiple test results. The availability of ABR, with its excellent performance, made the need for tests like SISI or ABLB less evident.

Implicit in the test battery concept are three assumptions: (a) additional tests provide additional information, (b) the audiologist can effectively use this additional information, and (c) the performance of the test battery is always superior to the performance of the best individual test.

For the test battery principle to be correct, these assumptions must be correct. For many years, these assumptions were not recognized, much less validated.

Clinical performance

The best method to validate the test battery principle is to demonstrate, using clinical data, that test battery performance is superior to the performance of individual tests. Surprisingly, this was not done, even though many studies evaluated the performance of the individual audiological tests. Turner, Frazer, and Shepard (1984) were able to find a few studies that presented sufficient raw data so as to permit the evaluation of selected test batteries.

A study by Owens (1971) determined the individual performance of ABLB, Bekesy, SISI, and TDT, but not their performance in combination. For many years, these tests formed the bases of the traditional audiological test battery. Using the raw data presented in this study, every combination of these four tests could be evaluated. The objective was to determine if any combination of these tests would have performed better than the individual tests. From the results in Table 14.9, we can see that the performance of the various combinations, even when using all four tests, was not much different than that of the individual tests. In fact, there was limited ability to manipulate hit rate or false alarm rate by combining tests. Maximum protocol hit rate was not much greater than that of TDT (79% vs. 73%). Minimum protocol false alarm rate was no lower than ABLB (4%). These results indicate a strong, positive correlation between tests.

The test battery can also be evaluated from the data of Johnson (1977). He determined the individual performance of Bekesy, SDS, and SISI for patients with retrocochlear disease. Because no cochlear diseased ears were studied, only hit rate could be calculated. It is possible to use his data to calculate performance for all combinations of the three tests, for a loose and strict criterion (Table 14.10). With a loose criterion, hit rate could be increased to 81% by combining all three tests; maximum individual HT was 66% for SISI. Also shown in Table 14.10 are predicted protocol hit rates assuming zero test correlation. These values are always larger, with a loose criterion, than actual performance. This indicates, like Owens's data, a positive test correlation.

Evaluation of principle

The concept of the audiological test battery is based on several assumptions. We can evaluate the legitimacy of the test battery principle by deter-

TABLE 14.9
Performance of Protocols Consisting of All Combinations of
ABLB, BEK, SISI, and TDT[a]

TEST	HT	FA		
ABLB (A)	66	4		
Bekesy (B)	59	8		
SISI (S)	69	9		
TDT (T)	73	12		

	Loose		Strict	
PROTOCOL	HTp	FAp	HTp	FAp
A*T	79	13	62	4
A*S	58	9	48	5
A*B	72	9	53	4
S*B	60	13	57	6
S*T	64	24	61	6
T*B	73	16	69	9
A*T*B	78	14	58	4
S*T*B	64	25	58	6
A*S*T	64	22	57	6
A*S*B	59	12	47	5
A*S*T*B	67	23	56	6

[a]Calculations based on data of Owens (1971). Tests are combined in parallel. Abbreviations are spelled out in Tables 14.1 and 14.4. Adapted from Turner, Frazer, & Shepard (1984).

mining the appropriateness of the assumptions. The first assumption is that additional tests provide new information. The clinical data presented above indicates a significant positive correlation between tests. This positive correlation limits the new information provided by additional tests. The second assumption is that the audiologist can effectively use the new information provided by additional tests. Combining tests is an extremely complex problem, as is probably painfully obvious to the readers of this chapter. It is unrealistic to evaluate multiple test results without a theoretical strategy and quantitative techniques. The third assumption is that the performance of the audiological test battery is always superior to that of the individual tests. We have shown that the performance of the battery can be inferior to that of the best individual tests.

The traditional concept of the audiological test battery is flawed because the underlying assumptions are simplistic or incorrect. There are,

TABLE 14.10
Hit Rate for Protocols Consisting of All Combinations
of Bekesy, Speech Discrimination, and SISI[a]

TEST	HT	
BEK (B)	56	
SDS (D)	54	
SISI (S)	66	
PROTOCOL	HTp—Loose	HTp—Strict
B*D	69 (80)	40 (30)
B*S	73 (85)	48 (37)
D*S	76 (84)	44 (36)
B*D*S	81 (93)	38 (20)

[a]Calculations based on clinical data of Johnson (1977). Protocol hit rate calculated for a loose and strict criterion. Tests are combined in parallel. Numbers in parentheses are predicted hit rate assuming zero test correlation. Abbreviations are spelled out in Tables 14.1 and 14.4. Adapted from Turner, Frazer, and Shepard (1984).

as discussed above, legitimate reasons for combining tests. Before a protocol is used, the performance of that protocol must be determined by some method. If the necessary clinical data are available, then protocol performance can be easily calculated. If data are not available, then some technique is needed to predict protocol performance.

Predicting protocol performance

Basic strategy

Often, appropriate clinical data may not be available for calculating protocol performance. Also, it may not be practical to collect the data through clinical studies. Is it possible to theoretically predict protocol performance? Yes, protocol performance can be predicted. The techniques are presented in detail by Turner (1988). We will review the basic strategy and equations that are used. Protocol performance can be predicted given sufficient information. It is necessary to know (a) the design of the protocol, (b) the performance of the individual tests in the protocol, and (c) the correlation between individual tests.

Protocol design is determined by the clinician; therefore, design is always known. Many combinations of tests are possible. For our discussion, protocol construction is initially limited to the basic design shown in Figure 14.14, Panel a. This protocol consists of blocks of tests connected in series. The patients begin with the test(s) in Block 1 (IN) and proceed through the tests until completed (OUT). A block can consist of a single test or several tests combined in parallel. For parallel tests, the criterion is limited to loose or strict. The blocks are combined in either series-positive or series-negative. One possible protocol is shown in Figure 14.14, Panel b. Block 1 contains three tests in parallel and Block 3 has two tests in parallel. Block 1 is combined to Block 2 in series-positive. All patients with positive results from Block 1 move to Block 2. The patients with negative results are defined as negative for the protocol and receive no more tests. Block 2 and Block 3 are combined in series-negative. All patients who test negative on Block 2 receive the tests in Block 3. All patients who test positive on Block 2 are defined as positive for the protocol and receive no more tests.

To determine protocol performance, the HT and FA of the individual tests in the protocol must be known. For audiological tests that distinguish

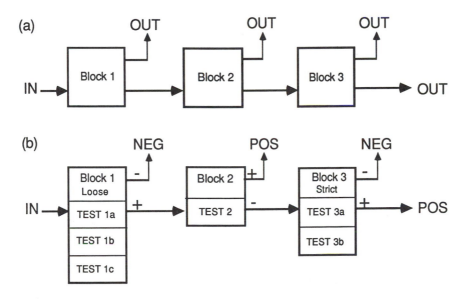

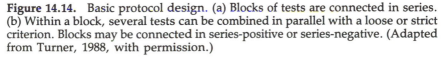

Figure 14.14. Basic protocol design. (a) Blocks of tests are connected in series. (b) Within a block, several tests can be combined in parallel with a loose or strict criterion. Blocks may be connected in series-positive or series-negative. (Adapted from Turner, 1988, with permission.)

cochlear from retrocochlear site-of-lesion, good estimates of performance are provided by Turner, Shepard, and Frazer (1984). For other tests, the performance measures may not be available.

To calculate protocol performance, it is necessary to know the performance of the individual tests in the protocol; however, this information is not sufficient. It is also necessary to know test correlation. For audiological tests, very limited data suggest a mid-pos correlation. That is, a test correlation that produces a protocol hit rate and false alarm rate that is halfway between the hit rates and false alarm rates produced by zero test correlation and max-pos correlation. These clinical data (Jerger & Jerger, 1983; Johnson, 1977) are summarized in Tables 14.11 and 14.12. Shown are a comparison of actual protocol hit rates and false alarm rates, calculated from clinical data, as compared to those predicted assuming mid-pos correlation. There is very good agreement between predicted and actual performance indicating an actual test correlation near mid-pos.

Mid-positive correlation

Protocol hit rate and false alarm rate for mid-pos correlation [HTp(m)/FAp(m)] is defined as the average of the protocol hit rates and false alarm rates for zero correlation [HTp(z)/FAp(z)] and max-pos correlation [HTp(+)/FAp(+)]. That is, protocol performance is first calculated assuming zero correlation and then recalculated assuming max-pos correlation. The protocol hit rates for the two correlations are averaged to obtain the protocol hit rate for mid-pos correlation. Protocol false alarm rate for mid-pos correlation is obtained in a similar way. For mid-pos correlation we have

$$HTp(m) = \frac{HTp(z) + HTp(+)}{2} \tag{17}$$

$$FAp(m) = \frac{FAp(z) + FAp(+)}{2} \tag{18}$$

Protocol hit rates and false alarm rates for max-pos correlation can be calculated using the equations discussed previously for calculating limits on protocol performance (Equations 9, 10, 11, and 12). To summarize, performance for parallel-strict (or series-positive) is given by $HTp(+) = HTm$ and $FAp(+) = FAm$, where HTm and FAm are the smallest hit rate and false alarm rate of the individual tests. For parallel-loose (or series-negative) the equations are $HTp(+) = HTx$ and $FAp(+) = FAx$, where HTx and FAx are the largest hit rate and false alarm rate of the individual tests.

TABLE 14.11
Comparison of Actual and Predicted Protocol Performance[a]

	HTp/FAp—Loose		HTp/FAp—Strict	
	Actual	Predicted	Actual	Predicted
ARC*PIPB	90/30	90/34	65/10	60/6
ARC*PIPB*BCL	100/45	92/43	55/0	56/5

[a]Calculations of actual HTp and FAp based on clinical data of Jerger and Jerger (1983). Mid-positive test correlation is assumed for calculating predicted HTp and FAp. Tests are combined in parallel to form protocol. Results are presented for both loose and strict criteria. Abbreviations are spelled out in Tables 14.1 and 14.4. Adapted from Turner (1988).

TABLE 14.12
Comparison of Actual and Predicted Protocol Hit Rates[a]

	HTp—Loose		HTp—Strict	
	Actual	Predicted	Actual	Predicted
BEK*SDS	69	68	40	42
BEK*SISI	73	70	48	46
SDS*SISI	76	75	44	45
BEK*SDS*SISI	81	80	38	37

[a]Calculations of actual HTp based on clinical data of Johnson (1977). Mid-positive test correlation is assumed for calculating predicted HTp. Tests are combined in parallel to form protocol. Results are presented for both loose and strict criteria. Abbreviations are spelled out in Tables 14.1 and 14.4. Adapted from Turner (1988).

These equations apply when all tests are combined in either parallel or series. Parallel protocols are limited to loose or strict criteria. Series protocols must be entirely series-positive or series-negative.

Zero correlation

Zero test correlation is a special case of some interest. Not only is performance for zero correlation needed to calculate mid-positive performance, but frequently the assumption is made that tests are independent or uncorrelated. The equations derived for zero correlation have general application.

There are two equations for zero correlation that must be considered. These are for loose and strict criterion with a parallel protocol, or series-positive and series-negative for a series protocol. Recall that the performance of a parallel protocol with a strict criterion is identical to that of a series-positive protocol; thus they can be considered equivalent when calculating performance. The same is true for parallel-loose and series-negative.

We will first consider the performance of a parallel protocol with strict criterion. Performance is given by

$$HTp(s/z) = \prod_{n=1}^{N} HTn \qquad (19)$$

$$FAp(s/z) = \prod_{n=1}^{N} FAn \qquad (20)$$

where N = number of individual tests, HTn and FAn are hit rate and false alarm rate of the nth test. The symbol Π means the product of the terms. Thus for three tests in a protocol (N = 3)

$$HTp(z) = HT1 \times HT2 \times HT3$$

$$FAp(z) = FA1 \times FA2 \times FA3.$$

The protocol hit rate and false alarm rate are just the product of the individual tests hit rates and false alarm rates.

Next we consider a parallel protocol with loose criterion. The equations are slightly more complex:

$$HTp(l/z) = HT1 + \sum_{n=2}^{N} HTn \times \prod_{m=1}^{n-1} (1 - HTm) \qquad (21)$$

$$FAp(l/z) = FA1 + \sum_{n=2}^{N} FAn \times \prod_{m=1}^{n-1} (1 - FAm) \qquad (22)$$

where N = number of individual tests, HTn and FAn are hit rate and false alarm rate of the nth test, HTm and FAm are hit rate and false alarm rate of the mth test. The symbol Σ means the sum of the terms. For three tests (N = 3),

$$HTp(z) = HT1 + HT2 \times (1 - HT1) + HT3 \times (1- HT1) \times (1 - HT2)$$

$$FAp(z) = FA1 + FAp \times (1 - FA1) + FA3 \times (1- FA1) \times (1 - FA2)$$

Example

The basic techniques for predicting performance will be illustrated by a simple protocol. Complex protocols require some additional techniques that will not be discussed here. Again, the reader is referred to Turner (1988). The protocol consists of three blocks of tests combined in series-positive (Figure 14.15, Panel a). The first block contains two tests combined in parallel with a loose criterion. The basic strategy is to determine the hit rate and false alarm rate of each block, and then combine the blocks to determine the performance of the total protocol. Protocol performance will be determined first for zero correlation and then for max-pos correlations. These results will be used to determine performance for mid-pos correlation.

We begin by assuming zero test correlation. The first step is to determine the hit rate and false alarm rate for each block. Block 1 has two tests combined in parallel with a loose criterion. The hit rate and false alarm rate of Block 1 (HB1/FB1) is determined by using Equations 21 and 22.

$$HB1 = HT1a + HT1b \times (1 - HT1a) = .60 + .76 \times (1 - .60) = .90 = 90\%$$

$$FB1 = FA1a + FA1b \times (1 - FA1a) = .10 + .22 \times (1 - .10) = .30 = 30\%$$

Block 2 and Block 3 contain just one test each; therefore, the performance of the test in the block is the performance of the block (Figure 14.15, Panel b). Now that an equivalent hit rate and false alarm rate has been calculated for each block, the three blocks can be combined using the equation for series-positive (Equations 19 and 20). Recall that series-positive is equivalent to parallel with a strict criterion. The resultant hit rate and false alarm rate are that of the total protocol for zero correlation (HTp(z)/FAp(z)).

$$HTp(z) = HB1 \times HB2 \times HB3 = .90 \times .80 \times .90 = .65 = 65\%$$

$$FAp(z) = FB1 \times FB2 \times FB3 = .30 \times .20 \times .16 = .01 = 1\%$$

We can think of reducing the protocol to a single test with a performance equal to that of the protocol (Figure 14.15, Panel c).

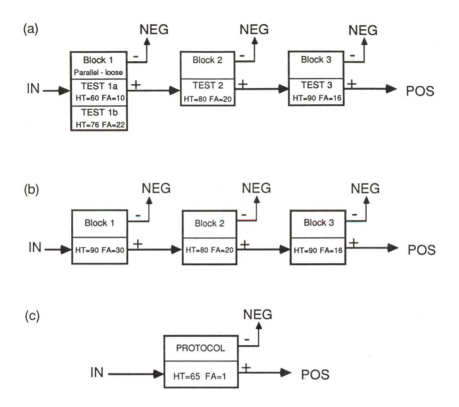

Figure 14.15. Basic strategy for predicting protocol performance. (a) Protocol design. (b) First step is to calculate the performance of each block. Protocol can then be represented as an equivalent protocol with one test in each block. (c) The blocks can be combined to calculate protocol performance. Protocol is represented as a single test with equivalent performance.

Next we determine protocol performance for max-pos correlation. Again, the first step is to determine the performance of each block. For max-pos correlation, the performance of Block 1 is given by Equations 9 and 10.

$$HB1 = MAX[HT1a, HT1b] = MAX[60,76] = 76\%$$

$$FB1 = MAX[FA1a, FA1b] = MAX[10,22] = 22\%$$

As before, the performance of the last two blocks equals that of the single test in each block. Protocol performance is determined by calculating the performance of the three blocks combined in series-positive (Equations 11 and 12).

$$HTp(+) = MIN[HB1, HB2, HB3] = MIN[76, 80, 90] = 76\%$$

$$FAp(+) = MIN[FB1, FB2, FB3] = MIN[22, 20, 16] = 16\%$$

The final step is to calculate protocol performance for mid-pos correlation (Equations 17 and 18).

$$HTp(m) = \frac{HTp(z) + HTp(+)}{2} = \frac{65 + 76}{2} = \frac{141}{2} = 71\%$$

$$FAp(m) = \frac{FAp(z) + FAp(+)}{2} = \frac{1 + 1}{2} \quad \frac{17}{2} = 8\%$$

The hit rate of the protocol is 71% and the false alarm rate is 8%, assuming a mid-positive correlation.

Audiological protocols

We can now use the techniques in this chapter to predict performance for two types of audiological protocols. First we will compare the performance of several protocols designed to distinguish cochlear from retro-cochlear site-of-lesion. Then we will evaluate one protocol designed to identify hearing loss in newborns. The detailed calculations will not be presented. In fact, these calculations were performed by a microcomputer; the data and diagram in Figures 14.16, 14.17, and 14.18 were computer-generated. The use of the computer greatly facilitates the evaluation of a large number of protocols.

Numerous audiological tests have been developed to identify retro-cochlear disease. The test battery principle says that these tests are not used in isolation but are combined into a protocol. The general strategy in developing this type of test protocol has been to combine audiological (and occasionally vestibular tests) with a definitive radiological test. Decisions concerning patient treatment are made on the basis of the definitive test. The financial cost, morbidity, and possible mortality have made it impractical to test every suspect patient with the definitive test. Other tests have served as a screening protocol to decide who receives the definitive test.

(a) Protocol Design

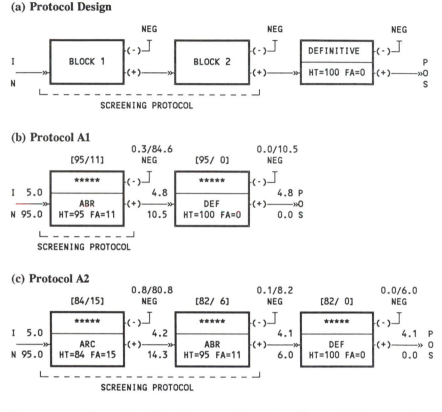

Figure 14.16. Protocols to identify retrocochlear site-of-lesion. Each protocol consists of a screening audiological protocol combined with a definitive test. This analysis is more complex than that in Figure 14.15. One hundred patients are tested; prevalence is 5%. The number of diseased and nondiseased patients are shown above and below, respectively, the arrow to the left of the first block. The number of misses and correct rejections for each block are shown, respectively, above the "NEG" for the block. The number of hits and false alarms for each block are shown above and below, respectively, the arrow to the right of each block. Protocol performance through each block is shown in brackets above each block. Test abbreviations are spelled out in Table 14.4. (From Turner, 1988, with permission.)

We will consider several protocols that have been proposed or used in clinical evaluation. These protocols are modeled as a screening protocol combined with a definitive test (Figure 14.16, Panel a). The general clinical approach has been to use a loose criterion for tests in parallel, and to use series-positive when combining tests in series. A loose criterion for parallel tests probably reflects a desire to increase the hit rate of the

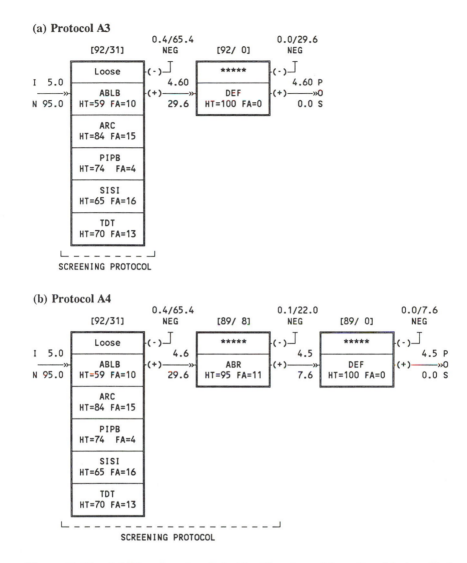

Figure 14.17. Additional protocols to identify retrocochlear site-of-lesion. Each protocol consists of a screening audiological protocol combined with a definitive test. This analysis is more complex than that in Figure 14.15. One hundred patients are tested; prevalence is 5%. The number of diseased and nondiseased patients are shown above and below, respectively, the arrow to the left of the first block. The number of misses and correct rejections for each block are shown, respectively, above the "NEG" for the block. The number of hits and false alarms for each block are shown above and below, respectively, the arrow to the right of each block. Protocol performance through each block is shown in brackets above each block. Test abbreviations are spelled out in Table 14.4. (From Turner, 1988, with permission.)

(a) Protocol Design

```
 NICU
                                                          NEG              NEG
 Pd=4%
 N=300                                         *****  (-)┐       *****  (-)┐
                                  NEG                                              P
                                   »  COG    (+)»  ABR        (+)———»O
 WBN          *****  (-)┐              HT=79 FA=20      HT=97 FA=11              S
                                       HT=79 FA=10
 Pd=0.2%    »  HHR     (+)┘
 N=2000       HT=65  FA=10
```

(b) Equivalent Protocol

```
                                 2.5/230.4              0.1/38.6
                        [79/20]   NEG      [78/ 7]       NEG
 NICU
                                 *****  (-)┐          *****  (-)┐
 I   12.0                                    9.5                    9.3
 ——————————————»  COG    (+)»  ABR      (+)┘
 N 288.0                          HT=79 FA=20  57.6   HT=97 FA=11  19.0
                                                                        HTp=73%

                                                                        11.6   P
                         1.4/1796.4            .3/89.8       <.1/8.9   ——————»O
             [65/10]      NEG      [58/ 6]      NEG    [57/ 5]   NEG    119.9  S
 WBN
              *****  (-)┐      *****  (-)┐      *****  (-)┐
 I   4.0               2.6              2.3              2.3           FAp=5%
 ————————»  HRR    (+)»  COG    (+)»  ABR    (+)┘
 N 1996    HT=65 FA=10 199.6  HT=79 FA=10 109.8  HT=97 FA=11 100.9
```

Figure 14.18. Protocol to identify hearing loss in newborns. NICU: Neonatal Intensive Care Unit; WBN: Well Baby Nursery; N: Number of infants in nursery; Pd: prevalence of disease. (a) Protocol design (b) Equivalent protocol to facilitate analysis. The number of misses and correct rejections for each block are shown, respectively, above the "NEG" for the block. The number of hits and false alarms for each block are shown above and below, respectively, the arrow to the right of each block. Protocol performance through each block is shown in brackets above each block. Test abbreviations are spelled out in Table 14.4. (From Turner, 1988, with permission.)

screening protocol, because with this type of protocol, a false alarm is usually considered preferable to a miss. The false alarm will be detected by the definitive test, the miss will be lost from the system. The screening protocol would be appropriately connected to the definitive test in series-positive. Tests within the screening protocol have typically been combined in series-positive, probably because series-positive is more "obvious" than series-negative. The use of series-positive will, in fact, decrease hit rate; this was, however, probably not evident to most clinicians.

For evaluating these protocols, we assume a mid-pos test correlation and a prevalence of 5%. Figures 14.16 and 14.17 present a detailed analysis of these four protocols for mid-pos correlation. This analysis is much more detailed than for the example protocol above. The hits, misses, false alarms, and correct rejections are calculated for each block. Also, the performance through each block is indicated above each block. This type of detailed analysis is necessary for most cost-benefit analyses; simply calculating total protocol performance is, in general, not sufficient.

The performances of all the evaluated protocols are summarized in Table 14.13. Included in this table are total protocol and screening protocol performance. These results reveal several interesting consequences of the particular protocol design shown in Figure 14.16, Panel b. Because all blocks of tests are connected in series-positive, all patients identified as positive by the screening protocol will receive the definitive test. These patients will consist of hits and false alarms. The definitive test will correctly sort these patients into hits and correct rejections. The hit rate of the total protocol (HTp) will equal the hit rate of the screening protocol (HTs). Any diseased patient not identified by the screening protocol will be lost from the system and not tested by the definitive test. The false alarm rate of the total protocol will be zero (FAp), even though the false alarm rate of the screening protocol (FAs) is not zero. All false alarms in the system will be correctly identified as nondiseased by the definitive test.

TABLE 14.13
Predicted Performance for Selected Audiological Protocols[a]

PROTOCOL	HTs/FAs	Pr[D/+]s	EFs	HTp/FAp	Pr[D/+]p	EFp
A1. ABR + DEF	95/11	31	89	95/0	100	99+
A2. ARC + ABR + DEF	82/6	41	93	82/0	100	99
A3. ABLB*ARC*PIPB* SISI*TDT + DEF	92/31	13	70	92/0	100	99+
A4. ABLB*ARC*PIPB* SISI*TDT + ABR + DEF	89/8	37	92	89/0	100	99+

[a]Mid-positive correlation assumed for predicting protocol hit rate and false alarm rate. Posterior probabilities and efficiency calculated using hit rate and false alarm rate. A + between tests indicates series-positive; an asterisk (*) between tests indicates tests in parallel with a loose criterion. EFs: efficiency of the screening protocol; EFp: efficiency of the total protocol. Other abbreviations are spelled out in Tables 14.1 and 14.4. Adapted from Turner (1988).

Other measures of protocol performance, posterior probabilities and efficiency, will be influenced by protocol design. Because FAp = 0, the probability of the total protocol being correct with a positive test result is 100%. There can be no false alarms. Because prevalence is small (5% for these calculations), efficiency and the probability of being correct with a negative result are >98% for the total protocol.

Performance measures for the screening protocols vary significantly with protocol design. HTs is important because that determines HTp. FAs largely determines the number of patients tested by the definitive test. Usually the definitive test is relatively expensive; thus FAs is correlated with the financial cost of the protocol.

Protocol A1.   This protocol was recommended by Turner, Frazer, and Shepard (1984) and uses ABR as the screening protocol (Figure 14.16, Panel b). All patients suspect for a retrocochlear lesion are screened by ABR. With this protocol, HTp is high (95%) and FAs is low (11%). This is currently a popular protocol for clinical use.

Protocol A2.   This protocol is a variation on Protocol A1 and uses ARC to determine which patients are tested with ABR (Figure 14.16, Panel c). This protocol has some appeal because the cost of ARC is generally much less than ABR. The use of ARC would reduce the number of patients receiving ABR and DEF. The problem with this protocol is that HTp is reduced to 82% because ARC and ABR are combined in series-positive, which reduces hit rate.

Protocol A3.   This protocol represents the audiological test battery concept (Figure 16.17, Panel a). Many of the traditional audiological tests are combined in parallel with a loose criterion to form the screening protocol. With the assumption of mid-pos correlation, this approach does increase HTs (92%) above that of the highest individual test (ARC = 84%). Some clinical data indicate that test correlation for the traditional tests might be greater than mid-positive, resulting in a smaller HTs (Turner, Frazer, and Shepard, 1984). The test battery produces a large FAs (31%). If a strict criterion was used, FAs would be reduced below 4% but HTs would also be reduced below 59%.

Protocol A4.   Is there some advantage to combining the traditional test battery with ABR? One approach is to use the test battery to determine who receives ABR (Figure 14.17, Panel b). This strategy reduces HTs below that for ABR alone (89% vs. 95%). In general, this is not a desirable effect.

Protocol A1 is probably the most popular protocol in use today. The protocol is simple with good performance (HTp = 95%, FAs = 11%), and it serves as a standard of comparison for the other protocols. Protocols A2 and A4 have a lower FAs than A1, but also a lower HTp. If the objective is to increase HTp and, thus, identify more disease, then these two protocols are not appropriate. Protocol A3 is the traditional test battery. This protocol has both a lower HTp and a higher FAs than A1. This protocol is clearly inferior to A1 and can be rejected.

Early identification of hearing loss

Various audiological protocols have been developed for use in hospitals to identify those children born with hearing loss. These early identification (EID) protocols can be expensive and difficult to evaluate because many children are typically lost from the program. The techniques presented in this chapter provide the means to easily evaluate the performance of many protocols. The application of these techniques will be illustrated with one theoretical EID protocol (Figure 14.18, Panel a). This is not a recommended protocol for clinical use. This protocol was designed to best demonstrate techniques.

As is frequently the case, the newborns are divided between the Neonatal Intensive Care Unit (NICU) and the Well Baby Nursery (WBN). All NICU babies are defined as "high-risk" for hearing loss and are tested by Crib-O-Gram (COG). The WBN babies are tested by a High-Risk Register (HHR). Those identified as "high-risk" receive COG. COG and ABR are combined in series-positive. Those babies that test positive on both are positive for the protocol.

The prevalence numbers and HT/FA for the tests come from several sources (Durieux-Smith, Picton, Edwards, Goodman, & MacMurray, 1985; Hosford-Dunn, Johnson, Simmons, Malachowski, & Kern, 1987; Murry, Javel, & Watson, 1985; Shepard, Turner, & Stein, 1982; Turner, Shepard, & Frazer, 1984). The accuracy of these numbers is not important for demonstrating the techniques; however, several facts should be noted. The prevalence of hearing loss is significantly different in the two nurseries; therefore, the two populations must be considered separately. The performance of the tests may be different for each population, as indicated for COG.

The basic strategy for evaluating this protocol is shown in Figure 14.18, Panel b. The two populations of babies are evaluated by separate subprotocols that are combined at the end to represent the actual protocol. The performance of each subprotocol is determined by the standard procedures developed previously. For the NICU babies, COG and ABR are combined in series-positive. For the WBN babies, HHR, COG, and ABR are all combined in series-positive. Mid-pos correlation is assumed, although there are little data to indicate the correlation between these types of tests. The total hits and false alarms of each subprotocol are combined to provide total hits and false alarms for the protocol. Total hits and false alarms are used to calculate HTp/FAp.

The performance of this protocol is not particularly good. Even though FAp is low (5%), HTp is very poor (73%). About one of every four hearing-impaired children would be missed. HTp is low because the hit rate of each subprotocol is poor (78% and 57%). The NICU subprotocol has a low hit rate because HT = 79% for COG. COG is combined with ABR in series-positive, which only reduces the hit rate even though ABR has a high HT. The situation with the WBN subprotocol is even worse. The HHR must be treated as a test with a hit rate and false alarm rate. The HT for the HHR is, in fact, poor. Because HHR, COG, and ABR are combined in series-positive, the hit rate of the subprotocol (57%) will be less than the lowest individual hit rate (65%).

Although the EID protocol shown in Figure 14.18, Panel a may have seemed reasonable, an analysis of performance revealed a poor hit rate. An evaluation of this type can indicate where in a protocol there is a problem and suggest changes in design. For example, COG could be removed from the NICU subprotocol. This would increase hit rate and increase the cost of the protocol. Because the prevalence (4%) in the NICU is relatively high, the increased cost may be justified. The hit rate of the WBN subprotocol could be increased by removing both the HHR and the COG. This may not be practical, however, because of the very low prevalence (0.2%) and the large number of children (2,000). Another alternative would be to remove the HHR and combine COG with ABR in series-negative.

Many EID protocols are possible and a variety have been used in hospital programs. There was no attempt in this chapter to determine the optimum EID protocol. Predicting protocol performance could, however, facilitate the evaluation of existing protocols and the design of more efficient protocols without years of clinical study.

Cost-benefit analysis

Overview

Cost-benefit analysis is the consideration of factors other than performance when selecting protocols for clinical use. Up to this point, we have been concerned with measures of performance. Cost-benefit analysis is necessary because the protocol with the best performance is not always the appropriate protocol to use. There may be significant financial cost or personal risk to the patient who makes the use of a particular protocol undesirable.

Subjective cost-benefit analysis is common in clinical practice. Ultimately, we must make decisions about patient care; we must decide what tests to administer. In lieu of formal, objective techniques we employ the subjective/intuitive strategy. We may not realize that we have performed a cost-benefit analysis, but we have. Whenever we decide not to use a test because it costs too much, it takes too long, the patients complain, no one uses the information, and so forth, we have conducted a cost-benefit analysis. We can avoid the sloppiness and bias of the subjective approach by using a more objective analysis.

The basic strategy of an objective cost-benefit analysis is to quantify the various costs and/or benefits of the protocols. Generally, costs are assigned to errors: misses and false alarms; benefits are assigned to correct decisions, hits, and correct rejections. The protocol with the greatest benefits and lowest cost is the one of choice.

Although conceptually simple, the cost-benefit analysis can be extremely difficult in practice. Most analyses are based on the number of hits, misses, false alarms, and correct rejections. To determine these numbers, we must know the performance of the protocol and the prevalence of the disease. Unfortunately, this necessary information may not be available from clinical data. The other major problem with cost-benefit analysis is quantifying costs and benefits. The financial cost of a procedure is easy to specify, but how is a number derived for patient suffering or death? Even financial cost can be difficult. For example, data may not be available to determine the long-term financial impact of an undetected disease on a patient or society.

All is not lost; even a simple cost-benefit analysis can be useful. The dollar cost of each protocol could be calculated based on the charge for each test. There would be no consideration of long-term financial or nonfinancial costs to a patient or society. Also, there would be no attempt to quantify subjective issues as morbidity or mortality. Protocols would be compared on the basis of cost (in dollars) per patient and cost per disease detected. This type of financial analysis is limited, but still important in today's health care environment.

Obviously, more complex cost-benefit analyses are needed, but even the simple financial analysis just described requires accurate measures of protocol performance that are not generally available. Fortunately, there is a procedure that can be used with limited performance data.

Ranking with cost ratios

Consider the following situation. We have several possible screening protocols that we wish to combine with a definitive test. We want to evaluate the performance of the screening protocols so as to determine the best protocol for clinical use. Patients that are positive on the screening protocol will receive the definitive test. Patients that test negative will not receive the definitive test and will, in most cases, be lost from the system. Patients who test positive on the screening protocol constitute the hits and false alarms. The definitive test will accurately sort these patients into the two groups. The patients who test negative are the misses and correct rejections. Because these patients do not receive the definitive test, we have no information as to the number in each group.

We would like to calculate the hit rate and the false alarm rate for the screening protocols, but we cannot because we do not have an accurate count of misses and correct rejections. If we had an exact measure of disease prevalence in the test population then the misses and correct rejections could be calculated from the hits and false alarms. In practice, the exact prevalence will not be known. Is the situation hopeless? No, Dobie (1985) provides a clever technique to rank order protocols by using only data on patients who test positive (the hits and false alarms). This technique requires that (a) a definitive test to be used to accurately determine hits and false alarms; and (b) we decide the relative costs of errors, that is, how many false alarms equal one miss.

The technique can be illustrated with this example. Three screening protocols are available for use with MRI to identify retrocochlear site-of-lesion. Protocol A1 is ABR alone, Protocol A2 is ARC combined in series positive with ABR, Protocol A3 is the traditional audiological test battery. (These are the first three protocols in Table 14.13.) We must choose a cost ratio, R; this is the maximum number of false alarms that we will accept for each miss. This decision is the cost-benefit component of this technique and can be somewhat subjective. In this case, we consider a false alarm preferable to a miss because of the danger of an undetected tumor. In other situations, we might consider a miss less costly than a false alarm. We decide to accept up to five false alarms for every miss, that is, R = 5.

The relative difference in the cost (CST) of two protocols is given by the following equation:

$$CST(X - Y) = (fsX - fsY) - R \times (hsX - hsY) \tag{23}$$

where hsX, fsX are the number of hits, false alarms of Protocol X; hsY, fsY are the number of hits, false alarms of Protocol Y. If CST is positive then the cost of Protocol X is greater than the cost of Protocol Y and, therefore, Protocol Y is superior. If CST is negative then Protocol X is superior.

To rank order our three protocols, we must compute the relative cost of the three pairs of protocols: CST(A1-A3), CST(A2-A3), CST(A1-A2). For this example, assume that 1,000 patients were tested with each protocol. With Protocol A1, 153 patients tested positive. MRI ultimately demonstrated that the 153 patients consisted of 48 hits and 105 false alarms. Protocol A2 was positive for 98 patients, of which 41 were hits and 57 were false alarms. For Protocol A3, there were 46 hits and 295 false alarms. Calculations of the cost differences are shown in Table 14.14. Note that CST(A1-A3) and CST(A2-A3) are both negative, indicating that Protocols A1 and A2 are both superior to Protocol A3. For R = 5, CST(A1-A2) is positive (+13), indicating that Protocol A2 is superior to Protocol A1. Thus we could rank order the three protocols as A2, A1, A3.

These results are somewhat surprising in that ABR was not the best protocol. This is a consequence of R, the cost ratio we selected. What would happen if we permitted 10 false alarms for each miss? The calculations for R = 10 are also shown in Table 14.14. In this case we see that CST(A1-A2) is negative, indicating that Protocol A1 (ABR) is superior. The rank orderings now would be A1, A2, A3. We see that the rank ordering of the protocols is highly dependent on our selection of R. If R is small, then protocols with low false alarm rates will be favored. If R is large, then protocols with high hit rates are favored.

The primary advantage of this technique is that protocols can be rank ordered using just hits and false alarms. These numbers are usually more available from clinical data than misses and correct rejections. The technique has, however, several disadvantages. The rank order is a strong function of the cost ratio we select; the orderings can change significantly with different ratios, as with our example. The selection of the cost ratio

TABLE 14.14
Calculations of Relative Difference in Cost of Three Protocols[a]

PROTOCOL	HTs/FAs	hs/fs
A1. ABR + DEF	95/11	48/105
A2. ARC + ABR + DEF	82/6	41/57
A3. ABLB*ARC*PIPB*SISI*TDT + DEF	92/31	46/295
RELATIVE COST	R = 5	R = 10
CST(A1−A2)	+13	−22
CST(A1−A3)	−200	−210
CST(A2−A3)	−213	−188

[a]Protocols are the same as in Table 14.13. A plus (+) sign between tests indicates series-positive. An asterisk (*) between tests indicates tests in parallel with a loose criterion. R: cost ratio. Other abbreviations are spelled out in Tables 14.1 and 14.4.

can be extremely arbitrary and subjective, and thus the resulting rank order will be equally arbitrary. This technique is only as good as the selection of the cost ratio. The second disadvantage is that these calculations provide a relative ranking, not an absolute measure of the performance of the different protocols. The protocols under consideration may all be terrible, the top ranked protocol may only be "less bad" than the others. Even with these limitations, this technique is still extremely valuable.

Future needs and applications

In this chapter, the techniques of clinical decision analysis have been applied to the audiological problem of identifying retrocochlear disease. This has been an important academic and clinical issue in audiology, and this problem is well suited to illustrate the concepts and methods of CDA. Today, however, this particular diagnostic issue is essentially moot. The development of ABR, CAT, and MRI have, for the most part, eliminated the use of tests like TDT, ABLB, SISI. The issue is not totally resolved, however. There is still the use of ABR as a screening protocol. When does it become cost effective to test all suspect patients with something like MRI instead of screening with ABR?

There are two other important applications of CDA to audiological issues. First, what is the optimum strategy for the early identification of hearing loss? With CDA, various protocols can be examined and their performance estimated. Problems with a particular protocol can be identified, as with the example protocol in this chapter. Cost-benefit analysis would be extremely useful to determine when it is cost effective to evaluate every newborn instead of just those at-risk for hearing loss.

The second application of CDA concerns the evaluation of the dizzy patient. Recently, two new instruments have been developed to compliment the ENG. The rotary chair is a computer controlled chair that provides precise stimulation of the vestibular system by rotating the patient. The dynamic postural platform evaluates the strategies used by patients to maintain posture under a variety of conditions. Each of these tests, as well as the ENG, contain a number of subtests. What is the optimum combination of these tests and subtests for the evaluation of patients with dizziness and other balance problems? This is an important issue because the newer tests are fairly expensive. Do the new tests provide additional information to the ENG? This is also a challenging problem for CDA because many vestibular tests have multiple outcomes, not just positive or negative for disease.

The application of clinical decision analysis to audiological decision making is relatively new. There are significant gaps in the clinical data and available techniques. The thrust of future research should be to provide the missing clinical data, advance theoretical knowledge, and develop practical procedures. There is little information on individual test performance except for tests designed to identify retrocochlear disease. There are almost no data on test correlation which may be different for different types of tests. The procedures presented in this chapter for predicting protocol performance must be validated by clinical data.

Most of the work in this chapter is based on simplifying assumptions. Tests were permitted to have only two outcomes: positive or negative for disease. We have already seen how that restriction is inappropriate for vestibular tests. We required that the criterion for parallel protocols be either loose or strict. Is there any advantage to using an intermediate criterion, such as three out of five tests positive for the protocol to be positive? What about weighting different tests in a protocol differently so that some tests count more than other tests? Additional theoretical work is needed to develop more powerful, less restrictive techniques.

From the perspective of practical methods, the greatest need is in the area of cost-benefit analysis. We are just beginning to develop cost-benefit strategies for clinical use. The cost-ratio approach is one of the few proposed for audiological tests. A cost-benefit analysis based on financial cost could be implemented using clinical or predicted measures of protocol performance.

References

Bauch, C. D., Rose, D. E., & Harner, S. G. (1982). Auditory brain stem responses from 255 patients with suspected retrocochlear involvement. *Ear and Hearing, 3*, 83–86.

Buxton, F. (1973). In J. Jerger (Ed.), *Modern developments in audiology* (Table 1, pp. 84). New York: Academic Press.

Dobie, R. A. (1985). The use of relative cost ratios in choosing a diagnostic test. *Ear and Hearing, 6*, 113–116.

Durieux-Smith, A., Picton, T., Edwards, C., Goodman, J., & MacMurray, B. (1985). The Crib-O-Gram in the NICU: An evaluation based on brain stem response audiometry. *Ear and Hearing, 6*, 20–24.

Egan, J. P. (1975). *Signal detection theory and ROC analysis*. New York: Academic Press.

Feldman, A. S. (1976). Diagnostic audiology. In J. L. Northern (Ed.), *Hearing disorders* (pp. 37–52). Boston: Little, Brown.

Hall, J. (1978, November). *Diagnostic audiology in sensori-neural loss: A critical survey.* Paper presented at the annual convention of the American Speech-Language-Hearing Association, San Francisco.

Hart, R. G., & Davenport, J. (1981). Diagnosis of acoustic tumors. *Neurosurgery, 9,* 450–463.

Hart, R. G., Gardner, D., & Howieson, J. (1983). Acoustic tumors: Atypical features and recent diagnostic tests. *Neurology, 33,* 211–221.

Hirsh, A., & Anderson, H. (1980). Audiologic test results in 96 patients with tumors affecting the eighth nerve. *Acta Oto-Laryngology, 369,* (Supplement), 1–26.

Hosford-Dunn, H., Johnson, S., Simmons, F. B., Malachowski, N., & Kern, L. (1987). Infant hearing screening: Program implementation and validation. *Ear and Hearing, 8,* 12–20.

Jerger, S. (1983). Decision matrix and information theory analysis in the evaluation of neuro-audiologic tests. *Seminars in Hearing, 4,* 121–132.

Jerger, S., & Jerger, J. (1983). The evaluation of diagnostic audiometric tests. *Audiology, 22,* 144–161.

Johnson, E. W. (1977). Auditory test results in 500 cases of acoustic neuroma. *Archives of Otolaryngology, 103,* 152–158.

Mikhael, M. A., Wolff, A. P., & Ciric, I. S. (1987). Current concepts in neuroradiological diagnosis of acoustic neuromas. *Laryngoscope, 97,* 471–476.

Moscicki, E. K. (1984). The prevalence of "incidence" is too high. *Asha, 26,* 39–40.

Murry, A., Javel, E., & Watson, C. (1985). Prognostic validity of auditory brainstem evoked response screening in newborn infants. *American Journal of Otolaryngology, 6,* 120–131.

Owens, E. (1971). Audiologic evaluation in cochlear versus retrocochlear lesions. *Acta Oto-Laryngology, 283,* (Supplement), 1–45.

Robinson, D. E., & Watson, C. S. (1972). Psychophysical methods in modern psychoacoustics. In J. V. Tobias (Ed.), *Foundations of modern auditory theory* (pp. 101–131). New York: Academic Press.

Rosenberg, P. E. (1978). Differentiating cochlear and retrocochlear disfunction. In J. Katz (Ed.), *Handbook of clinical audiology* (pp. 159–178). Baltimore: Williams & Wilkins.

Schuknecht, H. (1974). *Pathology of the ear.* Cambridge, MA: Harvard University Press.

Shepard, N. T., Turner R. G., & Stein, L. (1982). *Evaluation of hearing in neonates and difficult-to-test patients.* Paper presented at the meeting of the ASHA North Central Regional Conference, Milwaukee, WI.

Swets, J. A. (1964). *Signal detection and recognition by human observers.* New York: John Wiley.

Turner, R. G. (1988). Techniques to determine test protocol performance. *Ear and Hearing, 9,* 177–189.

Turner, R. G., Frazer, G. J., & Shepard, N. T. (1984). Formulating and evaluating audiological test protocols. *Ear and Hearing, 15,* 321–330.

Turner, R. G., & Nielsen, D. W. (1984). Application of clinical decision analysis to audiological tests. *Ear and Hearing, 5,* 125–133.

Turner, R. G., Shepard, N. T., & Frazer, G. J. (1984). Clinical performance of audiological and related diagnostic tests. *Ear and Hearing, 15,* 187–194.

chapter fifteen

Vestibular system assessment

DAVID G. CYR

Contents

Introduction

The interaction between visual, vestibular, and somatosensory (proprioceptive) systems, and the control exercised from the brainstem and cerebellum is critical to the maintenance of equilibrium (balance) and posture. This interaction also is important for the development of motor milestones such as sitting unsupported, crawling, and walking. Vestibular end organs (utricle, saccule, and semicircular canals) contribute to the maintenance of balance by providing sensory information to the brain for the detection of both linear and angular acceleration, and by monitoring head position relative to gravity. The vestibular system also plays an integral role in the control of eye position and eye movement when the head is in motion, through the vestibular-ocular reflex (VOR), a neural pathway that connects the vestibular end organs with the extraocular muscles of the eyes.

Deficits in any one of the three sensory systems (vestibular, visual, somatosensory), or dysfunction within the corresponding motor systems may impose obstacles to environmental adaption and result in a sensation of imbalance and/or dizziness. These symptoms also may be caused by a wide range of multisystem lesions involving the cardiovascular, cerebrovascular, metabolic, or central nervous system.

Vertigo

Although pure vestibular system lesions may produce a feeling of unsteadiness or imbalance, the primary sensation is one of dizziness and/or vertigo. The sensation of *dizziness* is often difficult to delineate. Patients complaining of dizziness describe lightheadedness, dysequilibrium, imbalance, presyncope, floating, whooziness, giddiness, confusion, visual distortion, ataxia, or a variety of other sensations. In contrast, the term *vertigo*, a specific type of dizziness, is definable and easier for the patient to describe. Derived from the Latin word *vertere* meaning "to turn," vertigo is a specific sensation of environmental motion, usually rotation or spinning. Vertigo is classified into two types (DeJong, 1979): objective (the person remains still while the environment moves) and subjective (the patient spins while the environment remains fixed). Although the two types are common, there does not appear to be a consistent relationship between the type of vertigo and a specific type or site-of-lesion. Nevertheless, differentiating between vertigo and general dizziness is important because the symptom of vertigo is seen more commonly in peripheral vestibular system lesions than in cardiovascular, cerebrovascular, metabolic, or central nervous system disease.

Partially because of the physical proximity between the vestibular and auditory systems, otolaryngologists (ear, nose, and throat physicians) traditionally have been responsible for the medical evaluation of patients with dizziness and/or dysequilibrium. Audiologists have become involved in the assessment of the dizzy patient primarily because of their professional relationship with otolaryngologists. If this arrangement is to be effective, it is imperative that audiologists be familiar with the methods used to evaluate these patients, although diagnosis remains the responsibility of the physician.

Brief history of ENG

Flourens (1830) was one of the first to observe that a connection exists between vestibular stimulation and eye movements. He noted that when one of the inner ear semicircular canals was destroyed in pigeons and rabbits, an uncontrollable movement of the eyes occurred along with a significant change in the animal's body posture. Several years later, Du Bois-Reymond (1849) discovered an electrical potential difference between the cornea (front part of the eye) and the retina (back part of the eye). This corneo-retinal potential (CRP) continues to serve as the basis for monitoring eye movements in general, and for recording eye movements generated by stimulation of the vestibular system in particular.

Raehlmann (1878) used the corneo-retinal potential to develop a procedure for recording the degree and direction of eye movement. His method consisted of placing a needle electrode into the cornea of the eye while measuring the changes in electrical polarity when the eye moved from side to side. Not until 21 years later, however, was the procedure repeated by Hogyes (1899) for the obvious reason that Raehlmann's technique was so highly invasive. This type of measurement was modified for clinical use in the field of ophthalmology with the development of a contact lens electrode. The technique eventually was designated electro-oculography (EOG), a safe, noninvasive method for recording a variety of eye movements including those recorded during the standard electronystagmographic procedure.

Preceding the emergence of the contact lens electrode, the initial electro-oculographic procedure was modified by Jung (1939) for the purpose of evaluating vestibular function in patients with dizziness. Jung's method, proposed initially by Schott (1922), consisted of applying surface electrodes around the periphery of the eyes. With the electrodes strategically placed, he was able to use the corneo-retinal potential for recording nystagmus and other eye movements in response to stimulation of the vestibular end organs.

Jung's noninvasive technique led directly to the development of modern-day clinical electronystagmography (ENG). With the development of more sophisticated stimulus delivery systems and recording devices, it is now possible to measure this electrical potential routinely. As a result, the ENG procedure is capable of recording the same types of eye movements obtained earlier with implanted corneal electrodes.

The primary purpose of this chapter is to familiarize the reader with the standard vestibular test methods used to assess the dizzy patient by describing the subtests that constitute the traditional test battery. The chapter describes primarily the traditional ENG technique. More recent clinical procedures (computerized rotation and dynamic posturography) also are reviewed. References are provided for the reader who desires more in-depth information that is beyond the scope of this chapter. Before detailing specific test procedures, a brief, basic review of vestibular anatomy and physiology is needed.

Vestibular anatomy and physiology

The vestibular system, acting partly through the VOR, serves to stabilize the visual environment when the head is in motion. Therefore, a compensatory eye movement occurs each time the vestibular system is stimulated by movement of the head. In order to achieve this compensatory goal, the eye movement should occur at the same speed but in the opposite direction as the head movement. How is the head direction and movement velocity detected and forwarded to the eye muscles to produce this compensatory eye movement?

The peripheral vestibular system consists of five sensory organs located within the petrous portion of each temporal bone (Figure 15.1). The organs include three semicircular canals (SCC) that are responsive to angular acceleration, and two otolith organs that are responsive to linear acceleration and static head position relative to gravity, referred to as "tilt." The semicircular canals are labeled relative to their orientation in space. They include the horizontal (lateral), posterior vertical, and superior vertical, also referred to as the anterior canal. The canals are positioned at right angles to each other. Imagine the canals placed on the floor in the corner of a room with the horizontal canal flat on the floor and the two vertical canals resting parallel against each wall, the latter two perpendicular to each other. When the head is in an upright position, the SCC system is tilted 30° from parallel to the floor. The horizontal semicircular canals in the right and left ears, respectively, form a synergic pair and are in a parallel plane with each other. The parallel canal for the right anterior canal is the left posterior canal, whereas the left anterior canal is parallel to the right posterior canal. Each SCC connects to the larger of the two otolith organs, the utricle. The other otolith organ, the saccule, is smaller and positioned below the utricle. Arising from the saccule is a small drainage tube for endolymph called the endolymphatic duct extending to and terminating in a ballooned area referred to as the endolymphatic sac. The auditory and vestibular systems are connected by the ductus reuniens that is positioned between the saccule and the scala media of the cochlea.

Within the membranous labyrinth are the cristae of the semicircular canals and the maculae of the utricle and saccule. These structures serve as the sensory system for the peripheral vestibular end organs. Both of these structures contain hair cells that translate mechanical information into neural impulses by way of a sheering action of the vestibular hair cells. In the maculae, each hair cell consists of one large projection, called the kinocilium, and many smaller projections called stereocilia (Figure 15.2). When the head moves in a direction that deflects the smaller

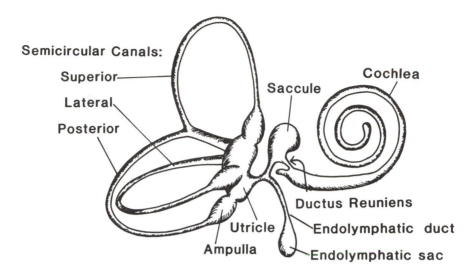

Figure 15.1. Structures of the inner ear apparatus showing semicircular canals and otolith organs. Each of the three semicircular canals has an ampulla although only the posterior canal ampulla is labeled.

stereocilia toward the kinocilium, a stimulation of the hair cell occurs (depolarization). When the stereocilia are deflected in the opposite direction (away from the kinocilium), a neural inhibition occurs (hyperpolarization). The hair cells of the macula of the utricle and saccule are imbedded in a gelatin-like material that rests immediately below a conglomerate of calcium carbonate crystals called otoconia. When the head moves in a linear fashion, or when the head position changes relative to gravity, the otoconia move within the gelatinous layer, thus bending the cilia, which trigger either a neural inhibition or facilitation of the hair cells.

Likewise, the cristae of the semicircular canals rest immediately below a dome-shaped structure called the cupula. The cupulae (one for each SCC), are situated in a widened area of each canal known as the ampulla (Figure 15.3). With the head at rest, the cupula remains upright with equal endolymphatic pressure on either side (3A). When the head turns in an angular path, the endolymph within the semicircular canal lags behind the head movement and moves initially in the opposite direction, thus bending the cupula so as to stimulate the hair cells. Bending the cupula toward the utricle (3B) causes an increase in neural activity (ampullopetal pull), whereas bending the cupula away from the utricle (3C) causes an inhibition of neural activity (ampullofugal pull). Because each semicircular canal has a synergic canal on the opposite side, a neural imbalance is set

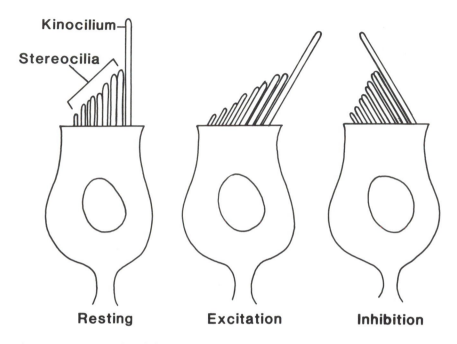

Figure 15.2. Macula of the utricle illustrating the single, large kinocilium and smaller stereocilia. Neural excitation occurs when the stereocilia are deflected toward the kinocilium. When the stereocilia are deflected away from the kinocilium, neural inhibition occurs.

up each time the head is turned in a major plane. Eye and head movements occur in the same plane as the stimulated canal and in the same direction as the flow of endolymph (Ewald's First Law). For example, when the head is turned to the right, the right horizontal SCC induces endolymph flow to the left (toward the center of the head), and the left horizontal SCC induces fluid flow away from the center of the head. The right horizontal SCC cupula is deviated toward the utricle and a neural increase occurs. The left horizontal SCC cupula is deviated away from the utricle (toward the side of the head), thus decreasing neural activity from that side (Ewald's Second Law). In the vertical canals, the opposite occurs where ampullopetal flow of endolymph produces a neural decrease while ampullofugal flow produces an increase in neural activity.

Each of the five sensory structures within the peripheral vestibular system is connected to a nerve that courses through the internal auditory canal (Figure 15.1) where they merge to form two distinct vestibular nerve branches, the superior and inferior. The superior branch of the vestibular

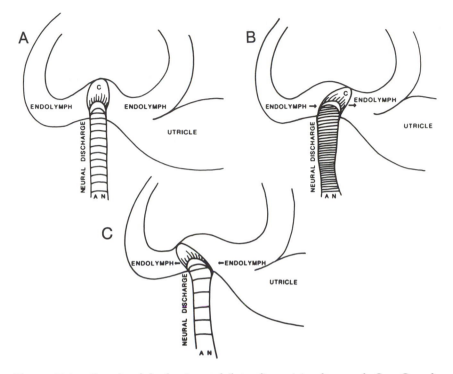

Figure 15.3. Cupula of the horizontal (lateral) semicircular canal. C = Cupula; AN = ampullar nerve. Horizontal stripes along AN illustrate the rate of neural discharge when the cupula is at rest (A), deflected toward the utricle (B), and deflected away from the utricle (C). Cupular deflection toward the utricle (ampullopetal of utriculopetal pull) creates a neural excitation, whereas cupular deflection away from the utricle (ampullofugal or utriculofugal pull) creates a neural inhibition.

nerve innervates the anterior and horizontal semicircular canals, the utricle, and part of the saccule. The inferior branch of the vestibular nerve innervates the posterior SCC and the major portion of the saccule (Baloh, 1984). The nerves merge at Scarpa's ganglion in the internal auditory canal and then pass medially through the cerebellopontine angle, entering the brainstem just above the medulla and immediately below the pons. The vestibular nerve afferent fibers transverse either directly to the cerebellum and to the spinal canal (vestibulo-spinal afferants), which constitutes the vestibulo-cervical reflex (VCR), or to one or more of the four major vestibular nuclei positioned on the floor of the fourth ventricle. The neural transmission then proceeds to the extraocular muscles via the medial longitudinal fasciculus (MLF) through the ocular motor nuclei (III, IV, and VI). This is, in essence, the vestibular-ocular pathway (VOR) for the horizontal SCC system and is illustrated in Figure 15.4A.

When the head is turned to either side, creating a neural imbalance between the right and left vestibular systems, the neural imbalance is transmitted via the vestibular nerves, through Scarpa's ganglion, to the vestibular nuclei and subsequently to the extraocular muscles that pull both eyes opposite the direction of the head turn (Figure 15.4B). The slow, compensatory deviation of the eyes represents the slow component of a vestibular nystagmus. The second phase, a rapid jerk in the direction opposite the slow eye movement makes up the remainder of a nystagmic beat. The fast phase (saccade) is generated most probably in the paramedian pontine reticular formation (PPRF) of the brainstem, whereas the

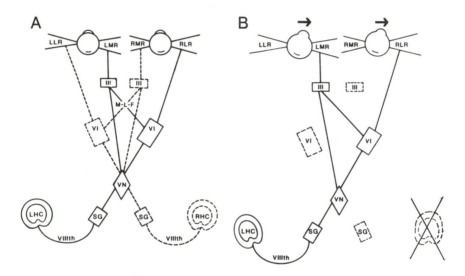

Figure 15.4. Vestibular-ocular reflex (VOR) of the horizontal semicircular canal to extra-ocular muscles. LHC = left horizontal SCC; RHC = right horizontal SCC; SG = Scarpa's ganglion; VN = vestibular nuclei; VI = nuclei of the 6th cranial nerve; III = nuclei of the 3rd cranial nerve; LLR = left lateral rectus muscle; LMR = left medial rectus muscle; RMR = right medial rectus muscule; RLR = right lateral rectus muscle; M-L-F = medial longitudinal fasciculus. Equal neural discharge shown in Panel A. Panel B illustrates the neural pathway to the extra-ocular muscles following an acute destruction of the right peripheral vestibular horizontal semicircular canal. The eyes will be pulled (slow phase) toward the side of the weaker neural discharge, whereas the fast phase of the nystagmic response will be in the direction opposite the weaker neural output. This would represent a left-beating nystagmus (slow phase to the right and fast phase to the left).

slow phase usually is generated within the vestibular end organs. Even though the vestibular (slow) phase of the nystagmus is of primary interest to the clinician, it is the fast phase that determines the direction in which the nystagmus is said to "beat." For example, an acute, right, peripheral vestibular lesion that creates a spontaneous nystagmus with the slow phase to the right and fast phase to the left (Figure 15.4B) is considered a left-beating spontaneous nystagmus. A deflection of the cupula toward the utricle creates an excitation voltage that is higher than the corresponding inhibited voltage created by the opposite cupula deflecting away from the utricle.

For the reader who desires a more in-depth discussion of vestibular/ocular motor anatomy and physiology, the work of Leigh and Zee (1983), Baloh and Honrubia (1982), and Barber and Stockwell (1980) are recommended highly.

Electronystagmography

Overview

Electronystagmography (ENG) is unquestionably the test used most commonly for the evaluation of patients with dizziness, vertigo, dysequilibrium, and various types of recordable eye movements. It consists of a battery of standard clinical neuro-otologic tests that have been used by physicians for many years (Coats, 1975). The primary difference between these two methods is that the eye movements elicited during the ENG are recorded either on a strip chart recorder or by a computer for more precise analysis. This method increases the sensitivity of the response measurement and enhances the effectiveness of each test. In addition, the ENG procedure records eye movements behind closed lids, thus eliminating the effect of visual suppression.

Electrodes are placed on the forehead (Figure 15.5), at the outer and inner canthi (for horizontal recordings), and above and below one eye (for vertical recordings). The electrodes should be positioned (as close to the eyes as possible) so that straight lines can be drawn to intersect at the center of the pupil. As the eyes move horizontally or vertically, the positive pole (cornea) of one eye moves closer to or further from the electrodes. The change in polarity is detected by the electrodes, transmitted to the strip-chart recorder, and the recorder pen is deflected in a manner that corresponds to the degree and direction of eye displacement (Figure 15.6). In this example, when the eyes are straight ahead,

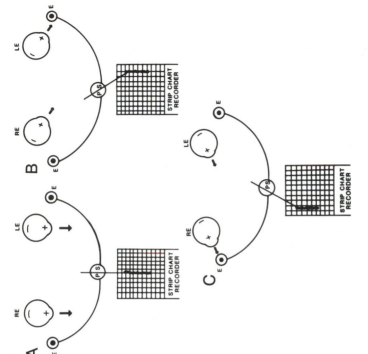

Figure 15.6. Eye-to-recorder connection. A = center gaze; B = gaze to patient's left; C = gaze to patient's right. The pen is deflected as the positive/negative pole of the eyes moves further from or closer to the electrodes. This is the principle of the EOG recording used for most ENG procedures.

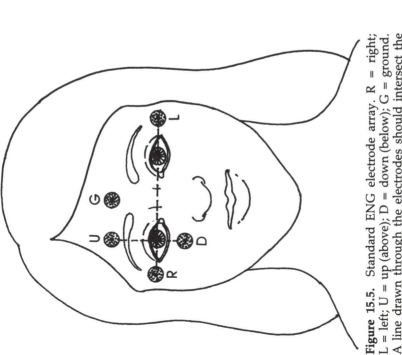

Figure 15.5. Standard ENG electrode array. R = right; L = left; U = up (above); D = down (below); G = ground. A line drawn through the electrodes should intersect the center of the pupil.

the position of the pen is in the center of the chart (Figure 15.6A). When the eyes move either to the right or left (Figure 15.6B and 15.6C), the pen moves to either side of the center position. For horizontal eye movements, upward pen deflections reflect rightward eye movements and downward pen deflections reflect leftward eye movements. For vertical eye movements, the eye and pen deviation occurs in the same direction.

The effectiveness of ENG as a clinical test depends on several factors. Recognizing the limitations of the test is prerequisite to understanding its diagnostic contributions. ENG deals primarily with only one of the major vestibular tracts, namely, the vestibular-ocular reflex pathway (VOR). The various subtests that comprise the clinical ENG essentially ignore the vestibular-spinal tracts. In addition, stimulation of the vestibular end organs, either by temperature change (caloric test) or by head/body acceleration (rotary chair test) is limited to the horizontal semicircular canals and superior branch of the vestibular nerves. The remaining semicircular canals (anterior and posterior), otolith organs (utricle and saccule), and the inferior branch of the vestibular nerves are not stimulated directly with standard ENG subtests. As a result, ENG is capable of providing limited information about total vestibular system function. This fact, accompanied by considerable variability in test administration and interpretation, has negated some of the overall effectiveness and general acceptance of ENG.

The purpose of ENG is not to diagnose or identify specific pathologies. Rather, the test is applied (a) to the detection of organic pathology within at least a portion of the vestibular system, (b) to the monitoring of change in vestibular function, and, to a degree, (c) to the identification of a general site-of-lesion limited to the central or peripheral vestibular pathways. The standard ENG test battery can be divided (conveniently, although not always accurately) into two groups of subtests. These subtests are:

Central ENG Subtests	and	*Peripheral ENG Subtests*
Gaze test		Positional tests
Saccade test		Dix-Hallpike test
Pursuit test		Caloric test
Optokinetic test		
Failure of Fixation		
Suppression		
(FFS) test		

The boundary between these two groups is porous, however, because peripheral vestibular lesions can affect results obtained during the central ENG subtests and vice versa. Nevertheless, the central subtests deal primarily with the ocular pathways of the brainstem and cerebellum, including the vestibular nuclei, MLF, ocular motor nuclei, and extraocular muscles (VOR), whereas the peripheral subtests deal primarily with the peripheral vestibular organs and vestibular nerves.

The central subtests include the assessment of gaze (fixation), saccades (refixation), smooth pursuit, and optokinetics. Failure of fixation suppression (FFS), also referred to as visual suppression, is considered a central subtest, although it is assessed during the peripheral subtests of the ENG battery, usually during the caloric test. The peripheral subtests consist of the assessment of spontaneous and positional nystagmus behind closed eyes, the Dix-Hallpike maneuver for benign paroxysmal vertigo, and the caloric test.

Unlike classical audiology where an end organ (cochlear) lesion is classified as peripheral and a lesion of the auditory nerve is considered retrocochlear, vestibular lesions involving the vestibular end organs *and* the vestibular nerve are classified as peripheral. Central vestibular lesions consist of abnormalities from the vestibular nuclei through the brainstem and cortex. In other words, an internal auditory canal (IAC) acoustic neuroma (intracanalicular) would be considered retrocochlear from an audiological standpoint but peripheral for vestibular test purposes. With reference to ENG, test results from a patient with an IAC acoustic neuroma might be no different from those of a patient with Ménière disease; one a neural lesion, the other an end organ lesion.

Central subtests

Gaze (fixation) test. The function of the gaze system is to maintain visual fixation of an object on the fovea of the eye (area on the retina of greatest visual acuity) during fixed, visual gaze. The purpose of the gaze test is to identify the presence of spontaneous eye motion during visual fixation. The spontaneous eye motion consists of nystagmus normally, although other types of eye movements may be observed, such as ocular flutter (a burst of horizontal, rapid, spontaneous eye movement), disconjugate eye position and drift, and square waves (larger, horizontal, spontaneous eye movements with a pattern slower than ocular flutter). A patient with normal gaze ability should be able to maintain a steady ocular fixation when looking at fixed targets in the visual field.

During the gaze test, the patient is asked to fixate visually on a stationary target placed directly in front, 20° or 30° to either side of center gaze, and 20° or 30° above and below the central fixation point (Figure 15.7). If gaze fixation ability is affected, either by an acute, unilateral, peripheral vestibular lesion such as Ménière disease or vestibular neuronitis, or by a lesion in the brainstem/cerebellum such as multiple

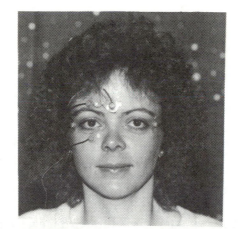

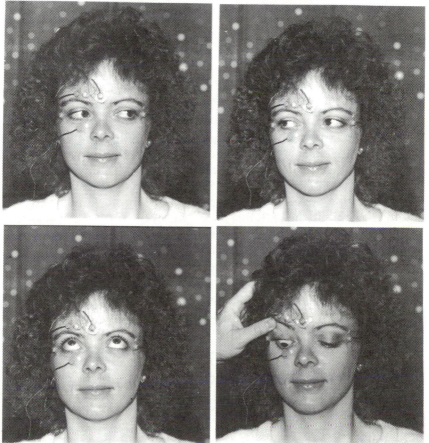

Figure 15.7.   Five directions of gaze used during ENG testing. Corner gaze is also used (not shown) during physical examination.

sclerosis, a brainstem infarction, or a large acoustic neuroma or other space-occupying lesion, a noticeable eye movement often results. As was noted earlier, the eye movement usually takes the form of a nystagmus, although other ocular movements also may be seen. If a gaze nystagmus is present, and its direction changes when the patient changes the direction of the gaze (e.g., right-beating nystagmus with right-lateral gaze, left-beating nystagmus with left-lateral gaze, up-beating nystagmus with upward gaze, etc.), it is likely that the lesion is isolated in the brainstem/cerebellum and not in the peripheral vestibular system. This is referred to as direction-*changing* gaze nystagmus (Figure 15.8A). In this case, the gaze nystagmus will beat (determined by the fast phase of the nystagmus) in the direction of the gaze. In addition, the right-beating nystagmus will be most intense the further the eyes are deviated to the right. The left-beating gaze nystagmus will be most intense the further the eyes are deviated to the left. This phenomenon is a function of Alexander's Law where the nystagmus beats most intensely when the eyes are deviated toward the side of the fast phase of the nystagmus. In the example given in Figure 15.8A, the left-beating gaze nystagmus is stronger with left lateral gaze compared to a weaker right-beating gaze nystagmus with right lateral gaze.

If the gaze nystagmus beats in only one direction (right-beating or left-beating), and horizontally, irrespective of the patient's direction of gaze, the cause likely is due to an acute, unilateral, peripheral vestibular lesion. This is referred to as a direction-*fixed* gaze nystagmus and is caused by the fact that one peripheral vestibular system is weaker in its neural output than the opposite side (Figure 15.8B). The asymmetry creates a neural imbalance in the VOR that causes the eyes to be pulled (slow phase of the nystagmus) toward the weaker ear, followed by a rapid saccade (fast phase of the nystagmus) directed toward the stronger ear. In other words, a peripherally based vestibular nystagmus will beat away from the weaker ear in most cases. Note in Figure 15.8B that a left-beating nystagmus is present in all positions of gaze (center, left, and right), although the nystagmus is strongest when the eyes are deviated to the left, in the same direction as the fast component of the nystagmus (Alexander's Law). In addition, a gaze nystagmus of peripheral origin should increase in intensity and amplitude when visual fixation is eliminated by eye closure or in darkness.

Even though the purpose of the ENG is to document the eye movement/nystagmic pattern by transferring the pattern to a strip-chart recorder or other recording device, during the gaze test, as well as for all other ENG subtests (excluding positional and caloric testing), visual inspection of the patient's eyes by the clinician is essential. Nystagmus velocity of less than 2° or 3° per second is difficult to identify on most

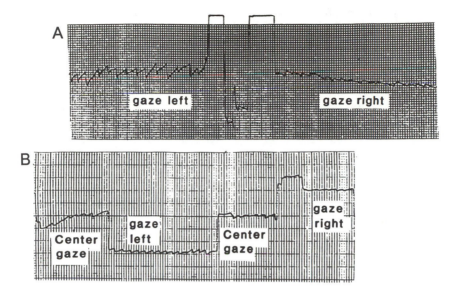

Figure 15.8. Direction-changing gaze nystagmus. Panel A: left-beating nystagmus with leftward gaze and right-beating nystagmus with rightward gaze. Panel B illustrates a direction-fixed gaze nystagmus. The left-beating nystagmus is present in all directions of gaze (center, right, and left) although the nystagmus is greatest when the eyes are deviated toward the side of the fast phase (left) and weakest when deviated toward the side of the slow phase (right).

standard ENG strip-chart recorders due primarily to the limited frequency response of the recorder and to the small amplitude changes of the signal. Most commercially available ENG recorders are designed with a limited frequency range so that extraneous neural and muscular activity will not interfere significantly with detection of the EOG response obtained through the corneo-retinal potential. However, a gaze-evoked nystagmus velocity of considerably less than 1° per second can be visualized by the human eye. If detection of gaze nystagmus is limited to the strip-chart recording alone, low-velocity gaze nystagmus often will not be identified. In addition, true rotary gaze nystagmus (i.e., nystagmus that rotates around its own horizontal axis without horizontal or vertical deviation) will not register on a strip chart recorder, irrespective of the number of surface electrodes around the eye, because the positively-charged cornea does not move toward or away from any of the electrodes in the array.

Although gaze-evoked nystagmus generally can be separated into central versus peripheral on the basis of it being either direction-fixed or direction-changing, horizontal, rotary or vertical, the specific side or site-of-lesion (cortical vs. brainstem for direction-changing; and end organ vs. nerve for direction-fixed) is difficult to determine. However, a few generalizations might be considered.

Rotary gaze nystagmus usually is consistent with a brainstem lesion, often involving the vestibular nuclei (Cogan, 1977). It is observed in such disease processes as multiple sclerosis, fourth ventricle cysts, and space-occupying lesions that distort the fourth ventricle where the vestibular nuclei are housed. Rotary gaze nystagmus has been reported in cerebellar disease as well (Zee, 1987). In very early stages of an acute, unilateral, peripheral vestibular lesion, a rotary component to the predominantly horizontal nystagmus may be present, and this should be considered whenever a patient is in an acute stage of vertigo.

Vertical gaze nystagmus is caused almost invariably by CNS disease, usually in the brainstem. Up-beating gaze nystagmus is fairly common in brainstem lesions and usually is present when the eyes are deviated upward. Down-beating gaze nystagmus, especially with lateral gaze (side-pocket nystagmus), is observed frequently in lesions of the cervico-medullary junction (Barber & Stockwell, 1980). This type of nystagmus has been noted in base-of-brain lesions such as Arnold Chiari malformation where the cerebellar tonsils are pushed down into the foramen magnum, or with a basilar artery impression at the junction of the skull base and spinal column. Down-beating gaze nystagmus has been reported also with lesions of the vestibular nuclei (Cogan, 1977) and with lesions in the flocculus of the cerebellum. This latter condition usually causes a down-beating gaze nystagmus when the eyes are in the primary gaze position as opposed to the lateral gaze position.

Periodic alternating nystagmus (PAN) is a form of gaze nystagmus that usually is present in the primary (center) gaze position (Kestenbaum, 1930). This nystagmus changes direction every 2 to 6 min and includes a null period each half cycle. That is, without the patient changing his or her direction of gaze, the nystagmus beats in one direction for a couple of minutes, stops, and then beats in the opposite direction before stopping only to repeat the cycle indefinitely. This condition often is secondary to a cerebellar lesion, although it can be seen also in patients with space-occupying or vascular lesions of the brainstem and midbrain and in many patients, no evident pathology is found. This type of nystagmus should not be confused with positional alcohol nystagmus (PAN I and PAN II).

Spontaneous ocular square waves observed during the gaze test often are caused by lesions of the brainstem/cerebellum, although this type of eye movement sometimes is characteristic of a tense or nervous patient as well. Figure 15.9A is a recording from an anxious patient who had difficulty fixating on the target. Figure 15.9B is a recording from a patient recovering from a recent brainstem infarction. The square-wave pattern

**Square waves during attempt at center gaze
(Horizontal Channel)**

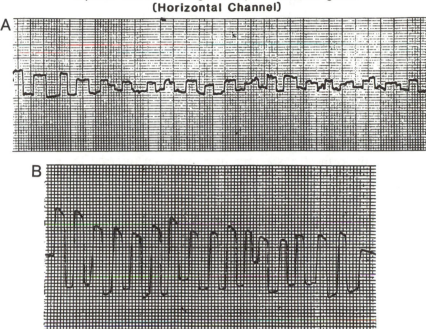

Figure 15.9. Square wave gaze pattern from an anxious patient (Panel A) and from a patient with a recent brainstem stroke (Panel B).

for this patient was present throughout the remainder of the ENG subtests, including pursuit and saccades.

During the gaze test, the presence of antiseizure medication such as Phenobarbitol, Dilantan, or Tegretol, and the presence of barbituates and alcohol should be considered since these compounds can create direction-changing gaze nystagmus and poor ocular fixation. In addition, when testing for gaze nystagmus, the eyes should not be deviated more than 30° from center gaze. Extending the eye deviation beyond this point, especially in elderly patients, can result in a physiologic ''end point'' nystagmus that does not represent actual vestibular or ocular motor disease. Patients always should be tested under a condition of best corrected vision. Eyeglasses are preferred over contact lenses because contact lenses can induce slippage and excessive eye blinking, thus creating difficulty with the detection of subtle, abnormal eye movement.

When disconjugate eye movement is present (the two eyes do not move as one), each eye should be recorded individually. This can be accomplished by connecting the electrodes of one eye to the horizontal channel of the strip-chart recorder and the electrodes of the other eye to the vertical channel. An additional electrode must be placed at the inner canthus (side of the nose bridge and eye) of each eye, and a two-channel recorder is required. Figure 15.10 illustrates the eye movement recording from a patient with dissociated nystagmus, a form of disconjugate eye movement, secondary to multiple sclerosis in this case. A left-beating nystagmus is present with leftward gaze, although it is considerably stronger in the left eye. The reverse is true with rightward gaze where the nystagmus in the right eye is much greater than in the left eye. At center gaze and during the calibration saccades, the gaze nystagmus is absent. This form of nystagmus has also been referred to as "ataxic" nystagmus (Wybar, 1952) where the gaze nystagmus in the abducted eye beats more intensely than in the adducted eye.

Saccade (refixation) test. The function of the saccadic eye movement system is to redirect the eyes from one target to another in the shortest possible time. It also corrects the retinal position error by bringing the object to the fovea of the eye as fast as possible and thus serves a refixation function. Saccadic eye movements are stereotypical and their pattern and velocity cannot be modified voluntarily once initiated.

During the saccade test, also known as the Calibration Overshoot test, the patient is asked to look between targets (usually small lights) on either side of center gaze for inspection of horizontal saccades, and above and below center gaze for vertical saccades. The targets usually are spaced 10° from center gaze, although this can vary depending on the purpose

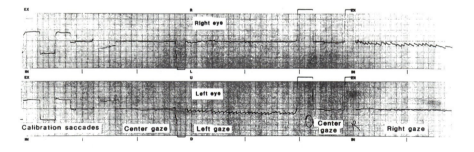

Figure 15.10. Dissociated nystagmus. Nystagmus in the right eye (top tracing) beats stronger than the left eye (bottom tracing) when the eyes are deviated to the right. The nystagmus in the left eye beats stronger than in the right eye when the eyes are deviated to the left. No nystagmus was recorded with center gaze or during the calibration saccade test.

of the test. The computerized version of this test that is described later employs the analysis of random saccades of varying amplitude. As the patient's eye movements are recorded on the strip chart, the gain (sensitivity of the recorder) is adjusted so that a 10°-eye movement is equal to a pen deflection of 10 mms on the recorder paper. The patient then is asked to look rapidly between the lights, and the examiner inspects for eye movement accuracy. Inaccurate eye movements, where the eyes either undershoot or overshoot the target is referred to as ocular dysmetria. Consistent undershoot (hypometric saccades) and overshoot (hypermetric saccades) is abnormal and seen frequently in patients with cerebellar dysfunction (Stockwell, 1979). In certain instances, hypometric saccades may be seen in normal subjects (Barber & Stockwell, 1980), although a consistent finding of hypo- or hypermetric saccadic eye movement deserves further consideration.

Once again, patients should wear eyeglasses if their vision warrants. If possible, ENG recorders should be set to the D/C mode unless the A/C mode has a time constant of at least 2 and preferably 3 s. Recorders with short A/C time constants (less than 2 s) make it difficult to separate hypermetric saccadic eye movements from eye blinks (unless vertical electrodes are used) or from the normal A/C function of the recorder returning the pen to the center of the strip chart following deviation of the eyes. Recordings from the saccade test are illustrated in Figure 15.11. A normal saccadic eye movement test should produce rapid and accurate eye movements that appear on the recorder as a clean square wave pattern (Figure 15.11A). Consistent overshooting of the target (Figure 15.11B) is seen commonly in patients with brainstem pathology, most often with involvement of the cerebellum as well. This patient overshoots primarily to the right, whereas the patient in Figure 15.11C overshoots in both directions. Figure 15.11D illustrates small catch-up eye movements in both directions in order for the eyes to reach the target. This is referred to as hypometric saccadic eye movement and is seen also in brainstem/cerebellar disease. The examiner should be aware of disconjungate eye movements, particularly internuclear ophthalmoplegia where the adducting eye moves slower and later than the abducting eye during rapid eye movements, generally with limited range of motion as well. If such a condition exists, the eyes should be recorded individually as described in the previous section on the gaze test.

Ocular pursuit test. The function of the ocular pursuit system is to stabilize a slowly moving object on the fovea of the eye by matching the angular velocity of the eye with that of the moving object. During this test, the patient is asked to watch a target that moves in a slow, sinusoidal manner (Figure 15.12A). Once again, the examiner should watch the

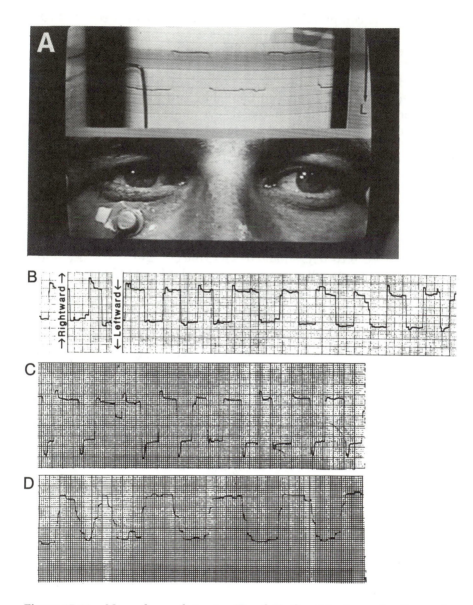

Figure 15.11. Normal saccade tracing (Panel A). Consistent overshooting to the right (Panel B) and to both sides (Panel C). Panels B and C represent hypermetric saccadic movements. Hypometric (undershooting) saccadic eye movements are illustrated in Panel D.

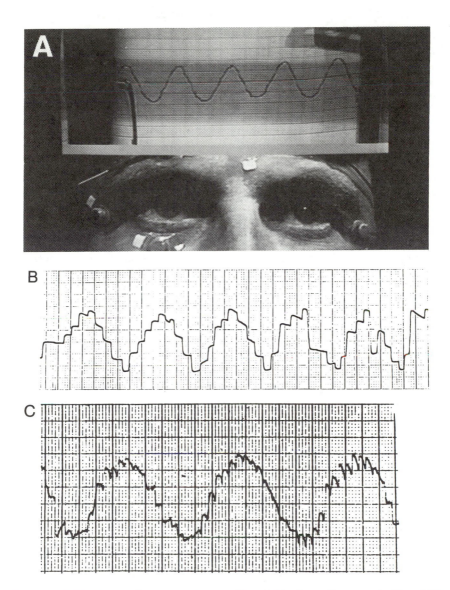

Figure 15.12. Normal pursuit tracing (Panel A). Saccadic pursuit (Panel B). Superimposed congenital nystagmus during pursuit test (Panel C).

patient's eyes during this test in addition to recording the eye motion on the strip-chart recorder. The patient should be tested under a condition of best corrected vision as is the case with all other ocular tests. When the pursuit system is impaired (Figure 15.12B), small corrective saccadic movements replace the smooth pursuit movement so the eye can "catch up" with the moving target—so-called, saccadic pursuit.

The pursuit test, or pendular tracking test as it also is known, can be affected by a variety of conditions including patient age and alertness, examiner instructions, and various medications. At times, an overriding gaze nystagmus can make it difficult to determine what portion of the abnormal smooth pursuit tracing is secondary to abnormal pursuit function per se, and what part is due to the overriding nystagmus. Figure 15.12C illustrates the effects of a superimposed congenital, ocular nystagmus. The pursuit system may be normal in this case, although the pursuit tracing is certainly not as smooth as in Figure 15.12A. Break-up of the pursuit tracing may be due to the spontaneous nystagmic activity rather than to dysfunction within the actual pursuit system.

Visual pursuit abnormalities may be caused by lesions in the brainstem, cerebellum or cortex. In addition, acute, peripheral vestibular lesions that cause a spontaneous nystagmus also may affect the smooth pursuit test and must be considered, although the intensity of the spontaneous nystagmus would have to be quite strong to have a significant effect. It is important to note that the smoothness of the pursuit tracing may be dependent on visual clutter or distraction behind the pursuit target. As a result, a clear, clutter-free background should be made available to eliminate extraneous visual cues to the patient. Nevertheless, even when several test artifacts are taken into account, sinusoidal tracking provides useful information for detection of ocular motor or central vestibular lesions. In fact, it may be the most sensitive subtest in the ENG battery for the detection of brainstem/cerebellar disorders.

With the emergence of microprocessor-based stimulus presentation and analysis systems, the ocular pursuit and saccade tests have been improved markedly over the past few years. Pursuit movements now can be assessed for gain (eye velocity/stimulus velocity), whereas saccadic eye movements can be evaluated for latency, velocity, and accuracy. This has resulted in more sensitive detection of various central vestibular system pathologies such as demyelinating disease, vascular insults, and space-occupying lesions.

A computerized version of the pursuit test is illustrated in Figure 15.13. Normal rightward and leftward pursuit is noted for frequencies ranging from .2 through .7Hz, (Figure 15.13A) where the shaded (abnormal) area represents 2 SDs. The normal/abnormal range is determined based on sex and age. Figure 15.13B is taken from a patient with a

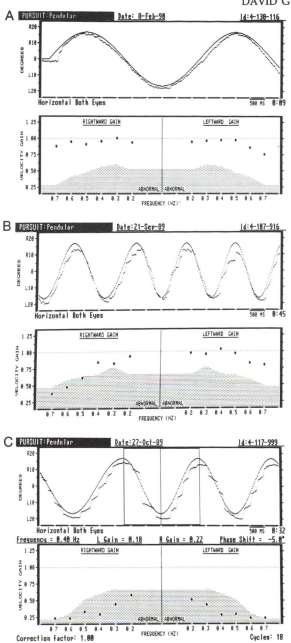

Figure 15.13. Computerized pursuit test results. Panel A: Normal patient. Panel B: Abnormal pursuit to the right and normal pursuit to the left in a patient with a right-sided brainstem lesion. Shaded (abnormal) area represents 2 SDs. Panel C: Abnormal pursuit in both directions in a patient with a large, midline brainstem tumor.

meningioma involving only the right side of the brainstem, which demonstrates normal pursuit to the left and abnormal pursuit in the high frequencies with rightward pursuit. Note the visual difference during rightward versus leftward pursuit on the top half of Panel B. Figure 15.13C illustrates abnormal pursuit in both directions from a patient with a large, midline brainstem glioma. This type of computer-assisted method eliminates much of the subjectivity in determining normalcy as is the case with the older method. Age and sex-related norms can be obtained easily with the computerized version for a more direct and accurate interpretation of pursuit function.

Computerized analysis of saccadic eye movements is illustrated in Figure 15.14. Normal saccadic velocity, accuracy, and latency is displayed in Figure 15.14A where the shaded, abnormal range represents 2 SDs. Figure 15.14B illustrates the results from a patient with spino-cerebellar degeneration with normal saccadic latency and accuracy but with a marked saccadic slowing in both directions.

Optokinetic test (OKN). The function of the optokinetic system is to maintain visual fixation when the head is in motion. This system compliments the vestibular system in this regard but functions primarily at frequencies lower than those of the vestibular system. The optokinetic test is performed by having the patient fixate visually on horizontal and vertical-moving stripes or objects. This task creates a nystagmus similar to that obtained during head rotation or following caloric irrigation. Optokinetic abnormalities may include an asymmetrical nystagmic response, a low-amplitude response, or poor nystagmic waveform morphology.

Isolated optokinetic abnormalities are said to be cortical although when they appear in conjunction with a direction-changing gaze nystagmus, the lesion is said to be in the brainstem or cerebellum (Coats, 1975). This can be expanded on somewhat in that an abnormal optokinetic response (when the lesion is in the brainstem) may be more commonly asymmetrical because of the presence of the gaze nystagmus as opposed to involvement of the cortical optokinetic pathways. In addition, a spontaneous nystagmus generated from an acute unilateral, peripheral vestibular lesion can cause an optokinetic asymmetry that is dominant in the direction of the peripheral spontaneous nystagmus. Figure 15.15A illustrates a normal OKN tracing, whereas Figures 15.15B and 15.15C show an OKN asymmetry secondary to an acute, unilateral (left), peripheral vestibular lesion. The degree of asymmetry increases with the OKN target speed. The optokinetic stimulus adds to the right-beating spontaneous nystagmus in one direction and subtracts from it in the opposite direction, thus creating or contributing to the asymmetry. Unfortunately,

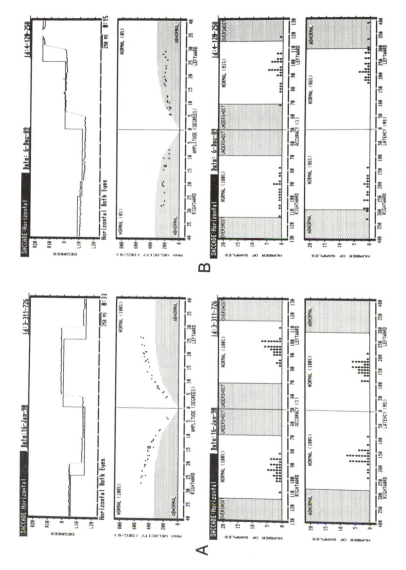

Figure 15.14. Computerized saccadic eye movement test results. Panel A: Normal saccadic velocity, accuracy, and latency for rightward and leftward eye movements. Panel B: Saccadic slowing for rightward and leftward saccades in a patient with brainstem/cerebellar disease. Saccadic accuracy and latency is normal. Shaded (abnormal) area represents 2 SDs.

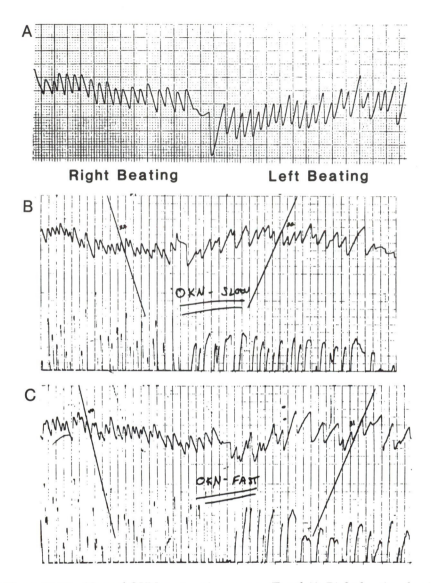

Right Beating   **Left Beating**

Figure 15.15. Normal OKN nystagmic response (Panel A). Right-beating dominant OKN response with OKN target moving at slow (Panel B) and fast (Panel C) speeds. The asymmetry of the response increases as the OKN target velocity increases. The asymmetry in this patient's recording was secondary to an acute, left, unilateral vestibular insult that caused a direction-fixed, right-beating spontaneous nystagmus.

this finding is not always consistent, and simple mathematical manipulation of the spontaneous nystagmus velocity is not always helpful.

Optokinetic abnormalities are noted in lesions affecting the visual pathways of the brainstem and cortex. Although most OKN abnormalities are secondary to slow phase (pursuit) deficits, they also can be caused by fast phase (saccade system) pathology. Instructions given to the patient often are critical in order to achieve the best possible tracing. Over-instruction, such as "follow each stripe as it moves in front of you and then follow the next stripe," may lead to a poorly formed nystagmic response, although the reverse may be true as well. As a result, various levels of instruction (beginning with brief explanations and moving to more exhaustive ones) should be considered. Often, simple instructions like "stare at the stripes" is most effective. Like the pursuit test, OKN test results may be affected by patient cooperation, and thus it is important to keep the patient on task and alert.

A potential problem to consider when performing the optokinetic test is the type of stimulus used to elicit the OKN response. The small hand-held optokinetic drums commercially available may not actually evaluate the optokinetic system. For a true test of this system, all or a majority of the visual field must be filled. If not, the patient may pursue the stimulus relative to a fixed reference point located around the periphery of the target. As a result, the OKN test may actually evaluate the ocular pursuit system as opposed to the optokinetic system. If a small stimulus is used (in the case of a digital light bar), the room should be darkened so that the only stimulus available in the patient's visual field is the optokinetic stimulus itself. This method seems to produce stronger and better-formed optokinetic responses. Once again, it is imperative that the patient have his or her glasses on during the test. Strong, measurable OKN responses are highly dependent on good functional vision and normal contrast sensitivity. These two factors may contribute to the fact that OKN responses in the elderly are occasionally weak and poorly formed. A lighted stimulus (Figure 15.16) might be more efficient for elderly patients or others whose visual acuity and contrast sensitivity may be decreased. Nevertheless, the OKN test at present is probably not specific and is replete with interpretation problems.

Peripheral subtests

Positional tests.   The static positional tests are conducted to determine if changes in head position cause or modify nystagmus. The test is conducted with the patient's head and body placed in various positions and with eyes closed, as is illustrated in Figure 15.17. The purpose of eye closure is to eliminate the effects of visual suppression on potential

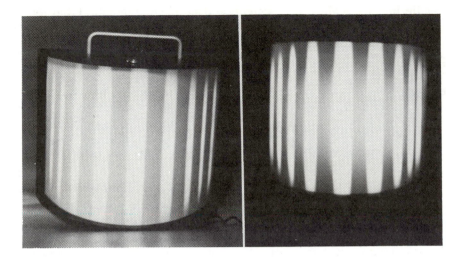

Figure 15.16. Lighted OKN stimulus used with patients who have poor visual acuity or decreased contrast sensitivity. When the room is dark, the stimulus fills most of the patient's visual field (right panel).

nystagmus. Nystagmus that is present with eyes closed during static head positions (sitting, supine, supine-head-right, supine-head-left, and supine-head-hanging) may indicate either a peripheral or central vestibular lesion; that is, positional nystagmus traditionally is considered to be nonlocalizing. A direction-fixed, positional nystagmus (the nystagmus beats in only one direction irrespective of the patient's head position) is seen more commonly in peripheral (end organ or nerve) vestibular lesions, although this type of nystagmus has been noted in a small percentage of central lesions as well. The direction-changing, ageotropic positional nystagmus (a nystagmus that changes direction when the head position changes and beats away from the down ear in the supine-head-left and supine-head-right positions) has been observed more commonly in central (vestibular nuclei and above) lesions and in bilateral, peripheral vestibular lesions (Figure 15.18). The above comments are only generalizations, however, and either type can be seen in central or peripheral vestibular pathology.

When a nystagmus is present in the sitting position and persists in other head positions without changing direction or intensity, it is referred to as a spontaneous nystagmus. If the spontaneous nystagmus changes (intensifies or changes direction) when the head is moved into other positions, the patient is said to have a spontaneous *and* positional nystagmus.

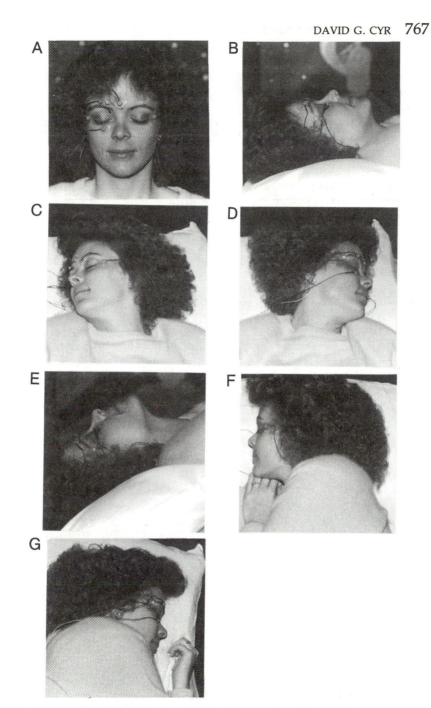

Figure 15.17. Position test. A = sitting; B = supine; C = supine-head-right; D = supine-head-left; E = supine-head-hanging; F = lateral right; G = lateral left. Eyes are closed and patient is kept mentally alert.

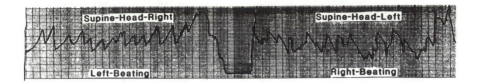

Figure 15.18. Direction-changing, ageotropic positional nystagmus. The nystagmus beats to the left in the supine-head-right position and beats to the right in the supine-head-left position. The nystagmus is present as long as the patient remains in each position.

When a nystagmus is present only in head positions other than sitting, the patient is said to have a positional nystagmus alone and it should be determined if the positional nystagmus is direction-fixed or direction-changing, geotropic (fast phase of the nystagmus beats toward the undermost ear) or ageotropic.

During the static positional tests, it is important to keep the patient in each position for at least 30 s. If a positional nystagmus is present, it should be present as long as the head is in the position, that is, nonfatiguing. If a head-lateral position (Figure 15.17C and 15.17D) causes a nystagmus, the patient should be turned on his or her side (Figure 15.17F and 15.17G) to rule out neck involvement (so-called cervical vertigo).

During all positional tests, and during rotation and caloric tests as well, it is extremely important to keep the patient mentally alert. It may be just as important, however, to use various levels of mental alerting with each patient. Although most adult subjects produce the strongest nystagmus during active alerting such as performing a mathematics task, some subjects respond better to questions, some better to tactile stimulation, and some better to no overt task. In other words, using only one specific mental alerting task (e.g., mathematics) for all patients may be as inappropriate, in some cases, as not tasking at all. Mental tasks that are too difficult can cause facial tension, eye blinking, and random, excessive eye motion that can affect the purity of the nystagmic response, thus making it difficult to identify and quantify.

Low-velocity positional nystagmus has been reported in "normal" patients (Barber & Stockwell, 1980; Coats, 1975). If the slow-phase velocity of nystagmus does not approach a certain level (6°-8°/s), it often is considered clinically insignificant. Although it may be true that many "normal" people have mild, static spontaneous and/or positional nystagmus, even a low-velocity nystagmus should be reported by the individual conducting the ENG so that the patient can be followed at the discretion of the referring physician. In cases where a low-velocity spontaneous and/or positional nystagmus is secondary to a peripheral vestibular lesion, the nystagmus is likely caused by the fact that one inner ear system is discharging at a rate different from that of the opposite side. If both peripheral vestibular systems are in fact neurologically equal, a nystagmus should not be present, regardless of velocity. When the nystagmus is secondary to a central vestibular lesion, organic dysfunction likely exists as well. In both cases, it is appropriate to note the presence of the nystagmus and its direction and velocity in each position, irrespective of how minimal the slow-phase velocity may be. Low-velocity spontaneous and/or positional nystagmus is not uncommon in early demyelinating disease, medulloblastomas and gliomas of the brainstem in children, and several other CNS lesions.

Vertical electrodes may be used during static position tests, although vertical nystagmus behind closed eyes has little apparent localizing value. On occasion, this phenomenon has appeared as an initial test finding in early multiple sclerosis and other CNS pathology, although most of the time a specific diagnosis is not made when this is the only objective test abnormality. Vertical electrodes for the detection of eye blinks is helpful because blinks often resemble nystagmic beats on the horizontal recorder channel, particularly if the recorder is set in the AC mode.

Dynamic positioning test. The dynamic positioning maneuver (Dix-Hallpike test for benign paroxysmal vertigo) is an important part of the ENG test battery, especially when patients complain of motion-related vertigo. This subtest is considered to be position*ing* rather than position*al*. Although the final position of the head is important, it is the maneuver that places the patient's head into the position that creates the response.

The phenomenon of benign paroxysmal positioning vertigo (BPPV) was described by Barany (1921) and popularized several years later by Dix and Hallpike (1952). They discovered that by moving certain patients rapidly from a sitting to a head-hanging lateral position (Figure 15.19), they were able to create a burst of nystagmus accompanied by vertigo a few seconds after the final head position was reached. Repeat maneuvers caused the response to lessen (fatigue). When a positive response was noted, the patient was said to have benign paroxysmal vertigo provided certain criteria were met. The criteria used today for a "classic" Dix-Hallpike response include a latency period of from 1 s to 10 s once the patient's head is in the position, subjective vertigo, a transient nystagmic burst, and a gradual lessening in the severity of the nystagmus and vertigo with repeat maneuvers (fatigue). If the response is determined to be classic, a benign peripheral vestibular lesion in the undermost ear is suspected. If the response is "nonclassic" (one or more of the above conditions are absent), the lesion can be either peripheral or central. Although

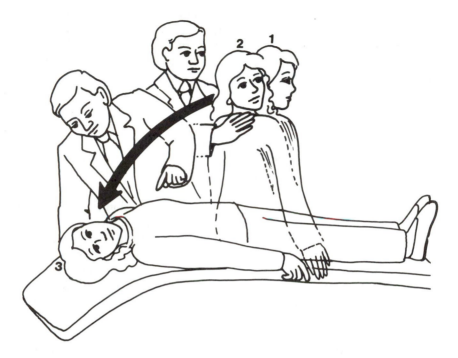

Figure 15.19. Dix-Hallpike test for benign paroxysmal vertigo. The patient is moved from the sitting to the supine-head-hanging (right and left) position. The head is turned before the patient is moved vertically.

the pathophysiology remains in question, one common theory suggests that otoconia become dislodged and fall from the utricle into the ampulla of the posterior SCC, thus stimulating mechanically the cupula of the posterior SCC when the patient performs a specific head movement such as rolling over in bed, looking upward, or bending down. This type of vertigo is arguably the most common in patients from 40 to 70 years old.

In a review of more than 1,200 patients with classical BPPV, Cyr and Brookhouser (1984) reported that a "pure" rotary nystagmus without horizontal or vertical components was present in 35% of the patients. Keeping in mind the fact that a true rotary nystagmus cannot be detected on a strip-chart recorder even with electrodes surrounding the eyes, it is imperative that the patient's eyes be monitored visually during the Dix-Hallpike maneuver. The optimal method is to observe the eyes behind lighted Frenzel lenses. If the lenses are not available to the clinician, the next favorable option would be to perform the test with the patient's eyes open and fixed. Even using this procedure, a positive nystagmic response will almost always occur with little or no effect of visual suppression, if the patient indeed has benign paroxysmal vertigo. The least favorable method is to test with the patient's eyes closed and rely on the recorder to determine a nystagmic response, given that this method will fail to identify those patients with pure rotary nystagmus. Conversely, if the nystagmic response consists of a horizontal, vertical, or diagonal component, the abnormality can be recorded behind closed eyes as is noted in Figure 15.20. Mental tasking is sometimes effective although rarely required during this test because the response is usually quite strong and unsuppressed.

During the Dix-Hallpike test, the patient's head should be turned to the side prior to movement into the down-left or down-right position. This procedure eliminates the several beats of righting nystagmus that are seen periodically even in normal patients. Neck strain is usually less with this procedure as well. True benign paroxysmal vertigo usually is present in only one head-hanging direction, although bilateral responses are noted periodically. A burst of nystagmus in the reverse direction may occur when the patient is moved back to the sitting position, although the nystagmic burst may be somewhat less intense.

It is important to perform the Dix-Hallpike test prior to the static position tests in case head-turning into the various positions fatigues the BPPV response. It is advisable to warn the patient before initiating the maneuver. Motion-induced vertigo can be frightening to many patients, and they may be more cooperative if they know about the potential response. Reassuring the patient that the response will dissipate quickly often helps to alleviate strong patient reaction as well. Speed of the maneuver is only mildly important. A moderate speed of positioning should be sufficient, especially in elderly patients and those with neck/spine problems.

Caloric tests. The bithermal caloric test has been the mainstay of the ENG battery for many years. The caloric test is a nonphysiologic procedure

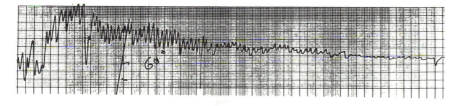

Figure 15.20. Positive nystagmic response following the Dix-Hallpike maneuver. Burst of nystagmus is followed by decay of the response. Repeat maneuvers will fatigue the overall response in a "classic" case.

used to induce endolymph flow in the semicircular canals (primarily the horizontal canal) by creating a temperature gradient from the lateral to the medial part of the canal. The standard procedure stimulates only one labyrinth at a time and the test results can be compared only within the same patient (one ear compared to the other).

The test consists of having the patient lay on a table with his or her neck ventroflexed 30° (Figure 15.21). This position places the horizontal semicircular canals in a vertical plane. A thermal stimulus, usually water, flows into the external ear canal. Water temperatures of 30° and 44° C are used with approximately 250 ccs delivered over a 30-s period. When cold water is used, the temperature is transmitted to the wall of the horizontal canal, cooling the endolymph and causing the fluid to become dense as it falls in the vertically positioned canal. This sets up a fluid motion in the canal that bends the cupula away from the utricle. The deflected cupula causes the resting neural discharge to drop relative to the opposite ear, creating a neural imbalance and resulting in a nystagmus with the slow phase toward the side of irrigation and the fast phase away from the irrigated side. The opposite occurs when warm water is used, causing the nystagmus to beat toward rather than away from the irrigated ear.

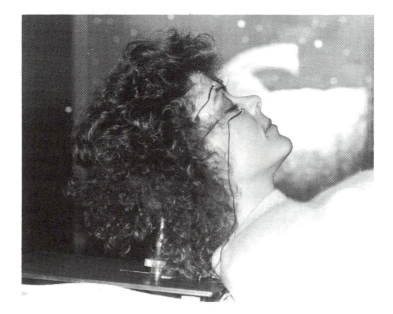

Figure 15.21. Caloric head position. The neck is ventroflexed 30° to place the horizontal SCC in a vertical plane.

The period of maximum nystagmic activity is identified (usually occurring approximately 60–90 s after the irrigation begins) and measured. The right ear warm and right ear cool responses are summed and compared to the left ear warm plus left ear cool responses to determine if a unilateral weakness (UW) exists. Right-beating (right warm + left cool) responses are compared to left-beating (left warm + right cool) responses to determine if a directional preponderance (DP) is present. Measurements of unilateral weakness (UW) and directional preponderance (DP) are made based on the following two formulas:

$$\text{UW} = \frac{(RW + RC) - (LC + LW)}{RC + RW + LC + LW} \times 100 \qquad (1)$$

$$\text{DP} = \frac{(RW + LC) - (RC + LW)}{RC + RW + LC + LW} \times 100 \qquad (2)$$

where RW = right ear warm irrigation response, RC = right ear cool irrigation response, LC = left ear cool irrigation response, and LW = left ear warm irrigation response.

In most clinics, an inter-ear difference of 20% or greater is considered abnormal for UW, and 30% or greater is considered abnormal for DP. Several methods are used to measure the slow phase velocity of the nystagmus (Coats, 1971). A simple method is illustrated in Figure 15.22 (Teter, 1983). After locating the region where the nystagmus is strongest, a line (dashed in this case) is drawn to extend the slow phase of several nystagmic beats. Another line is extended 10 mms horizontally from where it touches any vertical line. Because the paper is marked in 1 mm squares, and because the chart paper moves at 10 mms/s, 10 mms on the chart is equal to 1 s. The number of mms then is counted vertically until it reaches the originally diagonally extended line of the slow phase of the nystagmic beat. The number of mms on this vertical line determines the slow phase velocity of that beat. Figure 15.23 illustrates four caloric irrigations. Using the method described, measure the four responses to determine the percentage of UW and DP. If you perform this task correctly, you should arrive at approximately a 10% UW and 26% DP for this set of recordings.

Water caloric delivery systems have improved over systems 20 years ago. Yet the caloric test remains highly variable between and within patients for several reasons. The rather large normal range for UW (20% or greater) and DP (30% or greater) may be the result of several factors, including small but significant stimulus temperature and duration

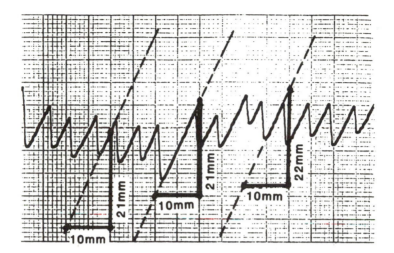

Figure 15.22.   One method used to measure the slope of the slow phase of the nystagmic response. Two beats measure 21°/s and one beat measures 22°/s.

changes, mental alerting procedures, size and shape of the external ear canal, aeration pattern of the mastoid, type of stimulus (water, air, closed loop), and operator competence. As a result, the variability of the caloric test makes it difficult to monitor subtle changes in vestibular function.

Caloric abnormalities (unilateral or bilateral weaknesses) usually reflect peripheral lesions. In a small percentage of patients, a caloric abnormality also may reflect a brainstem lesion, although this is rare. Directional preponderance is considered a nonspecific finding. In fact, most cases of directional preponderance simply represent either a spontaneous nystagmus or a positional nystagmus that is present in the caloric head position. Some have suggested that the spontaneous nystagmus be measured prior to the caloric test and figured into the caloric responses. In actuality, it is more appropriate to record and measure the nystagmus that is present when the patient's head is in the caloric position because a spontaneous nystagmus (sitting position) may have a different velocity or may beat in a direction opposite the nystagmus in the caloric position. The caloric-position nystagmic velocity is the figure that should be taken into account when calculating the caloric scores.

As was noted in the section on static position tests, a flexible approach to mental alerting also is important during the caloric test. In addition, a calibration factor (obtained prior to each irrigation) must be applied individually to each caloric response measurement (Coats, 1971). This ensures that all irrigations are compared under the same electrode impedance and

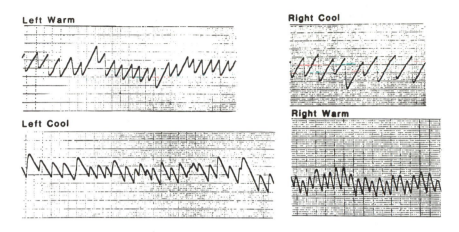

Figure 15.23. Four caloric-induced nystagmic responses. Copy the tracings and measure the responses using the method described. See text for directions.

sensitivity. Above all, each clinic should develop a set of caloric norms with whatever type of irrigator and with whatever test protocol is used. Depending on the experience of the examiner and the type of irrigator (water, air, loop), normal range in one clinic may be as low as a 10%–15% inter-ear difference, whereas another clinic may have a considerably higher range of normal caloric values. In addition, regardless of what the caloric irrigator temperature gauge reads, the examiner should check the temperature of the water at the probe tip, especially if the nystagmic responses are considerably stronger or weaker than those of other clinics.

Failure of fixation suppression (central). During the caloric test, normal patients and those with peripheral vestibular disease should be able to suppress nystagmus by opening their eyes and fixating visually on a target. Patients with CNS pathology show little difference between caloric-induced nystagmus when their eyes are open or closed (failure of fixation suppression). This ability is evaluated during the caloric test.

After the peak portion of the caloric-induced nystagmus has passed, the patient is instructed to open his or her eyes and fixate on a target at least 18 in. away (to prevent ocular convergence). Once again, this test should be conducted under optimum visual acuity conditions. Figure 15.24, Panel A, illustrates results from a patient with normal fixation suppression of a caloric-induced nystagmus. Figure 15.24, Panel B, is a recording from a patient with a brainstem medulloblastoma. There appears to be a slight reduction in the nystagmic activity when his eyes are open

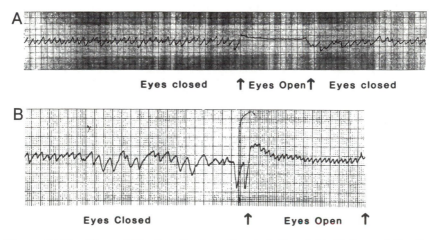

Eyes closed ↑ Eyes Open↑ Eyes closed

Eyes Closed ↑ Eyes Open ↑

Figure 15.24. Normal Fixation Suppression test (Panel A). Failure of Fixation Suppression (FFS) is illustrated in (Panel B). Nystagmic velocity remains virtually unchanged when the eyes are opened, although there is a reduction in the amplitude of the response.

and fixed, although not to the extent we would expect if this patient had a clear-cut peripheral vestibular lesion. A reduction in the nystagmus velocity of at least 40% should be achieved when the patient's eyes are open and fixed for fixation suppression to be considered normal. Failure of fixation suppression (FFS) is a strong indication of CNS (cerebellar/brainstem) disease, although the examiner should ensure that the patient has the functional visual acuity required to perform the test effectively.

Computer-assisted analysis of positional and caloric-induced nystagmus is also being used extensively. For a more thorough review of computerized ENG, see Stockwell (1988), and for additional information on nystagmus and ocular motor systems, the reader is referred to Cogan (1977), Leigh and Zee (1983), Zee (1985), Daroff and Del-Osso (1976) and Robinson (1964, 1965).

Table 15.1 provides a general guideline as to type of ENG abnormalities broken down into (a) peripheral vestibular, (b) central vestibular, and (c) abnormal but nonlocalizing. The table is meant to be a *general* guideline only because many exceptions are noted for each category.

Rotational tests

In addition to stimulation of the vestibular system by temperature change within the inner ear fluid (caloric test), a similar nystagmic response can

TABLE 15.1
Summary Table of ENG Abnormality and Suspected Site-of-Lesion.
This Must Be Used With Caution as Exceptions to the Rule May Occur.

Test	Type of Abnormality	Suspected Site-of-Lesion
Saccade	Ipsilateral dysmetria	Cerebellopontine angle
	Bilateral dysmetria	Cerebellum
	Decreased velocity	Throughout the CNS, muscle weakness or peripheral nerve palsy
	Internuclear ophthalmoplegia	Medial longitudinal fasciculus
Pursuit	Break-up	Brainstem or cerebrum
	Saccadic	Cerebellum
Gaze	Direction-fixed and horizontal	Peripheral vestibular
	Direction-changing and vertical	Brainstem
	Up-beating	Brainstem or cerebellum
	Down-beating	Cervico-medullary junction or cerebellum
	Rotary	Vestibular nuclei/brainstem
FFS	Less than 40% decrease	Brainstem or cerebellum
Positional	Direction-fixed	Non-localizing or peripheral
	Direction-changing	Non-localizing or central
Dix-Hallpike	Classic	Peripheral vestibular-undermost ear
	Nonclassic	Nonlocalizing
Caloric	Unilateral or bilateral weakness	Peripheral vestibular
	Directional preponderance	Nonlocalizing

be elicited by rotation of the head. In 1907, Barany described a manually driven rotary chair that produced observable nystagmic eye movements. Barany turned the patient, seated in the chair, in a rotating fashion and observed the patient's eye movements after the rotation stopped (post-rotary nystagmus). The test was performed with clockwise and counter-clockwise rotation. Numerous problems were noted during the early development of the test, including difficulty controlling the manually driven stimulus and the inconsistent effects of visual suppression and enhancement whenever postrotation nystagmus was assessed in light, with open eyes. Both problems contributed to excessively high variability between and within subjects.

The clinical use of the rotation test fell from grace somewhat because of its inability to produce repeatable results based on the stimulus/ response problems (Brown et al, 1983) and also because of the emergence of the ENG/caloric procedure. Renewed interest appeared in the 1970s (Mathog, 1972; Reder, Mathog, & Capps, 1977; Wolfe, Engelken, & Kos, 1978; Wolfe, Engelken, Olson, & Kos, 1978) based in part on the emergence of microprocessors and improved hardware. The torque-driven motors used to control the rotary chair improved dramatically, as did the computer software that controlled the stimulus and measured the perrotary nystagmic response, a more sensitive parameter than the postrotary nystagmus used earlier. Because the acceleration and deceleration of a chair could be controlled more accurately, the subsequent compensatory eye movements could be measured more effectively. In addition, the strong, accurate motors were able to compensate for weight differences between patients, a problem with earlier spring-driven torsion swing chairs.

Caloric versus rotation

Several advantages exist to the rotational chair systems when compared to the standard caloric test: (a) the rotational stimulus is less bothersome to the patient because it does not create the vertigo and vagal symptoms often associated with the caloric test; (b) the mechanical artifacts associated with delivering the caloric stimulus to the inner ear (size and shape of the external ear canal, scarring, thickness, and cross-sectional area of the tympanic membrane, aeration of the mastoid, thermal transmission through bone and soft tissue, small but significant temperature changes in the caloric stimulus, and operator experience and skill) are not factors with the rotational stimulus. As a result, a more accurate stimulus/ response relationship is possible; (c) the rotational stimulus is more natural than caloric irrigation because it attempts to simulate natural environmental motion. In addition, the nystagmic response can be measured at various acceleration levels, enabling the vestibular system to be tested over a wider portion of its operating range; (d) multiple gradations of the stimulus can be presented in a short time period; and (e) because the rotational stimulus is controlled more accurately and the response measured irrespective of the external ear canal and middle ear geometry, small changes within the vestibular-ocular reflex can be monitored more effectively.

The primary disadvantage of the rotary chair test is that it stimulates both labyrinths (horizontal semicircular canals and superior vestibular nerves) simultaneously. For example, when the patient is rotated to the right, an ampullopetal pull occurs in the right horizontal SCC (right cupula is deflected toward the center of the head) causing an increase in neural discharge from the canal. In the left horizontal SCC, an ampullofugal pull produces a decrease in neural discharge as the cupula is deflected away from the center of the head (Ewald's Second Law). The resultant neural asymmetry between the right and left horizontal canals causes the eyes to deviate slowly in the same direction as the horizontal SCC cupula deflection (towards the side of weaker neural discharge), and opposite the direction of rotation. Thus both right and left SCC systems respond mechanically and neurologically with rotation in each direction (left-to-right and right-to-left), although this situation holds for the horizontal semicircular canals only. Because of the bilateral response, each vestibular system cannot be tested independently. In order to determine the relative strength of the right and left horizontal semicircular canals, a caloric test must be performed.

Low-frequency rotary chair test

The low-frequency rotary chair test is the most commonly used rotational test in the United States. It is performed with the patient seated in a computer-driven chair that rotates around the earth's vertical axis (Figure 15.25). The chair is turned by a torque motor capable of accurate, sinusoidal acceleration and deceleration. The patient's head is tilted $30°$ forward so that rotation occurs in the plane of both horizontal semicircular canals. The chair is situated in an enclosure so that no light is present from within when the door is closed. Standard electro-oculographic (EOG) recordings are made of the compensatory nystagmic eye movements during rotation at acceleration frequencies generally ranging from 0.01Hz to 0.16Hz. Because the semicircular canal systems act as angular accelerometers, a range of acceleration frequencies is used to evaluate vestibular output over a wider portion of its operating range. The chair reaches a maximum velocity of $50°$/second for each test frequency, which results in acceleration rates from $3°/S^2$/degrees/second/second at 0.01Hz to $50°/S^2$ degrees/second/second at 0.16 Hz.

The rotary chair test protocol consists of several cycles of sinusoidal rotation at each of five test frequencies. Cyr, Brookhouser, Valente, and Grossman (1985) described a test protocol that consists of two cycles of rotation at 0.01 Hz, four cycles of rotation at 0.02 to 0.08 Hz, and eight cycles of rotation at 0.16 Hz. Total test time for all five frequencies using this protocol is approximately 12 min, a reduction in the original number

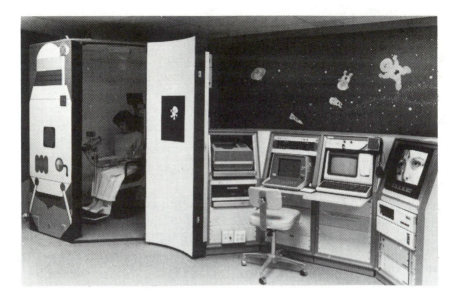

Figure 15.25.   Rotary chair test set-up. Patient is seated in the chair (in enclosure), neck bent forward to place the horizontal SCC in the horizontal plane. Infrared camera permits visual monitoring of the head and eye position and movement during the test. (Note monitor on right.)

of cycles by approximately one half. The reduction in test time negated some of the problems encountered in keeping the patient alert for long periods of time. In addition, the complaints of nausea, sometimes associated with the original, longer test protocol, were all but eliminated with the shorter test.

During the rotary chair test, the patient is kept mentally alert using a procedure that is also employed during the caloric and positional subtests of the standard ENG. Mental alerting tasks are selected that are appropriate for the age and sophistication level of the patient. Contact lenses are removed to prevent excessive blinking, thereby preventing an artificial reduction of the spectral purity of the nystagmic response. Suppressive medication is stopped 48 hours prior to the test, as would be the recommendation prior to an ENG. An infrared camera mounted to the chair allows monitoring of eye movement, head position, and patient status during the test. The infrared monitoring system is critical to the test because maximum patient alertness and cooperation must be maintained in order to produce the strongest and purest nystagmic response possible.

As the chair and patient begin to rotate, a slow, compensatory eye movement is observed in the direction opposite the rotation. The saccadic (fast) eye movement used to return the eye to the central position is eliminated via a fast Fourier transform (FFT). The slow-phase compensatory eye movement velocity is then averaged over all test cycles and compared to the average velocity of the rotating chair for rightward and leftward chair oscillations.

Rotary chair test parameters

Phase

Phase of the rotation-induced compensatory eye movement is the temporal relationship between the velocity of the head (chair) and that of the slow-phase component of the rotation-induced nystagmus. At high frequencies of head movement, the eyes move in a precise compensatory manner, although 180° out of phase. At lower acceleration frequencies, the eye movement velocity leads in reference to the chair velocity. The earlier rotary chair systems used chair acceleration as a reference when measuring phase. In this case, the eye acceleration typically lagged behind the acceleration of the chair. The more recent rotary chair systems use chair velocity as the reference for measuring phase. In this case, the eye velocity usually leads the chair velocity for sinusoidal motion. This latter presentation of test results has become the more common of the two. Figure 15.26A illustrates the phase parameter. The solid line indicates the chair velocity from right (positive) to left (negative). The dotted line represents the slow-phase movement velocity. Note that there is a phase shift (lag in this case, although phase leads are more common) for the eye velocity (R) compared to the chair velocity (S). The degree of phase shift varies as a function of acceleration frequency.

Phase leads are inversely related to rotational frequency. As the acceleration frequency decreases, the phase lead increases. A low-frequency phase lead is exaggerated in many patients with central or peripheral vestibular pathology and this phase lead will likely remain, even following compensation of unilateral vestibular lesions (Jenkins, 1985; Wolfe & Kos, 1977). This, however, may be the case only with complete loss of unilateral vestibular function. Phase probably is the most stable and repeatable parameter measured during the low-frequency rotary chair test, although it is affected strongly by gain changes and its clinical significance is still somewhat obscure.

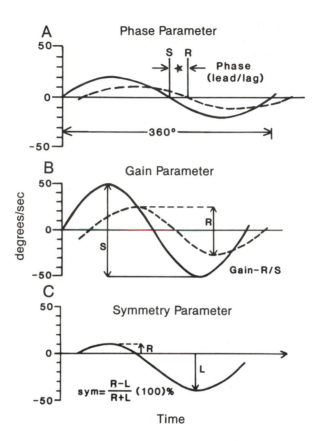

Figure 15.26. Rotary chair test parameters: phase (A), gain (B), and symmetry (C). R = response; S = stimulus for Panels A and B. For Panel C, R = rightward response, L = leftward response.

Gain

The gain parameter of the rotary chair test is the amplitude of maximum slow-phase velocity of the nystagmic eye movement compared with the amplitude of the maximum velocity of the rotating chair. In other words, the gain response is a ratio between the maximum eye velocity over the maximum chair velocity. At "natural" head movement frequencies (1–5 Hz), a gain of 1 indicates that the compensatory slow-phase eye movement velocity is equal and opposite the chair/head movement velocity. At lower chair/head velocities, the compensatory eye movement gain generally is less than the chair/head movement velocity. In other words, slow-phase eye movement velocity (in darkness) decreases when head velocity decreases. Figure 15.26B illustrates the gain parameter. The solid line (S) represents the chair rotation moving clockwise and counterclockwise at a maximum velocity of 50°/second. The dotted line (R) represents the resultant eye velocity. Because the peak eye movement velocity is approximately 25°/second, it represents a gain of 0.5 relative to the maximum velocity of the chair (50°/second). A gain of 0 is found when no eye movement occurs in response to chair/head motion.

Because gain is a performance parameter, abnormally low gain may indicate a pathological condition. Of all the parameters measured during the low-frequency rotary chair test, however, gain appears to be the most unstable because it is closely related to the patient's state of mental alertness. Because adequate gain is needed for the analysis algorithm used to calculate phase and symmetry, every effort must be made to keep the patient mentally alert. A consistent and appropriate level of mental alertness may be more critical during the rotary chair test than during the caloric test. As a result, several mental tasks should be considered for each patient depending on the patient's age and sophistication level. When the task is too simple, thus causing boredom or mental lethargy, gain may be decreased artificially. Conversely, if the task is too difficult, facial tightness (adding unwanted EMG interference), eye blinking, and random or excessive eye movements may decrease the purity of the nystagmic response, thus reducing its overall gain. If gain falls below normal levels, phase and symmetry data should be interpreted cautiously. Like the caloric procedure, however, each clinic should obtain their own normative data across a wide range of patient ages for all parameters of the rotary chair test.

In patients with acute, unilateral, peripheral vestibular lesions, gain is likely to be depressed. This finding has been noted following disease and labyrinthectomy (Jenkins, 1985; Wolfe & Kos, 1977). Following central compensation, gain appears to recover somewhat, provided appropriate mental alertness is maintained.

In bilateral, peripheral vestibular lesions secondary to ototoxicity, gain decreases as the drug-induced damage increases, although changes in phase also may be a sensitive parameter for monitoring purposes (Cyr, Moore, & Moller, 1989). Baloh, Jenkins, Honrubia, Yee, & Lau (1979) noted excessively high gain associated with cerebellar atrophy. Because the flocculonodular lobe of the cerebellum is involved in the inhibition of the VOR, it has been suggested that the high gain may be secondary to decreased cerebellar inhibition, possibly involving the vestibular nuclei. In these patients, slow-phase nystagmic velocity from caloric stimulation may be normal or even depressed.

Symmetry

With rotation to the right, a leftward compensatory eye movement occurs. A rightward eye movement occurs when the chair turns to the left. The symmetry parameter of the rotary chair test reflects the peak slow-phase eye velocity when the patient turns to the right, versus the peak slow-phase eye velocity when the patient turns to the left. This parameter is often expressed as a percentage and is illustrated in Figure 15.26C.

It must be stressed that the symmetry measure is not a definite indication of laterality (side of the lesion); rather, it is similar to directional preponderance on the caloric test. In both cases, the cause is often secondary to a spontaneous and/or positional nystagmus. In acute, unilateral, peripheral vestibular disease, the fast phase of the spontaneous nystagmus usually beats away from the weaker ear. In this situation, the rotary chair symmetry will indicate accurately a weakness on the impaired side. In unilateral, peripheral vestibular lesions where the spontaneous nystagmus beats toward the side of the disease (so-called irritative lesions), the rotary chair symmetry parameter mistakenly will indicate that the normal ear is in the involved side. A similar situation can occur also with certain chronic, unilateral, vestibular lesions such as acoustic neuroma or labyrinthine fistula, and occasionally, in early attacks of Ménière disease.

Because the symmetry parameter seems to reflect central compensation to some degree, it often is normal in compensated, unilateral, peripheral vestibular lesions. This observation is based on clinical evidence that shows the degree of asymmetry decreases as central compensation occurs. The improvement in symmetry in these cases likely reflects a decrease in the intensity of the spontaneous nystagmus, resulting in a decreased directional preponderance, another possible indication of central, physiological compensation following unilateral, peripheral vestibular disease. In addition, a spontaneous nystagmus caused by a central brainstem/cerebellar lesion may reflect an asymmetry that is unrelated to a peripheral vestibular imbalance.

Spectral purity

As was noted earlier, both the phase and symmetry measures depend to a large degree on the overall gain at each frequency of rotation (acceleration). That is, phase and symmetry measures become less accurate as gain decreases. In addition to sufficient gain, symmetry and phase depend on the spectral purity of the rotation-induced nystagmus, which is a measure of the integrity of the response. For example, excessive, random eye movements produce a significant decrease in the purity of the measured nystagmic eye movement because they introduce energy at frequencies other than that of the rotation frequency. Poor spectral purity may affect symmetry and phase measures even if gain is normal. Conversely, if gain is low and spectral purity is high, a reasonable amount of confidence can be placed in the symmetry and phase scores although caution still must be taken (Cyr et al., 1989). Consequently, every effort must be made to elicit the highest gain and purest nystagmic output possible at each test frequency if the phase/gain/symmetry pattern is to be used to monitor changes in vestibular function.

Figure 15.27 shows a Bode plot of the phase/gain/symmetry pattern of a normal patient. Responses are plotted for rotation frequencies ranging from 0.01 to 0.16 Hz. The right portion of the graph shows all symmetry responses (in percentages) are within one standard deviation of the mean. On the left side of the graph, phase (o) scores (in degrees) also are within one standard deviation on either side of the mean. Normal phase lead varies from approximately 45° at 0.01 Hz, to 6° at 0.16 Hz. The gain curve (diamond) shows that the nystagmic output (velocity) is approximately 1 SD above the mean at frequencies 0.02 and 0.04 Hz, 2 SDs above the mean at 0.01 Hz and 1 SD below the mean at frequencies 0.08 and 0.16 Hz.

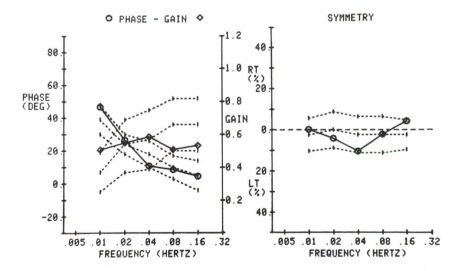

Figure 15.27. Bode plot of a normal rotary chair test at five test frequencies (0.01 Hz through 0.16 Hz). Symmetry (right side of graph), phase and gain (left side of graph). Dashed lines represent one standard deviation.

Attempts have been made to identify the site of a vestibular lesion based on the phase/gain/symmetry pattern. Although certain trends may appear, low-frequency phase leads, asymmetries, and depressed gain can be seen both in peripheral and central vestibular lesions (Baloh, 1984). As a result, it is difficult to determine site-of-lesion on a consistent basis from the parameter pattern generated during the low-frequency rotary chair test.

Clinical application

The primary strength of the computerized rotary chair test appears to be its sensitivity to monitor change within the vestibular system, particularly in the early detection of bilateral, peripheral vestibular disease (Cyr et al., 1989). Although disagreement continues about the low-frequency rotary chair test's ability to monitor physiologic compensation following a sudden, unilateral vestibular insult, some points are worth reviewing. For example, in an acute, unilateral vestibular weakness, an asymmetry usually will be present in the direction of the spontaneous nystagmus. In addition, gain may be depressed (primarily in the low frequencies) and a large phase lead should be seen. As central compensation occurs, the degree of asymmetry usually will decrease or resolve completely (probably secondary to a decrease in the spontaneous nystagmus), and gain may improve to a degree as well. In contrast, the low-frequency phase lead appears to persist in many patients (Hirsch, 1986). Our clinical experience suggests that total loss of unilateral vestibular function whether by lesion or surgical ablation, results in a permanent low-frequency phase lead, even after complete compensation has occurred. In patients with less than total loss of unilateral vestibular function, phase often returns to normal as compensation proceeds. In other words, a chronic low-frequency phase lead in compensated unilateral vestibular dysfunction, likely is related to the amount of residual function from the impaired side, although this has not been confirmed to date. Recall that the symmetry measure (degree of asymmetry) is likely to be a representation of a spontaneous nystagmus or directional preponderance, whereas gain can be affected by patient alertness and other extravestibular factors during low-frequency acceleration. For these reasons, the clinical significance of gain and asymmetry (as well as phase) during low-frequency rotation remains somewhat tenuous.

Because the rotary chair is extremely sensitive to bilateral, peripheral vestibular lesions, it is suited for monitoring the effects of vestibulotoxic medications (Cyr et al., 1989). If patient alertness is maintained, both low-frequency phase and gain can be used to monitor this type of bilateral vestibular dysfunction.

Another effective application of the rotary chair test is its use with special populations, especially infants and young children in whom caloric testing cannot be completed effectively (Cyr et al., 1985). The test is easy to administer, takes a minimal amount of time, and is not adversive to most patients unless claustrophobia is present.

Even though the low-frequency rotary chair test has specific limitations (e.g., inability to consistently identify site-of-lesion or side of involvement), it has demonstrated a significant clinical usefulness. It must be stressed, however, that the rotary chair results should be treated with a degree of caution. Our knowledge of the visual/vestibular system is limited to date, and the low-frequency rotary chair test monitors only a fraction of the VOR. We must take into account other factors such as the otolith organs (that may influence the response), the remaining semicircular canals, the brainstem integration of the response, and cognitive processes, such as prediction, that also may affect the test results (Larsby, Hyden, & Odkvist, 1984). As is appropriate with all clinical assessments, the rotary chair results, as well as those obtained with the standard ENG, should always be interpreted in conjunction with patient history, symptoms, and other test findings.

Figure 15.28 illustrates results from another type of commercially available rotary chair test system. This system includes test frequencies from 0.01 through 0.64 Hz with the shaded (abnormal) area representing 2 SDs from the mean. Panel A demonstrates normal symmetry, phase and gain at the four frequencies tested. Panel B is a fairly typical pattern of a patient with an old, compensated, unilateral vestibular weakness following a total labyrinthectomy of the left ear 8 months earlier. Note that symmetry and gain are normal, suggesting that central compensation has occurred, yet, as noted earlier, the phase lead remains in the low frequencies as is usually the case following total elimination of unilateral vestibular function. Panel C illustrates normal gain and phase although a rightward asymmetry is present. This patient also has a 12° spontaneous nystagmus and a directional preponderance on the caloric test with no unilateral weakness. The rotary chair asymmetry is the result of the spontaneous nystagmus and does not indicate a unilateral vestibular weakness. Panel D demonstrates results from a patient with a bilateral, peripheral vestibular weakness secondary to gentamicin. A caloric test showed no response in this patient, even with iced water. While nystagmic output (gain) is depressed in the low and middle rotation frequencies, the higher rotation frequencies produced normal gain. This condition is explored further in Figure 15.29. These results are taken from a patient with a gradually decreasing, bilateral, peripheral vestibular lesion of unknown etiology. Note the gradual decrease in gain over time in the higher frequencies of rotation (0.16 through 0.64 Hz) as she began to

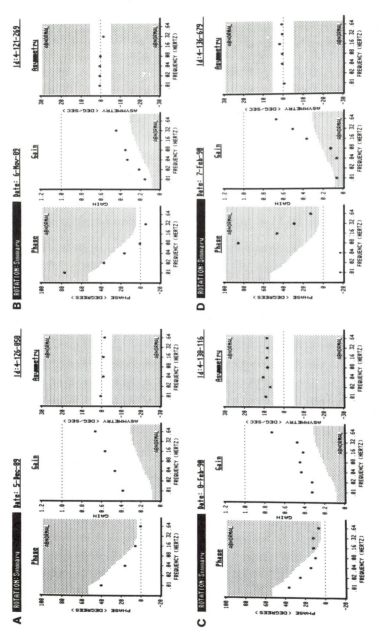

Figure 15.28. Computerized rotary chair test results. Panel A: Normal symmetry, phase and gain for all frequencies. Panel B: Low-frequency phase lead abnormality although gain and symmetry are normal. Panel C: Normal phase and gain with a rightward asymmetry secondary to a spontaneous nystagmus. Panel D: Normal symmetry, but with abnormal phase lead and low gain in the low and mid frequencies. High-frequency gain is normal although phase at those frequencies continues to show an abnormal lead.

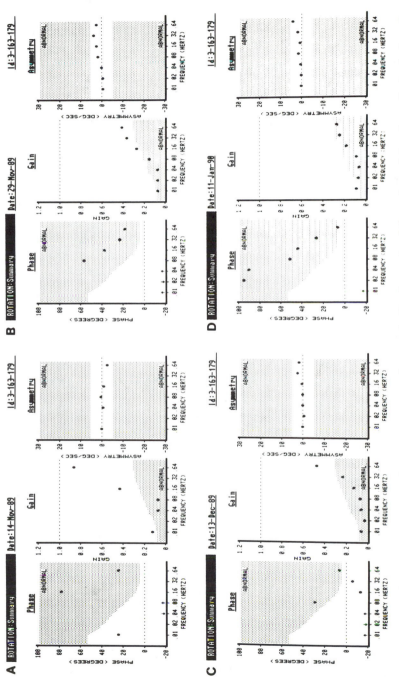

Figure 15.29. Rotary chair test results in a patient with a gradually-decreasing bilateral, peripheral vestibular lesion. Panels A through D show a gradual drop in gain in the high frequencies of rotation over time to the point where all frequencies eventually are abnormal (Panel D).

slowly lose vestibular output. This gradual loss of vestibular function was reflected also by increasingly poor on-feet balance and oscillopsia. These results further suggest that changes in vestibular output can be monitored effectively by measuring gain changes during rotation at higher frequencies, particularly when phase measurements are not available.

Computerized dynamic posturography

Overview

Dynamic equilibrium (balance and stability while in motion) is an automatic reflex consisting of both sensory and motor components (Figure 15.30). As the body moves or encounters a situation where imbalance occurs, sensory input from the vestibular, visual, and somatosensory systems is transmitted to the brain. The brain selects the accurate input(s) and attempts to ignore the input(s) that may be inaccurate. The appropriate sensory input is then selected with reference to the body position at that moment. This constitutes the sensory portion of equilibrium. Almost instantaneously, a motor response is initiated that selects the type and degree of muscle response (based on the sensory information) and generates coordinated muscle movements that allow the patient to remain stable. These corrective movements are made in a very short period of time (less than 100 ms). Motion (of a sufficient intensity) can be detected by the labyrinths in approximately 10 ms while the visual system reacts somewhat slower via retinal processing (70 ms). Still, a corrective postural movement occurs in sufficient time to keep the subject from falling, even though the brain must wait for sensory input arriving at different times.

For the patient to remain balanced with normal posture, both sensory and motor systems must be intact. As was noted earlier, human balance and posture depend on the coordinated integration of sensory input from vestibular receptors, the visual system, and pressure sensors (proprioceptors) in the feet, ankles, knees, hips, trunk, and neck. Dysfunction within any one of these three sensory systems (or the corresponding motor systems) will produce varying degrees of unsteadiness or imbalance. Although many of the patients referred for ''dizziness'' may have straightforward vestibular disease, others may have multisystem lesions. Standard vestibular tests such as electronystagmography (ENG) and computerized rotation may be insufficient for these patients, given that these tests deal almost exclusively with the vestibular-ocular reflex. The effects of vision and somatosensation are not effectively considered

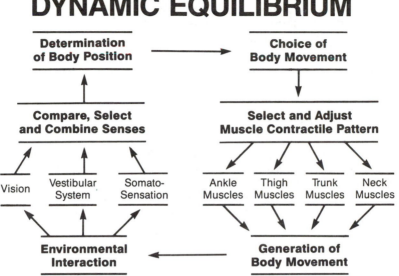

Figure 15.30. Flow chart of typical pattern of dynamic posture and balance. (From Nashner, 1987, with permission.)

with VOR tests that, as was noted earlier, assess primarily the horizontal semicircular canals and the superior branch of the vestibular nerves. The otolith organs (utricle and saccule), posterior and superior semicircular canals, and the inferior vestibular nerves are not evaluated effectively with rotation tests or ENG.

Distortion or total loss of function from any one of the three sensory balance systems can result in unsteadiness, dysequilibrium and often, a sensation of spatial disorientation. The contribution of each system is not necessarily equal. For example, in older children and adults, loss of proprioception will have a greater effect on overall balance than will loss of vision. The same may be true for young children, although this has yet to be confirmed in a controlled investigation. Whereas complete loss of vision only minimally affects equilibrium, visual distortion can have a significant effect on balance, even more so than total vestibular loss or vestibular distortion.

The impact of distorted visual input can be illustrated by the example of an individual sitting in a car at a stop sign, whose visual system notices a bus or car slowly moving nearby (so-called linear vection). The individual's reaction may be to suddenly slam on the brakes because his or her brain was falsely led to believe by the visual system that he or she was moving, rather than the nearby vehicle. Because of the numerous combinations of inappropriate sensory input the brain can receive, such as with the example noted above, it becomes advantageous to consider more than the VOR system when evaluating patients whose chief complaint is imbalance or unsteadiness as opposed to dizziness or vertigo per se.

Nashner and Berthoz (1978) and Nashner (1987) described a clinical test system (Equitest) to measure dynamic posture and balance, known generically as Computerized Dynamic Posturography or Computerized Stabilometry. The test system attempts to ferret out the effects of various sensory inputs to the brain and relate them to overall "on-feet" balance and stability. Because the effect of sensory input must be measured via a motor reaction, the coordinated muscle response also must be considered in the assessment of balance and posture. That is, the brain must not only receive appropriate input from the sensory balance systems in order for the subject to remain stable, it also might be able to integrate the inputs and initiate a coordinated motor response. As a result, both sensory and motor components of balance must be accounted for when assessing stability.

Computerized dynamic posturography (CDP) (Figure 15.31) uses a computer-controlled, menu-driven, moveable platform and visual surround. Both the platform and the visual surround are "sway referenced." That is, the platform and visual surround move to track the anterior/posterior (AP) sway of the patient as he or she stands on the platform surface. The patient's body sway is monitored by pressure-sensing strain gauges located in each quadrant of the platform. As the patient sways around his or her center of balance, the platform and/or visual surround track the patient's motion, providing an objective measure of actual AP sway. The surface platform also is able to operate independently of the visual surround. The test is conducted with eyes open and closed, creating both visual distortion as well as total elimination of visual cues. In addition, the platform can be jerked suddenly front-to-back and back-to-front to measure the patient's motor response to sudden loss of balance. The platform also performs a "toes-up" and "toes-down" movement. These latter computer-induced platform movements evaluate motor responses that include the strength (force), symmetry, and latency of muscle response. In addition, movement adaptation is evaluated with repeat platform rotations. A safety harness is attached to the patient to prevent injury should a fall occur.

The test is divided into two general areas: Sensory Organization (SO) and Movement Coordination (MC). The sensory portion of the test battery manipulates visual and proprioceptive inputs while determining the

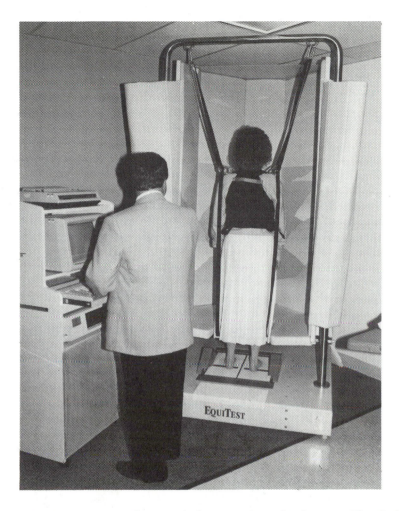

Figure 15.31. Patient standing on platform wearing safety harness. The platform contains pressure-sensing strain gauges to monitor anterior/posterior (AP) sway of the patient. The visual surround is capable of movement, as is the platform.

effect on equilibrium. The motor portion of the battery evaluates the muscle response to various computer-induced platform perturbations. In order for the effects of sensory system manipulation to be interpreted accurately, an intact motor system must be present.

Sensory organization

Six 20-s subtests are used in the SO portion of the test battery. Those six sensory conditions are shown in Figure 15.32 and Table 15.2. The first

SO condition measures patient stability while the patient stands on the platform with eyes open, hands at sides, and feet apart a comfortable distance. Both the platform and the visual surround are stationary. A baseline measure of stability is obtained, with 100% representing no body sway and 0% representing maximum sway or a patient fall. Under SO Condition 1, all three sensory systems are operational, and a high equilibrium score should be obtained. Under SO Condition 2, the test is repeated with eyes closed. Again, a high equilibrium score should be obtained, because the absence of visual cues will have little effect on balance if the vestibular and proprioceptive systems are functional.

SO Condition 3 provides orientationally inaccurate visual cues. The patient is in the same position as with SO Condition 1 (eyes open); however, in SO 3, the visual surround moves to track the AP sway of the patient. The sway is detected by the strain gauges in the platform,

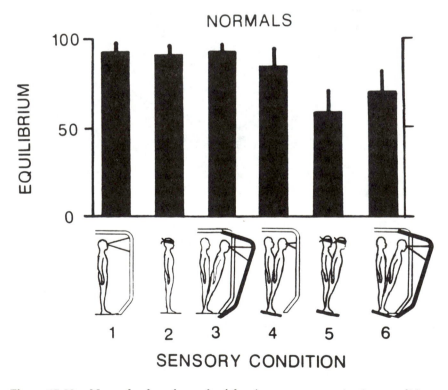

Figure 15.32. Normal values for each of the six sensory organization conditions. (From L. Nashner, NeuroCom, Intl., Portland, Ore., with permission.)

TABLE 15.2
Summary of Six Sensory Organization Conditions Reflected in Figure 15.28

Condition	Eyes	Platform	Visual Surround
No. 1	Open	Fixed	Fixed
No. 2	Closed	Fixed	Fixed
No. 3	Open	Fixed	Moving
No. 4	Open	Moving	Fixed
No. 5	Closed	Moving	Fixed
No. 6	Open	Moving	Moving

and the visual surround moves in response to the patient's sway while the platform remains fixed. Under this condition, the brain is asked to ignore the inaccurate visual input and rely on the orientationally accurate vestibular and proprioceptive inputs. Because the patient's stance is fairly wide-based, equilibrium should remain fairly normal under this condition, particularly if the vestibular system is normal as well. Condition 4 provides inaccurate proprioceptive input to the brain as the patient stands on the platform (eyes open) and the visual surround remains fixed. The platform moves in response to the patient's AP sway so that the ankle joints do not bend in response to the sway. As a result, the proprioceptive input to the brain is inaccurate, and balance must be maintained by the visual and vestibular systems. Condition 5 isolates the vestibular system more than any other condition does. This condition is identical to SO Condition 4 except the eyes are now closed. Because vision is absent and proprioception is somewhat compromised by the moving platform, balance and equilibrium must be maintained by the vestibular system. This test is more difficult than the preceding conditions because only one of three sensory systems is fully operational. Condition 6 also isolates the vestibular system but to a lesser degree than does SO 5. Under SO Condition 6, the patient stands on the platform with open eyes. The AP sway is detected by the strain gauges, and both the visual surround and platform track the AP sway. Under this condition, both vision and proprioception are compromised, and once again, the brain must ignore two inaccurate systems and rely on the orientationally accurate vestibular system. A normal sensory test is shown in Figure 15.33A.

In addition to obtaining equilibrium scores, balance strategies are measured. Under normal conditions, most people move about the ankle joint as a fixed point. This is referred to as ankle strategy, and it is the strategy of choice, provided the degree of body sway does not exceed certain limits. When body sway is increased beyond what the ankle move-

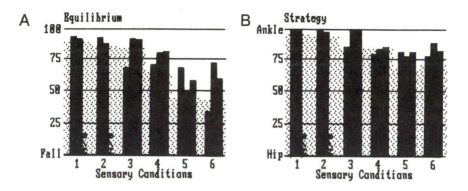

Figure 15.33. Patient results showing normal sensory organization test. Shaded area reflect 2 SD from the mean (Panel A). Normal ankle strategy for all six sensory organization conditions (Panel B).

ment can handle, the person must incorporate corrective movements by bending at the hip and/or using upper body and arm movements. This strategy would be normal for a large amount of body sway; however, it is usually considered inappropriate for the degree of body sway induced by the six SO conditions. A bar graph of normal ankle strategy is shown in Figure 15.33B.

Movement coordination

Movement coordination is the second portion of the CDP battery. During this part of the test, the platform performs sudden front-to-back and back-to-front perturbations. Three small, medium, and large forward and backward perturbations are made. The motor response to platform movement is measured to determine (a) if the patient's weight distribution during the platform perturbation was equal (static symmetry); (b) if the patient applied equal force to both feet during the platform movement (dynamic symmetry); (c) if the muscle reaction time (latency) was appropriate given the size of the platform movement; and (d) if the appropriate amount of force was applied given the magnitude of each platform perturbation (amplitude scaling). For the first determination (a & b), equal weight and force should be applied over both feet for all conditions unless an orthopedic or neurological problem is present. For the second determination (c), muscle reaction time should decrease as the platform perturbations move from small to large. For the third determination (d), the amount of force the patient applies to the platform should increase as the platform perturbations increase. As was the case with the sensory organization conditions, a balance strategy also is obtained for the movement coordination subtests.

The final subtest of the MC portion of the test battery consists of the platform performing five sudden "toes-up" and five "toes-down" movements. Under normal conditions, the amount of force applied to the platform should decrease with each toes-up or down movement. This is referred to as "adaptation," and as the patient becomes familiar with the platform movement, he or she should be able to decrease the motor response needed to maintain balance. Figure 15.34 shows a normal movement coordination test where the patient has normal weight and force symmetry and normal muscle response latencies. Figure 15.35A illustrates test results from a patient whose weight and applied force are shifted dramatically to the left. This patient is post-CVA (stroke) and was hemiparetic on the right side. Figure 15.35B shows results from a patient with an orthopedic problem on the right side (artificial hip). During weight bearing (static symmetry) he is shifted outside normal range to the left. Over time, however, this patient has learned to apply force over both feet to maintain balance as noted by the normal dynamic symmetry scores, even though his weight remains shifted to the left.

Clinical application

Computerized dynamic posturography is used for (a) patients with histories of imbalance and unsteadiness, (b) children with delayed motor development or "clumsiness," (c) neurologically impaired patients, and (d) patients with suspected organic disease where the standard VOR tests are noncontributory (Cyr, Moller, & Moore, 1988). In addition, the effects of various therapies (medical, surgical, and physical) are monitored in patients with known or suspected vestibular and or neurological disease/ dysfunction. Thus the test results can assist in planning remediation strategies for these groups of patients. In many cases, dynamic posturography is of great value in the evaluation of patients where standard VOR testing was noncontributory (Cyr & Moller, 1988).

CDP was designed to assess functional balance, not for the specific purpose of improving diagnosis via site-of-lesion detection. Nevertheless, in some cases, specific patterns have emerged that correspond to specific types of lesions. As an example, Figure 15.36 illustrates the sensory organization test results from a patient with a bilateral, peripheral vestibular weakness secondary to ototoxicity. Note the normal performance on SO Conditions 1–4 compared to SO Conditions 5 and 6 where the patient fell during each trial. Recall that SO Conditions 5 and 6 isolate the vestibular system by eliminating and/or distorting the effects of vision

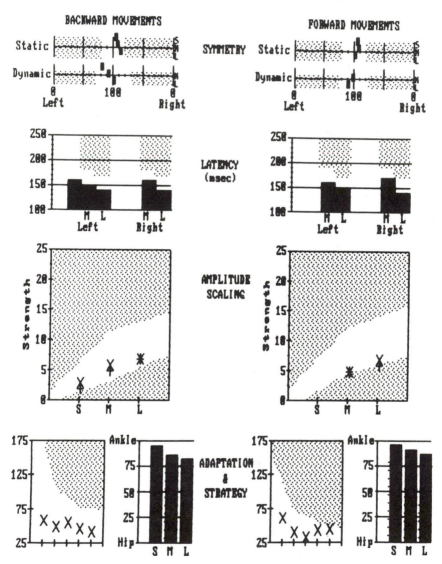

Figure 15.34. Patient results showing normal movement coordination (motor) scores for symmetry (top), latency (second from top), amplitude scaling (second from bottom), and adaptation/strategy (bottom). Shaded areas reflect 2 SDs from the mean.

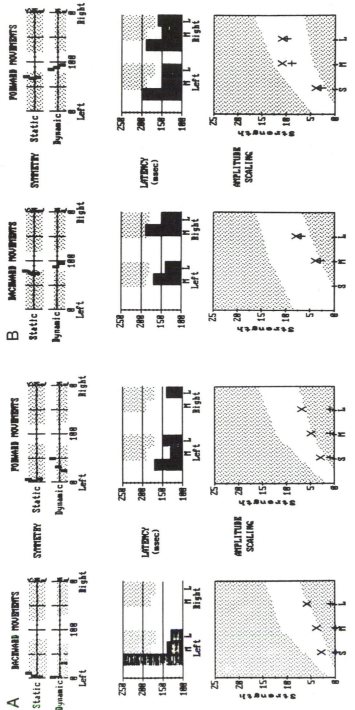

Figure 15.35. Movement coordination results from a patient who is hemiparetic following a stroke (Panel A) where weight and force are almost entirely on the left side (patient has a right hemiparesis). Test results from a patient with an artificial hip on the right side (Panel B). Note shift of weight to the left (static symmetry) although active force applied during platform motion is normal (dynamic symmetry).

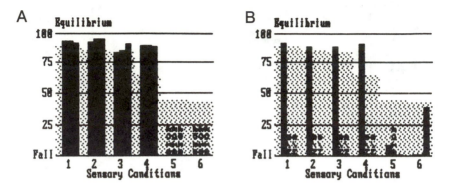

Figure 15.36. Patient with a bilateral, peripheral vestibular weakness secondary to gentamicin (Panel A). "STOP" on all three trials of sensory organization Conditions 5 and 6 indicates that the patient fell each time the test was attempted. Scores for patient with an acute, unilateral, peripheral weakness (Panel B) indicate abnormal although present function for sensory organization conditions 5 and 6. As central compensation proceeds, scores on Conditions 5 and 6 likely will return to normal levels provided all other systems are normal.

and by distorting the effects of proprioception. This pattern is observed classically in patients with bilateral, peripheral vestibular loss, although it can be observed also in central vestibular lesions. Figure 15.36B illustrates test results from a patient with an acute, unilateral, peripheral vestibular lesion (vestibular neuronitis). Again, note that SO Conditions 1–4 are normal although the patient has extreme difficulty on Conditions 5 and 6 where the vestibular system is asked to maintain balance when vision is absent or distorted and proprioception is compromised. The primary difference between these two types of patients is that those with bilateral peripheral vestibular loss will be unable to perform on SO Conditions 5 and 6, whereas those with unilateral, peripheral vestibular loss (even in an acute stage) will be able to perform to a degree on SO Conditions 5 and 6 although their equilibrium score will be abnormal. A point to note is that in older, compensated, unilateral vestibular lesions, the SO conditions (including 5 and 6) likely will be normal because functional balance returns along with physiologic compensation in most cases. These patterns depend on several factors, however, including status of the visual and proprioceptive systems, neurological deficits, orthopedic problems, duration of the condition, and prior physical therapy.

Although the primary value of this test is its ability to describe the functional aspects of balance, it is in the early stages of development at the time this chapter was written. Future consideration is being geared toward its potential diagnostic value and this may prove fruitful in time.

Computerized dynamic posturography can add significantly to the evaluation of patients with dizziness and various forms of dysequilibrium and imbalance. The test is easy to administer, requires very little time (approximately 15–20 minutes), and does not create discomfort. Although learning may be a small factor in repeated measurements, the test results appear to be repeatable, and change in on-feet stability can be monitored over time. Because of the reported high test-retest reliability, the effect of physical therapy and improvement noted following medical or surgical intervention can be quantified.

Conclusion

The purpose of so-called vestibular tests, including ENG, rotary chair, and dynamic posturography, is not to diagnose specific pathologies, but rather, to identify organic causes for the patient's symptoms. In doing so, various patterns and test findings can provide information related to which sensory or motor system may be involved, or to a general site-of-lesion within that system(s). Applying the test results in a careful, controlled manner, and considering the patient's pertinent history and symptoms, a physician may find that these clinical tests provide useful information when evaluating patients with a variety of complaints related to dizziness and/or imbalance. Granted the tests have numerous limitations. Nonetheless, they have been shown to assist in the identification of peripheral and central lesions of various types.

Acknowledgment

I wish to thank my friend and colleague Claes Moller, MD, PhD, for his many valuable suggestions and comments related to this manuscript. I would also like to thank the Mayo Clinic audiology and otorhinolaryngology staff for their comments during the preparation of this chapter.

References

Baloh, R. (1984). *The essentials of neurotology*. Philadelphia: F. A. Davis.
Baloh, R., & Honrubia, V. (1982). *Clinical neurophysiology of the vestibular system*. Philadelphia: F. A. Davis.

Baloh, R., Jenkins, H., Honrubia, V., Yee, R., & Lau, C. (1979). Visual–vestibular interaction and cerebellar atrophy. *Neurology, 29,* 116–119.

Barany, R. (1907). *Physiologie und pathologie des bogengangapparates biem menschen.* Vienna: Franz Deuticke.

Barany, R. (1921). Diagnose von Krankheitserschernungen in Bereiche des Otolithenapparates. *Acta Oto-Laryngology, 2,* 434–437.

Barber, H., & Stockwell, C. (1980). *Manual of electronystagmography.* St. Louis: C. V. Mosby.

Brown, B., Haegerstrom-Portnoy, G., Yingling, C., Herron, J., Galin, D., & Marcus, M. (1983). Dyslexic children have normal vestibular responses to rotation. *Archives of Neurology, 40,* 370–373.

Coats, A. (1971). *Manual of electronystagmographic technique.* Houston, TX: Life-Tech.

Coats, A. (1975). Electronystagmography. In L. Bradford (Ed.), *Physiological measures of the audio-vestibular system* (pp. 37–85). New York: Academic Press.

Cogan, D. (1977). *Neurology of the ocular muscles.* Springfield, IL: Charles C. Thomas.

Cyr, D., & Brookhouser, P. (1984). Diagnostic significance of ENG. Paper presented at the 7th Annual Military Audiology Conference, San Antonio, Texas.

Cyr, D., Brookhouser, P., Valente, M., & Grossman, A. (1985). Vestibular evaluation of infants and preschool children. *Otolaryngology: Head and Neck Surgery, 93,* 463–468.

Cyr, D., & Moller, C. (1988). Vestibular assessment: Case studies. *Hearing Journal, 41*(11), 50–53.

Cyr, D. G., Moller, C., & Moore, G. (1988, September). Clinical application of computerized dynamic posturography. *Ear, Nose and Throat Journal* (Supplement), 36–48.

Cyr, D. G., Moore, G., & Moller, C. (1989). Clinical experience with the low-frequency rotary chair test. *Seminars in Hearing, 10,* 171–189.

Daroff, R., & Del-Osso, L. (1976). The control of eye movements. *American Academy of Neurology,* 143–170.

DeJong, R. (1979). *The neurologic evaluation.* New York: Harper & Row.

Dix, M., & Hallpike, C. (1952). Pathology, symptomatology and diagnosis of certain disorders of the vestibular system. *Proceedings of the Royal Society of Medicine, 45,* 341–354.

Du Bois-Reymond, E. (1849). *Untersuchungen uber thiersche elektrizitat.* Verlag von G. Reimer.

Flourens, M. (1830). Experiences sur les cannaux semicirculairese de l'oreille dans les oiseaux. *Mem. Academy of Royal Sciences.* Paris, 455.

Hirsch, B. (1986). Computed sinusoidal harmonic acceleration. *Ear and Hearing, 7,* 198–203.

Hogyes, A. (1899). Neure experimentelle beitrage zur kenntnis der reflex-beziehungen zwischen ohr und auge. *Mathematikai es terme szettudo manz. Ertezito.*

Jenkins, H. (1985). Long-term adaptive changes of vestibulo-ocular reflex in patients following acoustic neuroma surgery. *Laryngoscope, 95,* 1224–1234.

Jung, R. (1939). Eine elektrische methode zure mehrfachen registrierung von augenbewegungen und nystagmus. *Klin. Wochenschr, 1,* 21–31.

Kestenbaum, A. (1930). Periodisch umschlagender nystagmus [Periodic alternating nystagmus]. *Klin. Monatsbl. f. augenh, 84,* 552.

Larsby, B., Hyden, D., & Odkvist, L. (1984). Gain and phase characteristics of compensatory eye movements in light and darkness: A study with a broad frequency-band rotatory test. *Acta Oto-Laryngologica* (Stockholm), *97*, 223–232.

Leigh, R., & Zee, D. (1983). *The neurology of eye movement.* Philadelphia: F. A. Davis.

Mathog, R. (1972). Testing of the vestibular system by sinusoidal angular acceleration. *Acta Oto-Laryngologica* (Stockholm), *74*, 96–103.

Nashner, L. (1987, October). *A systems approach to understanding and assessing orientation and balance disorders.* Paper presented at the conference on Advances in Diagnosis and Management of Balance Disorders. Boston, MA.

Nashner, L., & Berthoz, A. (1978). Visual contribution to rapid motor responses during postural control. *Experiments in Brain Research, 150,* 403–407.

Raehlmann, E. (1878). Uber den nystagmus und seine aetiologie. *Archives of Ophthalmology, 24,* 237–250.

Reder, M., Mathog, R., & Capps, M. (1977). Comparison of caloric and sinusoidal tests in the vestibulotoxic cat. *Laryngoscope, 87,* 2008–2015.

Robinson, D. (1964). The mechanics of human saccadic eye movement. *Journal of Physiology, 174,* 245–264.

Robinson, D. (1965). The mechanics of human smooth pursuit eye movement. *Journal of Physiology, 180,* 569–591.

Schott, E. (1922). Uber die registrierung des nystagmus und anderer augenbewegungen vermittels und saitengalvanometers. *Dtsch. Arch. Klin. Med., 140,* 79–90.

Stockwell, C. (1979). Electronystagmography. In W. Rintelmann (Ed.), *Hearing assessment* (459–486). Baltimore: University Park Press.

Stockwell, C. (1988). Computerized vestibular-function tests. *The Hearing Journal, November,* 20–29.

Teter, D. (1983). The electronystagmography test battery and interpretation. *Seminars in Hearing, 4,* 11–21.

Wolfe, J., Engelken, E., & Kos, C. (1978). Low frequency harmonic acceleration as a test of labyrinthine function: Basic methods and illustrative cases. *Transactions of the American Academy of Ophthalmology and Otolaryngology, 86,* 130–142.

Wolfe, J., Engelken, E., Olson, J., & Kos, C. (1978). Vestibular responses to bithermal caloric and harmonic acceleration. *Annals of Otology, 87,* 861–867.

Wolfe, J., & Kos, C. (1977). Nystagmus responses of the Rhesus monkey to rotational stimulation following unilateral labyrinthectomy. *Transactions of the American Academy of Opthalmology and Otolaryngology, 84,* 38–45.

Wybar, K. (1952). Ocular manifestations of disseminated sclerosis. *Proceedings of the Royal Sciences of Medicine, 45,* 315.

Zee, D. (1985, November). Mechanisms of nystagmus. *American Journal of Otology* (Supplement), 30–34.

Zee, D. (1987, March). Eye movement disorders in cerebellar disease. *ICS Medical ENG Report,* 1–3.

chapter sixteen

Instrument calibration

WILLIAM MELNICK

Contents

The sensation of hearing is a private experience. Audiologists can only infer indirectly what a person is experiencing by observing structured responses to specific sounds. If the inference concerning the hearing of a subject or a patient is to have any value, it must be based on accurately controlled signals. Validity and reliability of hearing assessment depend on several variables. Accuracy of the equipment used in the evaluations is one of the major variables. Although all students of the science of hearing would agree that this is completely obvious, still it is common to find audiometric equipment in clinical use whose performance has never been verified and for which there has been no provision for maintenance. Almost 20 years ago, Thomas, Preslar, Summers, and Steward (1969)

805

reported that 98% of the audiometers they surveyed did not meet the standard specifications for audiometer performance.

Problems with audiometer performance are not restricted to those attributable to aging and use. The author's own experience with audiometers that were delivered "new" for the Pittsburgh study of hearing in children was documented by Eagles and Doerfler (1961). Of five audiometers delivered by the manufacturer, none met the standard specifications for audiometers in use at that time (ASA-Z24.5, 1951). Problems were found with the tone frequency, the sound pressure output, transient audible clicks in the switching circuit, problems with tone onset and decay, harmonic distortion, attenuator linearity, and earphone failure. These were *new* audiometers!

Over the intervening few decades, clinical audiologists have been made aware of the need and importance of equipment calibration. The Occupational Safety and Health Administration regulations list periodic calibration as a requirement for acceptable industrial hearing conservation programs (OSHA, 1983). The American Speech-Language-Hearing Association criteria for adequate clinical service programs include regular calibration of audiometric testing equipment (ASHA, 1983). With the increased emphasis on the importance of equipment care and function, the calibration problems reported in the late 1960s and early 1970s should have been reduced considerably, if not eliminated. But as Wilber noted as recently as 1985, "Nothing in the current literature suggests that conditions have improved substantially" (p. 116).

The audiologist makes judgments concerning the hearing status of people that may influence medical diagnosis, subsequent medical and surgical treatment, and audiologic management of the hearing-impaired person. How these judgments can be made without assurance that the equipment is functioning as specified is incomprehensible.

The sound signal presented to the person being tested should be that indicated by the clinical instrument. The sound should be at the intensity and frequency selected by the tester. The signal should be presented to the listener in the temporal pattern dictated by the test procedure. The signal should be free from distortion and extraneous noise. The signal should be delivered only to the earphone, bone vibrator, or loudspeaker selected by the tester and not available to the listener by any other pathway. These are the reasons for calibration. Only when the audiologist is confident about the accurate performance of the equipment being used in the clinical program can appropriate judgments be made regarding the status of a person's hearing.

Calibration of equipment has come to mean testing instrument performance to assure that these devices meet designated specifications. If these specifications are not met, then the equipment should be repaired or modified to provide the required performance. Many audiologists do not have the expertise or the time to perform the electrical or mechanical repairs. Regardless of who makes the actual repairs, it is the audiologist's responsibility to ensure that the equipment is functioning properly. This chapter is concerned with providing basic information about the calibration of audiologic equipment and the acoustic environment in which audiologic measurements are made.

Standards program

The performance specifications for audiometric instruments are developed in the national voluntary standards program coordinated by the American National Standards Institute (ANSI). The standards of most interest to audiologists are developed in the American National Standards Committee, S3, Bioacoustics. This committee is supported in its work by the Acoustical Society of America. The standards are developed and written by professionals, manufacturers, and consumers for the standard. Audiologists are actively involved in the development of standard specifications for audiometers, test environments, and hearing aid performance. Note that the standards program is voluntary. There is no intent or method to force the use of the standards. If they are used it is usually with the approval of everyone concerned. Only when standards are written into legislation do they have the force of law. Standards are not static. They are constantly being reviewed and revised to reflect new information, new equipment, and new procedures.[1] In fact, ANSI requires that

---

[1] On May 23, 1989, ANSI approved a major revision of S3.6-1969 (R1973) while this book was in press. This revision will be designated S3.6-1989. Changes contained in the revision are significant and substantive and may alter some of the specifications contained in this chapter. The reader may be puzzled about why this chapter discusses material that was soon to be changed by a new standard. Revision of the audiometer standard has been in process for more than a decade. At the time of the first edition of this book, it was anticipated that the proposed revision would achieve consensus and replace the existing standard in 1979. That did not happen. Again while this revised chapter was being prepared, the new version of the audiometer standard was said to be imminent. Publication of this book could no longer be delayed, and the fact is that the publication of the revised standard could not be predicted with certainty. The decision was made to publish the chapter in its present form. Not all of the material contained in the chapter has been outmoded. Because of the unusual publication situation, an appendix to this chapter provides a brief discussion of the major features of the new standard S3.6-1989, and the important relationships to S3.6-1969 (R-1973).

each standard be reviewed every 5 years. At that time, it may be reaffirmed, revised, or abandoned. The interested audiologist should keep informed about the latest applicable standards.[2]

Core calibration equipment

Basic equipment needed for calibration of audiologic instrumentation includes (a) a voltmeter, (b) an oscilloscope, (c) a sound analyzer, (d) an electronic counter, (e) a graphic level recorder, (f) an acoustic coupler (artificial ear), (g) condenser microphones, and (h) an artificial mastoid. A typical arrangement of equipment is illustrated in Figure 16.1. This core of equipment can be prohibitively expensive for a small clinical operation. The person responsible for the audiometric equipment may choose to purchase calibration services from service laboratories or the equipment manufacturer. These services usually can be located by contacting colleagues in the area or in the larger regional university and hospital clinics.

Specific suggestions and recommendations regarding procedures for using the equipment for calibration are normally provided by the manufacturers of the test equipment and the audiometric instruments. Manufacturers have been helpful in preparing manuals for equipment users. Reading these manuals is informative concerning proper equipment use. Also, because the equipment used for calibration is electronic, these devices must be calibrated and serviced periodically as well. The equipment salesperson or the manufacturer's representative should be able to provide information concerning repair and maintenance facilities.

Voltmeter

Earphones and loudspeakers transduce electrical energy to sound. If these devices are operating within their specified physical limits, then the sound pressure wave generated will follow the waveform of the voltage applied to the transducer. Perhaps more important, from the standpoint of calibration, the output sound pressure level from the earphone or loudspeaker is directly proportional to the input voltage. Voltmeters can be used to establish whether a problem with audiometer output is an earphone problem or a problem with the electronics of the instrument. The voltmeter is used to measure the performance of the attenuator, especially at the

---

[2]Information may be obtained by writing the Standard Secretariat, the Acoustical Society of America, 335 E. 45th St., New York, NY 10017.

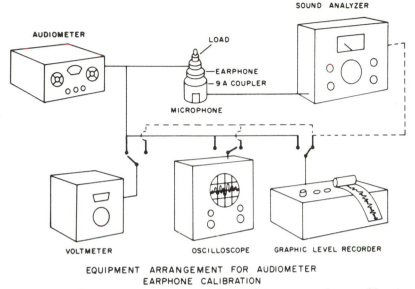

EQUIPMENT ARRANGEMENT FOR AUDIOMETER
EARPHONE CALIBRATION

Figure 16.1. Equipment arrangement for audiometer earphone calibration.

lower range of hearing level, where the acoustic signal exceeds the sensitivity of the sound measuring devices.

The voltmeter used in calibration should have a high-input impedance, usually in the megohm (million ohm) range so as not to affect the load of the circuit it is measuring. A meter that reads true root-mean-square (rms) voltage is most desirable because effective sound pressure is closely related to rms value of the sound pressure wave.[3] Another desirable feature is having a decibel scale on the meter because decibel differences in voltage are proportional to decibel changes in sound pressure. To encompass the range of voltages encountered with audiometers, the voltmeter should be able to measure voltages as much as the line voltage of 120 V to as little as 0.1 mV.

Oscilloscope

The oscilloscope is versatile and can be used as a voltmeter, timer, distortion detector, or frequency monitor. Because of its ability to follow rapidly

---

[3]The root-mean-square (rms) provides an estimate of average sound energy in an alternating sound wave. For pure tones the rms value is 0.707 times the peak value of the sine wave. RMS is essentially the square root of the square of the instantaneous voltages averaged over a given time.

changing voltages, the oscilloscope is especially useful in detecting switching abnormalities, faulty rise and decay times, pulse duration, click detection, signal overshoot, and amplitude distortion. Oscilloscopes are capable of measuring very low voltages and often are the only devices that can provide evidence of ineffective signal isolation, resulting in signal leaks or "crossover." This instrument is indispensable if a facility is to undertake electronic repair as well as calibration.

Oscilloscopes available on the market vary in operational characteristics and expense. Selection of an instrument depends on the intended use as well as budget restrictions. For audiometer calibration, desirable features would be: a bandwidth extending from DC to at least 100 kHz; voltage sensitivity ranging from 10 V/unit deflection to 0.5 mV/unit; a time base encompassing a range from 1 s/unit to 1 ms/unit; dual independent channels for comparing input and output signals; a triggering circuit capable of external as well as internal triggering. These features can be found in general purpose oscilloscopes, which are moderately priced. Oscilloscopes with signal storage capabilities are desirable. This storage facility is particularly useful for measuring temporal properties of the signal such as switching, rise-fall, overshoot, and so forth. Increasing the voltage sensitivity to handle signals in the microvolt range also would be useful, especially for detecting low-level signal leaks. However, this added sensitivity significantly increases the cost. A less expensive solution would be to preamplify the low-level input signal to the oscilloscope. There are many inexpensive preamplifiers available that would perform quite adequately when used with an oscilloscope of limited sensitivity.

Sound analyzer

The sound analyzer is basically an rms voltmeter calibrated to give measures of sound pressure level. Sometimes these devices are called audio spectrometers. Sound analyzers combine a sound pressure microphone (usually a condenser microphone), an amplifying circuit, filter networks, and a meter. Sound analyzers can be used as sound level meters for measuring basic sound levels in the test environment or noise levels in general. Usually, for this purpose, the analyzer incorporates three frequency-weighting networks, the A, B, and C scales, which simulate the 40-, 70-, and 100-phon equal-loudness contours. The A scale has become particularly useful as an index of noise levels. The sound analyzer used in calibration of audiometers also has other bandpass filter networks, which divide the sound spectrum into octave or one-third octave bands. These filters permit a finer, more precise analysis of the sound to be measured and are particularly useful in measuring harmonic distortion. When the sound analyzer is used in conjunction with specified acoustic couplers, the equipment serves as an "artificial ear" for calibrating earphone signals (e.g., air-conducted pure tones). When used with an accelerometer designed to replicate the impedance of the human mastoid, this system forms the basis for an "artificial mastoid" suitable for calibrating bone-conduction transducers.

Electronic counter

Electronic counters provide accurate measurements of time and frequency. The counter makes a comparison of an unknown frequency or time interval with a stable standard oscillation, usually from a vibrating crystal. These instruments are capable of measuring frequency to within ± 1 cycle and time intervals in the range of nanoseconds.

Graphic level recorder

Electrical events frequently occur too fast to be observed by eye or measured using a meter. Measuring devices have been developed that record the event in a more permanent form. Usually some sort of writing system is attached to a voltage-sensitive device. Chart paper is moved past the marker at specified, controlled rates so that time is represented on the chart as the horizontal axis. These devices are called graphic level recorders. The recorders are frequently designed to work logarithmically, thereby permitting the electronic magnitude to be graphed on a decibel scale. Graphic level recorders are used in conjunction with sound analyzers, providing records of sound intensity as a function of time or as a function of frequency, and are particularly useful in measuring switching characteristics of the audiometer, including onset and decay, as well as overshoot.

Artificial ear

A standard, convenient way of indicating the sound generated by an earphone is to measure, using a precision microphone, sound pressure produced in a precisely machined cavity of specified dimensions. This is accomplished by "coupling" the earphone to the measuring microphone by an enclosed volume of air, which is dictated by the volume of the cavity of the "coupler." In earphone calibration for audiometry, a coupler enclosing a volume of 6 cc is used. The 6-cc coupler was chosen because it approximates the volume of air enclosed between the earphone diaphragm and the tympanic membrane of the ear when the earphone is placed on the ear.

ANSI S3.6-1969 Standard Specifications for Audiometers designates the National Bureau of Standards (NBS) 9A coupler as standard for this purpose (see Figure 16.2). This coupler provides for making measurements of an earphone mounted in supra-aural cushions (e.g., MX41/AR). The NBS 9A coupler used in conjunction with a sound analyzer for measuring earphone response is called an artificial ear. The 9A coupler does not replicate the impedance of the human ear and so, in that sense, it is not truly an "artificial ear." Also, this coupler is not suitable for measuring earphones mounted in circumaural-cushion configurations. Thus far, no standard coupler has been proposed for measuring circumaural earphones. However, earphone configurations have been developed that incorporate a supra-aural earphone-cushion array in a circumaural enclosure. The earphones in these devices can be calibrated using the standard coupler, while the circumaural enclosure provides additional isolation from the ambient background noise (Villchur, 1970).

Until acceptable couplers for measuring sound pressure output of other kinds of circumaural earphones have been developed and standardized, the coupler method for calibration of this type of earphone for

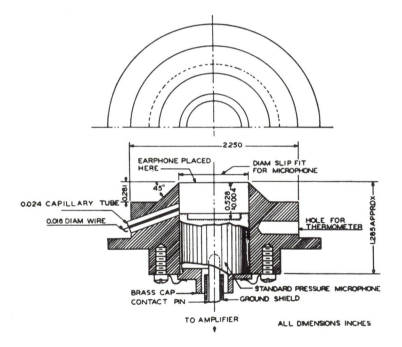

Figure 16.2. National Bureau of Standards 9A, 6-cc coupler for use in calibration of supra-aural earphones with MX41/AR or similar cushions. (From ANSI S3.6-1969, with permission of the Acoustical Society of America.)

audiometry is inappropriate (Benson et al., 1967). When the audiologist is faced with the task of assessing the output of these earphones, the loudness balancing techniques described later in this chapter can be used effectively.

Insert earphones are being used increasingly with audiometric equipment. The.9-A coupler is not appropriate for assessing performance of this type of earphone. The coupler usually specified for this purpose is the 2-cc coupler described as HA-1 in ANSI S3.7-1979, American National Standard for Coupler Calibration of Earphones (see Figure 16.3). Be aware, the output measured with a 2-cc coupler cannot be compared directly with that measured on a 6-cc coupler (Wilber, 1985). Neither of these devices represents the acoustic conditions found on real ears, nor are they equivalent to each other.

Coupler for bone vibrators

Specifications for mechanical couplers for calibrating bone vibrators used in audiometry and for making measurements on vibrators used with bone-conduction hearing aids have been published by the American National Standards Institute as ANSI Standard S3.13-1987. In this standard, design requirements are given for a mechanical coupler to be used in measuring threshold force levels corresponding to normal threshold of hearing as contained in ANSI Standard S3.26-1981, American National Standard

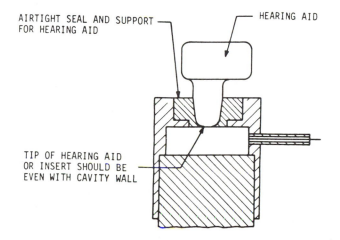

AIRTIGHT SEAL AND SUPPORT FOR HEARING AID

HEARING AID

TIP OF HEARING AID OR INSERT SHOULD BE EVEN WITH CAVITY WALL

Figure 16.3.   HA-1 2-cc coupler for calibrating insert earphones. (From ANSI S3.7-1979, with permission of the Acoustical Society of America.)

Reference Equivalent Threshold Force Levels for Audiometer Bone Vibrators. For this purpose, the bone vibrator is required to have a plane circular tip area of 175 ± 25mm² that corresponds to the characteristics of the B-71 bone vibrator, now widely used for bone-conduction audiometry. ANSI S3.13-1987 further specifies the application force to be used when coupling the vibrator to the mechanical coupler (5.4 ± 0.5 newtons). The coupler for bone vibrators would be used with equipment similar to that employed with the artificial ear, including appropriate amplifiers, filters, and sound level meters (sound analyzer). A schematic diagram of the mechanical coupler is shown in Figure 16.4.

Condenser microphone

A microphone is an integral part of most sound-measuring systems. There are many types of microphones, but a condenser microphone has several characteristics that recommend it as appropriate for calibration. These microphones have low internal noise levels, have a flat frequency response over a wide frequency range, and operate linearly over a wide range of intensities. The condenser microphone, however, has some disadvantages. It is sensitive to temperature and humidity changes. It has a high impedance and, therefore, should not be separated from the input of the amplifier by more than a few inches. The amplifier used is usually a cathode follower, an electronic circuit useful for matching high to low impedances. Frequently the microphone and cathode follower are assembled as a single unit or are housed in a single container. Other types of microphones, such as the ceramic microphone, are available and may be suitable for calibration of clinical audiometric equipment. The audiologist should be aware of the performance specifications and limitations of the microphone before selection and purchase. This information can be obtained from manufacturers' manuals and brochures.

Audiometric calibrators

There are commercially available devices that combine several instruments into one unit dedicated to calibrating audiometers. These instruments are combination "artificial ears," sound analyzers, counters, timers, and distortion analyzers in a single package designed to be operated relatively simply. This type of device may be preferable to combining several separate components into a single system, if the user does not mind sacrificing some flexibility in how the components can be used. The audiologist should be aware of the capabilities and limitations of integrated calibration systems before making a purchase. With the explosive development of computers, these devices, appropriately programmed, are being used increasingly in acoustic measurement and calibration systems.

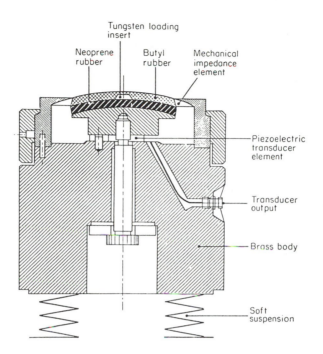

Figure 16.4. Mechanical coupler to be used for calibrating bone vibrators. (From ANSI S3.13-1987, with permission of the Acoustical Society of America.)

Pure tone audiometers

Biologic check

Although the previous section listed some expensive electronic equipment for calibration of audiometers, an audiologist can learn much about the operational status of clinical instruments by using his or her own ears and eyes and those of other clinical staff members or employees. A daily check of the equipment before clinical use will help ensure acceptable performance. A vulnerable part of the audiometer subject to the stress of handling and wear is the earphone cord. These cords should be visually inspected for cracked and worn insulation. Defects can also be detected by listening to a tone from an earphone serviced by the earphone cord while twisting and flexing the cord. A defective earphone cord will produce static or intermittent tones. Sometimes these symptoms will result because the cord is not tightly connected to the earphone, and the problem can be remedied by tightening the screws in the earphone. If this does not fix the problem, the earphone cord should be replaced. In cases where the problem still persists even when the cord has been replaced, the problem might be with the earphone itself.

Faulty performance can be detected by listening to the audiometer earphone output while manipulating the attenuator, frequency dial, and interrupter switch. Static or clicks other than those expected from switch contacts of the discrete step attenuator or the frequency selector indicate a problem that could influence hearing test results. Static when turning the attenuator could indicate dirty or worn contact points. Clicks or distorted onset or offset of the tone when the interrupter switch is depressed may mean a defective switching circuit with on-off times too abrupt to meet ANSI standards. Many of the functions previously accomplished mechanically are now performed electronically. The problem of transients introduced by mechanical switching has been reduced significantly. Hum or distracting background noise at high intensity levels both when the tone is presented and when it is off should warn the audiologist of faulty operation and a potential source of error. As the attenuation is gradually changed, the clinician should listen for gradual, systematic increases and decreases in the loudness of the signal. Abrupt shifts in loudness or no change in the tone may mean a break in the wiring of the attenuator or a faulty switch.

Listening to each tone at a comfortably loud level will provide clues about the tone purity. A raspy, brassy tone quality is an indication of tone distortion and a problem with the transducer (earphone) or the tone source in the audiometer. The clinician can isolate the cause of the problem by plugging another earphone into the suspected channel. If the distorted quality disappears, the original earphone was the culprit; if the distortion persists, the problem is probably in the oscillator.

Interchanging earphones is a good technique also when the output from one of the earphones is noticeably less than from the other earphone (right more than left or vice versa). The clinician can simply reverse the earphone connections to the audiometer. If the same channel is low, despite a different earphone, then the problem is with the audiometer circuit for that channel and not the earphone; if the same earphone continues to sound softer even when plugged into the second channel, then the problem is with that earphone.

Audiometer manufacturers go through considerable effort to isolate the output of one channel from that of any of the other channels. Nevertheless, this isolation can be faulty and a signal directed to one earphone may be heard in the contralateral earphone. This condition is sometimes called "cross-talk" or the circuit is said to "leak." This situation could produce misleading test results, especially when the hearing loss being evaluated is unilateral. Cross-talk can be detected by directing the signal to one earphone, disconnecting the earphone jack to the intentionally activated earphone, and listening for the signal in the supposedly inactive earphone. The possibility for these signal leaks exists where electrical connections for the earphones occur, at the audiometer, or at the connections to the test room. The clinician can isolate the problem by systematically plugging and replugging the earphone jacks in the several possible connections, starting with a direct connection to the audiometer.

The clinician can also conduct a periodic "biologic calibration" of the sound output of the audiometer. These relatively simple and fast checks can be made monthly or preferably at more frequent intervals and especially whenever there is a suspected problem. The method involves measuring thresholds of one or more people with previously known hearing levels in the normal range. If the threshold hearing levels change by 10 dB or more in one or both earphones, then the audiometer should be suspect and a thorough electroacoustic calibration should be considered.

Electroacoustic calibration

Electroacoustic calibration of pure tone audiometers should be made in accordance with the ANSI-S3.6-1969, "American National Standard Specifications for Audiometers," for air conduction and the ANSI-S3.13-1987, "American National Standard for a Mechanical Coupler for Measurement of Bone Vibrators" in conjunction with ANSI S3.26-1981, "Reference Equivalent Threshold Force Levels for Audiometric Bone Vibrators." It is important to note that these specifications only apply to signals transduced by an earphone or hearing aid bone vibrator. No standards currently exist for making sound field calibration measurements; however, a special section is devoted to this topic later in this chapter.

Output sound pressure level. Although there are procedures for using "real ears" to calibrate earphone output levels, these methods are cumbersome, and thus are used only in those research applications where it is necessary to specify the sound pressure level at some point (e.g., eardrum) in a "real ear" canal. Earphone calibration is most commonly accomplished electroacoustically using an "artificial ear." Standard reference equivalent threshold sound pressure levels generated by supraaural earphones fitted with MX41/AR cushions in an NBS-9A coupler are published in ANSI-S3.6-1969. This standard presents reference sound pressure levels (re audiometric zero) for the Western Electric 705A earphone and, in addition, provides equivalent levels for other commonly used earphones in an appendix. These reference threshold sound pressure levels are presented in Table 16.1.

TABLE 16.1
Reference Threshold Levels for Various Earphones

Frequency (Hz)	Western Electric 705A	Telephonics TDH-39	Telephonics[b] TDH-49 & 50	Telex 1470[c]
	Reference Threshold Levels re 20 $_m$Pa (0.0002 dynes/cm^2)[a]			
125	45.5	45.0	47.5	47.0
250	24.5	25.5	26.5	27.5
500	11.0	11.5	13.5	13.0
1000	6.5	7.0	7.5	6.5
1500	6.5	6.5	7.5	5.0
2000	8.5	9.0	11.0	8.0
3000	7.5	10.0	9.5	7.5
4000	9.0	9.5	10.5	8.5
6000	8.0	15.5	13.5	17.5
8000	9.5	13.0	13.0	17.5

[a]Adapted from ANSI-S3.6-1969.
[b]Michael and Bienvenue, 1977, and in proposal revision of ANSI S3.6-1969.
[c]Michael and Bienvenue, 1980.

The measurement of sound pressure output using the artificial ear is simple. The earphone is carefully positioned on the coupler with a 500-g load. To be sure the earphone is located properly, it should be moved slightly while on the coupler until maximum voltage (or decibel output) is read on the meter of the accompanying sound analyzer when the audiometer is set for 250 Hz at 70 dB hearing level (HL).

Measurements of threshold sound pressure levels (SPL) are not made at the zero level attenuator setting. These sound pressure levels exceed the lower limits of most sound measuring microphones. It is also difficult to find environments with ambient noise levels low enough to measure the small sound magnitude specified as normal audiometric zero. Consequently, the convention has been adopted that reference sound pressure levels are measured at a setting of 70 dB HL. For example, the standard reference threshold level for a TDH-39 earphone at 1000 Hz is specified as 7 dB SPL (see Table 16.1). With the audiometer at 70 dB HL, the sound analyzer should indicate 77 dB SPL generated in the coupler.

The standard specifications for audiometers recognize the variation of performance that exists in these acoustic instruments. Compromises have been made between the variation in output precision and the cost of the equipment. This judgment reflects professional opinion of what would constitute a significant clinical variation. The acceptance of the reality of equipment variance is evidenced by tolerances specified for each aspect of audiometer performance. In sound pressure output the present standard permits variation of ± 3 dB for the frequencies up to 3000 Hz, ± 4 dB at 4000 Hz, and ± 5 dB for frequencies higher than 4000 Hz. Based on these accepted tolerances, one should recognize that the right earphone could vary as much as 10 dB from the left earphone on a given audiometer and still meet the standard requirements for high frequencies. This tolerance should be kept in mind when assigning precision to audiometric test results and deciding what constitutes a significant change in hearing level.

As stated earlier in this chapter, standard coupler measurement for audiometers is only possible for supra-aural earphones fitted with earphone cushions like the MX41/AR. There is no approved standard for coupler measurements of circumaural earphones. At this time, the only calibration procedure for circumaural earphones is one of loudness balance (Wilber, 1985). A clinician can obtain a reasonable idea of performance by having a sample of (not fewer than six) normal hearing people make threshold comparisons and equal-loudness judgments at levels 20 to 40 dB above the subject's threshold for each test frequency. The comparison should be between the output produced by the circumaural earphone assembly and that produced by calibrated supra-aural earphones.

Attenuator linearity. Checking attenuator linearity merely means checking the accuracy of the attenuator as indicated by the demarcations on the hearing threshold level dial. This function may be checked either electrically or acoustically. The hearing threshold level dial should be adjustable in steps of 5 dB or less for pure tone signal. If the earphone can be assumed to operate linearly (output directly proportional to input) over the voltage range of the audiometer, then measuring changes in voltage applied to the earphone will provide an accurate indication of earphone sound pressure output. Changes of sound pressure level in decibels will be exactly the same as decibel changes in voltage under these conditions.

Assessing attenuator linearity is a simple matter using a voltmeter that includes a decibel scale. When measurements are made electrically the audiometer line should be loaded by the earphone itself or by a dummy load, which simulates the earphone electrically. The audiologist might prepare a special earphone cord arrangement that would allow the probes of a voltmeter to be connected conveniently to the earphone line with the earphone attached. This can be done by splicing access wires to the two wires leading to the earphone connection.

Attenuator performance is determined by comparing succeeding voltages as the hearing threshold level dial is moved through its range.

The measurement usually begins with the output at maximum and then attenuated taking measurements at each level until the entire range is sampled.

The audiologist may want to check the sound pressure output acoustically at more than just the 70 dB HL. If attenuator linearity is measured only electrically then there is the risk of missing nonlinearity of the earphone even though tests of harmonic distortion should provide clues to the existence of earphone malfunction. It is wise to measure acoustic output at as many hearing levels as the calibration equipment will permit, at least for one test frequency. This measurement will not be a problem at levels higher than 70 dB HL. Problems usually arise at lower intensities. Acoustic measures of output linearity are easier to accomplish at 250 Hz because of the higher reference threshold sound pressure levels. If the equipment calibration includes a sound analyzer with octave or one-third octave filters, it will be possible to measure almost the entire attenuator range acoustically.

The specifications in ANSI S3.6-1969 state that the actual change in attenuation measured should be within 0.3 of the indicated interval or 1.0 dB, whichever is larger. For a 5-dB step, then, an attenuator would meet the specification if the measured change is between 3.5 and 6.5 dB. The cumulative error of the attenuator cannot exceed the tolerances for sound pressure output, that is, $\pm$ 3 dB for 3000 Hz and lower frequencies, $\pm$ 4 dB for 4000 Hz, and $\pm$ 5 dB for higher frequencies.

The Bekesy-type automatic recording audiometer adds an additional complication in measuring attenuator performance. The attenuator of the automatic audiometer must meet the same specifications for linearity as a manual audiometer. The added concern with these devices is the rate at which hearing level is changed. There is no standard for this operation at this time. However, the preferred rate of change is proposed to be 2.5 dB/s. To measure performance of automatic or motor-driven attenuators, the device should be able to be stopped in operation at specific levels at the discretion of the operator. Using a timing device (stopwatch) together with measures of the amount of change in output, the audiologist can calculate easily the rate of attenuation. For example, a change of 10 dB in 4 s would indicate an attenuation rate of 2.5 dB/s.

Frequency.   The frequency of the test tone from the audiometer can be measured using an electronic counter or an oscilloscope. By using suitable connector cables, the signal from an audiometer can be connected to the counter and a measure of the frequency output can be obtained almost immediately with an accuracy of $\pm$ 1 cycle. This is by far the most convenient way to obtain the necessary information. Using an oscilloscope provides an estimate of the period of the sine wave, and the frequency of the test tone then can be calculated using the reciprocal relationship of frequency to period of the wave. The accuracy of this estimate depends on the individual's ability to estimate the period from the oscilloscopic trace and the time range of the scope. The standard for audiometers permits tolerances of ± 3% of the stated frequency in fixed or discrete frequency audiometers and ± 5% in an audiometer capable of continuous frequency change.

Bekesy-type automatic audiometers may provide continuously changing frequency or "sweep" frequency presentation. Again, there are no current standards that specify the rate of frequency change. The preferred rate for diagnostic audiometers is 1 octave/min. Some automatic audiometers offer discrete frequency testing. In these devices each frequency should be presented for a minimum of 30 s. These suggested performances can be checked easily with a timing device and a method for measuring frequency.

Harmonic distortion. Harmonic distortion may be expressed as a percentage of the output of the fundamental frequency or may be specified in terms of measured sound pressure level at higher harmonics. ANSI S3.6-1969 requires that the level of any harmonic be at least 30 dB below the output of the fundamental frequency. This specification may be checked using a sound analyzer with narrowband or third-octave filters. The harmonic distortion must be measured at the maximum limits of audiometer output for test frequencies (i.e., 125 Hz—70 dB HL, 250 and 6000 Hz—dB HL, 500 through 4000 Hz—100 dB HL, and 8000 Hz—80 dB HL). To accomplish this measurement, one selects the appropriate filter on the analyzer to measure the output at the fundamental frequency (by convention the fundamental frequency also is defined as the first harmonic). Next, the analyzer is shifted to the filter appropriate for the second harmonic (twice the fundamental), and the output should be at least 30 dB less than that measured for the fundamental. This procedure is repeated for the higher harmonics. Although the standard specification states "any harmonic," as a practical matter, only the second and perhaps the third harmonic needs to be checked. It is highly unlikely that higher harmonics will cause distortion problems if the second and third harmonics fall within the accepted tolerances.

Tone-switching characteristics. Manual audiometers are provided with tone switches for presentation or interruption of test tones. Specifications have been developed for switching characteristics that help ensure that the person being tested is responding to the test tone rather than to an audible transient or extraneous noise. These characteristics include rise time, fall time, and overshoot. Rise time is the time required for a tone to increase from the level measured when the switch is in the "off" position until it reaches the steady-state level, achieved when the tone is switched "on." Fall time is the time taken for a tone to decrease to the level measurable when the switch is turned off. When a tone is turned on it will sometimes temporarily exceed its steady-state level. This condition is known as overshoot. Verifying the recommended performance generally requires the use of an oscilloscope. Figure 16.5 is a diagrammatic representation of an oscilloscopic trace of a tone pulse illustrating the switching properties. The peak amplitudes in the diagram are connected with a solid line to emphasize the "envelope" of the tone pulse. A storage oscilloscope or a graphic level recorder will simplify the task of measuring the temporal switching patterns.

The current ANSI requirement is that the signal voltage level in the "off" position be at least 50 dB below that measured in the "on" position, or 10 dB below the reference threshold hearing level, whichever is larger. This requirement can be measured electrically with the voltmeter or acoustically with the artificial ear. The calibrated voltage and time scale of the oscilloscope will enable the audiologist to measure other time specifications for switching. These require that the sound pressure level rise (rise time) from -20 dB to -1 dB re its steady output between 20 and 100 ms. When the tone is turned off the sound pressure level should drop (fall time) 20 dB in not less than 5 ms nor more than 100 ms. Only 1 dB of overshoot is to be tolerated when the tone switch is operated.

Some audiometers incorporate the use of a tone-pulse train for the mode of tone presentation. The preferred pulse duration is 200 ms on, 200 ms off, with rise-fall requirements similar to those required for the manual tone switch. There are some clinical tests that employ tone pulses of shorter duration. The temporal properties of these signals should be verified using the oscilloscope. Some electronic counters have circuits that will permit measuring of time intervals. These devices also may be used to verify pulse duration. The counter-timers are not suitable for measuring rise-fall times.

Masking.   The clinical audiologist is well aware of the importance of masking in audiometry. The standard specifications for audiometers now in effect present minimal requirements for the masking noise. Masking is required for audiometers capable of measuring bone conduction and speech. A particular type of masking noise is not required, but ANSI S3.6-1969 suggests narrow-band masking noise in the frequency region of the test tones and/or a broad-band signal encompassing the frequency range 250-4000 Hz. Narrow-band noises are more efficient maskers for pure tones, but a broad-band noise must be used with complex test signals, such as speech. The levels of masking should be sufficient to mask

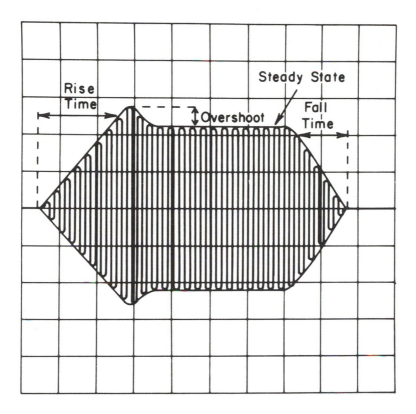

Figure 16.5. Diagram of an oscilloscope trace for a tone pulse. Solid outline emphasizes the signal envelope. Illustrated are the rise and fall time, steady state level, and overshoot.

a 250 Hz tone at 40 dB HL, a 500 Hz tone at 50 dB, and tones 1000 Hz and above at 60 dB. This performance can be verified by actually measuring the masking obtained on at least six otologically normal ears with the masking noise and the test tone being electronically mixed and applied to the same earphone. Some audiometers have this capability through the design of their switching circuitry. In audiometers where this arrangement is not available, the audiologist will need to have auxiliary electronic mixing components available (see Sanders & Rintelmann, 1964). Sometimes this requires consultation with an electronics technician.

The masking noise is not to exceed 120 dB SPL at its maximum level. This output can be established using the coupler method for measuring earphone output. The masking noise should be adjustable in levels over a range of at least 40 dB in steps of 5 dB or less. The audiologist can determine the accuracy of masking noise attenuators in the same manner as that used for pure tone signals. One deficiency of masking S3.6-1969 is the absence of a specification for accuracy of the attenuator for noise. The output for masking reasonably can be expected within ± 5 dB of the stated value.

The standard requirements and specifications for masking noise are "loose." Revisions of the standard for audiometers should include a more detailed consideration of masking noise. Nevertheless, the audiologist should be concerned with knowing how the clinical test equipment is functioning whether or not a standard calls for a specific operation. If the audiometer has broad-band white noise, this noise should have a relatively uniform (± 5 dB) spectrum level over the test frequency range and the range of the earphone. Spectrum level is the sound energy contained in a portion of the noise band 1 cycle wide. The spectrum level can be estimated by measuring the output of the white noise using the 6-cc coupler and an octave or one-third octave band analyzer. The level of the noise chosen for measurement should be sufficiently intense to avoid the effects of ambient noise and be read easily on the calibrating equipment. Spectrum level can be calculated by subtracting the contribution by the bandwidth of the particular octave or third-octave band from the measured output of noise in that band. If the white noise were truly of equal amplitude for all frequencies, then the octave band levels should increase by 3 dB as the octave bands increase in frequency. Each successive octave bandwidth doubles in frequency range. If each frequency in an octave contributes an equal amount of sound energy, the intensity should double. Doubling the sound intensity should result in a 3-dB increase in level (dB = 10 log 2). By the same calculation, each increase of a third octave should result in approximately a 1-dB increase in sound intensity when measuring white noise. This relationship of octave and one-third octave bandwidth of the sound pressure level of a white noise is illustrated simplistically by the graph in Figure 16.6.

The bottom graph in the figure represents a segment of the spectrum of white noise. The intensity is uniform for all frequencies. The intensity (I) at a given frequency defines the spectrum level (L_s) of the noise. The top graph illustrates the increase in level as the bandwidth of the noise is increased, thereby increasing the sound energy in the noise band. The audiologist should keep in mind that this relationship only holds when the spectrum level is uniform throughout the noise band. Not only can the noise vary in its spectrum but also the earphone response varies as a function of frequency. Adjustments will have to be made to account for spectral variation.

For complex weighted random noises or narrowband noises, the filter characteristics of the noise should be checked using a narrow-band wave

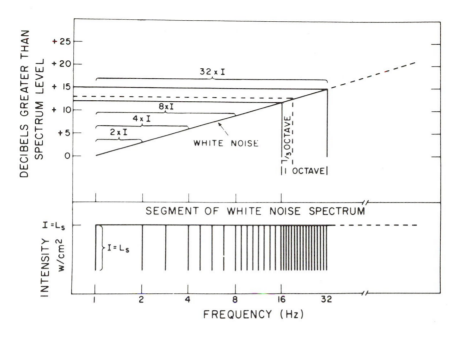

Figure 16.6. Bottom—Simplification of a segment of a broad-band white noise as a line spectrum. Top—Graph indicating increase in intensity as a noise of uniform amplitude increases in bandwidth. An increase of bandwidth by 1 octave increases the intensity by 3 dB; an increase of one-third octave increases the intensity by 1 dB. I = intensity; L_s = spectrum level.

analyzer. A reasonable approximation of the noise characteristics can be obtained with a third-octave analyzer. The noise output should be such that for 0 dB masking the sound pressure level in the appropriate band is equal to the standard reference threshold level of the noise being tested. For narrow-band noise, the recommended bandwidths change with frequency and are illustrated in Table 16.2 (Scharf, 1970).

The masking noise should be specified by effective masking. This concept corresponds to the amount of change in threshold hearing level that should be expected if the tone were to be detected in the presence of the noise when both are presented simultaneously to the test ear.

In situations where maximum isolation between the test and nontest ear is necessary, masking noise is delivered to the ear by insert receivers. These devices cannot be evaluated using a 6-cc coupler. A 2-cc coupler has been developed for use with insert earphones, and is designated an HA-1 coupler by ANSI S3.7-1973 (R1979), "Standard Method for Coupler Calibration of Earphones" (Figure 16.3). The 2-cc volume of the coupler

TABLE 16.2
Recommended Bandwidths for Narrow-Band Noise

Test Tone Frequency	Bandwidths (Hz)
125 Hz	100
250 Hz	100
500 Hz	115
750 Hz	145
1 kHz	160
1.5 kHz	225
2 kHz	300
3 kHz	470
4 kHz	700
6 kHz	1130
8 kHz	1500

Adapted from Scharf (1970).

was chosen as a first approximation to the volume of air between the tip of the insert receiver and the tympanic membrane.

Bone transducer. The standard specifications for audiometers in ANSI S3.6-1969 are vague about calibration of transducers used for measuring bone-conduction thresholds for hearing. This problem has been remedied by the publication of ANSI S3.26-1981 "American National Standard Reference Equivalent Threshold Force Levels for Audiometric Bone Vibrators" and S3.13-1987 (1987a), which, as mentioned earlier, specifies the requirements for a mechanical coupler to be used for measuring the performance of these vibrators. The purpose of ANSI S3.26-1981 is to specify bone-conduction thresholds that will correspond to threshold hearing levels adopted as standard in ANSI S3.6-1969 for the test frequencies between 250 and 4000 Hz. The published force levels are for bone vibrators with defined properties and dimensions; these specifications are met by the Radioear B-71 vibrator, now generally being supplied with audiometers. These levels are indicated in Table 16.3.

The values listed in Table 16.3 were derived on unoccluded ears using contralateral masking. The values, therefore, assume that masking of the contralateral ear will be used when obtaining the desired threshold measure. The mechanical coupler also can be used to measure harmonic distortion. With the relatively low mass of the hearing aid bone vibrator, harmonic distortion is particularly a problem at low frequencies. The

TABLE 16.3
Reference RMS Equivalent Threshold Force Levels (dB re 1 N)
for B-71 Vibrator Used With a P-3333 Headband (ANSI S3.26-1981)

Frequency	Threshold Force Level
250	61.0
500	59.0
1000	39.0
2000	32.5
3000	28.0
4000	31.0

output level accuracy of the attenuator can be verified with the output of the coupler or electrically and should follow the specifications for earphones.

Bone vibrators may present another problem that should be evaluated as part of the total calibration. Because of its construction, the bone vibrator may radiate acoustic energy. ANSI S3.6-1969 states that there should be no perceived radiation for frequencies 8000 Hz and lower. The standard specifies that threshold by bone conduction should be at least 5 dB lower than threshold resulting from air conduction of the acoustically radiated signal. This condition can be established by first measuring bone-conduction threshold and then measuring threshold with the vibrator separated from the listener's head and loaded by the finger of the tester.

Special tests

Short increment sensitivity index (SISI). This test is being used less frequently but nevertheless is still conducted by some clinics for categorizing a sensorineural loss as cochlear or retrocochlear. Although there are no standard specifications for the increments in intensity used in the SISI, Jerger, Shedd, and Harford (1959) made specific recommendations regarding the stimulus parameters for the SISI. Intensity increments of 1 dB (50 ms rise time, 200 ms duration at maximum amplitude, and 50 ms decay time) are superimposed on a steady carrier tone at 5-s intervals. For further details of the SISI refer to Chapter 13. The accuracy of these units, particularly the 1 dB increment, is of major importance to the results of the test. The increments should be checked at each test frequency at a level convenient for measurement. The measures can be made electrically and acoustically using the artificial ear. The signal can be displayed on the oscilloscope to detect switching problems or other signs of distortion as well as rise-fall times of the tone pulses. A graphic level recorder will be particularly useful for examining not only the intensity increments but the overall timing of the increments. The audiologist should listen for clicks or frequency distortion, which could serve as extraneous clues and affect the validity of the test results.

Alternate binaural loudness balance (ABLB). Alternate binaural loudness balancing requires separate control of two channels activating the two earphones and a method for switching between the two channels. This test requires a second hearing level control, which allows the manipulation of intensity for the reference tone level. The requirements for this second channel with respect to frequency accuracy, distortion, rise and decay times, on-off ratio, and output hearing level are just as stringent as those of the primary channel and should be measured in precisely the same fashion. Switching between the two channels can be accomplished manually by the audiologist or automatically by the electronics of the audiometer. Although the stimulus parameters for automatic switching have not been standardized, Jerger (1962) has proposed that the alternating tones be 500 ms and that the rise-fall times be 50 ms. These specifications have been adopted by a number of clinical programs. Chapter 14 provides the reader with more information concerning the ABLB procedure.

Speech audiometers

The speech audiometer and pure tone audiometer have many performance characteristics in common (i.e., intensity of the signal, attenuator linearity, harmonic distortion, and masking noise). The nature of the test signal poses some additional problems. Speech fluctuates in amplitude and in its temporal properties. The speech source can be either live voice, magnetic tape, or what is less frequently used, a phonograph record. Speech involves a much more complex frequency spectrum. These properties dictate other calibration procedures to assure performance meeting standard specifications for speech audiometers.

Sound pressure level of speech

Speech audiometers are required to have meters to monitor the input intensity of the test signal. These meters are called volume unit (VU) meters and must meet specifications published in ANSI/IEEE 152-1953,

"Volume Measurements of Electrical Speech and Program Waves." The VU meter is a type of voltmeter that is calibrated in decibels referred to the power of 1 mW through 600 ohms. The VU meter was designed to indicate power levels that avoid amplifier distortion and overloading the sound transmission system. In a speech audiometer the meter is placed into the circuit ahead of the attenuator so that a constant input level may be monitored despite changes in the level presented to the person being tested.

To accommodate the fluctuating properties of speech, the output sound pressure level for the speech signal is defined by a pure tone. Specifically, ANSI S3.6-1969 defines this output as the rms sound pressure level of 1000 Hz adjusted so that the VU meter deflection is equal to the average peak meter deflections produced by the speech signal. The standard reference threshold hearing level for speech is 19 dB SPL. This standard level applies to the Western Electric 705A earphone measured in a NBS 9A coupler. A more general specification has been recommended that would apply to other earphones as well. This recommendation states the reference level as 12.5 dB more than the standard reference threshold sound pressure level (audiometric zero) for a 1000-Hz tone in the earphone being measured. Thus for a TDH-39 earphone, which has a standard reference level of 7 dB SPL (see Table 16.1), the reference level for speech is 19.5 dB SPL.

Use of a 1000-Hz tone for calibrating the output for speech signals is a reasonable, expedient method when the transducers are earphones. Certainly this method is not as accurate as integrating energy in a long speech sample, but it is less time-consuming and requires a smaller equipment investment. When the speech signal is transduced by loudspeakers or by several transducers that differ considerably in frequency response, a more stable estimate of the speech signal would be provided by a broadband noise than by the 1000-Hz pure tone (Dirks, Morgan, & Wilson, 1976). Tillman, Johnson, and Olsen (1966) felt that a thermal noise shaped to simulate the long-term speech spectrum (Licklider & Miller, 1951) provided a more acceptable estimate of speech intensity. Nevertheless, since the use of a 1000-Hz calibrating tone is specified in ANSI S3.6-1969, this method should be followed when speech is transduced by an earphone.

For the live-voice mode, the source of the 1000-Hz tone can be an oscillator, amplifier, and loudspeaker combination, which produces an acoustic sine wave field. The test sound should be approximately 74 dB SPL at the microphone of the speech audiometer (ANSI S3.6-1969). The test sound source should be at the distance and orientation to the microphone (e.g., proper angle of incidence) recommended by the manufacturer. Records of speech test material, either tape or disc, should include a calibrating signal of 1000 Hz at the same level as the speech material to be used in adjusting the input level to the appropriate meter deflection on the VU meter. This signal can be used to verify the calibration output of the speech audiometer.

The output sound pressure level should be within ± 3 dB of the indicated value. Measurement of the output level should be made acoustically at the dial setting of 60 dB HL (ANSI S3.6-1969). Output at other levels can be deduced from the acoustic measure at this level and by electric measure of voltage at other settings of the attenuator.

The attenuator for speech audiometry should encompass a range from 0 dB to 100 dB in steps of 2.5 dB or less. These steps should not differ by more than 1 dB from the indicated value. The standard specifies that attenuator linearity should be checked at 1000 Hz electrically when the circuit is loaded by the earphone attached to a coupler or by a dummy load that simulates the earphone (ANSI S3.6-1969).

Frequency response

The speech signal encompasses a wide range of frequencies. Calibration of the speech audiometer should include a check of the frequency response of the device. This can be done by subjecting the microphone of the audiometer to a sound field of 74 dB SPL, with the distance and orientation of the sound source to the microphone being that recommended by the manufacturer. The sound pressure level generated by the earphone in the coupler at 200, 300, 400, 700, 1500, 2000, 3000, and 4000 Hz should not differ from the output at 1000 Hz by more than ± 5 dB and should not rise by more than 10 dB for frequencies outside this range. This measurement can also be carried out at the dial reading of 60 dB HL (ANSI S3.6-1969).

The recorded speech circuit should be checked for frequency response by using test recordings of sine waves. The manufacturer of the speech audiometer should be able to supply these test recordings or should provide information about where they can be obtained. The output from the test records can be used to check the frequency response of the equipment and also can be used to determine the speed of the tape or disc transport system. The frequency response specifications for the recording circuit is the same for the live-voice circuit. If the frequency of the test pure tone is measured using an electronic counter, problems with the recording speed will become apparent. Turntable speed for phonographs (becoming outmoded) also can be determined using a time disc and a stroboscopic light. The recommended speeds are (a) phonographs: 33⅓ rotation/min; (b) reel-to-reel tape recorders: 7½ in/s; (c) cassette tape: 1⅞ in/s. These speeds are common for such playback systems and are being considered by the standards work group responsible for revising the present standard for audiometers.

Harmonic distortion

Harmonic distortion of the speech audiometer must be determined using a pure tone signal. All harmonics of the input test signal should be at least 40 dB below the fundamental frequency. Tests for harmonic distortion must be made at the maximum output of the speech audiometer. The input signal should be set so that the VU meter needle deflection is 6 dB higher than the standard 0 VU reference point. The test frequencies can be 200, 400, 700, 1000, 2000 and 4000 Hz or 250, 500, 1000, 2000 and 4000 Hz. The output signal at the earphone can be monitored for harmonic distortion using the same procedure described for pure tone audiometers. The standard specification for speech audiometers (ANSI S3.6-1969) states that the sound level of the fundamental frequency shall be at least 25 dB greater than that for any higher harmonic.

Masking noise

Two types of masking sound are suggested for use with speech tests: a broad-band noise, covering a minimum range of 250 to 4000 Hz, or a noise patterned after the average long-term spectrum for speech (Licklider & Miller, 1951), with a 3 dB/octave increase in level over the range 250 to 1000 Hz and a 12 dB/octave decrease for the range 1000 to 4000 Hz. These spectra can be checked using the coupler and the sound analyzer. The masking sound for speech should have a sufficient intensity range to mask speech sounds of 60 dB HL (ANSI S3.6-1969).

Recorder maintenance

In addition to the performance checks described, tape recorders and phonographs require additional care. Tape recorders that are used frequently in testing should have the recording heads cleaned with a solvent and demagnetized weekly. Carbon tetrachloride, acetone, or alcohol can be used as solvents. Head-cleaning cassettes are available for cassette tape players. The heads may be demagnetized using a degaussing tool, which consists of a coil with an electric current running through it. Because the degausser can magnetize as well as demagnetize the heads, the user should be careful to follow the manufacturer's instructions.

Phonograph discs are being used less and less frequently as a source of speech. If they are used, phonograph records and the phonograph stylus should be cleaned weekly, if not daily, to ensure proper performance. Phonograph records do not have infinite life. Information about the functional life of these records should be obtained from the producer. Recorded speech helps reduce the variation in presentation of speech signals. However, the instruments used to reproduce these signals must not be ignored in the care and calibration of clinical equipment.

Sound field

The audiologist should be concerned with the sound field for at least two reasons: (a) assuring that the ambient background noise levels are adequate for audiometry, and (b) specifying the sound conditions for measuring hearing for speech and for pure tones in a sound field rather than with earphones. Measurement of the sound field for both of these purposes requires the use of a sound level meter with the capabilities of octave, or even better, one-third octave filters.

Sound level meters

The sound analyzer has already been discussed in calibration of earphones and bone vibrators. Frequently these sound analyzers can be used as sound level meters by simply eliminating the associated couplers and using the microphone as a device for measuring sound pressure in the environment. In order to function in a calibration network for audiometers, the precision of the sound level meter should be that specified in the ANSI S1.4-1983, "Specification for Sound Level Meters as Type 0, Laboratory Sound Level Meter, or Type 1, Precision Sound Level Meter." This standard also provides specifications for a Type 2, General Purpose, and Type 3, Special Purpose Sound Level Meter. As the type number increases the tolerances become less stringent. In order to be called a sound level meter, an instrument must be able to measure the rms level of sound pressure, meet specifications of response and specifications for linearity and accuracy of an associated attenuator, and should contain the weighting networks labeled A, B, and C. The meter should offer the option of two responses (differing ballistics), "fast" and "slow." The slow response is particularly helpful when measuring noise levels that fluctuate in level by 4 dB or more. These fluctuations would make the meter difficult to read because of the rapid needle movement if the "fast" response were used. The fast response can be used for measuring sounds accurately that do not change appreciable in periods of less than 0.2 s.

Selection of a type of sound level meter depends on the need for accuracy as well as the frequency and temporal characteristics of the sounds to be measured. For sound environments that can be characterized as steady-state and with spectral components mainly below 3000 Hz, the Type 2 sound level meter may be sufficient. When the acoustic environment involves sounds with significant spectral content above 3000 Hz, or consists of rapidly varying temporal properties, or both, then either a Type 0 or Type 1 instrument may be required.

Sound level meters also need to be calibrated. Acoustic calibrators are available that can be used to verify the sensitivity of a sound measuring system. Specifications for acoustical calibrators are contained in ANSI Standard S1.40-1984. Typically, these calibrators generate a known sound pressure level in a coupler into which the microphone of the sound measuring system is inserted. Acoustic calibrators may provide two or more sound pressure levels at two or more frequencies. Multiple levels and multiple frequencies are useful in checking the linearity of the sound level meter and, to some extent, its frequency response. Most sound level meters have internal adjustments available to offset changes in meter sensitivity.

Background noise level

If hearing test results are to be true estimates of hearing sensitivity and not measures of masked thresholds caused by noise in the environment, then the background noise levels should be such that no masking will occur. This applies to testing conducted with earphones or with loudspeakers in a sound field. The American National Standards Institute has published ANSI S3.1-1977, "Criteria for Permissible Ambient Noise During Audiometric Testing." This document lists octave and third-octave band levels that should produce no more than 1 dB of masking for the monaural threshold hearing levels specified in ANSI 3.6-1969. Criterion noise levels are specified for testing with a supra-aural earphone-cushion array and also for sound field testing. Permissible octave band noise levels are listed in Table 16.4.

The difference in allowable octave band levels between covered and uncovered testing simply reflects the attenuation of ambient sound that results from a supra-aural earphone-cushion combination, TDH-39 with MX41/AR cushions (Appendix, ANSI S3.1-1977). If other earphone-cushion combinations (i.e., circumaural) were used, then these permissible ambient noise levels would be altered to account for the differing attenuation properties of the particular earphone-cushion array.

The sound level meter-analyzer combination must not have internal noise greater than 3 dB below the specified levels (ANSI S3.1-1977). If the internal noise exceeds this level, then the equipment is inappropriate.

TABLE 16.4
Maximum Allowable Octave Band SPL for No More Than 1 dB Masking re Reference Hearing Threshold Levels as Specified in ANSI-S3.6-1969

	Test Frequency (Hz)										
Test Condition	125	250	500	750	1000	1500	2000	3000	4000	6000	8000
Soundfield or bone conduction	28.0	18.5	14.5	12.5	14.0	10.5	8.5	8.5	9.0	14.0	20.5
Earphone with MX41/AR cushion	34.5	23.0	21.5	22.5	29.5	29.0	34.5	39.0	42.0	41.0	45.0

Adapted from ANSI 3.1-1977.

It is preferable, however, that the internal meter noise is 10 dB less than the levels to be measured.

The background noise measurements should be made under the noisiest environmental conditions in which an actual hearing test is conducted. The same number of people should be inside and outside the test room as are present during testing. Air conditioning and ventilation equipment should be operating. The noise measurements should be made at the time of day when the noise from exterior sources is greatest. Additional measures should be taken to assess the noise levels caused by intermittent sources, such as typewriters, telephone bells, or footsteps. The measurements can be made with the person doing the measuring in the test room as long as that person assumes a position that will not reduce the level of ambient noise reaching the microphone. The microphone should be placed at the center of the possible location of the head of the person to be tested audiometrically in the sound field and should be oriented in the direction yielding the highest sound pressure levels. Sufficient measures should be taken so that the audiologist is confident that the results are representative of the ambient noise conditions. If the environment is found adequate for pure tone testing, it is reasonable to assume that the noise conditions will not interfere with measurement of the speech reception threshold.

Sound field testing

Audiologic practice frequently requires conducting speech audiometry in a sound field. This is particularly true in hearing aid evaluation or in assessing the status of hearing in young children. Several factors will affect the results of this testing, including the acoustic properties of the test room, the location of the loudspeakers, the intensity of the speech, background noise level, and the differences measured for minimum audible field (sound field) and minimum audible pressure (earphones).

Most test rooms used for hearing testing are not anechoic. Because pure tones introduced in the sound field of the typical test rooms will generate standing waves, use of "speech noise" is recommended for calibrating the sound output of the loudspeakers (Dirks et al., 1976). The location of the microphone for the sound level meter should be in the center of the position occupied by the listener's head when being tested. Because this position varies from listener to listener, the audiologist should make measurements at several locations comprising a geometric space that will encompass most head locations. The average level of this space should be fairly representative of the test sound field. The overall level can be read using the C scale or using the linear scale on a sound level meter. Measures should be made at sound levels sufficiently intense so that the meter readings are not affected by background noise level (approximately at 80 dB HL). Linearity of the attenuator can be checked electrically using the method described for earphones.

The frequency response of the loudspeaker can be checked using the same procedure and test tones as specified for measuring the frequency response of the speech audiometer through earphones. The recommended tolerance is less stringent under these conditions. The output of the calibrating frequencies should not vary by more than ± 10 dB from that measured at 1000 Hz. Levels for frequencies outside the range of 200 to 4000 Hz should not rise more than 15 dB above the level measured at 1000 Hz. The microphone should be oriented in the same direction as the listener's head in relation to the loudspeakers.

The orientation of the listener's head to the sound source will influence the sound level available at the listener's ear. This variation in the sound field results because of the diffraction properties of the listener's head as an obstacle in the sound field (Dirks, Stream, & Wilson, 1972; Wiener & Ross, 1946). Although at the time of this writing there is no standard, if the sound source is a single loudspeaker, it should be located so that the listener will be facing the loudspeaker (0° azimuth). When two loudspeakers are used, the preferable speaker location is at 45° angles to either side of the center of the listener. The person being tested should be located at a distance of at least 1 m from the sound source (see Figure 16.7).

The sound room should be arranged in the same way as would be the case if a person were being tested, with the exception of the absence of the person himself or herself. Introduction of other furniture or other

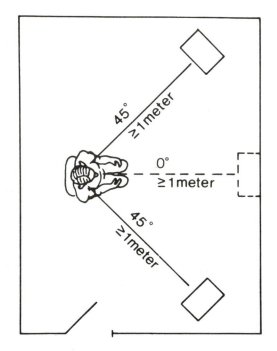

SPEAKER–MICROPHONE ARRANGEMENT
FOR MEASURING SOUND FIELD

Figure 16.7.   Speaker-microphone arrangement for measuring sound field.

equipment would very likely change the sound field. For this reason, the sound measuring equipment should not be in the room if at all possible. The microphone should be attached to the sound analyzer by an extension cable and should be supported in the sound field by a method that would disturb the field minimally. This can be accomplished by using a tripod or by suspending the microphone from the ceiling of the room by its attached cable.

Hearing thresholds measured using earphones (minimum audible pressure, MAP) require more sound pressure than when threshold is measured in a sound field (minimum audible field, MAF). Sivian and White (1933) reported differences amounting to approximately 6 dB for pure tone signals. A difference also exists between earphone and sound field speech reception thresholds (Tillman et al., 1966). There are at least three sources for this difference: (a) head diffraction effects, (b) change in impedance in the ear canal between an open canal and one closed by an earphone, and (c) physiologic masking. When calibrating a sound field for testing speech, the MAF-MAP difference must be taken into account. As noted previously, the threshold for hearing under sound field conditions has not been standardized by ANSI. Tillman et al. (1966) recommended that sound field threshold hearing levels for spondees be 7 dB less than the threshold sound pressure level for speech measured with an earphone. Dirks et al. (1972) suggested a level of 3.5 dB lower for 0° azimuth and a level of 7.5 dB lower for a 45° azimuth. These corrections can be used in sound field calibration until a standard for sound field threshold level exists.

Loudspeakers

Calibration of loudspeakers should be accomplished in an anechoic chamber. Given that not many facilities have anechoic rooms, most audiologists will depend on the equipment manufacturer or an independent acoustics test laboratory for this service. The standard method for measuring loudspeaker response was described in ANSI S1.5-1963, but this document is no longer accepted as an ANSI standard. However, for discussion of loudspeaker calibration the interested reader is referred to Dirks et al. (1976).

Acoustic impedance or admittance devices

Electroacoustic equipment designed to measure acoustic impedance or admittance at the tympanic membrane has become indispensable for the practice of clinical audiology. Large numbers of these instruments are being used today. Specifications and recommended calibration procedures for these devices are contained in ANSI S3.39-1987, "American National Standard Specifications for Instruments to Measure Aural Acoustic Impedance and Admittance" (ANSI, 1987b, Aural Acoustic Immittance). The specifications provided are those that are applicable to a probe tone of the frequency 226 Hz, the only probe tone required by the standard. If other probe frequencies are provided, tolerances and specifications should be provided by the manufacturer.

In ANSI S3.39-1987, four types of instruments are classified according to the kinds of measurements that can be made, according to the features available on an instrument, and according to the tolerances and ranges specified by the standard. As was the case for sound level meters, as the numerical value for a given type of device increases, the required precision decreases and, in this standard, the number of available functions also decrease. Instruments that provide the greatest range of functions and capabilities are classified as Type 1, whereas no minimum requirements are specified for Type 4 instruments.

The immittance standard contains, among others, specifications for the measurement of system, the probe signal, the pneumatic system, and the acoustic reflex-activating system. A detailed description of these specifications is beyond the scope of this chapter. However, a general description of the contents of the standard in these various areas with an indication of a few of the important requirements is appropriate. Audiologists who use acoustic immittance devices clinically (certainly, those who are responsible for equipment calibration) should obtain a copy of the ANSI S3.39-1987 standard for reference.

Acoustic-immittance measurement system

ANSI S3.39-1987 specifies a range of measurement capabilities for instruments designed for measuring either admittance (in $m^3/Pa.s$ and in acoustic mmho) or impedance (in $Pa.s/m^3$ and acoustic ohms). These values could also be expressed in terms of the admittance or impedance of an equivalent volume of air. Specifications are provided both for devices designed to assess immittance at the frontal surface of the probe (measurement plane) and devices that correct for the immittance of the external auditory canal (compensated acoustic immittance). The accuracy for these measures should be within ±5% of the indicated immittance value. The manufacturer is responsible for specifying the response time (and tolerances) of the measuring devices, characteristics that are particularly important in evaluating the temporal characteristics of the middle-ear muscle reflex.

Probe signal

The only required probe signal is a sinusoid of 226 Hz. Other probe signals may be provided, but it is the responsibility of the manufacturer to describe the acoustic characteristics of these additional signals. The probe signal is to be calibrated using a standard HA-1, 2 cm³ coupler. The frequency output shall be within ±3% of the expected value. Harmonic distortion should not exceed 5% of the fundamental frequency. The manufacturer should specify the output sound pressure level and tolerances of the probe, but the level must not exceed 90 dB and the tolerances should not exceed ±3 dB. If the instrument provides pulsed probe signals, the temporal characteristics of the tone pulses and the procedures for measuring these characteristics should be indicated by the manufacturer.

Calibration cavities

ANSI S3.39-1987 requires the manufacturer to provide with Type 1, 2, and 3 devices at least three calibration cavities for calibration of acoustic immittance and air pressure. These cavities should have volumes of 0.5, 2.0, and 5 cm³. The accuracy of the volumes for these cavities should be within ±2%.

Pneumatic system

Devices designated as Type 1, 2, or 3 must have the capabilities to change and to indicate air pressure in the external ear canal as well as in the calibration cavities. The minimum range of air pressures depends on the type of device. For Type 1 and 2 devices, the range should be at least −600 to +200 decapascals (daPa), whereas for a Type 3 instrument, the minimum range should be −300 to +100 daPa. Regardless of the type of device, the maximum limits of pressure is specified as −800 to +600 daPa as measured in the provided 0.5 cm³ test cavity. The actual air pressure should not deviate from the indicated air pressure by more than ±10% for Type 1 and 2 instruments, and ±15% for Type 3 devices.

Acoustic-reflex activating signals

Type 1 instruments must provide (at least) tones of 500, 1000, 2000, and 4000 Hz for both contralateral and ipsilateral reflex measurements. Type 2 devices must provide 500, 1000, and 2000 Hz for either contralateral or ipsilateral measures. The requirements for accuracy of level, frequency, linearity, and harmonic distortion are essentially those required for pure tone audiometers in ANSI S3.6-1969. Typically, reflex activating sounds are delivered by supra-aural earphones, and therefore, performance measurements should be made using an NBS 9A coupler. If insert earphones are used by a particular instrument for evoking the reflex, the appropriate coupler would be the HA-1.

If an instrument provides noise stimuli for reflex activation, the power spectrum of the noise should be measured using a coupler. Broad-band noises should have a uniform spectrum, within ±5 dB relative to the level at 1000 Hz, over the frequency range from 250 through 6000 Hz for supra-aural earphones, and from 400 through 4000 Hz for insert phones. If other noises are provided, the manufacturer must specify their characteristics.

Acoustic immittance devices have achieved widespread use. The information derived with these instruments plays a major role in audiologic assessment. The calibration of these instruments is just as important as that of the clinical audiometer and deserves similar attention.

Auditory evoked potentials

Measurement of evoked auditory potentials including electrocochleography (ECochG), the auditory brainstem response (ABR), middle latency response (MLR), and the late cortical response has become an important diagnostic activity in the practice of audiology. There are no ANSI standards available for the equipment used in making these measurements. The standards community has recognized the need for standardization in this area and has initiated this activity (Working Group S3-72, Accredited Standards Committee on Bioacoustics, S3).

With these methods of audiologic assessment, not only must there be concern for equipment that generates and presents the acoustic signal but also the characteristics of the equipment for detecting and processing the appropriate evoked neurologic electrical activity. Although the important parameters of the auditory signal are the same as those of interest in pure tone audiometry (namely: intensity, frequency, and time), these procedures involve some unique problems as well. Calibration of the acoustic signal is particularly a problem for electrocochleography and for measurement of the auditory brainstem response, both of which require the use of short transients. There are no standard threshold levels for these signals and there is no universal agreement on the method for specifying the physical intensity of these sounds. The measurement of evoked responses is treated in detail in Chapter 6 by Durrant and Wolf. Chapter 6 includes a comprehensive consideration of signal definition and equipment function.

Conclusion

This chapter will not assure the audiologist expertise in calibration of clinical equipment; however, the clinician should be aware of the many possibilities for faulty equipment that can influence clinical test results. Clearly, one cannot be complacent about equipment function. Audiologic equipment should be checked carefully and frequently. Calibration not only involves measuring equipment performance, but also requires proper equipment repair and adjustment when indicated. Most audiologists are capable of making some "first-line" repairs. They should, however, recognize their limitations and have access to laboratory facilities capable of performing major electronic repairs. With appropriate calibrating equipment and proper knowledge of calibration procedures, there is no reason for any audiologist to lack confidence in the electronic devices that are so vital to accurate hearing assessment.

Appendix: ANSI S3.6-1989

ANSI S3.6-1989 replaces American National Standard S3.6-1969. This standard describes the minimum test capabilities of six types of audiometers. Instruments are classified according to the types of test signals they generate, according to the mode of operation, according to their complexity, or according to the range of auditory functions they test. Audiometers with which a diagnostic assessment is possible and which, at the very least, are capable of measuring both air and bone conduction are classified as Types 1, 2, and 3. Instruments with only facilities for measuring air conduction are classified as Types 4 and 5. No minimum facilities are listed for the Type 6 instrument.

Importantly, the reference threshold levels for the Western Electric 705A earphone remain the same as those contained in ANSI S3.6-1969. In the new standard, reference threshold values are specified for the Telephonics earphones TDH-39, TDH-39P, TDH-49, TDH-49P, TDH-50, TDH-50P, and the Telex earphone 1470A. These values are now in the body of the standard. (These values are the same as those contained in Table 16.1 of this chapter.) Reference threshold levels for the Etymotic ER-3A Insert earphone are available in an appendix to the standard.

The output level, frequency, and attenuator linearity tolerances for pure tone signals are essentially those listed in ANSI 3.6-1969. The only change in level tolerances in S3.6-1989 is for 4000 Hz. Previously this tolerance was $\pm$ 4 dB and now it is $\pm$ 3 dB. The frequency and hearing level ranges vary according to the type of instrument. Harmonic distortion requirements are specified in terms of percentages for individual test frequencies. Specification for harmonic distortion is more detailed in the new standard.

For speech testing the response characteristics of the channel are similar to those published in the old standard. The 1989 revision considers not only disk-recording specifications but also those for reel-to-reel and cassette magnetic tape recordings. Again, harmonic distortion is stated in terms of percentages. The reference threshold sound pressure level for speech has remained the same.

A major change in the new standard is a detailed description and specification for masking sounds. Upper and lower cutoff frequencies for narrow-band maskers are tabularized for each pure tone test frequency. Specifications are provided for broad-band noise, weighted random noise for masking pure tones and for masking of speech. The new standard specifies masking output tolerances and performance differences tolerated between channels in two-channel devices.

Another major addition in the new standard is a section devoted to recommended reference tone facilities. This section considers instruments that provide the capabilities of alternating or simultaneous presentation of some auditory standard as, for example, in loudness balancing. This section specifies frequencies to be provided, reference tone level control, level increments, and output tolerances.

There are other differences and additions in the new standard S3.6-1989, including consideration of the bone vibrator configuration, acceptable earphone cushions, rates of attenuation change, frequency change in Bekesy-type audiometers, and others. In addition, there are seven appendices that consider sound field testing, subjective tests for verification of audiometer performance, procedure for transfer of reference equivalent threshold values, recordings for speech audiometers, audiogram format, audiometer design and construction, and interim reference threshold levels for insert earphones.

The new standard represents a major revision of the audiometer standard. Copies can be obtained from the Standards Secretariat, Acoustical Society of America, 355 East 45th Street, New York, New York 10017-3483.

References

American National Standards Institute. (1977). *American National Standard criteria for permissible ambient noise during audiometric testing* (ANSI S3.1-1977). New York: Author.

American National Standards Institute. (1981). *American National Standard reference equivalent threshold force levels for audiometric bone vibrators* (ANSI S3.26-1981). New York: Author.

American National Standards Institute. (1983). *American National Standard specifications for sound level meters* (ANSI S1.4-1983). New York: Author.

American National Standards Institute. (1984). *American National Standard specification for acoustical calibrators* (ANSI S1.40-1984). New York: Author.

American National Standards Institute. (1987a). *American National Standard specification for a mechanical coupler for measurement of bone vibrators* (ANSI S3.13-1987). New York: Author.

American National Standards Institute. (1987b). *American National Standard specifications for instruments to measure aural acoustic impedance and admittance* (ANSI S3.39-1987). New York: Author.

American National Standards Institute. (1969). *American National Standard specifications for audiometers* (ANSI S3.6-1969; R1973). New York: Author.

American National Standards Institute. (1973). *American National Standard method for coupler calibration of earphones* (ANSI S3.7-1973). New York: Author.

American Speech-Language-Hearing Association. (1983). *Professional Service Board standards for accreditation of professional service programs in speech-language pathology and audiology.* Rockville, MD: Author.

American Standards Association. (1951). *American standard specifications for audiometers for general diagnostic purposes* (Z24.5-1951). New York: Author.

Benson, R., Charan, K., Day, J., Harris, J., Niemoller, A., Rudmose, W., Shaw, E., & Weissler, P. (1967). Limitations on the use of circumaural earphones. *Journal of the Acoustical Society of America, 41,* 713–714.

Dirks, D. D., Morgan, D. E., & Wilson, R. H. (1976). Experimental audiology. In C. A. Smith & J. A. Vernon (Eds.), *Handbook of auditory and vestibular research methods* (pp. 498–547). Springfield, IL: Charles C. Thomas.

Dirks, D. D., Stream, R. W., & Wilson, R. H. (1972). Speech audiometry earphones and sound field. *Journal of Speech and Hearing Disorders, 37,* 162–176.

Eagles, E. L., & Doerfler, L. G. (1961). Hearing in children: Acoustic environment and audiometer performance. *Journal of Speech and Hearing Research, 4,* 149–163.

Institute of Electrical and Electronics Engineers. (1953). *Volume measurements of electrical speech and program waves* (ANSI/IEEE 152-1953). New York: Author.

Jerger, J. (1962). Hearing tests in otologic diagnosis. *Asha, 4,* 139–145.

Jerger, J., Shedd, J., & Harford, E. (1959). On detection of extremely small changes in sound intensity. *Archives of Otolaryngology, 69,* 200–211.

Licklider, J. C. R., & Miller, G. A. (1951). The perception of speech. In S. S. Stevens (Ed.), *Handbook of experimental psychology* (pp. 1040–1074). New York: John Wiley.

Michael, P. L., & Bienvenue, G. R. (1977). Real-ear threshold level comparisons between the Telephonics TDH-39 earphone with a metal outer shell and the TDH-39, TDH-49, and TDH-50 earphones with plastic outer shells. *Journal of the Acoustical Society of America, 61,* 1640–1642.

Michael, P. L., & Bienvenue, G. R. (1980). Calibration data for the Telex 1470-A audiometric earphones. *Journal of the Acoustical Society of America, 67,* 1812–1815.

Occupational Safety and Health Administration. (1983). *Occupational noise exposure, hearing conservation amendment.* Final rule (Federal Register 48, No. 46). Washington, DC: U.S. Government Printing Office.

Sanders, J. W., & Rintelmann, W. F. (1964). Masking in audiometry. *Archives of Otolaryngology, 80,* 541–556.

Scharf, B. (1970). Critical bands. In J. V. Tobias (Ed.), *Foundations of modern auditory theory* (Vol. 1, pp. 157–202). New York: Academic Press.

Sivian, L. J., & White, S. D. (1933). On minimum audible sound fields. *Journal of the Acoustical Society of America, 4,* 288–321.

Thomas, W. G., Preslar, M. J., Summers, R., & Steward, J. L. (1969). Calibration and working condition of 100 audiometers. *Public Health Report, 84,* 311–327.

Tillman, T., Johnson, R., & Olsen, W. (1966). Earphone versus sound field threshold sound pressure levels for spondee words. *Journal of the Acoustical Society of America, 39*, 125–133.

Villchur, E. (1970). Audiometer-earphone mounting to improve inter-subject and cushion-fit reliability. *Journal of the Acoustical Society of America, 48*, 1387–1396.

Wiener, F. M., & Ross, D. A. (1946). The pressure distribution in the auditory canal in a progressive sound field. *Journal of the Acoustical Society of America, 18*, 401–408.

Wilber, L. A. (1985). Calibration: Pure tone, speech and noise signals. In J. Katz (Ed.), *Handbook of clinical audiology* (3rd ed., pp. 116–150). Baltimore: Williams & Wilkins.

Author Index

Page numbers in italics refer to figures. Page numbers followed by "t" refer to tables, and those followed by "n" refer to notes.

Subject Index

Page numbers in italics refer to figures. Page numbers followed by "t" refer to tables, and those followed by "n" refer to notes.

A' parameter, 690, *690*
Abnormal growth of loudness, 654
Accelerated speech test, 557–58, 583
Accredited Standards Committee on Bioacoustics, 840
Acoustic admittance, 181, 258–61, 263, 265, *266*, 267t, 280–81
Acoustic compliance, 197
Acoustic conductance, 258, 261
Acoustic immittance. *See also* Aural acoustic immittance
ANSI standard for instruments, 196–99
calculation of static acoustic immittance, 191–92
calibration of instruments, 198–99
change in, 287
of complex systems, 188–90, *189*
definition of, 181
description of, 183–86, *186*, 187t
design principles of instruments for, 193–96, *194*, *195*
in elderly, 532
equations pertaining to, 187t
frequency dependence of, 186–88
measurement of, 256
measurement units and terminology, 197–98
plotting formats, 198
pseudohypacusis and, 636, 642
Acoustic immittance instruments, 3, 191, 193–99, *194*, *195*
Acoustic-immittance measurement system, 838
Acoustic impedance, 181, 258, 260, 263–64, 265, 267t
Acoustic impedance or admittance devices
acoustic-immittance measurement system, 838
acoustic-reflex activating signals, 839–40
calibration cavities, 839
pneumatic system, 839
probe signal, 838–39
Acoustic neurilemmomas, 696
Acoustic neurinomas, 696
Acoustic neurofibromas, 696

Acoustic neuromas, 291, 386, 393, *394*, 396, 400, 403, 406, 410, 412–13, 696, 752, 784
Acoustic reflex
accuracy of, 667t, 668
anatomy and physiology of, 250, 252–55, *252*, *253*, *255–57*
brainstem lesions and, 585
cases concerning, 297–309, *298*, *300–303*, *305–308*, *310*
definition of, 247
elderly and, 533–35, *534*
history of study of, 247–50
life span changes of, 271–75, *274*
pseudohypacusis and, 636–37
retrocochlear dysfunction and, 672
suprathreshold measures of, 285–92, *288*, *290*
Acoustic-reflex activating signals, 839–40
Acoustic-reflex adaptation, 279–85, *280*, *281*, 283t, *285*
Acoustic-reflex arc, 250, 252–54, *252*, 275, 292, 297–309, *298*, *300–303*, *305–308*, *310*
Acoustic reflex-combined (ARC), 698t, 701, 710–12, 711t–13t, 734, 735t
Acoustic reflex decay (ARD), 698t
Acoustic-reflex growth functions, *256*, 262, 263, 264, 265, 266–67, *266*, 289–90
Acoustic-reflex latency, 286–88, *288*, 288n
Acoustic-reflex measurement,
acoustic-reflex amplitude, 288–92, *290*
acoustic-reflex latency, 286–88, *288*, 288n
history of, 248–50
methods of, 255–58, *259*
quantification of the amplitude of acoustic reflex, 258–64, *261*, *262*, *264*
suprathreshold measures, 285–92, *288*, *290*
Acoustic-reflex thresholds (ART)
abnormal reflex thresholds, 275–79, *276*, *277*
in aging adults, 273, *274*, 275
cases concerning, 297–309, *298*, *300–303*, *305–308*, *310*
definition of, 267
detection of hearing loss from, 292–97, *294–96*
in infants, 272–73
introduction to, 264–65

865